Infections of the Central Nervous System

Infections of the Central Nervous System: Pathology and Genetics

EDITORS

FABRICE CHRÉTIEN, MD, PhD
Department of Neuropathology, Sainte Anne Hospital, Paris;
Paris University, Paris;
Experimental Neuropathology Unit, Pasteur Institute, Paris, France

KUM THONG WONG, MBBS, MPath, FRCPath, MD
Department of Pathology, Faculty of Medicine, University of Malaya, Kuala Lumpur, Malaysia

LEROY R. SHARER, MD
Division of Neuropathology, Department of Pathology, Immunology, and Laboratory Medicine, Rutgers New Jersey Medical School and University Hospital, Newark, NJ, USA

SERIES EDITORS

CATHERINE (KATY) KEOHANE, MB, BCH, BAO, FRCPath, FFPath
Department of Pathology and School of Medicine, University College Cork,
Brookfield Health Science Complex, Cork, Ireland

FRANÇOISE GRAY, MD, PhD
Retired from Department of Pathology, Lariboisière Hospital, APHP, Paris;
University Paris Diderot (Paris 7), Paris, France

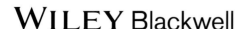

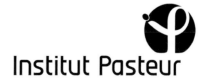

This edition first published 2020
© 2020 John Wiley & Sons Ltd

All rights reserved. No part of this publication may be reproduced, stored in a retrieval system, or transmitted, in any form or by any means, electronic, mechanical, photocopying, recording or otherwise, except as permitted by law. Advice on how to obtain permission to reuse material from this title is available at http://www.wiley.com/go/permissions.

The right of Fabrice Chrétien, Kum Thong Wong, Leroy R. Sharer, Catherine (Katy) Keohane and Françoise Gray to be identified as the author(s) of the editorial material in this work has been asserted in accordance with law.

Registered Office(s)
John Wiley & Sons, Inc., 111 River Street, Hoboken, NJ 07030, USA
John Wiley & Sons Ltd, The Atrium, Southern Gate, Chichester, West Sussex, PO19 8SQ, UK

Editorial Office
9600 Garsington Road, Oxford, OX4 2DQ, UK

For details of our global editorial offices, customer services, and more information about Wiley products visit us at www.wiley.com.

Wiley also publishes its books in a variety of electronic formats and by print-on-demand. Some content that appears in standard print versions of this book may not be available in other formats.

Limit of Liability/Disclaimer of Warranty
The contents of this work are intended to further general scientific research, understanding, and discussion only and are not intended and should not be relied upon as recommending or promoting scientific method, diagnosis, or treatment by physicians for any particular patient. In view of ongoing research, equipment modifications, changes in governmental regulations, and the constant flow of information relating to the use of medicines, equipment, and devices, the reader is urged to review and evaluate the information provided in the package insert or instructions for each medicine, equipment, or device for, among other things, any changes in the instructions or indication of usage and for added warnings and precautions. While the publisher and authors have used their best efforts in preparing this work, they make no representations or warranties with respect to the accuracy or completeness of the contents of this work and specifically disclaim all warranties, including without limitation any implied warranties of merchantability or fitness for a particular purpose. No warranty may be created or extended by sales representatives, written sales materials or promotional statements for this work. The fact that an organization, website, or product is referred to in this work as a citation and/or potential source of further information does not mean that the publisher and authors endorse the information or services the organization, website, or product may provide or recommendations it may make. This work is sold with the understanding that the publisher is not engaged in rendering professional services. The advice and strategies contained herein may not be suitable for your situation. You should consult with a specialist where appropriate. Further, readers should be aware that websites listed in this work may have changed or disappeared between when this work was written and when it is read. Neither the publisher nor authors shall be liable for any loss of profit or any other commercial damages, including but not limited to special, incidental, consequential, or other damages.

Library of Congress Cataloging-in-Publication Data
Names: Chrétien, Fabrice, editor. | Wong, Kum Thong, editor. | Sharer, Leroy R., editor. |
    Keohane, Catherine, editor. | Gray, Françoise, editor. | International Society of Neuropathology, issuing body.
Title: Infections of the central nervous system : pathology and genetics / edited by Fabrice Chrétien,
    Kum Thong Wong, Leroy R. Sharer, Catherine (Katy) Keohane, Françoise Gray.
Other titles: Infections of the central nervous system (Chrétien)
Description: Hoboken, NJ : Wiley-Blackwell, 2020. | Includes bibliographical references and index.
Identifiers: LCCN 2019033002 (print) | LCCN 2019033003 (ebook) | ISBN 9781119467762 (hardback) |
    ISBN 9781119467700 (adobe pdf) | ISBN 9781119467793 (epub)
Subjects: MESH: Central Nervous System Infections–pathology | Central Nervous System Infections–genetics
Classification: LCC RC359.5 (print) | LCC RC359.5 (ebook) | NLM WL 301 | DDC 616.8–dc23
LC record available at https://lccn.loc.gov/2019033002
LC ebook record available at https://lccn.loc.gov/2019033003

Cover Design: Wiley
Cover Images: Logo used with permission of Pasteur Institute, Main image, 1st and 6th images on right courtesy of Françoise Gray; 2nd image on right courtesy of Michael Farrell; 3rd and 4th images courtesy of Catherine (Katy) Keohane; 5th and 7th images courtesy of Gregory Jouvion

Set in 9.5/12pt Minion by SPi Global, Pondicherry, India

Printed and bound in Singapore by Markono Print Media Pte Ltd

10 9 8 7 6 5 4 3 2 1

Contents

List of Contributors, ix

1. Introduction and Classification of Infections of the CNS According to the Agent, 1
   Fabrice Chrétien, Kum Thong Wong, Leroy R. Sharer, Catherine (Katy) Keohane, and Françoise Gray

2. Sepsis-Associated Encephalopathy, 11
   Franck Verdonk, Aurelien Mazeraud, Fabrice Chrétien, and Tarek Sharshar

3. Variation of CNS Infections According to the Host, 21
   Leroy R. Sharer, Catherine (Katy) Keohane, and Françoise Gray

4. Clinical Approach to the Adult Patient with CNS Infection, 29
   Michel Wolff, Romain Sonneville, and Tarek Sharshar

5. Herpes Simplex Virus Infections of the CNS, 43
   Bette K. Kleinschmidt-DeMasters, Catherine (Katy) Keohane, and Françoise Gray

6. Varicella-Zoster Virus and Epstein-Barr Virus Infections of the CNS, 55
   Catherine (Katy) Keohane and Françoise Gray

7. Cytomegalovirus Infections of the CNS, 65
   Homa Adle-Biassette and Natacha Teissier

8. Adenovirus Meningoencephalitis, 77
   Harry V. Vinters and Xinhai R. Zhang

9. Polyomavirus Infections of the CNS, 83
   Susan Morgello

10. Measles Virus Infection of the CNS, 95
    Catherine (Katy) Keohane, Leroy R. Sharer, and Françoise Gray

11. Rubella Virus, 105
    Bette K. Kleinschmidt-DeMasters

12. Henipavirus Encephalitis, 113
    Kum Thong Wong and Kien Chai Ong

13. Rabies, 121
    Guilherme Dias de Melo, Perrine Parize, Grégory Jouvion, Laurent Dacheux, Fabrice Chrétien, and Hervé Bourhy

14. Flaviviruses 1: General Introduction and Tick-Borne Encephalitis, 131
    Herbert Budka

15. Flaviviruses 2: West Nile, St. Louis Encephalitis, Murray Valley Encephalitis, Yellow Fever, and Dengue, 147
    Edward S. Johnson and Juan M. Bilbao

16. Flaviviruses 3: Zika Virus Infection of the CNS, 163
    Leila Chimelli

17. Flaviviruses 4: Japanese Encephalitis, 169
    Shankar Krishna Susarla, Anita Mahadevan, Bishan Radotra, Masaki Takao, and Kum Thong Wong

Contents

18 CNS Disorders Caused by Hepatitis C and Hepatitis E Viruses, 177
Melissa Umphlett, Clare Bryce, and Susan Morgello

19 Alphaviral Equine Encephalomyelitis (Eastern, Western, and Venezuelan), 183
Kum Thong Wong

20 Chikungunya Virus, 189
Cássia Shinotsuka, Michael Blatzer, Grégory Jouvion, and Fabrice Chrétien

21 Poliovirus Infection and Postpolio Syndrome, 195
Catherine (Katy) Keohane, Leila Chimelli, and Aisling Ryan

22 Enterovirus A71 Infection, 205
Kum Thong Wong, Kien Chai Ong, Thérèse Couderc, and Marc Lecuit

23 Human Immunodeficiency Virus Infection of the CNS, 215
Françoise Gray and Leroy R. Sharer

24 HTLV-1 and Neurological-Associated Disease, 231
Antoine Gessain, Olivier Cassar, and Philippe V. Afonso

25 Parechovirus A, 243
Clayton A. Wiley

26 Acute Disseminated Encephalomyelitis and Acute Hemorrhagic Leukoencephalomyelitis, 251
Romana Höftberger and Hans Lassmann

27 Miscellaneous Inflammatory Disorders of the CNS of Possible Infectious Origin, 259
Mari Perez-Rosendahl, Jamie Nakagiri, Xinhai R. Zhang, and Harry V. Vinters

28 Mycoplasmal and Rickettsial Infections of the CNS, 267
Roy H. Rhodes

29 Pathogenesis and Pathophysiology of Bacterial Infections of the CNS, 279
Loic Le Guennec and Sandrine Bourdoulous

30 Pyogenic Infections of the CNS 1: Acute Bacterial Meningitis, 295
Loic Le Guennec and Sandrine Bourdoulous

31 Pyogenic Infections of the CNS 2: (Brain Abscess, Subdural Abscess or Empyema, Epidural Abscess, Septic Embolism, and Suppurative Intracranial Phlebitis), 309
Arnault Tauziede-Espariat, Alexandre Roux, Megan Still, Marc Zanello, Gilles Zah-Bi, Ghazi Hmeydia, Catherine Oppenheim, Michel Wolff, Johan Pallud, and Fabrice Chrétien

32 Pyogenic Infections of the CNS 3: Following Neurosurgical Procedures, 319
Alexandre Roux, Megan Still, Marc Zanello, Gilles Zah-Bi, Arnault Tauziede-Espariat, Ghazi Hmeydia, Catherine Oppenheim, Michel Wolff, Fabrice Chrétien, and Johan Pallud

33 CNS Involvement in *Tropheryma whipplei* Infection, 331
Emmanuèle Lechapt-Zalcman

34 Cerebral Actinomycosis, 337
Arnault Tauziede-Espariat

35 Cerebral Nocardiosis, 343
Arnault Tauziede-Espariat and Leroy R. Sharer

36 CNS Tuberculosis, 349
Michael A. Farrell, Eoin R. Feeney, and Jane B. Cryan

37 Non-Tuberculous Mycobacterial Infections, 357
Leroy R. Sharer

38 Spirochetal Infections of the CNS, 363
Françoise Gray and Catherine (Katy) Keohane

39 Neurobrucellosis, 379
Marine Le Dudal, Fabrice Chrétien, and Grégory Jouvion

40 Legionellosis, 383
Edward S. Johnson

41 Neurosarcoidosis, 393
Michael A. Farrell and Alan Beausang

42 Hypertrophic Pachymeningitis, 403
Françoise Gray and Leroy R. Sharer

43 Toxin-Induced Neurological Diseases, 411
Pierre L. Goossens, Cédric Thépenier, and Michel R. Popoff

44 Fungal Infections of the CNS, 419
*Michael Blatzer, Fanny Lanternier,
Jean-Paul Latgé, Anne Beauvais,
Stéphane Bretagne, Fabrice Chrétien,
and Grégory Jouvion*

45 Cerebral Malaria, 437
*Patrícia Reis, Vanessa Estato, and
Hugo Caire de Castro Faria Neto*

46 *Toxoplasma* Infection of the CNS, 449
*Stéphane Bretagne, Catherine (Katy) Keohane,
and Homa Adle-Biassette*

47 Other Protozoal Infections, 463
Leila Chimelli and Catherine (Katy) Keohane

48 Helminth Infections of the CNS, 475
*Marine Le Dudal, Stéphane Bretagne,
David Hardy, Fabrice Chrétien, and
Grégory Jouvion*

Appendix: CASE EXAMPLE: *Schistosoma mekongi* Neuroschistosomiasis, 500
Edward S. Johnson

49 Brain Myiasis, 503
Arnault Tauziede-Espariat

50 Emerging CNS Infections, 505
Kum Thong Wong

Index, 515

List of Contributors

Homa Adle-Biassette
Department of Pathology
Lariboisière Hospital
APHP, Paris;

Paris University, NeuroDiderot
INSERM F-75019
Paris, France

Philippe V. Afonso
Oncogenic Virus Epidemiology and
Pathophysiology
Department of Virology
Pasteur Institute
Paris, France

Alan Beausang
Department of Neuropathology
Beaumont Hospital
Dublin, Ireland

Anne Beauvais
Aspergillus Unit
Pasteur Institute
Paris, France

Juan M. Bilbao
Department of Pathology
University of Toronto
Toronto, Ontario, Canada

Michael Blatzer
Aspergillus and Experimental Neuropathology Units
Pasteur Institute
Paris, France

Sandrine Bourdoulous
Inserm, U1016, Institut Cochin, CNRS
UMR8104, Paris University
Paris, France

Hervé Bourhy
Lyssavirus Epidemiology and Neuropathology Unit
French National Reference Centre for Rabies
WHO Collaborating Centre for Reference and
Research on Rabies
Pasteur Institute
Paris, France

Stéphane Bretagne
Saint Louis Hospital
APHP, Paris;

University Paris Diderot
Sorbonne Paris Cité, Paris;

Molecular Mycology Unit
French National Reference Centre for Invasive
Mycoses and Antifungal Treatments
Pasteur Institute
Paris, France

List of Contributors

Clare Bryce
Department of Pathology, Neurology, and Neuroscience
Icahn School of Medicine
Mount Sinai, New York
NY, USA

Herbert Budka
Institute of Neurology
Medical University Vienna
Vienna, Austria

Olivier Cassar
Oncogenic Virus Epidemiology and Pathophysiology
Department of Virology
Pasteur Institute, Paris;

CNRS, UMR3569
Paris, France

Hugo Caire de Castro Faria Neto
Laboratory of Immunopharmacology
Oswaldo Cruz Institute, FIOCRUZ
Rio de Janeiro, Brazil

Leila Chimelli
Laboratory of Neuropathology and Molecular Genetics
State Brain Institute Paulo Niemeyer
Rio de Janeiro, Brazil;

Federal University of Rio de Janeiro (UFRJ),
Rio de Janeiro, Brazil

Fabrice Chrétien
Department of Neuropathology
Sainte Anne Hospital
Paris;

Paris University
Paris;

Experimental Neuropathology Unit
Pasteur Institute
Paris, France

Thérèse Couderc
Biology of Infection Unit
Pasteur Institute
Paris;

Inserm U1117
Paris, France

Jane B. Cryan
Department of Neuropathology
Beaumont Hospital
Dublin, Ireland

Laurent Dacheux
Lyssavirus Epidemiology and Neuropathology Unit
French National Reference Centre for Rabies
WHO Collaborating Centre for Reference and Research on Rabies
Pasteur Institute
Paris, France

Marine Le Dudal
Experimental Neuropathology Unit
Pasteur Institute
Paris;

Embryology, Histology and Pathology Unit
The National Veterinary School of Alfort
University Paris-Est
Maison-Alfort, France

Vanessa Estato
Laboratory of Immunopharmacology
Oswaldo Cruz Institute, FIOCRUZ
Rio de Janeiro, Brazil

Michael A. Farrell
Department of Neuropathology
Beaumont Hospital
Dublin, Ireland

Eoin R. Feeney
Department of Infectious Diseases
St. Vincent's Hospital
Dublin, Ireland

Antoine Gessain
Oncogenic Virus Epidemiology and Pathophysiology
Department of Virology, Pasteur Institute
Paris;

CNRS, UMR3569
Paris, France

List of Contributors

Pierre L. Goossens
Experimental Neuropathology Unit
Pasteur Institute
Paris;

Yersinia, Pasteur Institute
Paris, France

Françoise Gray
Retired from Department of Pathology
Lariboisière Hospital
APHP, Paris;

University Paris Diderot (Paris 7)
Paris, France

Loic Le Guennec
Inserm, U1016, Institut Cochin
CNRS, UMR8104
Paris University, Paris;

La Pitie-Salpetriere Hospital
APHP, Paris, France

David Hardy
Experimental Neuropathology Unit
Pasteur Institute
Paris, France

Romana Höftberger
Institute of Neurology
Medical University of Vienna
Vienna, Austria

Ghazi Hmeydia
Department of Neuropathology
Sainte-Anne Hospital
Paris, France

Edward S. Johnson
Department of Laboratory Medicine
and Pathology
University of Alberta
Edmonton, Alberta, Canada

Grégory Jouvion
Experimental Neuropathology Unit
Pasteur Institute
Paris, France

Catherine (Katy) Keohane
Department of Pathology and School of Medicine
University College Cork
Brookfield Health Science Complex
Cork, Ireland

Bette K. Kleinschmidt-DeMasters
Department of Pathology, Neurosurgery,
and Neurology
University of Colorado School of Medicine
Aurora, CO, USA

Fanny Lanternier
Molecular Mycology Unit
French National Reference Centre
for Invasive Mycoses and Antifungal Treatments
Pasteur Institute, Paris;

Paris University,
Paris;

Department of Infectious Diseases and
Tropical Medicine
Necker-Sick Children University Hospital
and Imagine Institute
APHP, Paris, France

Hans Lassmann
Center for Brain Research
Medical University of Vienna
Vienna, Austria

Jean-Paul Latgé
Aspergillus Unit
Pasteur Institute
Paris, France

Emmanuèle Lechapt-Zalcman
Department of Neuropathology
Sainte Anne Hospital
Paris, France

Marc Lecuit
Biology of Infection Unit
Pasteur Institute
Paris;

Inserm U1117, Paris;

Department of Infectious Diseases and
Tropical Medicine

List of Contributors

Necker-Sick Children University Hospital
and Imagine Institute
APHP, Paris;

Paris University
Paris, France

Anita Mahadevan
Department of Neuropathology
National Institute of Mental Health and
Neurosciences (NIMHANS)
Bangalore, India

Aurelien Mazeraud
Experimental Neuropathology Unit
Pasteur Institute, Paris;

Department of Anesthesiology and Intensive Care
Sainte Anne Hospital
Paris;

University Paris Diderot, Sorbonne Paris Cité
APHP, Paris, France

Guilherme Dias de Melo
Lyssavirus Epidemiology and Neuropathology Unit
French National Reference Centre for Rabies
WHO Collaborating Centre for Reference and
Research on Rabies
Pasteur Institute
Paris, France

Susan Morgello
Department of Pathology, Neurology, and
Neuroscience
Icahn School of Medicine
Mount Sinai, New York
NY, USA

Jamie Nakagiri
Department of Pathology and Laboratory Medicine
UC Irvine Medical Center
Orange, CA, USA

Kien Chai Ong
Department of Biomedical Science
Faculty of Medicine
University of Malaya
Kuala Lumpur, Malaysia

Catherine Oppenheim
Department of Neuroradiology
Sainte Anne Hospital
Paris;

Paris University
Paris;

Inserm U894, IMA-Brain
Psychiatry and Neurosciences Center
Paris, France

Johan Pallud
Department of Neurosurgery
Sainte Anne Hospital
Paris;

Paris University
Paris;

Inserm U894, IMA-Brain
Psychiatry and Neurosciences Center
Paris, France

Perrine Parize
Lyssavirus Epidemiology and Neuropathology Unit
French National Reference Centre for Rabies
WHO Collaborating Centre for Research
on Rabies
Pasteur Institute
Paris, France

Mari Perez-Rosendahl
Department of Pathology and Laboratory Medicine
UC Irvine Medical Center
Orange, CA, USA

Michel R. Popoff
Bacterial Toxins Unit
Pasteur Institute
Paris, France

Bishan Radotra
Department of Histopathology
Postgraduate Institute of Medical Education
and Research
Chandigarh, India

Patrícia Reis
Laboratory of Immunopharmacology
Oswaldo Cruz Institute, FIOCRUZ
Rio de Janeiro, Brazil

Roy H. Rhodes
School of Medicine
Department of Pathology
Louisiana State University
New Orleans, LA, USA

Alexandre Roux
Department of Neurosurgery
Sainte Anne Hospital
Paris;

Paris University
Paris;

Inserm U894, IMA-Brain
Psychiatry and Neurosciences Center
Paris, France

Aisling Ryan
Department of Neurology
Cork University Hospital
Cork, Ireland

Leroy R. Sharer
Division of Neuropathology
Department of Pathology, Immunology, and Laboratory Medicine
Rutgers New Jersey Medical School and University Hospital
Newark, NJ, USA

Tarek Sharshar
Experimental Neuropathology Unit
Pasteur Institute, Paris;

Department of Anesthesiology and Intensive Care
Sainte Anne Hospital
Paris;

University Paris Diderot
Sorbonne Paris Cité
Paris, France

Cássia Shinotsuka
Experimental Neuropathology Unit
Pasteur Institute
Paris, France

Romain Sonneville
Department of Anesthesiology and Intensive Care
Saint Anne Hospital
Paris;

Department of Intensive Care Medicine and Infectious Diseases
Inserm U1148, Bichat-Claude-Bernard Hospital
APHP, Paris;

University Paris Diderot
Sorbonne Paris Cité
Paris, France

Megan Still
Department of Neurosurgery
Sainte Anne Hospital
Paris, France

University of Texas Southwestern Medical Center
Dallas, TX, USA

Shankar Krishna Susarla
Department of Neuropathology
National Institute of Mental Health and Neurosciences (NIMHANS)
Bangalore, India

Masaki Takao
Department of Neurology
Saitama International Medical Center
Saitama Medical University
Hidaka, Japan

Arnault Tauziede-Espariat
Department of Neuropathology
Sainte Anne Hospital
Paris;

Paris University
Paris, France

Natacha Teissier
Department of Pediatric Otolaryngology
Robert Debre Hospital
APHP, Paris;

Paris University, NeuroDiderot
INSERM F-75019
Paris, France

Cédric Thépenier
Experimental Neuropathology Unit
Pasteur Institute
Paris, France

List of Contributors

Melissa Umphlett
Department of Pathology, Neurology, and Neuroscience
Icahn School of Medicine
Mount Sinai, New York, NY, USA

Franck Verdonk
Experimental Neuropathology Unit
Pasteur Institute
Paris;

Department of Anesthesiology and Intensive Care
Saint Antoine Hospital
Paris;

Sorbonne University
Paris, France

Harry V. Vinters
Department of Pathology and Laboratory Medicine (Neuropathology) and Neurology
David Geffen School of Medicine UCLA and Ronald Reagan UCLA Medical Center
Los Angeles, CA, USA

Clayton A. Wiley
Division of Neuropathology
UPMC Presbyterian Hospital
Pittsburgh, PA, USA

Michel Wolff
Department of Anesthesiology and Neurological Intensive Care
Sainte Anne Hospital
Paris;

Department of Intensive Care Medicine and Infectious Diseases
Bichat-Claude-Bernard Hospital
APHP, Paris, France

Kum Thong Wong
Department of Pathology
Faculty of Medicine
University of Malaya
Kuala Lumpur, Malaysia

Gilles Zah-Bi
Department of Neurosurgery
Sainte-Anne Hospital
Paris, France

Marc Zanello
Department of Neurosurgery
Sainte Anne Hospital
Paris;

Paris University
Paris;

Inserm U894, IMA-Brain
Psychiatry and Neurosciences Center
Paris, France

Xinhai R. Zhang
Department of Pathology
RUSH University Medical Center
Chicago, IL, USA

1

Introduction and Classification of Infections of the CNS According to the Agent

Fabrice Chrétien[1,2,3], Kum Thong Wong[4], Leroy R. Sharer[5], Catherine (Katy) Keohane[6], and Françoise Gray[7,8]

[1] Department of Neuropathology, Sainte Anne Hospital, Paris, France
[2] Paris University, Paris, France
[3] Experimental Neuropathology Unit, Pasteur Institute, Paris, France
[4] Department of Pathology, Faculty of Medicine, University of Malaya, Kuala Lumpur, Malaysia
[5] Division of Neuropathology, Department of Pathology, Immunology and Laboratory Medicine, Rutgers New Jersey Medical School and University Hospital, Newark, NJ, USA
[6] Deparment of Pathology and School of Medicine, University College Cork, Brookfield Health Science Complex, Cork, Ireland
[7] Retired from Department of Pathology, Lariboisière Hospital, APHP, Paris, France
[8] University Paris Diderot (Paris 7), Paris, France

Despite modern antimicrobial therapies and vaccines, infections of the CNS still have an unacceptably high mortality and may generate permanent neurologic deficits in survivors. The bony structures of the skull and vertebral column and the blood-brain barrier (BBB) afford strong protection for the brain and spinal cord from invading pathogens. However, once the pathogen enters the CNS, the host defense mechanisms are often inefficient in preventing severe, life-threatening infections. The clinical severity of infection results from complex interactions between the host and the invading pathogen, but it is clear that CNS infections differ fundamentally from those in other organs and are usually more serious, partly because of the CNS's immunological privilege.

The growing numbers of patients with immune deficiency together with the increased displacement of people (i.e. migrants or international travelers) has expanded the spectrum of infectious diseases and its range, making the pathological diagnosis of CNS infectious disease more difficult. On the other hand, important advances in molecular medicine have improved our knowledge of the genetics of both the pathogens and the immunological characteristics of the host.

For these reasons, the International Society of Neuropathology devotes a volume of the established series of Pathology and Genetics textbooks to the pathology and genetics of infections in the CNS.

This volume *Infections of the Central Nervous System: Neuropathology and Genetics* consists of 50 chapters describing the most important infections involving the CNS. Numerous agents may infect the CNS, including viruses, bacteria, fungi, parasites, and arthropods (myiasis), and sequential chapters describing them have been laid out in this order. An exceptional case of meningitis resulting from an alga *Prototheca wickerhamii* in a patient with severe immunodeficient acquired immunodeficiency syndrome (AIDS) has been reported [1] but does not warrant a special chapter.

This introductory chapter proposes a classification of the different pathogens affecting the CNS; Chapters 2–4 discuss inflammation and sepsis, genetic and other host variations in infections, and the clinical approach to CNS infectious diseases.

The section on viral infections starts with DNA viruses, beginning with the large herpesvirus group, including herpes simplex 1 and 2, varicella-zoster and Epstein-Barr viruses, and cytomegalovirus, followed by adenovirus and polyomavirus (Table 1.1). For the RNA viruses, there are chapters on measles, rubella, henipavirus, rabies, hepatitis C and E viruses, alphaviral equine encephalitis viruses, Chikungunya virus, poliovirus (including postpolio syndrome), enterovirus A71, human immunodeficiency virus (HIV), human T-lymphocytic/leukemia virus I, and parechovirus. The large important group of flaviviruses are dealt with in four chapters with a general introduction to flaviviral encephalitides and a description of tick-borne encephalitis, followed by encephalitides caused by yellow fever, West Nile, St. Louis, dengue and Murray Valley encephalitis viruses, Zika virus, and Japanese encephalitis virus. Chapter 26 describes entities long known to be associated with viral infections (e.g. acute disseminated encephalomyelitis); the subsequent chapter deals with encephalitides of uncertain origin but that may be associated with viral infection (e.g. Rasmussen encephalitis).

Descriptions of CNS bacterial infections (Table 1.2) include chapters on *Mycoplasma* and *Rickettsia*, pyogenic bacteria, *Actinomyces*, *Tropheryma whipplei* (Whipple disease), *Nocardia*, *Mycobacterium tuberculosis*, nontuberculous *Mycobacteria*, spirochetes, *Brucella*, and *Legionella*. In addition to a chapter on general pathogenesis and pathophysiology of bacterial infections, the different types of pyogenic bacteria are discussed according to the clinicopathological entities they commonly cause: acute meningitis and abscess or suppuration; additionally, a separate chapter is devoted to bacterial infections following neurosurgical procedures. Disease entities such as neurosarcoidosis and chronic immunoglobulin G4 (IgG4) pachymeningitis are included because they are often a major differential diagnosis of bacterial infections. Toxin-induced neurological diseases are discussed in a separate chapter.

Numerous fungi (Table 1.3) cause CNS infections; according to their morphology, fungal pathogens can be divided into three major groups: molds, yeasts, and dimorphic fungi. This categorization does not relate to the taxonomic groups, but it may be helpful in guiding diagnosis because each category shares similar clinical features.

Parasitic infections of the CNS caused by protozoa include infections by *Plasmodium*, *Toxoplasma*, and other protozoa such as amebae, trypanosomes, *Microsporidium*, and *Leishmania* (Table 1.4). Helminthic cestodes (i.e. *Taenia*, *Echinoccocus*, *Spirometra*), trematodes (i.e. Schistosoma, Paragonimus), and nematodes (i.e. Angiostrongylus, *Gnathostoma*, *Toxocara*, *Trichinella*, filaria, *Strongyloides*) infections and CNS myiasis resulting from fly larvae infestation of the CNS are also described.

Many factors determine the incidence of different CNS infections in disparate geographical regions. Endemic and emerging infections in susceptible human populations depend on the dynamic interactions between (or changes in) microbe-environment-host factors. The increasing virulence of CNS pathogens because of antimicrobial resistance is of huge importance, resulting in increased incidence of more severe infections. Environmental factors caused by poor sanitation and hygiene and absence of vector control, and so on, enable diseases to spread rapidly. Host factors including changes in human behavior and demography, immunosuppression, genetic predisposition, and many others conspire to increase host susceptibility to CNS infections. In recent years, acquired immunosuppression resulting from HIV infection or associated with therapeutic modalities, including newer immunomodulating treatments, has dramatically increased host susceptibility to numerous opportunistic agents. A separate chapter on emerging CNS infections discusses more details about this phenomenon.

This book aims to describe and illustrate the various lesions and entities that may be encountered in CNS infections to help in pathological diagnosis. These include meningitis, abscess, encephalitis, myelitis, demyelination, vasculopathy, infarction, or combinations thereof (e.g. meningoencephalitis and encephalomyelitis). The

Table 1.1 Main viruses involving the CNS.

Virus	Genus/Species	Main CNS neurological syndromes[a]	Characteristics[b]
DNA viruses			
Herpes virus	Herpes simplex I, II HHV-1 and -2	Encephalitis	Virus targets neurons
	Varicella-zoster virus HHV-3	Myelitis Vasculitis/infarcts Meningoencephalitis Etc.	Virus targets neuroglial and Schwann cells, blood vessels.
	Epstein-Barr virus HHV-4	Myelitis Meningoencephalitis	Associated with immunosuppression
	Cytomegalovirus HHV-5	Myelitis Ventriculoencephalitis Congenital neurological syndrome	Associated with immunosuppression
Adenovirus	Adenovirus species	Meningoencephalitis	Associated with immunosuppression
Polyomavirus	JC virus BK virus	Progressive multifocal leukoencephalopathy	Virus targets oligodendroglia mainly Associated with immunosuppression
RNA viruses			
Morbillivirus	Measles virus (rubeola)	Acute postinfectious encephalitis MIBE SSPE	Virus targets neuroglial cells and neurons in MIBE and SSPE MIBE mainly associated with immunosuppression SSPE associated with mutant virus
Rubivirus	Rubella virus	CRS (RE)	Cerebral blood vessel damage and microcephaly in CRS Neuronal degeneration in RE
Henipavirus	Hendra virus Nipah virus	Acute encephalitis Relapsing encephalitis	Virus targets cerebral blood vessels and neuroglial cells in acute encephalitis Virus targets only neuroglial cells in relapsing encephalitis
Lyssavirus	Rabies virus and other species	Encephalitis (Paralytic rabies; furious rabies)	Virus mainly targets neurons
Flavivirus	Tick-borne encephalitis virus	Encephalitis	Virus targets neurons
	West Nile virus	Encephalitis	Virus targets neurons
	St. Louis encephalitis virus	Encephalitis	Virus targets neurons
	Murray valley encephalitis virus	Encephalitis	Virus targets neurons
	Yellow fever virus	Encephalopathy	Mainly viscerotropic
	Dengue virus	Encephalopathy	Mainly viscerotropic
	Zika virus	Congenital Zika syndrome	Virus mainly targets neural progenitor cells
	Japanese encephalitis virus	Encephalitis	Virus targets neurons
	Hepatitis C virus	Neuropsychiatric-related (parainfectious) Meningoencephalitis/myelitis (rare)	Neurotropism unconfirmed
Hepevirus	Hepatitis E virus	Meningoencephalitis/myelitis (rare)	Neurotropism unconfirmed

(continued)

Infections of the Central Nervous System

Table 1.1 (Continued)

Virus	Genus/Species	Main CNS neurological syndromes[a]	Characteristics[b]
Alphavirus	Eastern equine encephalitis virus	Encephalitis	Virus targets neurons
	Western equine encephalitis virus		
	Venezuelan equine encephalitis virus		
	Chikungunya virus	Encephalopathy Encephalitis	Specific neuropathology unknown
Enterovirus	Enterovirus A71	Acute flaccid paralysis Encephalomyelitis	Virus targets mainly lower motor neurons
	Poliovirus	Poliomyelitis Polioencephalitis Postpolio syndrome	Virus targets mainly lower motor neurons
Retrovirus	HIV	HIV-induced encephalitis and other encephalopathy/disorders Opportunistic infections	Virus targets CD4 lymphocytes and macrophages/microglia
	HTLV	Tropical spastic paraparesis/HTLV-1–associated myelopathy	Virus targets CD4 lymphocytes Pathogenesis may be associated with immune factors
Parechovirus	Parechovirus A	Encephalitis	Virus targets cerebral blood vessels

[a] Commonly used terms for the neurological syndromes in the CNS; peripheral nervous system disease not included.
[b] Selected characteristics only; cellular tropism is not well established in a significant number of viral CNS infections.
CRS, congenital rubella syndrome; HHV, human herpes virus; HIV, human immunodeficiency virus; HTLV, human T cell leukemia/lymphoma virus; JC virus, John Cunningham virus; MIBE, measles inclusion body encephalitis; RE, rubella encephalitis; SSPE, subacute sclerosing panencephalitis.

Table 1.2 Mycoplasmal rickettsial and bacterial infections of the CNS.

Organisms	Genus/Species	Type of CNS infection	Characteristics
Mycoplasma	*M. pneumoniae*	Encephalitis	Intracellular bacteria
	M. hominis	Brain abscess Meningitis	Intracellular bacteria
Rickettsia	*R. rickettsii*	Encephalitis Chronic leptomeningitis Cerebral infarction	Intracellular bacteria Tick-borne
	R. conorii	Meningoencephalitis Cerebral infarction Polyneuropathy and polyneuritis	Intracellular bacteria Tick-borne
	R. prowazekii	Meningoencephalitis Peripheral neuropathy Transverse myelitis	Intracellular bacteria Louse-borne
	R. typhi	Meningoencephalitis	Intracellular bacteria Flea-borne

Table 1.2 (Continued)

Organisms	Genus/Species	Type of CNS infection	Characteristics
Orientia	*O. tsutsugamushi*	Meningoencephalitis Cerebral vein thrombosis Guillain-Barré syndrome Transverse myelitis Cranial neuropathy Polyneuropathy	Intracellular bacteria Mite-borne
Ehrlichia	*E. chaffeensis*	Lymphocytic meningitis Cranial neuropathy Demyelinating polyneuropathy	Intracellular bacteria Tick-borne
Anaplasma	*A. phagocytophilum*	(same as ehrlichiosis?)	Intracellular bacteria Tick-borne
Gram-positive pyogenic bacteria	*Streptococcus pneumoniae* *Staphylococcus* spp.	Meningitis Brain abscess	Diplococcus Cocci
Gram-negative pyogenic bacteria	*Neisseria meningitidis*	Meningitis	Waterhouse-Friderichsen syndrome
	Escherichia coli	Meningitis	
	Haemophilus influenzae	Meningitis	Vaccine available
	Pseudomonas spp.	Abscess, meningitis	Hemorrhagic
Actinomycetaceae	*Actinomyces israelii* *Actinomyces meyeri* *Actinomyces viscosus*	Brain abscess	Filamentous
Actinobacteria	*Tropheryma whipplei*	Multifocal encephalitic nodules	Accumulation of partially degraded bacteria in macrophages
Nocardiaceae	*Nocardia asteroides complex* *Nocardia brasiliensis complex*	Brain abscess	Filamentous
Mycobacteria	*M. tuberculosis*	Basal meningitis Tuberculoma Abscesses (HIV)	Acid-alcohol resistant
	Non-tuberculous mycobacteria: MAC *M. haemophilium* *M. kansasii*	Brain abscess	Opportunistic pathogens
Spirochaetaceae	*Treponema pallidum*	Neurosyphilis	Humans only known natural hosts
	Borrelia burgdorferi	Lyme disease	Tick-borne
	Borrelia recurrentis	Relapsing fever	Louse-borne
	Other *Borrelia* species	Relapsing fever	Tick-borne
	Leptospira interrogans	Meningitis Meningoencephalitis Meningomyelitis Polyradiculoneuropathy Intracranial hemorrhage	Rodents are reservoirs

(continued)

Infections of the Central Nervous System

Table 1.2 (Continued)

Organisms	Genus/Species	Type of CNS infection	Characteristics
Brucella	B. melitensis B. suis B. abortus	Neurobrucellosis	The most frequent zoonosis worldwide
Legionella	58 species, 30 of which are pathogenic for humans	Encephalopathy Transient focal neurological signs	Always associated with pulmonary disease

HIV, human immunodeficiency virus; MAC, *Mycobacterium avium-intracellulare complex*.

Table 1.3 Important fungal pathogens in the CNS.

Group/Genus	Species (common)	Types of CNS infections (common)	Distinct fungal characteristics
Molds (Filamentous fungi)			
Hyaline (not pigmented)			
Aspergillus	A. fumigatus	Brain abscess	Branching septate hyphae
	A. flavus	Skull-base syndromes	Angiophilic
	Other species	Stroke/infarction Disseminated infection	
		Hemorrhagic	
		Myelitis	
Fusarium	F. solani species complex	Meningoencephalitis Brain abscess	Branching septate hyphae
Mucorales			Branching nonseptate hyphae
Rhizopus	R. arrhizus	Brain abscess	Angiophilic
Rhizomucor	R. pusillus	Rhino-cerebral	
Mucor	M. indicus	Stroke/infarction Disseminated infection Hemorrhagic	
Lichtheimia	L. corymbifera	Brain abscess Rhino-cerebral	
Apophysomyces	A. elegans	Rhino-cerebral	
Pigmented molds (Dematiaceous)			
Cladophialophora	C. bantiana	Meningitis	Branching nonseptate pigmented hyphae
Exophiala	E. dermatitidis	Brain abscess	
Rhinocladiella	R. mackenziei		
Verruconis	V. gallopava		
Fonsecaea	F. pedrosoi		
	F. monophora		
Curvularia	C. spicifera		
	C. hawaiiensis		
	C. lunata		
Alternaria	A. Infectoria		

Table 1.3 (Continued)

Group/Genus	Species (common)	Types of CNS infections (common)	Distinct fungal characteristics
Yeasts			
Candida	C. albicans	Meningitis	Unicellular yeasts
	C. parapsilosis	Meningoencephalitis	
		Brain abscess	
		Disseminated infection	
Cryptococcus	C. neoformans	Meningitis	
	C. gattii	Meningoencephalitis	
		Myelitis	
		Cryptococcoma	
		Disseminated infection	
Trichosporon	T. asahii	Meningitis	Yeast-like, arthroconidia
		Brain abscess	
Dimorphic fungi			
Blastomyces	B. dermatitidis	Brain abscess	Yeast form in vivo and filamentous form in vitro
		Myelitis	
Histoplasma	H. capsulatum	Meningitis	
		Brain abscess	
		Disseminated infection	
Coccidioides	C. immitis	Meningitis	
	C. posadasii	Meningoencephalitis	
		Brain abscess	
		Myelitis	
		Disseminated infection	
Paracoccidioides	P. brasiliensis	Brain abscess	
		Disseminated infection	

Table 1.4 Main parasitic infections of the CNS.

Category/Genus	Species	Main CNS neurological syndrome/disease	Characteristics
Protozoa			
Plasmodium	P. falciparum	Cerebral malaria	Parasitized RBCs in cerebral blood vessels
	P. knowlesi	Cerebral malaria	Parasitized RBCs in cerebral blood vessels
Toxoplasma	T. gondii	Encephalitis/abscess	Associated with immunosuppression
		Congenital toxoplasmosis	
Amoeba	Entamoeba histolytica	Encephalitis/abscess	Non-free-living amoeba
	Naegleria fowleri	Primary meningoencephalitis	Free-living amoeba
	Acanthamoeba species	Granulomatous meningoencephalitis	Free-living amoeba
	Balamuthia mandrillaris	Granulomatous meningoencephalitis	Free-living amoeba
	Sappinia pedata		
Trypanosoma			
	T. brucei gambiense	African trypanosomiasis/ meningoencephalitis	Unicellular hemoflagellate
	T. brucei brucei		
	T. cruzi	South American trypanosomiasis/Chagas disease (acute, chronic, congenital)	Unicellular hemoflagellate
Microsporidia	Microsporidium spp.	Encephalitis	Associated with immunosuppression

(continued)

Table 1.4 (Continued)

Category/Genus	Species	Main CNS neurological syndrome/disease	Characteristics
Leishmania	L. donovani	Visceral leishmaniasis with CNS involvement (rare)	Nonflagellate amastigotes
Helminth (cestodes)			
Taenia	T. solium	Neurocysticercosis	Larva form (cysticerci) involved
	T. multiceps	Coenurosis	Larva form (coenurus) involved
Echinococcus	E. granulosus	Cerebral echinococcosis	Larva form (hydatid cysts) involved
Spirotmetra	S. mansoni	Cerebral sparganosis	Plerocercoid larva (spargana) involved
	S. mansonoides		
	S. poliferum		
Helminth (trematodes)			
Schistosoma	S. haematobium	Cerebral schistosomiasis	Ova involved
	S. mansoni	Cerebral schistosomiasis	Ova involved
	S. japonicum	Cerebral schistosomiasis	Ova involved
	S. mekongi	Cerebral schistosomiasis	Ova involved
Paragonimus	P. westermani and other species	Cerebral paragonimiasis	Immature flukes involved
Helminth (nematodes)			
Angiostrongylus	A. cantonensis	Neuroangiostrongylosis (eosinophilic meningitis)	Larva involved
Gnathostoma	Gnathosoma spp.	Cerebral gnathostomiasis	Larva involved
Toxocara	T. canis	Visceral larva migrans	Larva involved
	T. cati	Neurotoxocariasis	
	(other non-Toxocara spp.)		
Trichinella	T. spiralis	Neurotrichinosis	Larva involved
	Other species		
Filaria	Loa loa	CNS involvement not well established	Microfilaria involved
	Onchocerca volvulus		
Strongyloides	S. stercoralis	Cerebral strongyloidiasis	Larva involved

CNS, central nervous system; RBCs, red blood cells; spp., species.

different types of lesions and their distribution in various parts of the CNS may be dictated by the different routes of neuroinvasion (e.g. hematogenous or along peripheral nerves or olfactory bulb); spread from adjacent extracranial structures; the nature of the pathogen and its predilection for different cellular or tissue targets; the tempo of the infection whether acute, subacute, or chronic; and the host immune response

The typical inflammation observed in many viral CNS infections consists of perivascular cuffing and parenchymal infiltration by inflammatory cells, often with microglial nodule formation, neuronophagia, and necrosis. Most viruses infecting the CNS are neuronotropic and, therefore, could potentially affect all areas where neurons are found. However, preferred routes of CNS invasion or even a predilection for different neuronal populations may determine the topography of the inflammation (e.g. in herpes simplex 1 and enterovirus A71 infections). Viral inclusions in different cellular compartments (i.e. nucleus or cytoplasm) may be observed in many DNA viruses and a few RNA viruses (e.g. paramyxoviruses: measles and henipavirus) and can be useful diagnostic features. Although relatively rare, vasculopathy (e.g. vasculitis and thrombosis) is observed not only in henipavirus and varicella-zoster virus infections but may also be encountered in angioinvasive fungal and rickettsial infections and in CNS tuberculosis.

Abscesses are generally localized, circumscribed acute or subacute inflammations caused by pyogenic bacteria, fungi, and *Toxoplasma*. They may be found in most areas of the CNS. Certain bacteria such as *Streptococcus pneumoniae* and *Haemophilus influenzae* are the main culprits for acute pyogenic meningitis. Granulomatous inflammation in the CNS is most often associated with more chronic infections, notably *Mycobacteria*, fungi, and spirochetes and in some parasitic infections like amoebiasis. Sarcoidosis, although not regarded as an infection, is included as it is an important differential diagnosis in granulomatous CNS inflammation.

Despite recent advances in molecular diagnosis using polymerase chain reaction (PCR)-based methods, sequencing, and so on, light microscopy using routine hematoxylin and eosin (H&E) stains may still be quite useful to help identify pathogens in infected tissues and other biological specimens based on morphology alone, especially if combined with special histochemical stains, immunohistochemistry, and in situ hybridization. Familiarity with diagnostic morphological features of certain fungi and parasites are particularly helpful. Commercial or proprietary specific primary antibodies for immunohistochemistry, if available, could also help detect some viral, bacterial, fungal, and parasitic infections to enable a more rapid diagnosis.

This volume also highlights the major historical and epidemiological characteristics of the different diseases, their clinical presentation and difficulties in diagnosis, and their pathogenesis, including information from animal models. It also gives some information on the microbiological characteristics of the agents, although it is not intended to be a detailed microbiological book. Genetic characteristics of both the agents and the hosts are discussed with reference to how these can favor disease development in particular hosts.

This monograph will be of interest to a wide variety of medical doctors, postgraduate students, and scientists involved in studying, diagnosing, or treating infections involving the CNS. We hope that it will become a reference book in neurology departments and microbiology and pathology laboratories because it approaches the topic in a way not dealt with in other books.

We have been fortunate in benefiting from numerous international authors who have written about their own area of expertise in CNS infectious diseases. Collaborating with the authors has been productive, interesting, and useful, and we sincerely thank them all for their generosity.

Reference

1. Kaminski, Z., Kapila, R., Sharer, L.R. et al. (1992). Meningitis due to *Prototheca wickerhamii* in a patient with AIDS. *Clin Infect Dis* 15: 704–706.

2

Sepsis-Associated Encephalopathy

Franck Verdonk[1,2,3], **Aurelien Mazeraud**[1,2,4], **Fabrice Chrétien**[1,5,6], **and Tarek Sharshar**[1,2,4]

[1] Experimental Neuropathology Unit, Pasteur Institute, Paris, France
[2] Department of Anesthesiology and Intensive Care, Saint Antoine Hospital, Paris, France
[3] Sorbonne University, Paris, France
[4] University Paris Diderot, Sorbonne Paris Cité, Paris, France
[5] Paris University, Paris, France
[6] Department of Neuropathology, Sainte Anne Hospital, Paris, France

Abbreviations

AMPA	α-amino-3-hydroxy-5-methyl-4-isoxazolepropionic acid
APACHE	acute physiology and chronic health disease classification system II
AQP4	aquaporin 4
Bax	proapoptotic factors
BBB	blood-brain barrier
BCL	B-cell lymphoma
CLP	cecal ligation and puncture
CNS	central nervous system
DAMPs	damage-associated molecular pattern molecules
DSM-5	*Diagnostic and Statistical Manual of Mental Disorders*-5
EEG	electroencephalogram
ICU	intensive care unit
DIC	disseminated intravascular coagulopathy
IL	interleukin
MRI	magnetic resonance imaging
NMDAR	N-methyl-D-aspartate receptor
NOS	nitric oxide synthase
NSE	neuron-specific enolase
PAA	plasma anticholinergic activity
PAMPs	pathogen-associated molecular pattern molecules
SAE	sepsis-associated encephalopathy
TLR	toll-like receptor
TNF	tumor necrosis factor
ZO	zonula occludens

Infections of the Central Nervous System: Pathology and Genetics, First Edition. Edited by Fabrice Chrétien, Kum Thong Wong, Leroy R. Sharer, Catherine (Katy) Keohane and Françoise Gray.
© 2020 John Wiley & Sons Ltd. Published 2020 by John Wiley & Sons Ltd.

Infections of the Central Nervous System

Definition of the disorder, major synonyms, and historical perspective

Sepsis is defined as a life-threatening organ dysfunction caused by a dysregulated host response to infection [1]. Sepsis is the most common causes of mortality in intensive care units (ICUs) and ranges from 10 to 50% [2]. During sepsis, CNS dysfunction, called sepsis-associated encephalopathy (SAE), occurs in more than 30% of patients. It is clinically characterized by impaired consciousness, which ranges from dizziness to coma and delirium, but it is also associated with an increased risk of stroke or epilepsy. SAE is associated with increased ICU and in-hospital mortality and long-term cognitive decline [3].

Epidemiologic characteristics

The incidence of SAE has been calculated in prospective and retrospective cohorts. In one of the first large prospective studies of 1333 patients with severe sepsis, Sprung et al. reported that 307 (23%) developed cognitive and behavioral changes [4]. More recently, in a retrospective study, Zhang et al. found a lower incidence of 17.7% [5]. This discrepancy is because the diagnostic criteria for SAE have evolved over the last decade and remain controversial. They should combine both clinical and neurophysiological parameters. Electroencephalogram (EEG) changes suggesting SAE are present in up to 80% of bacteremia cases [6, 7]. Considering the estimated number of patients treated for sepsis worldwide, the number of patients affected by SAE could range from 5.3 to 25.2 million annually.

Predictive factors
The risk factors in SAE include patients' comorbidities, clinical and microbiological characteristics of septic shock, and intensive-care interventions. Age, comorbid illness (notably neuropsychiatric), severity of organ failure (notably renal and liver), sedation, and drug side effects are all risk factors. Antibiotic overdose has to be excluded in this context. Encephalopathy is more frequent in cases of bacteremia or of infection with *Staphylococcus aureus*, *Enterococcus faecium*, *Acinetobacter* spp., *Pseudomonas aeruginosa*, or *Stenotrophomonas maltophilia*.

Consequences for survival
SAE is associated with increased morbidity and mortality. Sepsis-related mortality rises from 26 to 49% when complicated by encephalopathy [4]. Delirium is associated with a threefold increase in mortality rate in the general population of patients who are critically ill [8].

Consequences for long-term cognitive dysfunction
About one-third of patients will have cognitive impairment 12 months after their ICU discharge [9], and the degree of impairment is proportional to the duration of delirium during their ICU stay [10]. Similar to mild Alzheimer disease, memory, attention, verbal fluency, and executive functions are mainly affected [11, 12]. Patients with sepsis seem particularly susceptible to cognitive decline. Iwashyna et al. reported that hospitalization for sepsis tripled the risk of developing moderate to severe cognitive decline [13].

Patients with sepsis are also at risk of suicide and of developing psychological disorders, including depression, anxiety, and post-traumatic stress disorder [14].

Clinical features including appropriate investigations

Clinical examination
The fundamental features of SAE are the combination of sepsis and impairment of consciousness, ranging from delirium to coma. Delirium can be either hyperactive (i.e. agitation) or hypoactive. But before encephalopathy occurs, patients with sepsis usually develop a "sickness behavior," which is a physiological response to any systemic inflammation and characterized by lethargy, depression, anxiety, loss of appetite, drowsiness, hyperalgesia, difficulty concentrating, and thermal regulation disorder [15].

Motor signs, such as paratonic rigidity, asterixis, tremor, or myoclonus are rarely observed compared to hepatic, uremic, or toxic encephalopathies.

Intensivists have validated clinical test scales at their disposal for the detection of SAE. These include the Confusion Assessment Method for Intensive Care Units (CAM-ICU) [16] or the Intensive Care

Delirium Screening Checklist Worksheet (ICDSC) [17] for the diagnosis of delirium. Because the clinical spectrum of SAE is extremely broad and not limited to delirium, no single clinical examination is sufficiently specific and sensitive to be systematically applied, particularly in less-severe and early forms of SAE. It should be noted that the majority of clinical studies conducted on SAE only target delirium for the sake of diagnostic simplicity.

Once SAE is suspected, a thorough neurological examination is required, including an assessment of neck stiffness, motor responses, muscle strength, and deep tendon and cranial nerve reflexes. Although the frequent use of sedatives in ICU may limit the clinical examination, assessment of brainstem responses appears useful and loss of responses in patients who are sedated is predictive of mortality and altered mental status [18].

SAE blood markers

Serum S100β protein and neuron-specific enolase (NSE) have been proposed as biomarkers for SAE [19, 20], but their usefulness for predicting, diagnosing, and monitoring SAE awaits confirmation.

EEG

In patients with sepsis, two types of electroencephalographic abnormalities are visible affecting either the background activity or superimposed epileptic features. Background activity changes range from slowing of the normal alpha rhythm with the onset of theta activity in patients with mild encephalopathy (i.e. confusion or delirium), to an increase in slow waves, the onset of delta waves, and even "burst suppression" in severe encephalopathy associated with coma. The latter indicate damage to deep brain structures such as the central gray nuclei and midbrain [21].

Epileptic features are the second type of anomaly observed and have recently been precisely defined. Electrographic seizures are associated with delirium, whereas lack of EEG reactivity is associated with mortality [22]. EEG changes can also be observed in patients with sepsis who are asymptomatic, making it an interesting method for detecting and monitoring SAE. EEG anomalies are also associated with radiologic findings [23]. We, therefore, recommend that an EEG should always be performed in cases of SAE or suspected SAE.

Brain imaging

Brain imaging is not systematically carried out, but to exclude the usual causes of neurological deterioration (i.e. ischemic or hemorrhagic stroke, subarachnoid hemorrhage, abscess, etc.), it is required when seizures, focal neurological signs, persistent delirium, or coma occur.

Imaging usually reveals white matter hyperdensities, mainly related to vasogenic edema, and ischemic stroke, mainly related to DIC [15]. However, it can be normal in half the cases [15]. Magnetic resonance imaging (MRI) is useful to assess secondary cognitive impairment associated with white matter changes and hippocampal atrophy [24].

Physiopathology

Systemic inflammation is the main basis for SAE pathophysiology. Sepsis induces a dramatic immune inflammatory response associated with the clinical manifestations of SAE. Circulating levels of proinflammatory markers (namely interleukin (IL)-1, IL-6 or tumor necrosis factor (TNF)-soluble receptor decreased matrix metalloproteinase-9 [MMP-9] and protein C concentrations) are associated with an increased risk of delirium [25–27]. More generally, it has been shown that cognitive impairment relates to systemic inflammation whether as a result of sepsis or occurring after surgery [28, 29].

SAE is historically viewed as an aseptic insult of the CNS, justifying the term "encephalopathy" rather than "encephalitis" [30]. However, a recent study questions this view. In a mouse model of sepsis using cecal ligation and puncture (CLP) [31], Singer et al. found that sepsis is associated with polymicrobial spread within the CNS by viable bacteria during the acute phase up to the fifth day. The authors showed an increased expression of neuroinflammatory markers in microglial cells. These findings gain some support from a human study reporting brain abscesses in about 10% of patients [32]. If a microbial process is involved, encephalopathy is mainly secondary to the systemic inflammation.

The consequences of systemic inflammation on the brain can be separated into three nonexclusive mechanisms: ischemic, neuroinflammatory, and epileptic processes. In combination, these processes result in impairment of neurotransmission and neurotoxicity. Particular structures are vulnerable to these phenomena: the frontal cortex and hippocampus, which accounts for acute and chronic neurological symptoms of sepsis, and central autonomic nuclei (i.e. amygdala, locus coeruleus, medullary nuclei), accounting for acute impairment of the response to stress [33].

Systemic or local inflammation is transmitted to the CNS via three major pathways [34]:
1. Circumventricular organs enable inflammatory mediators to pass directly into the brain parenchyma. They are thought to play a major role in the "humoral pathway" and induce neuroinflammation.
2. Blood-brain barrier (BBB) disruption increases the passage of inflammatory mediators to brain parenchyma, enabling their participation in micro- and macroangiopathy and neuroinflammation.
3. Neural pathways, notably via the vagus nerves, transfer the peripheral inflammatory signal to the medullary autonomic nuclei. The increased neuronal activity can produce excitotoxicity and is associated with neuroinflammation.

Ischemic processes

Macrocirculatory impairment

In addition to hypotension, hypovolemia, and cardiac dysfunction, impairment of autoregulation can compromise cerebral perfusion. Autoregulation is a physiological mechanism that aims to maintain a constant cerebral blood flow. In physiological conditions, the vessel diameter adapts to blood pressure. In patients with sepsis, this mechanism can be impaired. Schramm et al. showed that autoregulation is impaired in 60% at day 1 and 46% at day 4 [35]. Moreover, impaired autoregulation at day 1 was associated with delirium occurring at day 4, and this association was confirmed in a larger cohort of 50 patients with sepsis [36]. Interestingly, early decrease in cerebral flow correlates with long-term cognitive impairment [37].

Microcirculatory impairment

Sepsis frequently causes microvascular dysfunction that is considered an important mechanism in organ failure [38]. Microcirculatory dysfunction hampers diffusion of gases and induces a mosaic of tissue hypoxia and vascular shunts alongside well-oxygenated areas. Endothelial dysfunction, glycocalyx (pericellular matrix) changes, mechanisms inducing leukocyte translocation and platelet microthrombi, and pericyte dysfunction are its main mechanisms [39, 40]. This microcirculatory dysfunction can affect the brain, compromising its metabolism as oxygen demand and supply become unbalanced [41]. Microcirculation impairment impinges neurovascular coupling during sepsis [42]. So far, there are no preventive or therapeutic strategies for microcirculatory dysfunction.

Endothelial dysfunction

Endothelial activation at the early phase of sepsis results in increased permeability of the BBB, although tight junction proteins such as occludin, zonula occludens (ZO)-1 and ZO-2 [43], and claudin-3 and claudin-5 [44] seem preserved. Other factors contribute to BBB dysfunction, including astrocyte activation and overexpression of aquaporin 4 (AQP4). Endothelial activation contributes to the neuroinflammatory process by releasing inflammatory and neurotoxic factors or allowing their passage through an impaired BBB [45].

Ischemic lesions in sepsis

Ischemic lesions are constantly observed in patients who die from sepsis. They are found in areas of the brain sensitive to ischemia such as Ammon's horn, the lenticular nucleus, and frontal cortex but also and more specifically (in comparison to patients who died from causes other than sepsis) in autonomic nuclei involved in cardiovascular control (i.e. posterior and anterior hypothalamus, locus coeruleus). Pronounced neuronal apoptosis is also observed in these same areas. In addition, cerebral hemorrhages are found in 17–26% of patients who die of septic shock [32, 46]. Necrotizing multifocal leukoencephalopathy can also be found and correlates with brain expression of tumor necrosis factor alpha (TNF-α) and IL-1β and elevated circulating levels of TNF-α, IL-1β, IL-6, IL-8, IL-10, the soluble receptor for TNF II, and for IL-1 receptor antagonist [47]. Hypoxemia and hyperglycemia are frequent features of sepsis, which potentiate the deleterious effects of impaired cerebral perfusion. To date, there is no recommendation for monitoring and optimizing cerebral perfusion.

Neuroinflammatory process
The central player in neuroinflammation is the microglial cell. Microglial cells are involved in brain immune defense but also synaptic plasticity. As innate immune cells, they express receptors to pathogen-associated molecular pattern molecules (PAMPs) and damage-associated molecular pattern molecules (DAMPs) such as toll-like receptors (TLRs; especially TLR2 and TLR4) particularly involved in microglial activation. When activated, microglial cells release cytokines that promote the recruitment of circulating immune cells [48]. He et al. have demonstrated that natural killer (NK) cells penetrate into the brain early during sepsis and modulate microglia to recruit neutrophils [49].

The concerted action of all signaling pathways leads to a high production of proinflammatory cytokines via the induction of an M1 immunophenotype that can have several cytotoxic properties [50]. Activated microglia can also release large amounts of glutamate and, thus, induce neuronal dysfunction [51]. Excessive stimulation of N-methyl-D-aspartate receptors (NMDARs) could deregulate the calcium flow and lead to neuronal cell death [52].

Activated microglial cells also release free radicals that cause axonal damage or peroxidation of membrane lipids, resulting in neuronal loss [53]. Also, microglial cells' inducible nitric oxide synthase (iNOS) can produce nitric oxide and contribute to neuronal apoptosis [54, 55]. Conversely, microglia can also help in the "clearance" of free radicals (e.g. by regulating ceruloplasmin levels) and prevent neuronal death.

Various experimental studies aimed at modulating microglial activation to improve SAE phenotype. One promising research lead is minocycline, an antibiotic with anti-inflammatory and neuroprotective properties [56, 57]. In an experimental study, minocycline limited the expression of markers of oxidative damage such as carbonylated proteins and inflammation (particularly TNFα and IL-6) in the hippocampus 24 hours after sepsis and improved cognitive performance after sepsis [58]. These effects seem to be mediated through specific inhibition of M1 microglial polarization [59].

Other experimental studies showed that resveratrol decreases microglial activation and neuronal apoptosis with improvement in spatial memory. These effects are probably mediated by the inhibition of the *NLRP3*/IL-1β pathway in hippocampal microglia. Ketamine, an anesthetic drug acting as a N-methyl-D-aspartate (NMDA) antagonist, also holds promise in this field of microglial modulation. Numerous experimental [60] and clinical [61] studies showed an immune-modulatory effect of this molecule with benefit in the context of sepsis or aseptic inflammation [62]. A recent French study of continuous injection of ketamine in patients in the ICU, including patients with sepsis, resulted in a significant decrease in the incidence of delirium [63].

Finally, persistent microglial activation or microglial priming are thought to be involved in the cognitive decline following sepsis, even in neurodegenerative process. It has been hypothesized that decreased microglial cholinergic inhibition accounts for translation from delirium to cognitive impairment. However, rivastigmine administration failed to show any benefit for this purpose in a randomized clinical trial [64].

Neurotransmission impairment and neurotoxicity

Neurotransmission impairment
There is a body of evidence that neurotransmission is impaired during sepsis and may result in reduced or aberrant neural activity [65]. All neurotransmitters can be affected, but an imbalance between the cholinergic and dopaminergic systems has been particularly incriminated.

Several studies have shown a strong association between plasma anticholinergic activity (PAA) [66] and the incidence of delirium. During sepsis, global hypocholinergia is observed because of a lack of acetylcholine production (dependent on acetyl CoA) and pre-, per-, and postsynaptic cholinergic dysfunction. In addition, the cholinergic system is modulated by dopamine, noradrenaline, or serotonin whose neurotransmission is impaired by sepsis-related increase in plasma levels of amino acids such as tryptophan or tyrosine [67].

Dexmedetomidine, a selective alpha2-adrenergic receptor agonist of the locus coeruleus, has been proposed as a regulator of mono-aminergic transmission to prevent glutamate-dependent neuronal death [68]. However, a randomized clinical trial failed to show a benefit on incidence of SAE, and lorazepam was more effective than benzodiazepines, which are commonly used in sepsis and act as agonists of the gamma-aminobutyric acid-ergic (GABAergic) pathways [69].

Excitotoxicity
Increased neurotransmission, especially glutamatergic, augments the energy needs to maintain cell homeostasis. Inadequate supply for energy needs can induce mitochondrial dysfunction, which in turn can result in apoptosis and cell death via an oxidative mechanism. Several mechanisms increase neuronal activity: increased concentration of neurotransmitters or co-neurotransmitters in synaptic clefts or neurotransmitter receptor sensitization. During sepsis, the first observable phenomenon is neuronal hyperactivity, notably in the centers (such as amygdala) controlling the response to stress. A recent study has even shown that TNF-α can play a role as a co-transmitter and sensitize glutamate receptor during sepsis. Finally, cytokines can increase the expression of α-amino-3-hydroxy-5-methyl-4-isoxazolepropionic acid (AMPA) receptors and NMDARs on neurons, associated with cognitive and behavioral dysfunction [70]. Thus, neuronal activity is dramatically increased during sepsis, leading to energy failure, mitochondrial dysfunction, and cell death. Interestingly, it has been shown that hippocampal apoptosis can result from vagal signaling of the stretch-lung induced by invasive mechanical ventilation [71].

Consequences for cell status
Cell death
A neuropathological study of 23 patients who died from septic shock showed neuronal apoptosis in central autonomic nervous system nuclei [32]. The majority of necrotic neurons did not express caspase 3, suggesting a role for other proapoptotic factors. Later experimental studies confirmed that sepsis induces apoptosis in various region of the brain, notably the frontal cortex and the hippocampus [72].

Mitochondrial dysfunction and oxidative stress
Mitochondrial dysfunction and oxidative stress are considered to be major mechanisms of organ failure during sepsis. Neurons and microglial cells are liable to mitochondrial dysfunction and oxidative stress and consequently to apoptosis. These phenomena seem to occur early and to preferentially affect the hippocampus and CNS autonomic centers [73]. Hippocampal neurons have increased expression of the proapoptotic factor, BAX2, which induces apoptosis by stimulating cytochrome C release from mitochondria [74]. Decrease in the phosphorylation of cerebral mitochondrial complexes OXPHOS I, II, and III also supports mitochondrial brain dysfunction during sepsis [75]. It has also been shown that combined antioxidants (N-acetylcysteine and deferoxamine) reduce cell damage in the hippocampus six hours after sepsis induction [76]. Hyperglycemia and hypoxemia can aggravate mitochondrial dysfunction and oxidative stress. If blood glucose control reduces microglial activation and neuronal death in stressed animals [72], its benefit on neurological outcome has not been seen in patients who are critically ill or have had a stroke [77]. It must also be mentioned that hyperoxia can be neurotoxic [78].

Axonal damage
A recent translational neuropathological and neuroimaging study has shown that sepsis induces axonal damage [79]. The mechanism has not been proven and might be multifactorial, inflammatory, and metabolic. It is conceivable that along with ischemic damage and persistent neuroinflammation, axonal injury may account for long-term cognitive decline.

Treatment, future perspective, and conclusions

To date, there is no specific treatment for SAE. Its management relies essentially on the control of sepsis according to established recommendations, for instance, the Surviving Sepsis Campaign Guidelines for Management of Severe Sepsis and Septic Shock [80]. General recommendations for the prevention and treatment of delirium must also be applied (Table 2.1).

Table 2.1 Pharmacological and nonpharmacological measures for the management of severe sepsis and septic shock.

Pharmacological measures
Reduce use of benzodiazepines and opioids
Interrupt sedation daily
Use dexmedetomidine (vs midazolam or propofol) as sedative agents
Pain assessment
Sedation – analgesia – delirium protocol

Nonpharmacological measures
Prevention of metabolic disturbances (Severe hypoxemia, dysnatremia(s), prolonged hyperglycemia)
Sleep protocol
Reorientation and cognition-stimulating activities
Rehydration
Use of eyeglasses, magnifying lenses, and hearing aids
Avoid use of physical restraints
Early mobilization

- Cerebrospinal fluid (CSF) analysis should be performed when meningitis or encephalitis is suspected, and brain imaging should be done in cases with focal neurological signs, seizures, or severe/persistent encephalopathy.
- We regard EEG as mandatory to confirm SAE diagnosis and to exclude an epileptic process.
- Side effects of drug therapy must be systematically excluded, especially antibiotic overdose.
- Vitamin deficiency needs to be prevented or treated.
- Prevention and appropriate treatment of a secondary brain insult is required, knowing that tight blood glucose control has not been of proven benefit.
- Several drugs, which have been tested experimentally targeting BBB dysfunction, microglial activation, neurotransmitter imbalance, or oxidative stress tested, could be considered for use in patients with sepsis.

Unfortunately, the main limitation of intervention is the absence of noninvasive or reliable methods for monitoring the processes involved in SAE.

References

1. Singer, M., Deutschman, C.S., Seymour, C.W. et al. (2016). The third international consensus definitions for sepsis and septic shock (sepsis-3). *JAMA* 315: 801–810.
2. Tran, D.D., Groeneveld, A.B., van de Meulen, J. et al. (1990). Age, chronic disease, sepsis, organ system failure, and mortality in a medical intensive care unit. *Crit. Care Med.* 18: 474–479.
3. Eidelman, L.A., Putterman, D., Putterman, C., and Sprung, C.L. (1996). The spectrum of septic encephalopathy. Definitions, etiologies, and mortalities. *JAMA* 275: 470–473.
4. Sprung, C.L., Peduzzi, P.N., Shatney, C.H. et al. (1990). Impact of encephalopathy on mortality in the sepsis syndrome. The veterans administration systemic sepsis cooperative study group. *Crit. Care Med.* 18: 801–806.
5. Zhang, L., Wang, X.T., Ai, Y.H. et al. (2012). Epidemiological features and risk factors of sepsis-associated encephalopathy in intensive care unit patients: 2008–2011. *Chin. Med. J.* 125: 828–831.
6. Young, G.B., Bolton, C.F., Austin, T.W. et al. (1990). The encephalopathy associated with septic illness. *Clin. Invest. Med.* 13: 297–304.
7. Young, G.B., Bolton, C., Archibald, Y.M. et al. (1992). The electroencephalogram in sepsis-associated encephalopathy. *J. Clin. Neurophysiol.* 9: 145–152.
8. Ely, E.W., Shintani, A., Truman, B. et al. (2004). Delirium as a predictor of mortality in mechanically ventilated patients in the intensive care unit. *JAMA* 291: 1753–1762.
9. Pandharipande, P.P., Girard, T.D., and Ely, E.W. (2014). Long-term cognitive impairment after critical illness. *N. Engl. J. Med.* 370: 185–186.
10. Girard, T.D., Jackson, J.C., Pandharipande, P.P. et al. (2010). Delirium as a predictor of long-term cognitive impairment in survivors of critical illness. *Crit. Care Med.* 38: 1513–1520.
11. Semmler, A., Hermann, S., Mormann, F. et al. (2008). Sepsis causes neuroinflammation and concomitant decrease of cerebral metabolism. *J. Neuroinflammation* 5: 38.
12. Rothenhäusler, H.B., Ehrentraut, S., Stoll, C. et al. (2001). The relationship between cognitive performance and employment and health status in long-term survivors of the acute respiratory distress syndrome: results of an exploratory study. *Gen. Hosp. Psychiatry* 23: 90–96.

13. Iwashyna, T.J., Ely, E.W., Smith, D.M., and Langa, K.M. (2010). Long-term cognitive impairment and functional disability among survivors of severe sepsis. *JAMA* 304 (16): 1787–1794.
14. Boer, K.R., van Ruler, O., van Emmerik, A.A.P. et al. (2008). Factors associated with posttraumatic stress symptoms in a prospective cohort of patients after abdominal sepsis: a nomogram. *Intensive Care Med.* 34: 664–674.
15. Annane, D. and Sharshar, T. (2015). Cognitive decline after sepsis. *Lancet Respir. Med.* 3: 61–69.
16. Ely, E.W., Inouye, S.K., Bernard, G.R. et al. (2001). Delirium in mechanically ventilated patients: validity and reliability of the confusion assessment method for the intensive care unit (CAM-ICU). *JAMA* 286: 2703–2710.
17. Bergeron, N., Dubois, M.J., Dumont, M. et al. (2001). Intensive care delirium screening checklist: evaluation of a new screening tool. *Intensive Care Med.* 27: 859–864.
18. Sharshar, T., Porche, R., Siami, S. et al. (2011). Brainstem responses can predict death and delirium in sedated patients in intensive care unit. *Crit. Care Med.* 39: 1960–1967.
19. Hsu, A.A., Fenton, K., Weinstein, S. et al. (2008). Neurological injury markers in children with septic shock. *Pediatr. Crit. Care Med.* 9: 245–251.
20. Yao, B., Zhang, L.N., Ai, Y.H. et al. (2014). Serum S100β is a better biomarker than neuron-specific enolase for sepsis-associated encephalopathy and determining its prognosis: a prospective and observational study. *Neurochem. Res.* 39: 1263–1269.
21. Hosokawa, K., Gaspard, N., Su, F. et al. (2014). Clinical neurophysiological assessment of sepsis-associated brain dysfunction: a systematic review. *Crit. Care* 18: 674.
22. Azabou, E., Magalhaes, E., Braconnier, A. et al. (2015). Early standard electroencephalogram abnormalities predict mortality in septic intensive care unit patients. *PLoS One* 10: e0139969.
23. Polito, A., Eischwald, F., Maho, A.L. et al. (2013). Pattern of brain injury in the acute setting of human septic shock. *Crit. Care* 17: R204.
24. Gunther, M.L., Morandi, A., Krauskopf, E. et al. (2012). The association between brain volumes, delirium duration, and cognitive outcomes in intensive care unit survivors: the VISIONS cohort magnetic resonance imaging study*. *Crit. Care Med.* 40: 2022–2032.
25. Girard, T.D., Ware, L.B., Bernard, G.R. et al. Associations of markers of inflammation and coagulation with delirium during critical illness. *Intensive Care Med.* 38: 1965–1973.
26. Skrobik, Y., Leger, C., Cossette, M. et al. (2013). Factors predisposing to coma and delirium: fentanyl and midazolam exposure; CYP3A5, ABCB1, and ABCG2 genetic polymorphisms; and inflammatory factors. *Crit. Care Med.* 41: 999–1008.
27. van den Boogaard, M., Kox, M., Quinn, K.L. et al. (2011). Biomarkers associated with delirium in critically ill patients and their relation with long-term subjective cognitive dysfunction; indications for different pathways governing delirium in inflamed and noninflamed patients. *Crit. Care* 15: R297.
28. Terrando, N., Monaco, C., Ma, D. et al. (2010). Tumor necrosis factor-alpha triggers a cytokine cascade yielding postoperative cognitive decline. *Proc. Natl. Acad. Sci. U. S. A.* 107: 20518–20522.
29. Terrando, N., Rei Fidalgo, A., Vizcaychipi, M. et al. (2010). The impact of IL-1 modulation on the development of lipopolysaccharide-induced cognitive dysfunction. *Crit. Care* 14: R88.
30. Mazeraud, A., Bozza, F.A., and Sharshar, T. (2018). Sepsis-associated encephalopathy is septic. *Am. J. Respir. Crit. Care Med.* 197: 698–699.
31. Singer, B.H., Dickson, R.P., Denstaedt, S.J. et al. (2018). Bacterial dissemination to the brain in sepsis. *Am. J. Respir. Crit. Care Med.* 197: 747–756.
32. Sharshar, T., Annane, D., Lorin de la Grandmaison, G. et al. (2004). The neuropathology of septic shock. *Brain Pathol.* 14: 21–33.
33. Heming, N., Mazeraud, A., Vzerdonk, F. et al. (2017). Neuroanatomy of sepsis-associated encephalopathy. *Crit. Care* 21: 65.
34. Dantzer, R., O'Connor, J.C., Freund, G.G. et al. (2008). From inflammation to sickness and depression: when the immune system subjugates the brain. *Nat. Rev. Neurosci.* 9: 46–56.
35. Schramm, P., Klein, K.U., Falkenberg, L. et al. (2012). Impaired cerebrovascular autoregulation in patients with severe sepsis and sepsis-associated delirium. *Crit. Care* 16: R181.
36. Pfister, D., Siegemund, M., Dell-Kuster, S. et al. (2008). Cerebral perfusion in sepsis-associated delirium. *Crit. Care* 12: R63.
37. Pierrakos, C., Attou, R., Decorte, L. et al. (2017). Cerebral perfusion alterations and cognitive decline in critically ill sepsis survivors. *Acta Clin. Belg.* 72: 39–44.
38. Lelubre, C. and Vincent, J.L. (2018). Mechanisms and treatment of organ failure in sepsis. *Nat. Rev. Nephrol.* 14: 417–427.
39. Østergaard, L., Granfeldt, A., Secher, N. et al. (2015). Microcirculatory dysfunction and tissue oxygenation in critical illness. *Acta Anaesthesiol. Scand.* 59: 1246–1259.

40. De Backer, D., Orbegozo Cortes, D., Donadello, K., and Vincent, J.L. (2014). Pathophysiology of microcirculatory dysfunction and the pathogenesis of septic shock. *Virulence* 5: 73–79.
41. Taccone, F.S., Castanares-Zapatero, D., Peres-Bota, D. et al. (2010). Cerebral autoregulation is influenced by carbon dioxide levels in patients with septic shock. *Neurocrit. Care.* 12: 35–42.
42. Rosengarten, B., Krekel, D., Kuhnert, S., and Schulz, R. (2012). Early neurovascular uncoupling in the brain during community acquired pneumonia. *Crit. Care* 16: R64.
43. Yi, X., Wang, Y., and Yu, F.S. (2000). Corneal epithelial tight junctions and their response to lipopolysaccharide challenge. *Invest. Ophthalmol. Vis. Sci.* 41: 4093–4100.
44. Yang, C.H., Kao, M.C., Shih, P.C. et al. (2015). Simvastatin attenuates sepsis-induced blood-brain barrier integrity loss. *J. Surg. Res.* 194: 591–598.
45. Alexander, J.J., Jacob, A., Cunningham, P. et al. (2008). TNF is a key mediator of septic encephalopathy acting through its receptor, TNF receptor-1. *Neurochem. Int.* 52: 447–456.
46. Jackson, A.C., Gilbert, J.J., Young, G.B., and Bolton, C.F. (1985). The encephalopathy of sepsis. *Can. J. Neurol. Sci.* 12: 303–307.
47. Sharshar, T., Gray, F., Poron, F. et al. (2002). Multifocal necrotizing leukoencephalopathy in septic shock. *Crit. Care Med.* 30: 2371–2375.
48. González, H., Elgueta, D., Montoya, A., and Pacheco, R. (2014). Neuroimmune regulation of microglial activity involved in neuroinflammation and neurodegenerative diseases. *J. Neuroimmunol.* 274: 1–13.
49. He, H., Geng, T., Chen, P. et al. (2016). NK cells promote neutrophil recruitment in the brain during sepsis-induced neuroinflammation. *Sci. Rep.* 6: 27711.
50. Takeuchi, O. and Akira, S. (2010). Pattern recognition receptors and inflammation. *Cell* 140: 805–820.
51. Takeuchi, H., Jin, S., Wang, J. et al. (2006). Tumor necrosis factor-alpha induces neurotoxicity via glutamate release from hemichannels of activated microglia in an autocrine manner. *J. Biol. Chem.* 281: 21362–21368.
52. Zou, J.Y. and Crews, F.T. (2005). TNF alpha potentiates glutamate neurotoxicity by inhibiting glutamate uptake in organotypic brain slice cultures: neuroprotection by NF kappa B inhibition. *Brain Res.* 1034: 11–24.
53. Siesjö, B.K., Agardh, C.D., and Bengtsson, F. (1989). Free radicals and brain damage. *Cerebrovasc. Brain Metab. Rev.* 1: 165–211.
54. Zhang, Y.H., Chen, H., Chen, Y. et al. (2014). Activated microglia contribute to neuronal apoptosis in Toxoplasmic encephalitis. *Parasit. Vectors* 7: 372.
55. Heneka, M.T., Löschmann, P.A., Gleichmann, M. et al. (1998). Induction of nitric oxide synthase and nitric oxide-mediated apoptosis in neuronal PC12 cells after stimulation with tumor necrosis factor-alpha/lipopolysaccharide. *J. Neurochem.* 71: 88–94.
56. Schmitz, T., Krabbe, G., Weikert, G. et al. (2014). Minocycline protects the immature white matter against hyperoxia. *Exp. Neurol.* 254: 153–165.
57. Garrido-Mesa, N., Zarzuelo, A., and Gálvez, J. (2013). What is behind the non-antibiotic properties of minocycline? *Pharmacol. Res.* 67: 18–30.
58. Michels, M., Vieira, A.S., Vuolo, F. et al. (2015). The role of microglia activation in the development of sepsis-induced long-term cognitive impairment. *Brain Behav. Immun.* 43: 54–59.
59. Kobayashi, K., Imagama, S., Ohgomori, T. et al. (2013). Minocycline selectively inhibits M1 polarization of microglia. *Cell Death Dis.* 4: e525.
60. Takahashi, T., Kinoshita, M., Shono, S. et al. (2010). The effect of ketamine Anesthesia on the immune function of mice with postoperative Septicemia. *Anesth. Analg.* 111: 1051–1058.
61. Kettenmann, H., Hanisch, U.K., Noda, M., and Verkhratsky, A. (2011). Physiology of microglia. *Physiol. Rev.* 91: 461–553.
62. Hudetz, J.A., Iqbal, Z., Gandhi, S.D. et al. (2009). Ketamine attenuates post-operative cognitive dysfunction after cardiac surgery. *Acta Anaesthesiol. Scand.* 53: 864–872.
63. Sebastien, P., Franck, V., Thomas, G. et al. (2018). Low doses of ketamine reduce delirium but not opiate consumption in mechanically ventilated and sedated ICU patients: a randomised double blind control trial. *Anaesth. Crit. Care Pain Med.* 37: 589–595. https://doi.org/10.1016/j.accpm.2018.09.006.
64. van Eijk, M.M., Roes, K.C., Honing, M.L. et al. (2010). Effect of rivastigmine as an adjunct to usual care with haloperidol on duration of delirium and mortality in critically ill patients: a multicentre, double-blind, placebo-controlled randomised trial. *Lancet* 376: 1829–1837.
65. van Gool, W.A., van de Beek, D., and Eikelenboom, P. (2010). Systemic infection and delirium: when cytokines and acetylcholine collide. *Lancet* 375: 773–775.
66. Flacker, J.M., Cummings, V., Mach, J.R. Jr. et al. (1998). The association of serum anticholinergic activity with delirium in elderly medical patients. *Am. J. Geriatr. Psychiatry* 6: 31–41.
67. Pandharipande, P.P., Morandi, A., Adams, J.R. et al. (2009). Plasma tryptophan and tyrosine levels are independent risk factors for delirium in critically ill patients. *Intensive Care Med.* 35: 1886–1892.

68. Yang, L., Xu, J.M., Jiang, X. et al. (2013). Effect of dexmedetomidine on plasma brain-derived neurotrophic factor: a double-blind, randomized and placebo-controlled study. *Ups. J. Med. Sci.* 118: 235–239.
69. Pandharipande, P., Shintani, A., Peterson, J. et al. (2006). Lorazepam is an independent risk factor for transitioning to delirium in intensive care unit patients. *Anesthesiology* 104: 21–26.
70. Stellwagen, D. and Malenka, R.C. (2006). Synaptic scaling mediated by glial TNF-alpha. *Nature* 440: 1054–1059.
71. González-López, A., López-Alonso, I., Aguirre, A. et al. (2013). Mechanical ventilation triggers hippocampal apoptosis by vagal and dopaminergic pathways. *Am. J. Respir. Crit. Care Med.* 188: 693–702.
72. Sonneville, R., Derese, I., Marques, M.B. et al. (2015). Neuropathological correlates of hyperglycemia during prolonged polymicrobial sepsis in mice. *Shock* 44: 245–251.
73. Sharshar, T., Gray, F., Lorin de la Grandmaison, G. et al. (2003). Apoptosis of neurons in cardiovascular autonomic centres triggered by inducible nitric oxide synthase after death from septic shock. *Lancet* 3: 1799–1805.
74. Messaris, E., Memos, N., Chatzigianni, E. et al. (2004). Time-dependent mitochondrial-mediated programmed neuronal cell death prolongs survival in sepsis. *Crit. Care Med.* 32: 1764–1770.
75. Lyu, J., Zheng, G., Chen, Z. et al. (2015). Sepsis-induced brain mitochondrial dysfunction is associated with altered mitochondrial Src and PTP1B levels. *Brain Res.* 1620: 130–138.
76. Barichello, T., Machado, R.A., Constino, L. et al. (2007). Antioxidant treatment prevented late memory impairment in an animal model of sepsis. *Crit. Care Med.* 35: 2186–2190.
77. Fahy, B.G., Sheehy, A.M., and Coursin, D.B. (2009). Glucose control in intensive care unit. *Crit. Care Med.* 37: 1769–1776.
78. Hafner, S., Beloncle, F., Koch, A. et al. (2015). Hyperoxia in intensive care, emergency, and perioperative medicine: Dr. Jekyll or Mr. Hyde? A 2015 update. *Ann. Intensive Care* 5: 42.
79. Ehler, J., Barrett, L.K., Taylor, V. et al. (2017). Translational evidence for two distinct patterns of neuroaxonal injury in sepsis: a longitudinal, prospective translational study. *Crit. Care* 21: 262.
80. Rhodes, A. et al. (2017). Surviving sepsis campaign. *Crit. Care Med.* 45: 486–552.

3 Variation of CNS Infections According to the Host

Leroy R. Sharer[1], Catherine (Katy) Keohane[2], and Françoise Gray[3,4]

[1] Division of Neuropathology, Department of Pathology, Immunology, and Laboratory Medicine, Rutgers New Jersey Medical School and University Hospital, Newark, NJ, USA
[2] Department of Pathology and School of Medicine, University College Cork, Brookfield Health Science Complex, Cork, Ireland
[3] Retired from Department of Pathology, Lariboisière Hospital, APHP, Paris, France
[4] University Paris Diderot (Paris 7), Paris, France

Abbreviations

ADEM	acute demyelinating encephalomyelitis
AIDS	acquired immune deficiency syndrome
CNS	central nervous system
EBV	Epstein-Barr virus
EGF	Epidermal growth factor
EREG	epiregulin
HAART	highly active antiretroviral therapy
HHV	human herpes virus
HIV	human immunodeficiency virus
HIVE	HIV encephalitis
IL	interleukin
IRIS	immune reconstitution inflammatory syndrome
IUIS	International Union of Immunological Societies
JCV	JC virus
KSHV	Kaposi-sarcoma-associated virus
LPS	lipopolysaccharide
MS	multiple sclerosis
Mtb	*Mycobacterium tuberculosis*
OI	opportunistic infection
PL	phospholipase
PRR	pathogen recognition receptor
TB	tuberculosis
TLR	toll-like receptor
TNF	tumor necrosis factor
VZV	varicella-zoster virus
WHO	World Health Organization

Introduction

The clinical response to pathogens infecting the CNS depends on multiple factors interacting among microbes, the host, and the environment. These include microbial variation (qualitative or quantitative), environmental factors such as poverty, malnutrition and hygiene, route of infection, and host-specific factors mainly affecting the immune system. These host factors not only predispose the individual to particular infections but also modify their clinicopathological features. Figure 3.1 illustrates a proposed scheme to account for variation in individual clinical presentation,

---

Infections of the Central Nervous System: Pathology and Genetics, First Edition. Edited by Fabrice Chrétien, Kum Thong Wong, Leroy R. Sharer, Catherine (Katy) Keohane and Françoise Gray.
© 2020 John Wiley & Sons Ltd. Published 2020 by John Wiley & Sons Ltd.

Infections of the Central Nervous System

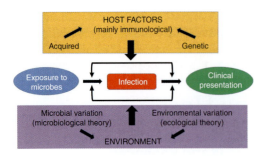

Figure 3.1 Scheme of overlapping factors influencing infectious diseases. In principle, variation in individual clinical presentation, ranging from asymptomatic to lethal infection, in individuals who are infected depends on different overlapping forces in the host and environment: Host factors mainly consist of alterations in the patient's immune status that may be acquired or innately genetic. Disease is attributed to microbial variation (qualitative or quantitative) in the microbiological theory and to environmental variation (other than for the pathogen concerned) in the ecological theory. All these factors are both complementary and overlapping. Source: Adapted and modified from [1].

ranging from asymptomatic to lethal infection, depending on several overlapping forces in the host and the environment. These correspond to acquired or genetic immunological factors in the host and microbiological and ecological variations in the environment. These four factors are both complementary and overlapping [1].

Patient age is an important modifying factor, mainly because of the variation in the maturity of the immune system, which is immature at birth and inefficient in people who are older. Environmental factors also play a part because young children are not exposed to the same number of agents as adults. Intrauterine infections on the one hand [2] and perinatal and postnatal CNS infection on the other [3] differ from CNS infections in children, adults, and patients who are older.

Rare anatomical abnormalities also favor specific infections. The most classical is the association of brain abscesses with cardiac malformations [4]. Another less frequent example is intracranial epidural abscess in patients who are young and are likely to have vascular diploic bone, which increases valveless bidirectional flow between the frontal sinus mucosa and dural veins emptying into the superior longitudinal sinus [5].

However, most variations result from alterations in the patient's immune status. These may be physiological, like immaturity of the immune system in neonates and young children, but most are pathological resulting from congenital or acquired deficiency of the host immune response.

In the past 20 years, the number of patients with immunodeficiencies has dramatically increased. This is partly because of better detection of inborn errors of immunity-based on new technologies [6] but largely because of the growing number of patients with acquired immunodeficiencies.

Primary and congenital immunodeficiency

In 1970, the World Health Organization (WHO) convened a committee to catalog primary immunodeficiencies. This group focused on understanding whether these disorders could be categorized as disorders of B or T cells [7]. Their initial report identified 16 distinct immunodeficiencies. Twenty years later, the International Union of Immunological Societies (IUIS) took the remit of this committee. Its last report (February 2017) categorized and listed 354 inborn errors of immunity with 344 different gene defects, classified according to their clinicopathologic phenotype into nine groups: (i) immunodeficiencies affecting cellular and humoral immunity, (ii) combined immunodeficiencies with associated or syndromic features, (iii) predominantly antibody deficiencies, (iv) diseases of immune dysregulation, (v) congenital defects of phagocyte number, function, or both, (vi) defects in intrinsic and innate immunity, (vii) autoinflammatory disorders, (viii) complement deficiencies, and (ix) phenocopies of primary immunodeficiencies [6, 8].

From these reports it appears that these diseases manifest mostly, but not invariably, in children and young adults, and that they mainly predispose to lymphoproliferative disorders (including Epstein-Barr virus [EBV] + B-cell lymphoproliferation), or autoimmune disorders.

Predisposition to specific infections may be found in the different groups, but recurrent bacterial infections (mainly pulmonary and gastrointestinal) are largely observed in the predominantly antibody deficiencies (PID) group, whereas specific susceptibility to mycobacterial disease, predisposition to severe viral infection (particularly herpes simplex encephalitis), predisposition to invasive fungal infections including *CARD9* deficiency favoring *Candida* CNS infection [9] and toll-like receptor (TLR) signaling pathway deficiency with bacterial susceptibility, are found in the defects in intrinsic and innate immunity group.

In the near future, single-gene inborn errors of immunity underlying infections are likely to be discovered as a result of technological advances, particularly in deep sequencing. This should allow us to understand the pathogenesis of specific infections in patients with known risks factors and to decipher the cellular and molecular mechanisms of immune anti-infectious agents. Studying primary immunodeficiencies that predispose to specific infections can serve both purposes, by elucidating genetic etiologies of unexplained infectious diseases and by improving our understanding of immunity in other settings to develop new therapies and preventive measures [9].

Acquired immunodeficiencies and opportunistic infections

Congenital and idiopathic immunodeficiency disorders, particularly those underlying CNS infections, are relatively rare and mainly relate to specific infections. However, this group may expand with the development of molecular technologies. Most immunodeficiencies underlying CNS infection are acquired. In the last 20 years, the number of affected patients has dramatically increased because of the aging population and the growing number and longer survival of patients with debilitating diseases such as diabetes, alcoholism, and lymphoid neoplasms. In addition, many patients are receiving immunosuppressive treatment for inflammatory and neoplastic diseases and for organ transplantation. Finally, the acquired immunodeficiency syndrome (AIDS) epidemic (cf. Chapter 23) represents a major cause of acquired immunodeficiency with numerous opportunistic infections (OIs).

By definition, an OI is an infection that takes the opportunity of a deficiency in the immune response of the host to develop. It may be a primary infection or a reactivated latent infection. Classically, OIs are due to saprophytic organisms that do not cause diseases in immunocompetent individuals and that have different characteristics to primary pathogens (Table 3.1). Primary pathogens have the following features: they induce specific diseases in immunocompetent hosts, have identifiable reservoirs and routes of infection, interact with specific cellular or humoral target molecules, share specific virulence or pathogenicity determinants, can be transmitted from host to host and induce the same disease (therefore potentially epidemic), have a clonal

Table 3.1 Differential characteristics of primary and opportunistic pathogens.

Primary pathogens	Opportunistic pathogens
- Induce specific diseases in hosts who are immunocompetent with identified reservoirs and routes of infection	- Induce atypical infections in patients who are immunocompromised; present in wide environmental reservoirs, in commensal (endogenous) flora, or latent in host
- Interact with specific cellular or humoral target molecules	- Lack defined cellular or humoral host receptors
- Share specific virulence/pathogenicity determinants	- May express potentially virulent and pathogenic molecules (constitutive or inducible), once they have colonized the host
- Can be transmitted from host to host and induce the same disease (potential for epidemics)	- Are acquired from the environment, from food sources, or from endogenous flora, and, for nosocomial infections, are communicable to susceptible contacts
- Clonal origin with limited genetic variability	- Genetic diversity and plasticity, which hamper indirect diagnosis and specific immunotherapies and vaccines
- Induce specific immune responses, enabling specific serological diagnoses and effective vaccines	- High frequency of genetic variations and rearrangements, allowing acquired resistance to antimicrobial agents

origin with limited genetic variability, and induce specific immune responses, enabling immunological (antibody) diagnoses and vaccine development. By contrast, saprophytic organisms induce atypical infections in patients who are immunocompromised, are widely present in environmental reservoirs, in commensal (endogenous) flora, or latent in the host. They lack defined cellular or humoral host receptors and may express potentially virulent and pathogenic molecules (constitutive or inducible) once they have colonized the host. They are acquired from the environment, from food sources, or from endogenous flora and, for nosocomial infections, are communicable to susceptible contacts. They have genetic diversity and plasticity that hamper indirect diagnosis and specific immunotherapies and vaccines, and they undergo frequent genetic variations and rearrangements, leading to acquired resistance to antimicrobial agents.

Infections by common pathogens such as tuberculosis, syphilis, measles, or varicella-zoster virus (VZV) tend to be included in this group because they may behave as OIs in patients with impaired lymphocyte function. The concept of OIs can be extended to some viral-related neoplasms that only develop in individuals who are immunocompromised. Examples are Kaposi sarcoma in patients with AIDS, related to infection by human herpes virus (HHV) type 8 (also known as Kaposi-sarcoma-associated virus [KSHV]), and primary brain lymphoma related to infection by EBV (or HHV type 4), occurring in patients with AIDS and recipients of organ transplants [10].

Different types of immunodeficiency may be associated with particular OIs involving the CNS as described in the following sections.

OIs of the CNS in patients with granulocytic disorders

Severe depletion of granulocytes is usually the consequence of decreased or absent production in the bone marrow. This may occur in myeloid leukemia or more often in the course of treatment with cytotoxic drugs. More rarely, severe granulocytopenia may result from peripheral sequestration in hypersplenism or as an idiosyncratic reaction to medication. In people with severe granulocytopenia, the most common OIs affecting the CNS are mycoses, particularly *Aspergillus* spp. [11, 12] and *Candida* spp. and certain bacterial infections, particularly *Pseudomonas aeruginosa*, *Listeria monocytogenes*, and *Nocardia asteroides*.

OIs of the CNS in patients with combined granulocytic and lymphocytic disorders

Immunodeficiency resulting from both granulocytic and lymphocytic impairment is the rule in recipients of both hematopoietic cell and solid organ transplants. It may also occur in patients with lymphoid neoplasms, other malignancies treated with chemotherapy, or in patients on prolonged, high-dose corticosteroid therapy.

In addition to mycoses (aspergillosis, cryptococcosis) and bacterial infections (listeriosis, nocardiosis), other cerebral OIs include toxoplasmosis [13], progressive multifocal leukoencephalopathy (PML), and cytomegalovirus infection. Primary malignant non-Hodgkin lymphomas of the brain, related to EBV infection, may also develop. It is of historical interest that primary brain lymphomas were first recognized as an opportunistic event in patients who had undergone renal transplantation [14].

OIs of the CNS in patients with lymphocytic disorders

This is particularly characteristic of AIDS. Before the introduction of highly active antiretroviral therapy (HAART) or combination therapy including a human immunodeficiency virus (HIV) protease inhibitor, OIs secondary to depletion in CD4+ T cells causing the cell-mediated immunodeficiency syndrome characteristic of AIDS were frequent and often the presenting illness. OIs usually occurred during the late stages in full-blown AIDS in people with depletion of CD4 cells and with high viral loads, and they included multiple parasitic (*Toxoplasma*), fungal (cryptococcal), bacterial (mycobacterial), and viral (cytomegalovirus, PML) infections, as well as primary brain lymphomas. Unlike the situation with granulocytopenia, by and large, patients with AIDS did not have frequent infections resulting from *Aspergillus* spp. Although bacterial infections are rare, it should be noted that brain abscess in patients with AIDS who do not have bacterial endocarditis is more likely to be a result of *Nocardia* spp. than to any other agent (cf. Chapter 35).

The type of infection also depends on the severity of immunodeficiency. Toxoplasmosis (a frequent presenting disease) occurs in patients with milder immunodeficiency (CD4 < 200) than PML, cytomegalovirus infection, and primary brain lymphomas, which are all found in patients who are severely immunodeficient (CD4 count <5).

Multiple OIs in patients with AIDS modify their presentations and make their diagnoses difficult because there is an increased range of organisms involved; a particular patient may have successive or simultaneous infections by different agents [15], several organs can be involved simultaneously, and there is generally a reduced inflammatory reaction.

Recently, multiple sclerosis (MS) has been treated by natalizumab, a humanized anti-alpha4-integrin antibody that binds to T cells, B cells, and monocytes, inhibiting their extravasation into the cerebrospinal fluid (CSF) [16], and by Fingolimod, a sphingosine 1-phosphate receptor modulator that prevents egress of T and B lymphocytes from lymph nodes and reduces the infiltration of autoaggressive cells into the CNS [17]. Both treatments have resulted in a T-cell mediated immunodeficiency syndrome and are significantly associated with PML (which is not a complication of MS) [17, 18].

Immune reconstitution inflammatory syndrome

An immune reconstitution disease defined as "an acute symptomatic or paradoxical deterioration of a (presumably) pre-existing infection that is temporally related to recovery of the immune system" was described in different types of immunodeficiency [19].

Introduction of HAART has dramatically modified the course and prognosis of HIV disease. In the developed world, where HAART is readily available and the management of OIs in general has improved, the incidence of CNS OIs has declined significantly since the 1980s [20]. The benefit is mainly because of a decreased HIV viral load and a restored functional immune system.

In parallel, in patients with AIDS with underlying OIs, after initiation of HAART, unusual clinical inflammatory syndromes have been increasingly reported. The name immune reconstitution inflammatory syndrome (IRIS) was proposed [21] for this entity, which clinically has four diagnostic criteria: (i) Patients with AIDS, (ii) efficiently treated by HAART, (iii) presenting symptoms consistent with an infectious or inflammatory condition that appeared while the patient was on antiretroviral therapy, with (iv) symptoms that could not be explained by a newly acquired infection, the expected course of a previously recognized infection, or side effects of therapy.

In the CNS, IRIS caused paradoxical exacerbation of tuberculosis (TB) and cryptococcal infection, as well as of cytomegalovirus (CMV) retinitis. In some patients with PML or HIV encephalitis (HIVE), the onset or deterioration of neurological signs following HAART institution was associated with contrast enhancement on magnetic resonance imaging (MRI), suggesting intense inflammation with impairment of the blood-brain barrier (BBB). Neuropathological studies confirmed intense inflammation with an influx of CD8+ lymphocytes, variably associated with acute deterioration of the underlying infection (HIV or John Cunningham virus [JCV]) and a nonspecific immunopathologic reaction resembling acute disseminated encephalomyelitis (ADEM) or MS. In most cases, IRIS correlated with prolonged survival, interpreted as a marker of both improved immune status and outcome; in rare instances, IRIS coincided with clinical and radiological aggravation and death [22].

IRIS has been reported in patients with other immunodeficiencies following reconstitution of the immune system or discontinuation of immunosuppressive treatment (for, review see [19]) in patients with Whipple disease [23], in patients with natalizumab-induced PML following withdrawal of natalizumab and plasma exchange [24], or in a patient with generalized TB secondary to treatment with the tumor necrosis factor alpha (TNF-α) antagonist adalimumab for rheumatoid arthritis, after receiving anti-TB therapy and discontinuing adalimumab [25].

Intrauterine infection

Infection during pregnancy can involve the mother, the placenta, and the fetus. Whether the fetus becomes infected, and the resulting effects depend on a variety of factors, including the specific infectious agent, the maternal immune response, the effectiveness of the placental barrier, and the fetal immune response. Because of changes in maternal, placental, and fetal physiology during the course of pregnancy, the effects of an infectious agent on the fetus often depend on when in gestation the infection occurs.

Adverse effects of intrauterine infections vary widely and include stillbirth and abortion, intrauterine growth restriction, premature birth, developmental anomalies, and congenital disease [2]. Congenital disease may manifest in utero or at birth or may not become apparent until weeks, months, or years after birth.

CNS infections in neonates and children

In neonates and children, overwhelmingly, a CNS infection may be the first evidence of an underlying congenital immune disorder (e.g. agammaglobulinemia).

In contrast to mature neonates protected by maternal antibodies, low-birth-weight or premature newborns have immature immunity and increased risk of infection, especially meningitis [26]. They have low maternal immunoglobulin and antibodies to bacteria, their neutrophils are functionally immature, and the immune response to bacteremia is also immature. They frequently have intravenous catheters; nasogastric or endotracheal tubes, which facilitate bacterial invasion; and metabolic acidosis, which compromises the host response [27].

Congenital immune deficiencies of T- and B-lymphocytes, of complement, and of phagocytes are severe and fortunately rare. They represent the tip of the iceberg in predisposition to infection [28]. Milder immune dysregulations probably remain unrecognized but are more common. In the human CNS, pathogen recognition receptors (PRRs) include TLRs expressed in meningeal macrophages, in the choroid plexuses, and in perivascular spaces [29]. Human TLR2 and TLR4 are activated by bacterial lipopolysaccharide (LPS). A retrospective study in 535 preterm infants investigating the role of polymorphic variants in genes that modulate the host response to infection including inflammatory cytokines (interleukin [IL]-6, IL-10, IL-1β, and TNF), cytokine receptors Il1 RN, TLRs (TLR2, TLR4, and TLR5), and cell surface receptors(CD14) found that polymorphisms in TLR2 (*rs3804099*), TLR5 (*rs5744105*), IL-10 (*rs1800896*), and Phospholipase A2 PLA2G2A (*rs1891320*) genes were associated with neonatal sepsis [30]. Allelic variants in PLA2G2A and TLR2 were associated with Gram-positive infections, whereas IL-10 was associated with Gram-negative infections.

A genome-wide expression study using *Mycobacterium tuberculosis (*Mtb*)*-stimulated macrophages, identified that human polymorphism in *epiregulin* (EREG), a TLR-dependent gene and a member of the epidermal growth factor (EGF) family involved in the macrophage response to *Mtb* infection, was associated with susceptibility to TB. TB risk was further increased in individuals who had EREG polymorphism *rs7675690* and were infected with the Beijing strain of *Mtb* [31]. Impaired interferon gamma (IFN-γ)–mediated immunity in children is found in atypical mycobacterial infection [32] and may also be a risk factor for herpes virus infection [33]. Mutations in the genes controlling TLR3 pathways may be a risk factor for some cases of childhood herpes simplex encephalitis [34].

The *World Malaria Report* of November 2018 reported there were 219 million cases of malaria in 2017, an increase from 217 million cases in 2016. The estimated number of malaria deaths was 435 000 in 2017. Children younger than five years are particularly susceptible to malaria infection; 70% of all malaria deaths occur in this age group, mainly in sub-Saharan Africa. Between 2000 and 2016, the younger-than-five-years malaria death rate fell from 444 000 to 285 000, translating into almost six million child lives saved. Host genetic mutations and polymorphisms are linked to malaria susceptibility in humans. These include the protective effect of sickle cell trait, alpha-thalassemia and glucose −6 phosphate dehydrogenase deficiency, and increased parasite density in children with different expression profiles in genes encoding for proinflammatory molecules as well as host gene responses *(HmOX1HSPCB* and *TNFRSF6)* [35].

Recognition of aberrant genes in chronic persistent infections explains the lack of clearance from the CNS and increases understanding of the pathogenesis. Elucidation of subtle differences in host and organism factors at a molecular level contributes to the understanding of infectious pathogenesis.

Acquired immunodeficiencies are less frequent in children than in adults but may occur following immunosuppressive treatment for neoplasms, chronic diseases, or following grafts. Childhood AIDS has been recognized in children for more than 30 years and an estimated 1.8 million children were living with HIV at the end of 2017, mostly in sub-Saharan Africa [36]. Children up to 13 years of age in general have a lower incidence of CNS OIs than adults, probably because children have had less time than adults to be exposed to opportunistic pathogens. This is especially true for toxoplasmosis, which is a less common cause of CNS mass lesion than primary brain lymphoma in children with AIDS. For this reason, it is recommended that children with AIDS who have a CNS mass lesion be biopsied at presentation, rather than after a trial of anti-*Toxoplasma* therapy [37]. Cryptococcal meningitis and PML are also rare in children with AIDS. CMV, which is often spread from child to child in childcare centers, continues to be the most common opportunistic pathogen in this age group, even in young children. In addition, children with AIDS are at risk for bacterial meningitis (including *Streptococcus pneumoniae*), as well as disseminated candidiasis, which often involves the CNS.

References

1. Casanova, J.L. and Abel, L. (2013). The genetic theory of infectious diseases: a brief history and selected illustrations. *Annu. Rev. Genomics Hum. Genet.* 14: 215–243.
2. Keohane, C. and Adle-Biassette, H. (2018). Intrauterine infections. In: *Developmental Neuropathology*, 2e (eds. H. Adle-Biassette, B.N. Harding and J.A. Golden), 500–502. Wiley Blackwell.
3. Keohane, C. (2018). Perinatal and postnatal infections. In: *Developmental Neuropathology*, 2e (eds. H. Adle-Biassette, B.N. Harding and J.A. Golden), 500–502. Wiley Blackwell.
4. Guy, J.M., Cerisier, A., Lamaud, M. et al. (1992). Cerebral abscess disclosing congenital heart disease. *Ann. Cardiol. Angeiol.* 41: 387–389.
5. Pradilla, G., Ardila, G.P., Hsu, W., and Rigamonti, D. (2009). Epidural abscess of the CNS. *Lancet Neurol.* 8: 292–300.
6. Picard, C., Bobby Gaspar, H., Al-Herz, W. et al. (2018). International Union of Immunological Societies: 2017 primary immunodeficiency diseases committee report on inborn errors of immunity. *J. Clin. Immunol.* 38: 96–128.
7. Fudenberg, H.H., Good, R.A., Hitzig, W. et al. (1970). Classification of the primary immune deficiencies: WHO recommendation. *N. Engl. J. Med.* 283: 656–657.
8. Bousfiha, A., Jeddane, L., Al-Herz, W. et al. (2015). The 2015 IUIS phenotypic classification for primary immunodeficiencies. *J. Clin. Immunol.* 35: 727–738.
9. Lanternier, F., Cypowyj, S., Picard, C. et al. (2013). Primary immunodeficiencies underlying fungal infections. *Curr. Opin. Pediatr.* 25: 736–747.
10. Chrétien, F., Jouvion, G., Wong, K.T., and Sharer, L.R. (2019). Infections of the central nervous system, Chapter 5. In: *Escourolle and Poirier Manual of Basic Neuropathology*, 6e (eds. F. Gray, C. Duyckaerts and U. de Girolami), 122–158. Oxford University Press.
11. Economides, M.P., Ballester, L.Y., Kumar, V.A. et al. (2017). Invasive mold infections of the central nervous system in patients with hematologic cancer or stem cell transplantation (2000–2016): uncommon, with improved survival but still deadly often. *J Infect* 75: 572–580.
12. Pagano, L., Caira, M., Falcucci, P., and Fianchi, L. (2005). Fungal CNS infections in patients with hematologic malignancy. *Expert Rev. Anti-Infect. Ther.* 3: 775–785.
13. Robert-Gangneux, F., Meroni, V., Dupont, D. et al. (2018). Toxoplasmosis in transplant recipients, Europe, 2010–2014. *Emerg. Infect. Dis.* 24: 1497–1504.
14. Mahale, P., Shiels, M.S., Lynch, C.F., and Engels, E.A. (2018). Incidence and outcomes of primary central nervous system lymphoma in solid organ transplant recipients. *Am. J. Transplant.* 18: 453–461.
15. Gray, F. and Sharer, L.R. (1993). Combined pathologies. In: *Atlas of the Neuropathology of HIV Infection* (ed. F. Gray), 162–172. Oxford, New York, Tokyo: Oxford University Press.
16. Niino, M., Bodner, C., Simard, M.L. et al. (2006). Natalizumab effects on immune cell responses in multiple sclerosis. *Ann. Neurol.* 59: 748–754.

17. Berger, J.R., Cree, B.A., Greenberg, B. et al. (2018). Progressive multifocal leukoencephalopathy after fingolimod treatment. *Neurology* 90: e1815–e1821.
18. Kleinschmidt-DeMasters, B.K. and Tyler, K.L. (2005). Progressive multifocal leukoencephalopathy complicating treatment with natalizumab and interferon beta-1a for multiple sclerosis. *N. Engl. J. Med.* 353: 369–374.
19. D'Arminio Monforte, A., Duca, P.G., Vago, L. et al. (2000). Decreasing incidence of CNS AIDS defining events associated with antiretroviral therapy. *Neurology* 54: 1856–1859.
20. Cheng, V.C., Yuen, K.Y., Chan, W.M. et al. (2000). Immunorestitution disease involving the innate and adaptive response. *Clin. Infect. Dis.* 30: 882–892.
21. Shelburne, S.A., Hamill, R.J., Rodriguez-Barradas, M.C. et al. (2002). Immune reconstitution inflammatory syndrome. Emergence of a unique syndrome during HAART. *Medicine* 81: 213–227.
22. Gray, F., Lescure, F.X., Adle-Biassette, H. et al. (2013). Encephalitis with infiltration by CD8+ lymphocytes in HIV patients receiving combination antiretroviral treatment. *Brain Pathol.* 23: 525–533.
23. Lagier, J.C., Fenollar, F., Lepidi, H. et al. (2010). Successful treatment of immune reconstitution inflammatory syndrome in Whipple's disease using thalidomide. *J. Infect.* 60: 79–82.
24. Wüthrich, C., Popescu, B.F., Gheuens, S. et al. (2013). Natalizumab-associated progressive multifocal leukoencephalopathy in a patient with multiple sclerosis: a postmortem study. *J. Neuropathol. Exp. Neurol.* 72: 1043–1051.
25. Tanaka, T., Sekine, A., Tsunoda, Y. et al. (2015). Central nervous system manifestations of tuberculosis-associated immune reconstitution inflammatory syndrome during adalimumab therapy: a case report and review of the literature. *Intern. Med.* 54: 847–851.
26. Smith, A.J. and Haas, J. (1991). Neonatal bacterial meningitis. In: *Infections of the Central Nervous System* (eds. W.M. Scheld, R.J. Whitley and D.T. Durack), 313–333. New York: Raven Press.
27. Edwards, M.S. and Baker, C.J. (2003). Bacterial infections in the neonate. In: *Principles and Practice of Pediatric Infectious Diseases*, 2e (eds. S.S. Long, L.K. Pickering and C.G. Prober), 536–542. Philadelphia: Churchill Livingstone.
28. Somech, R., Amariglio, N., Spirer, Z., and Rechvi, G. (2003). Genetic predisposition to infectious pathogens: a review of less familiar variants. *Pediatr. Infect. Dis. J.* 22: 457–461.
29. Deckert, M. (2015). Bacterial infections, chapter 20. In: *Greenfield's Neuropathology*, 9e (eds. S. Love, H. Budka, J.W. Ironside and A. Perry), 1197. New York: CRC Press.
30. Abu-Maziad, A., Schaa, K., Bell, E.F. et al. (2010). Role of polymorphic variants as genetic modulators of infection in neonatal sepsis. *Pediatr. Res.* 68: 323–329.
31. Thuong, N.T.T., Hawn, T.R., Chau, T.T.H. et al. (2012). Epiregulin (EREG) variation is associated with susceptibility to GE tuberculosis. *Genes Immun.* 13: 275–281.
32. Levin, M., Newport, M.J., D'Souza, S. et al. (1999). Familial disseminated atypical mycobacterial infection in childhood; a human mycobacterial susceptibility gene? *Lancet* 345: 79–83.
33. Dorman, S.E., Uzel, G., Roesler, J. et al. (1999). Viral infections in interferon-gamma receptor deficiency. *J. Pediatr.* 135: 640–643.
34. Sancho-Shimizu, V., Pérez de Diego, R., Lorenzo, L. et al. (2011). Herpes simplex encephalitis in children with autosomal recessive and dominant TRIF deficiency. *J. Clin. Invest.* 121: 4889–4902.
35. Driss, A., Hibbert, J.M., Wilson, N.O. et al. (2011). Genetic polymorphisms linked to susceptibility to malaria. *Malar. J.* 10: 271.
36. UNAIDS (2018). *Global HIV& AIDS statistics—2018 fact sheet*. http://www.unaids.org/en/resources/factsheet (accessed 22 January 2019).
37. Epstein, L.G., DiCarlo, F.J., Joshi, V.V. et al. (1988). Primary lymphoma of the central nervous system in children with acquired immunodeficiency syndrome. *Pediatrics* 82: 355–363.

4

Clinical Approach to the Adult Patient with CNS Infection

Michel Wolff[1,2]**, Romain Sonneville**[3,4,5]**, and Tarek Sharshar**[4,5,6]

[1] Department of Anesthesiology and Neurological Intensive Care, Sainte Anne Hospital, Paris, France
[2] Department of Intensive Care Medicine and Infectious Diseases, Bichat-Claude Bernard Hospital, APHP, Paris, France
[3] Department of Intensive Care Medicine and Infectious Diseases, Inserm U1148, Bichat-Claude-Bernard Hospital, APHP, Paris, France
[4] University Paris Diderot, Sorbonne Paris Cité, Paris, France
[5] Department of Anesthesiology and Intensive Care, Sainte Anne Hospital, Paris, France
[6] Experimental Neuropathology Unit, Pasteur Institute, Paris, France

Abbreviations

ABM	acute bacterial meningitis
ADC	apparent coefficient diffusion
AIDS	acquired immunodeficiency syndrome
BBB	blood-brain barrier
CNS	central nervous system
CSF	cerebrospinal fluid
DWI	diffusion-weighted imaging
EEG	electroencephalography
HHV-6	human herpesvirus-6
HIV	human immunodeficiency virus
HSV-1	herpes simplex virus 1
ICP	intracranial pressure
ICU	intensive care unit
LP	lumbar puncture
MRA	magnetic resonance angiography
MRI	magnetic resonance imaging
TBM	tuberculosis meningitis
VZV	varicella-zoster virus

Introduction

Microorganisms entering the CNS are diverse and have the propensity to affect all parts of the nervous system, causing distinct clinical syndromes. From a simple but clinically convenient classification, the "big three" CNS infections are acute bacterial meningitis (ABM), encephalitis, and brain abscess.

Although the definition of brain abscess is clear-cut (i.e. a focal infection of the brain), "meningitis," "encephalitis," "meningoencephalitis," and "aseptic meningitis" are used to describe a wide spectrum of diseases. With a strictly pathological definition, meningitis is an inflammation of the meninges, and encephalitis an inflammation of the brain parenchyma, resulting mainly from infectious and immune-mediated causes. Aseptic meningitis definition is clinical, consisting of symptoms of meningism with increased cells in cerebrospinal fluid (CSF) and a sterile bacterial culture [1].

Infections of the Central Nervous System: Pathology and Genetics, First Edition. Edited by Fabrice Chrétien, Kum Thong Wong, Leroy R. Sharer, Catherine (Katy) Keohane and Françoise Gray.
© 2020 John Wiley & Sons Ltd. Published 2020 by John Wiley & Sons Ltd.

We have chosen a pragmatic approach: ABM is defined as an infection of the CNS with pyogenic bacteria with or without abnormal consciousness. Acute encephalitis (or meningoencephalitis) is defined as an infection of the CNS by viruses, non-pyogenic bacteria (i.e. *Mycobaterium tuberculosis*, *Mycoplasma pneumoniae*), or fungi. Brain abscess is a focal bacterial, fungal, or parasitic infection of the brain that begins as a localized area of cerebritis and progresses into a collection of pus surrounded by a well-vascularized capsule.

This chapter will focus on community-acquired infections in adults who are immunocompetent and immunocompromised.

Community-Acquired ABM

Epidemiology

The incidence of ABM varies throughout the world (also see Chapter 30). In France and Western Europe, the incidence is 1–2 cases per 100 000 people per year, but can be 500- to 1000-fold higher in the Sahel region of Africa. A dramatic reduction has occurred over the past few decades, partly explained by herd protection by pediatric conjugate vaccines. In the Netherlands, the incidence of ABM declined from 1.72 cases per 100 000 adults per year in 2007–2008, to 0.94 per 100 000 per year in 2013–2014 [2]. A similar trend has been observed in United States, where the incidence of *Streptococcus pneumoniae* and *Neisseria meningitidis* have declined threefold and sixfold, respectively, between 1997 and 2010 [3] (see Chapter 30).

These trends have not substantially modified the prevalence of the causative pathogens. *S. pneumoniae* and *N. meningitidis* (serogroup B in the majority of cases) are isolated in more than 80% of ABM in adults [2]. *S. pneumoniae* is by far the most frequent bacterium, especially in patients older than 40 years of age, whereas *N. meningitidis* is predominant in younger adults. *Listeria monocytogenes* (5%), streptococci (5%), and *S. aureus* are much less frequently isolated.

Classical risk factors for *S. pneumoniae* are alcoholism, comorbidities (cancer, diabetes), previous splenectomy, and otitis or sinusitis. Neurolisteriosis occurs mainly in patients older than 65 years of age; 86% have at least one immunosuppressive comorbidity according to a nationwide study in France [4].

ABM is still a severe infection resulting in a high mortality (nearly 20%) and morbidity worldwide. The overall case fatality rate is sixfold higher in *S. pneumoniae* than in *N. meningitidis* infection. Sequelae, hearing disability, or neurologic deficits are reported in 30–50% of patients [5]. A Dutch study in 1412 patients identified the following factors giving an unfavorable outcome (death or sequelae): older age, absence of otitis or sinusitis, alcoholism, tachycardia, impaired consciousness, cranial nerve palsy, a CSF white blood cell count of <1000 cells/µl, and a positive blood culture [2]. Many studies highlighted the delay in initiation of antibiotic therapy [2, 5, 6], and absence of adjunctive steroids as additional adverse prognostic factors in this setting [2].

Clinical features and appropriate investigations

Data from meta-analyses and large cohort studies indicate that the classic triad of fever, altered mental status, and neck stiffness is present in only 40–45% of cases. However, 95% of the patients with ABM have at least one of the following: headache (77%), fever (87%), neck stiffness (83%), or impaired consciousness (69%). Focal neurologic signs and seizures are present, respectively, in 25% and 5% of patients. A rash is noted in 8% of cases; nearly all patients with purpura are infected with *N. meningitidis* [2, 7].

Lumbar puncture (LP) for the analysis of CSF is the cornerstone of ABM diagnosis. Most international guidelines indicate that focal neurological signs, moderate to severe impairment of mental status, immunocompromised state, and new onset seizures are contraindications to immediate LP because they can be associated with an increased risk of a cerebral mass lesion and raised intracranial pressure (ICP) [8]. The risk of delaying diagnosis and the lack of firm evidence for some contraindications for prompt LP resulted in the Swedish guidelines being revised, so that moderate to severe impairment of mental status and new-onset seizures were deleted as contraindications to initial LP. The new guidelines were significantly associated with earlier antibiotic therapy and a favorable outcome [5]. The CSF white blood cell count is higher than 1000 cells/μl in 75% of the cases, between 100 and 1000 in 18%, and <100 in 7% [2]. CSF-to-blood glucose ratio is <0.40 in most patients, and protein is higher than 0.40 g/l, between 2 and 6 g/l in the majority of cases. Sensitivity and specificity of Gram coloration are 67–97% and 100%, respectively, when the examination is performed before antibiotic treatment. When LP is performed after the onset of antibiotics, the sensitivity is only 40–60%, depending on the inoculum. The sensitivity of antigen detection in the CSF with the immune-chromatographic method (BinaxNOW *S. pneumoniae*®) is 95–100% and the specificity is 100%. Multiplex polymerase chain reaction (PCR) assays may be useful, especially for patients with negative direct examination. Cultures from blood (positive in 70–80% of cases) and from CSF are of utmost importance to isolate the causative bacteria and to test for antibiotic sensitivity.

Histologic examination, standard cultures, or PCR in samples from skin lesions may also be useful in meningococcal sepsis. Two other tests can help to distinguish bacterial from viral meningitis; several studies have shown that CSF lactate had the highest accuracy for discriminating bacterial from viral meningitis, with a cutoff set at 3.5 mmol/l providing 100% sensitivity, specificity, and positive and negative predictive values [9]. Similarly, the highly accurate value of serum procalcitonin is suggested by a number of studies and confirmed by a recent meta-analysis of nine studies (725 patients) [10].

Most patients undergo neuroimaging (i.e. computed tomography [CT] scan or magnetic resonance imaging [MRI]) during the course of meningitis. Neuroimaging should be done before LP only in patients who have clinical signs that might suggest brain shift. Later in the course of the disease, neuroimaging may help detect some complications (e.g. empyema, cerebral infarct, thrombophlebitis, sinusitis, or otitis), especially in those patients who have an unfavorable outcome [11].

Pathophysiology of ABM

The mechanisms that bacteria have developed to cross the CNS barriers have been extensively studied in recent years [12]. See Chapter 29 for details of CNS invasion by *S. pneumoniae*, *N. meningitidis*, and other bacteria.

Many patients with ABM experience coma, focal neurologic signs, or seizures. Cerebral edema is a hallmark of bacterial meningitis and a common cause of deteriorating consciousness. It is caused by a combination of vasogenic, cytotoxic, and interstitial edema, which may be worsened by systemic hypotension. Neuroimaging abnormalities consistent with diffuse cerebral edema include a loss of differentiation between gray and white matter, loss of sulcal markings, and absence of visualization of perimesencephalic, suprasellar, or quadrigeminal cisterns. Acute ischemic complications are observed in up to 15% of cases in patients with pneumococcal ABM. Increased cerebral blood flow velocity on transcranial Doppler, defined as peak systolic values above 150 cm/s, is detected in more than 40% of patients with bacterial meningitis and conveys an increased risk of stroke and unfavorable outcome. Finally, seizures occur in 20–22% of adult patients with ABM and are associated with CNS and systemic inflammation, acute structural CNS lesions, and pneumococcal meningitis [13].

Treatment

The winning combination for the management of ABM is early appropriate antibiotic therapy, early administration of adjunctive dexamethasone, and optimal neurocritical care.

Early antibiotic treatment is associated with better outcomes [6]. All efforts should be made to administer the first dose of antibiotic within one hour of hospital admission. If CT scan is deemed necessary before LP, antibiotics in combination with adjunctive dexamethasone (i.e. 10 mg four times daily (QID), for four days) must be given immediately after obtaining a blood culture. It is beyond the scope of this paragraph to review all aspects of antibiotic therapy, which are detailed in recent guidelines such as those published in Europe [8] and summarized in Table 4.1. Increased drug entry into the CSF and its delayed

Table 4.1 Antibiotic therapy for community-acquired meningitis in adults.

Presumed or documented microorganisms	Empiric (context and CSF direct Gram stain)	After documentation
Streptococcus pneumoniae	Cefotaxime[a] or ceftriaxone[b] plus vancomycin or rifampin[c]	MIC of cefotaxime/ceftriaxone ≤0.5 mg/l • MIC AMOX ≤ 0.5 mg/l: AMOX: 200 mg/kg/day • MIC AMOX > 0.5 mg/l: continue cefotaxime (200 mg/kg/day) or ceftriaxone (75 mg/d) MIC cefotaxime/ceftriaxone >0.5 mg/l cefotaxime (300 mg/kg/day) or ceftriaxone (100 mg/d) • Severe allergy to beta-lactams: meropenem or vancomycin[d] + rifampicin[e] • Duration: 10 (if good outcome and fully susceptible strain)–14 days
Neisseria meningitidis	Cefotaxime[a] or ceftriaxone[b]	MIC AMOX[d] ≤0.125 mg/l: amoxicillin: 200 mg/kg/day MIC AMOX[d] >0.125 mg/: continue cefotaxime (200 mg/kg/day or ceftriaxone 75 mg/kg/day) Duration: 7 days
Listeria monocytogenes	Amoxicillin[f] + gentamicin (5 mg/kg/day)	AMOX[f]: duration: 3 weeks + gentamicin (3–5 days) Severe allergy to beta-lactams: trimethoprim-sulfamethoxazole 6–8 mg/kg/day or 30–40 mg/kg/day in four injections.
Enterobacteriacae	Cefotaxime[a] or ceftriaxone[b]	Cefotaxime[a] or ceftriaxone[b]: duration: 14 days
Streptococci	Amoxicillin[f]	AMOX[f]
Direct examination of CSF negative and age > 50 years or age > 18 and < 50 years plus risk factors for L. monocytogenes[g]	Amoxicillin + cefotaxime or ceftriaxone Idem S. pneumoniae	Comment: in the absence of bacterial identification in CSF parameningeal infection (brain abscess, infective endocarditis with cerebral complications, epiduritis) should be looked for as well as a pathogens responsible for encephalitis (Table 4.3)

[a] Cefotaxime: 300 mg/kg/day in four to six injections (200 mg/kg/d for N. meningitidis).
[b] Ceftriaxone: 100 mg/kg/day in two injections.
[c] In countries with low incidence level of strains with reduced susceptibility to penicillin G (i.e. France) monotherapy with either cefotaxime or ceftriaxone is recommended.
[d] Vancomycin: 15 mg/kg over 1 h as loading dose then 40–60 mg/kg as continuous infusion.
[e] Rifampin: 600 mg every 12 h.
[f] Amoxicillin: 200 mg/kg/d in six injections.
[g] Diabetes mellitus, use of immunosuppressive drugs, cancer, and other conditions causing immunocompromise.
AMOX, amoxicillin; CSF, cerebrospinal fluid.

removal by reducing CSF bulk flow, and by inhibiting activity of efflux pumps, synergistically lead to elevated CSF antibiotic concentrations. This is particularly true for drugs like beta-lactam antibiotics that have poor entry into the CSF in the absence of meningeal inflammation [14].

Adjunctive dexamethasone significantly reduces hearing loss and neurologic sequelae but does not reduce overall mortality. Data support the use of corticosteroids (initiated with the first antibiotic dose) in patients with ABM in countries with a high level of medical care, and when S. pneumoniae is suspected [15].

Recommendations for optimal neurocritical care in patients with severe ABM are not uniform, but some general measures are of utmost importance: head-of-bed elevation 30–45°, maintaining a mean arterial pressure of ≥65 mm Hg, using

Table 4.2 Adjunctive measures other than adjunctive steroids: ESCMID guidelines [8].

Measures	Guidelines
Routine paracetamol	Not recommended (grade D)
Routine mannitol	Not recommended (grade D)
Prophylactic antiepileptic drugs	Not recommended (grade D)
Hypertonic saline	Not recommended (grade D)
Glycerol	Contraindicated (harmful) (grade C)
Hypothermia	Contraindicated (harmful) (grade C)
Use of intracranial pressure /cerebral perfusion pressure monitoring	Can be life-saving in selected patients; cannot be recommended as routine management because solid evidence is lacking and may cause harm (grade C)

ESCMID, European Society of Clinical Microbiology and Infectious Diseases.

norepinephrine as the initial vasopressor for hypotension after correction of hypovolemia, early treatment for suspected or proven seizures, prevention of excessive hyperthermia, and maintenance of normal respiratory and metabolic parameters (i.e. partial pressure of arterial carbon dioxide ($PaCO_2$), natremia, glycemia). The potential role of other adjunctive therapies is summarized in Table 4.2.

Encephalitis

Specific definition and epidemiology

Infection constitutes approximately 50% of identifiable cases and is the most commonly recognized cause of encephalitis. The epidemiology of encephalitis has changed considerably over the past decade with the discovery of new pathogens and the development of new diagnostic tools such as multiplex PCR. However, the proportion of encephalitis of unknown cause still remains higher than that for any specifically identified etiology.

According to the International Encephalitis Consortium [16], probable or confirmed encephalitis requires:

1. The presence of a major criterion: patients with altered mental status (defined as decreased or altered level of consciousness, lethargy, or personality change) lasting ≥24 hours with no alternative cause identified.

2. Three of the following minor criteria: documented fever ≥38 °C (100.4 °F) within 72 hours before or after presentation; generalized or partial seizures not fully attributable to a preexisting seizure disorder; new onset of focal neurologic findings; CSF white blood cell count ≥5/mm³; abnormality of brain parenchyma on neuroimaging suggestive of encephalitis that is either new (not present on prior studies) or appears acute in onset; abnormality on electroencephalography (EEG) that is consistent with encephalitis and not attributable to another cause.

Although these criteria have not been validated, this definition fits for both infectious and autoimmune etiologies.

The spectrum of causative agents is very large and depends on immune status, geographical factors, season, and exposure. In three large epidemiologic studies in industrialized countries (United States, England, and France), the main etiological agents were herpes simplex virus 1 (HSV-1), enterovirus, *M. pneumoniae*, varicella-zoster virus (VZV), and *M. tuberculosis* [17–19]. The percentage of cases of unknown cause was 63% in the oldest study, but only 37% in the most recent study. This likely reflects the increased recognition of immune-mediated encephalitis. In a series of 279 patients requiring intensive care unit (ICU) admission, causes of encephalitis (excluding AIDS-defining CNS diseases) were infections (53%), immune-mediated causes (15%), and undetermined (32%). *M. tuberculosis*, HSV-1, VZV, and *L. monocytogenes*, accounted for 23%, 14%, 5%, and 7%, respectively, of all cases [20].

Clinical features and appropriate investigations

A diagnostic algorithm for initial evaluation of encephalitis should take the aforementioned factors and specific signs and symptoms into account (Table 4.3) as well as neuroimaging and laboratory features [16].

MRI is the most sensitive neuroimaging test (vs. CT scan) to evaluate patients with encephalitis, provided that appropriate sequences are performed. Diffusion-weighted imaging or fluid attenuated inversion recovery (FLAIR) may allow detection of early signal abnormalities. MRI can help distinguish HSV-1 from other infections. In a study of 251 cases of temporal lobe encephalitis, bilateral temporal lobe involvement and lesions outside the temporal lobes, insula, or cingulate were associated with lower odds of HSV-1 encephalitis. Bilateral temporal lobe involvement is more frequent in autoimmune encephalitis [21], whereas lesions of the thalamus and basal ganglia may suggest respiratory viruses or flaviviruses. In patients with vasculitis detected by magnetic resonance angiography (MRA), the following pathogens should be considered: VZV, *Treponema pallidum*, *M. tuberculosis*, and in patients who are immunocompromised, filamentous fungi, especially *Aspergillus* spp. The four main patterns of CNS tuberculosis are meningitis, brain tuberculomas, brain ischemic lesions, and hydrocephalus (see Chapter 36). MRI is the key imaging for the diagnosis of acute disseminated encephalitis (ADEM), when localized or diffuse white matter lesions are present and when common infectious causes have been reasonably excluded.

EEG is recommended and has three main purposes:
1. To assist diagnosis: periodic discharges and focal slowing are suggestive of HSV-1 encephalitis; the extreme delta brush pattern is in favor of autoimmune encephalitis.
2. To rule out nonconvulsive seizures.
3. To assist with prognosis [22].

The classical laboratory tests include serology, routine blood cultures, Gram stain, and bacterial cultures of CSF, plus India ink in patients who are immunocompromised, and specific PCR according to the context: HSV-1 or -2, VZV, enterovirus, *M. pneumoniae*, and *M. tuberculosis*. Multiplex PCR and next-generation sequencing are valuable new diagnostic tools and may increase the number of successful investigations of encephalitis cases [23, 24].

HSV and VZV encephalitis

HSV-1 is the most common infectious cause of sporadic encephalitis; the estimate incidence worldwide is between 2 and 4 cases/1 000 000 (see Chapter 5). Most patients are immunocompetent and extraneurologic signs are absent, except for nonspecific prodromal signs suggestive of upper respiratory tract or gastrointestinal infection. The most likely routes to the CNS include retrograde transport through the olfactory or trigeminal

Table 4.3 Causative microorganisms according to clinical signs and symptoms or biological abnormalities.

Signs, symptoms, and biological abnormalities	Main microorganisms or diseases
Hepatitis	*Coxiella burnetii*
Lymph nodes	EBV, CMV, measles, rubeola, West Nile virus, *Bartonella* spp., *Mycobaterium tuberculosis*
Parotitis	Mumps
Cutaneous lesions	VZV, HHV-6, West Nile virus, rubeola, enterovirus, *Mycoplasma pneumoniae*, *Rickettsia*, *Borrelia burgdorferi*, *Ehrlichia chaffeensis*, arbovirus
Respiratory signs, pneumonia	Influenza A, adenovirus, *M. pneumoniae*, *C. burnetii*, *M. tuberculosis*
Retinitis	West Nile virus
Cerebellar ataxia	VZV (children), EBV, mumps, *Tropheryma whipplei*
Cranial nerves palsies	HSV-1, EBV, *Listeria monocytogenes*, *M. tuberculosis*, *B. burgdorferi*, *T. whipplei*
Face or limb myoclonus	*T. whipplei*

CMV, cytomegalovirus; Epstein-Barr virus; HHV-6, human herpesvirus 6; HSV-1, herpes simplex virus 1; VZV, varicella-zoster virus.
Source: adapted from [16].

nerves. The exact pathogenic mechanism is still uncertain but includes reactivation of latent HSV-1 in the trigeminal ganglia with subsequent spread of infection to the temporal and frontal lobes or reactivation of latent virus within the brain parenchyma itself [25].

The most common manifestations include headache, fever, cognitive disorders, impaired consciousness, seizures, and focal neurological deficits. On EEG, patients with HSV-1 are significantly more likely to have periodic discharges and focal slowing in the frontotemporal and occipital areas, compared with patients with encephalitis of other etiologies. Diffusion restriction on diffusion-weighted imaging (DWI) is more sensitive than FLAIR in the early phase of infection [26]. PCR is the gold standard for the diagnosis of HSV-1 encephalitis with a sensitivity of 96% and a specificity of 99% [25]. Because PCR can be falsely negative in the very early stage of infection, it is wise to continue acyclovir therapy in this setting and to test a repeat sample within three to five days. Overall, 10–15% patients have absence of fever or absence of CSF pleocytosis at admission. Conventional CT may be normal in the first few days in 33% of patients. Several uncommon or atypical forms have been reported in patients who are immunocompromised, including absence of fever, minimal neurological signs and symptoms, normal cell count in the CSF, and atypical brain MRI lesions [27].

Intravenous acyclovir is the first-line treatment for HSV-1 encephalitis and should be continued for 14–21 days. There is no benefit in continuing oral antiviral therapy after 21 days, and the potential benefit of steroids has not been demonstrated so far. Although, the mortality is less than 10%, only 40–50% of patients have a favorable outcome (absence of sequelae) [28]. In the subset of patients requiring ICU admission only one third has a favorable outcome [29]. Autoimmune post-HSV-1 encephalitis has been reported recently [30].

VZV encephalitis may present as acute nonspecific encephalitis, preferentially affecting patients who are older and have comorbidities, [18] or as vasculopathy, often in patients who are immunocompromised (see Chapter 6). Complications range from gray or white matter infarcts to aneurysms and subarachnoid hemorrhages. The CSF profile generally shows a lymphocytic pleocytosis with normal CSF glucose levels.

Encephalitides in patients who are immunocompromised
Cryptococcosis

Patients with human immunodeficiency virus (HIV) who have CD4 cell counts <100 cells/mm^3 have the highest risk, but with the decline of HIV infection, the prevalence of patients with non-HIV immunosuppression and solid-organ transplant is increasing [31].

Cryptococcosis commonly presents as subacute meningitis with or without secondary encephalopathy features that are usually due to raised ICP. The opening pressure in the CSF may be elevated; pressure ≥18 cm H$_2$O occurs in more than 60% of patients. CSF analysis demonstrates mildly elevated protein levels, low-to-normal CSF glucose levels, and moderate lymphocytic pleocytosis. Patients with HIV may have little CSF inflammation, but staining with India ink and cultures of CSF demonstrate encapsulated yeasts in 60–90% of cases, whereas CSF cryptococcal antigen is positive in nearly all cases.

The combination of amphotericin B deoxycholate (1.0 mg/kg/day) or lipid formulations of amphotericin B (3–4 mg/kg/day) with flucytosine is associated with both improved survival and more rapid sterilization of CSF, compared to the same dose of amphotericin B without flucytosine. After two weeks of successful induction therapy, a switch to fluconazole is recommended. Early ICP elevation (>25 mm H$_2$O) following diagnosis is associated with mortality, and its diagnosis and management is of paramount importance. Protocols using serial LP for ICP management in resource-limited settings suggest a reduction in mortality compared to historical controls. When required, shunting (preferably ventriculo-peritoneal) may provide sustained relief from intracranial hypertension symptoms.

Tuberculous encephalitis and meningitis

The most common presentation includes headache, fever, altered mental status, focal signs, and cranial nerve palsies.

CSF shows pleocytosis with lymphocyte predominance, high protein levels, and low glucose levels. However, this CSF profile is non-specific and polymorphonuclear cells can predominate. New commercial molecular diagnostic tests, such as GeneXpert MTB/RIF, have an important role in tuberculous meningitis diagnosis, but as with all other available tests, they lack sensitivity and cannot exclude the disease. The most common neuroimaging findings include meningeal enhancement, hydrocephalus, basal exudates, infarcts, and tuberculomas.

Treatment of tuberculosis meningitis (TBM) includes a four-drug regimen, with isoniazid, ethambutol, rifampin, and pyrazinamide for an induction phase of two months. After the induction phase, isoniazid and rifampin should be continued for 10 months. A recent Cochrane Review supports the use of adjunctive intravenous dexamethasone (0.4 mg/kg/day), with a reduced risk of death at least in the short term [32]. However, corticosteroids may have no effect on the number of people who survive tuberculous encephalitis with disabling neurological deficit. The benefits in terms of reduced mortality in patients coinfected with HIV are uncertain.

Good outcomes depend on careful management of the common complications and controlling ICP. Hydrocephalus is detected in up to 65% of patients at presentation and is independently associated with visual impairment, cranial nerve palsy, and basal exudate. Hyponatremia is one of the most common acute complications of tuberculous encephalitis, occurring in 45% of patients. It is mainly a result of cerebral salt wasting and relates to disease severity. The outcome for patients requiring invasive mechanical ventilation is poor (<30% survival at three months) [33].

Viral encephalitides

In addition to VZV and more rarely HSV-1, other viruses can be associated with encephalitis in patients who are immunocompromised.

Progressive multifocal leukoencephalopathy, caused by reactivation of John Cunningham virus (JCV) is a feared complication of HIV infection, lymphoproliferative disorders, and the treatment of autoimmune conditions (see Chapter 9).

Human herpesvirus 6 (HHV-6) encephalitis is mainly a complication of allogeneic hematopoietic cell transplantation. Symptoms are characterized by memory loss, loss of consciousness, and seizures. MRI typically shows bilateral signal abnormalities in the limbic system. Although no controlled trial has evaluated the clinical efficacy of ganciclovir and foscarnet, these molecules are recommended to treat HHV-6 encephalitis [34].

Cytomegalovirus, which is an extremely infrequent cause of encephalitis, manifests as impairments in cognition, attention, and arousal. Typical patterns of MRI are periventricular enhancement, infarcts, or hemorrhages (see Chapter 7).

Table 4.4 Exotic and emergent viruses.

Virus	Geographical areas
West Nile	Worldwide
Toscana	Italy, Spain, Portugal, France
Japanese encephalitis	Asia
Ebola	Africa
Zika virus	Americas, French Polynesia
Enterovirus 71	Worldwide (children)
Rabies	Asia, Africa, Americas
Chikungunya	Asia, South Pacific, French West Indies Reunion, India, Indonesia
Nipah and Hendra	Australia, Asia
Lyssavirus	Australia, Europe

Exotic and emerging agents

Viral infections are considered "emergent" when new hosts are involved, if they occur in new geographic areas, or if they are caused by newly recognized pathogenic viruses (see Chapter 50). Encephalitis caused by these viruses may affect residents or travelers in tropical regions. The main responsible agents are indicated in Table 4.4.

Community-Acquired brain abscess

Epidemiology and microbiology

The epidemiology of brain abscess differs markedly depending on the immunologic status of the host.

Patients who are immunocompetent
The incidence of brain abscess in the general population has been estimated at 0.3–0.9 per 100 000 inhabitants per year in developed countries. A systematic review of 9699 cases of brain abscess reported between 1935 and 2012 found the most common predisposing conditions were contiguous foci of infection: otitis or mastoiditis (33%), sinusitis (10%), and meningitis (6%). Brain abscess was deemed to be due to hematogenous spread in 33% of cases, mostly with endocarditis (13%), pulmonary infection (8%), or dental infection (5%) as the primary causes. Others were attributed to recent neurosurgery (9%) or cranial trauma (14%), but the source could not be identified in 19% of cases, so-called "cryptogenic brain abscess" [35].

Of 6663 patients with brain abscesses who had samples submitted for cultures during the years 1935–2012, 4543 (68%) yielded at least one potential pathogen, of whom 902 (23%) were polymicrobial. Streptococci predominated ($n = 2000$; 34%), mostly oral streptococci, including the *milleri* group and anaerobic streptococci, whereas *S. pneumoniae* was isolated from only 2.4% of patients. Staphylococci were second ($n = 1076$; 18%); 84% were *S. aureus*. Gram-negative bacilli came third ($n = 861$; 15%) and were mostly *Enterobacteriaceae* [35]. Anaerobic bacteria are frequently involved, including *Bacteroides* spp. not isolated through conventional cultures. Molecular biology and genome sequencing have demonstrated the gap between bacterial species identified through conventional cultures and bacterial genetic material that can be amplified from brain abscess samples. The systematic use of multiple 16S ribosomal DNA sequencing on samples obtained from 71 patients with brain abscess increased the proportion of patients with documented microbial agents from 66 to 83%, with the identification of 186 strains, as compared to only 58 with conventional cultures [36]. However, the clinical significance of these large numbers of bacteria (as many as 16 distinct species in a single brain abscess), identified only by metagenomics but not by conventional cultures, remains to be proven.

Patients who are immunocompromised
The epidemiology of CNS opportunistic infections (OIs) differs, depending on the type and etiology of immunosuppression. In patients infected with HIV, the most prevalent OI responsible for cerebral abscess is toxoplasmosis. In patients requiring chronic immunosuppressant therapy after solid-organ transplantation or for other reasons, OIs depend on the level of immunosuppression and typically occur within one year following transplantation. The most frequent etiologies are CNS aspergillosis, endemic fungi, and other molds, including *Mucorales* and *Nocardia* [37].

Pathogenesis
In patients who are immunocompetent, bacteria are responsible for >95% of brain abscess and enter the brain either through contiguous spread (e.g. following otitis, mastoiditis, sinusitis, neurosurgical procedures, or brain trauma) in 40–50% of cases. Bacteria may also reach the brain through hematogenous dissemination in 30–40% of cases, especially in cases of infective endocarditis, in patients with predisposing conditions associated with pulmonary circulation shunts (e.g. congenital heart disease, pulmonary arteriovenous fistulas, hereditary hemorrhagic telangiectasia), or as a consequence of distant infectious foci (e.g. dental infection, pulmonary abscess).

In patients who are immunocompromised, the pathogenesis of infection depends on the host context and the microorganism. *Aspergillus* spp. reaches the brain either from direct spread from paranasal sinuses or through hematogenous dissemination. Cerebral toxoplasmosis is caused by the protozoan *Toxoplasma gondii*, attributed to reactivation of latent tissue cysts. *Nocardia* spp. brain infection usually complicates pulmonary infection.

Neuroimaging
At the capsule stage, CT contrast-enhancement in brain abscess typically shows a peripheral ring-enhancing lesion with a hypodense center (central necrosis), surrounded by a variable hypodense area (edema). In most cases, a brain abscess is single on CT and located in the frontal or temporal lobes. MRI offers many advantages over contrast-enhanced

CT. The combined use of morphological sequences, proton MR spectroscopy, DWI, and the calculation of apparent coefficient diffusion (ADC) has improved the sensitivity and specificity of MRI in differentiating abscess from tumor to 94% and 95%, respectively [37].

Pyogenic abscess appears as a mass with a continuous capsule, hyperintense on T1- and hypointense on T2-weighted sequences, with regular enhancement postgadolinium injection. The necrotic center is hypointense on T1-weighted sequence, hyperintense on T2-weighted sequence, and hyperintense on DWI. Moreover, it typically presents with low values of ADC and peaks corresponding to lipids, lactate, and amino acids in MR spectroscopy.

The neuroimaging pattern of OIs in patients who are immunocompromised may be somewhat different.

In brain aspergillosis spreading from paranasal sinuses, MRI typically demonstrates a peripheral invasive lesion adjacent to the nasosinusal cavities. The lesion is multilobulated with a well-defined rim enhancement after gadolinium. In brain aspergillosis resulting from hematogenous dissemination, all brain areas may be involved with a predilection for the cortico-medullary junction in supratentorial white matter, basal nuclei-thalamus, and infratentorial structures. A hemorrhagic component may be present. Vascular lesions characterized by proximal or distal aneurysms are relatively frequent [38].

Brain imaging of neuro-toxoplasmosis typically shows multiple ring-enhancing lesions in cortical gray matter or basal ganglia with associated edema and mass effect [39].

Nocardia spp. brain abscesses in patients with solid-organ transplants are supratentorial and multiple in the vast majority of cases [40].

Diagnostic approach to brain abscess

The diagnosis of brain abscess should be based on a systematic approach, including:

1. The characteristics of the host, immunocompetent or immunocompromised (for the latter, type of immunosuppression, HIV, solid organ or bone marrow transplantation, other). In individuals with HIV, the risk of CNS OI depends on the CD4-cell count and is low in patients with counts >200 CD4-cells/mm^3. The peak period for CNS OIs in transplant recipients is one to six months after transplant. In these patients, the anti-infective prophylaxis must be taken into account when considering the diagnosis (e.g. cotrimoxazole prevents *Listeria*, *Nocardia,* and *Toxoplasmosis*);
2. The search for a portal of entry (sinusitis, otitis, lung, left-side endocarditis)
3. If present, clinical extraneurological signs may point toward a specific etiology and indicate specific microbiological tests or biopsy.
4. Clinical neurologic signs: Clinical signs and symptoms of CNS infections in patients who are immunocompromised may be confounded by the effects of immunosuppressive therapy or by renal or hepatic dysfunction and associated metabolic disturbances or drug accumulation. Of note, fever may be absent.
5. Brain imaging features (see text discussion)
6. CSF analysis whenever possible. Experts recommend that brain imaging should be performed before LP in all patients who are severely immunocompromised and presenting with suspected CNS infection.
7. Optimal microbiological investigation of samples taken from blood, CSF, or tissues according to the context (i.e. bronchoalveolar lavage, skin biopsy). For example, detection of *T. gondii* by PCR in CSF has high specificity but low sensitivity (50%), giving a high false-negative rate in patients with HIV[41]. Blood or CSF levels of β-D-glucan and galactomannan and pan-fungal or specific-fungal PCR are useful tools for the diagnosis of aspergillosis or other filamentous infections of CNS, but their sensitivity and specificity remain to be determined [38].
8. Brain biopsy should be considered for patients with HIV who fail to respond to specific anti-*Toxoplasma* therapy and for patients presenting with focal lesion(s) with significant mass effect and risk of brain herniation. In patients with hematological disorders or in recipients of solid-organ transplants, stereotactic brain biopsy and neurosurgical resection of brain lesions followed by identification and resistance testing of the causative organisms should be considered for all patients presenting with focal parenchymal abnormalities (e.g. brain abscess) without extraneurological involvement (see text discussion) [42].

Table 4.5 Anti-infective therapy for community-acquired brain abscess.

	Primary regimen	Alternative regimen	Duration
Suspected portal of entry: dental, sinusitis, otitis, lung	Cefotaxime 2 g IV q 4 h or ceftriaxone 2 g IV q 12 h + metronidazole 500 mg IV q 6–8 h	Cefepime 2 g IV q 8 h (if mastoiditis *Pseudomonas aeruginosa* is possible) + metronidazole	6–8 weeks. Shorter duration possible if abscess is drained
Staphylococcus aureus suspected (e.g. post-trauma, suspected hematogenous spread)	Cloxacillin 2 g IV q 4 h + rifampin 600 mg IV PO q 12 h	Cloxacillin 2 g IV q 4 h + levofloxacin 500 mg IV PO q 12 h	6–8 weeks
Aspergillus spp.	Voriconazole: 6 mg/kg IV PO q 12 h on day 1; then 6 mg/kg IV PO q 12 h	Liposomal Amphotericin B 3–5 mg/kg IV	≥8 weeks
Nocardia spp.	Trimethoprim-sulfamethoxazole: 15 mg/kg/day IV PO 75 mg/kg/j in four injections + Imipenem: 2 g/d	Linezolid: 600 mg IV PO q 12 h + meropenem 2 g IV q 8 h	After 3–6 weeks of IV therapy switch to PO therapy. Total duration: At least one year for patients who are immunocompromised
Toxoplasmosis	Pyrimethamine 200 mg at D1 then 75 mg PO d + sulfadiazine 4–6 g + folinic acid	Pyrimethamine 200 mg at D1 then 75 mg PO d + clindamycin 600 mg PO IV q 6 h	Minimum 6 weeks followed by suppressive therapy

d, day; D1, day 1; h, hour; IV, intravenous; PO, by mouth; q, every.

Table 4.6 Guidelines for processing surgical samples (stereotactic aspiration or craniotomy).

Laboratory	Samples	Targets, comments
Bacteriology	10 ml to be directly inoculated in blood culture bottles (aerobic/anaerobic)	Streptococci, staphylococci, anaerobes (blood culture bottles increase the yield, especially if previous use of antibacterials)
	Two separate dry tubes At least 5 ml in each tube	– Gram staining – Cultures on routine media – Molecular biology to be performed if cultures sterile after 48 h – Tests for mycobacteria if risk factors for tuberculosis
Histology	One dry tube for fluid sample If tissue, to be sent in sterile water	Differential diagnosis (cancer)
Mycology, parasitology	Dry tube	Only if immunocompromised (HIV, immunosuppressive agents, organ transplant, malignant hemopathy) Specific tests for *Toxoplasma*, invasive mycosis (*Aspergillus* spp.)

Basic rules
To be sent within 1 h to the microbiology laboratory, for immediate processing, 24/24
Two sets of blood cultures should be obtained, before and just after surgery, optimally prior to antibiotic administration.
Patient's characteristics and clinical suspicion to be documented on the laboratory form

HIV, human immunodeficiency virus.
Source: from [44] with permission.

Anti-Infective therapy

The main anti-infective regimens are summarized in Table 4.5

Neurosurgery

Progress in neurosurgical techniques is one of the key factors contributing to improved prognosis over recent decades. Stereotactic surgery enables aspiration of even small brain abscesses ≥1 cm and is well tolerated, regardless of its location. Neuronavigation assistance in neurosurgery allows an optimal trajectory to be planned for entry to the abscess, to avoid damaging critical areas [43].

Consequently, the neurosurgical approach has dramatically changed: (i) total resection through craniotomy is now rarely considered first, except for patients with a large multilobulated abscess and severe cranial hypertension; (ii) stereotactic aspiration by neuro-navigation, either CT or MRI guided, is indicated for all patients with microbiologically undocumented brain abscess ≥1 cm; (iii) an abscess size ≥2.5 cm is considered as a stand-alone indication for drainage, even in patients with microbiological documentation (e.g. through positive blood cultures; and (iv) drainage should be considered for periventricular lesions with a high risk of intraventricular rupture and in difficult-to-treat bacterial or fungal infections, especially in patients who are immunocompromised.

Other indications for neurosurgery include placement of an external ventricular catheter for drainage and monitoring of ICP in all cases of intraventricular abscess rupture and in selected cases of large cerebral or cerebellar abscess with hydrocephalus. Guidelines for processing stereotactic or craniotomy samples are indicated in Table 4.6 [44].

Conclusions

CNS infections have diverse etiologies and a high risk of mortality and morbidity. The systematic approach includes assessment of risk factors, clinical examination, neuroimaging, and modern laboratory tests. Early appropriate anti-infective treatment combined with critical care may contribute to improved outcome.

References

1. McGill, F., Heyderman, R.S., Michel, B.D. et al. (2016). The UK joint specialist societies guideline on the diagnosis and management of acute meningitis and meningococcal sepsis in immunocompetent adults. *J. Infect.* 72: 405–438.
2. Bijslma, M.W., Brouwer, M.C., Kasanmoentalib, E.S. et al. (2016). Community-acquired bacterial meningitis in adults in the Netherlands, 2006–14: a prospective cohort study. *Lancet Infect. Dis.* 16: 339–347.
3. Castelblanco, R.L., Lee, M., and Hasbun, R. (2014). Epidemiology of bacterial meningitis in the USA from 1997 to 2010: a population-based observational study. *Lancet Infect. Dis.* 14: 813–819.
4. Charlier, C., Perrodeau, E., Leclercq, A. et al. (2017). Clinical features and prognostic factors of listeriosis: the MONALISA national prospective cohort study. *Lancet Infect. Dis.* 17: 510–519.
5. Glimaker, M., Johansson, B., Grinborg, O. et al. (2015). Adult bacterial meningitis: earlier treatment and improved outcome following guideline revision promoting prompt lumbar puncture. *Clin. Infect. Dis.* 60: 1162–1169.
6. Auburtin, M., Wolff, M., Charpentier, J. et al. (2006). Detrimental role of delayed antibiotic administration and penicillin-nonsusceptible strains in adult intensive care unit patients with pneumococcal meningitis: the PNEUMOREA prospective multicenter study. *Crit. Care Med.* 34: 2758–2765.
7. van de Beek, D., de Gans, J., Spanjaard, L. et al. (2004). Clinical features and prognostic factors in adults with bacterial meningitis. *N. Engl. J. Med.* 351: 1849–1859.
8. van de Beek, D., Cabellos, C., Dzupova, O. et al. (2016). ESCMID guideline: diagnosis and treatment of acute bacterial meningitis. *Clin. Microbiol. Infect.* 22 (Suppl 3): S37–S62.
9. Giulieri, S., Chapuis-Taillard, C., Jaton, K. et al. (2011). CSF lactate for accurate diagnosis of community-acquired bacterial meningitis. *Eur. J. Clin. Microbiol. Infect. Dis.* 34: 2049–2055.
10. Vikse, J., Henry, B.M., Roy, J. et al. (2015). The role of serum procalcitonin in the diagnosis of bacterial meningitis in adults: a systematic review and meta-analysis. *Int. J. Infect. Dis.* 38: 68–76.
11. Weisfelt, M., van de Beek, D., Spanjaard, L. et al. (2006). Clinical features, complications, and outcome in adults with pneumococcal meningitis: a prospective case series. *Lancet Neurol.* 5: 123–129.
12. Coureuil, M., Lecuyer, H., Bourdoulous, S., and Nassif, X. (2017). A journey into the brain: insight into how bacterial pathogens cross blood–brain barriers. *Nat. Rev. Microbiol.* 15: 149–159.
13. Sonneville, R., Citerio, G., and Meyfroidt, G. (2016). Understanding coma in bacterial meningitis. *Intensive Care Med.* 42: 1282–1285.
14. Nau, R., Sorgel, F., and Eiffert, H. (2010). Penetration of drugs through the blood-cerebrospinal fluid/blood-brain barrier for treatment of central nervous system infections. *Clin. Microbiol. Rev.* 23: 858–883.
15. Brouwer, M.C., McIntyre, P., Prasad, K., and van de Beek, D. (2015). Corticosteroids for acute bacterial meningitis. *Cochrane Database Syst. Rev.* 12 (9): CD004405.
16. Venkatesan, A., Tunkel, A.R., Bloch, K.C. et al. (2013). Case definitions, diagnostic algorithms, and priorities in encephalitis: consensus statement of the international encephalitis consortium. *Clin. Infect. Dis.* 57: 1114–1128.
17. Hasbun, R., Rosenthal, N., Balada-Lliasat, J.M. et al. (2017). Epidemiology of meningitis and encephalitis in the United States, 2011–2014. *Clin. Infect. Dis.* 65: 359–363.
18. Mailles A, Stahl JP, Steering Committee and Investigators Group (2009). Infectious encephalitis in France in 2007: a national prospective study. *Clin. Infect. Dis.* 49: 1838–1847.
19. Granerod, J., Ambrose, H.E., Davies, N.W.S. et al. (2010). Causes of encephalitis and differences in their clinical presentations in England: a multicentre, population-based prospective study. *Lancet Infect. Dis.* 10: 835–844.
20. Sonneville, R., Gault, N., de Montmollin, E. et al. (2015). Clinical spectrum and outcomes of patients with encephalitis requiring intensive care. *Eur. J. Neurol.* 22: 6–16.
21. Chow, F.C., Glaser, S.H. et al. (2015). Use of clinical and neuroimaging characteristics to distinguish temporal lobe herpes simplex encephalitis from its mimics. *Clin. Infect. Dis.* 60: 1377–1383.
22. Claasen, J., Taccone, F.S., Horn, P. et al. (2013). Recommendations on the use of EEG monitoring in critically ill patients: consensus statement from the neurointensive care section of the ESICM. *Intensive Care Med.* 39: 1337–1351.
23. Leber, A.L., Everhart, K., Balada-Lliasat, J.M. et al. (2016). Multicenter evaluation of BioFire FilmArray meningitis/encephalitis panel for detection of bacteria, viruses, and yeast in cerebrospinal fluid specimens. *J. Clin. Microbiol.* 54: 2251–2261.

24. Wilson, M.R., Naccache, S.N., Samayoa, E. et al. (2014). Actionable diagnosis of neuroleptospirosis by next-generation sequencing. *N. Engl. J. Med.* 370: 2408–2417.
25. Bradshaw, M.J. and Venkatesan, A. (2016). Herpes simplex Virus-1 encephalitis in adults: pathophysiology, diagnosis, and management. *Neurotherapeutics* 13: 493–508.
26. Renard, D., Nerrant, E., and Lechiche, C. (2015). DWI and FLAIR imaging in herpes simplex encephalitis: a comparative and topographical analysis. *J. Neurol.* 262: 2101–2105.
27. Poissy, J., Wolff, M., Dewilde, A. et al. (2009). Factors associated with delay to acyclovir administration in 184 patients with herpes simplex virus encephalitis. *Clin. Microbiol. Infect.* 15: 560–564.
28. Mailles, A., de Broucker, T., Constanzo, P. et al. (2012). Long-term outcome of patients presenting with acute infectious encephalitis of various causes in France. *Clin. Infect. Dis.* 54: 1455–1464.
29. Jacquet, P., de Montmollin, E., Dupuis, C. et al. (2009). Functional outcomes in adult patients with herpes simplex encephalitis admitted to the ICU: a multicenter cohort study. *Intensive Care Med.* 45: 1103–1111.
30. Schein, F., Gagneux-Brunon, A., Antoine, J.C. et al. (2017). Anti-N-methyl-D-aspartate receptor encephalitis after herpes simplex virus-associated encephalitis: an emerging disease with diagnosis and therapeutic challenges. *Infection* 45: 545–549.
31. Bratton, E.W., El Husseini, N., Chastain, C.A. et al. (2012). Comparison and temporal trends of three groups with Cryptococcosis: HIV-infected, solid organ transplant, and HIV-negative/non-transplant. *PlosOne* 7: e43582.
32. Prasad, K., Singh, M.B., and Ryan, H. (2016). Corticosteroids for managing tuberculous meningitis. *Cochrane Database Syst. Rev.* (4): CD002244.
33. Misra, U.K., Kalita, J., Betai, S., and Bhoi, S.K. (2015). Outcome of tuberculous meningitis patients requiring mechanical ventilation. *J. Crit. Care* 30: 1365–1369.
34. Ogata, M., Oshima, K., Ikebe, T. et al. (2017). Clinical characteristics and outcome of human herpesvirus-6 encephalitis after allogeneic hematopoietic stem cell transplantation. *Bone Marrow Transplant.* 52: 1563–1570.
35. Brouwer, M.C., Coutinho, J.M., and van de Beek, D. (2014). Clinical characteristics and outcome of brain abscess: systematic review and meta-analysis. *Neurology* 82: 806–813.
36. Al Masalma, M., Lonjon, M., Richet, H. et al. (2012). Metagenomic analysis of brain abscesses identifies specific bacterial associations. *Clin. Infect. Dis.* 54: 202–210.
37. Server, A., Bargalló, N., Fløisand, Y. et al. (2017). Imaging spectrum of central nervous system complications of hematopoietic stem cell and solid organ transplantation. *Neuroradiology* 59: 105–126.
38. Marzolf, G., Sabou, M., Lannes, B. et al. (2016). Magnetic resonance imaging of cerebral aspergillosis: imaging and pathological correlations. *PlosOne* 11: e0152475.
39. Sonneville, R., Ferrand, H., Tubach, F. et al. (2011). Neurological complications of HIV infection in critically ill patients: clinical features and outcomes. *J. Infect.* 62: 301–308.
40. Coussement, J., Lebeaux, D., van Delden, C. et al. (2016). Nocardia infection in solid organ transplant recipients: a multicenter European case-control study. *Clin. Infect. Dis.* 63: 338–345.
41. Tan, I.L., Smith, B.R., von Geldern, G. et al. (2012). HIV-associated opportunistic infections of the CNS. *Lancet Neurol.* 11: 605–617.
42. Wright, A.J. and Fishman, J.A. (2014). Central nervous system syndromes in solid organ transplant recipients. *Clin. Infect. Dis.* 59: 1001–1011.
43. Meng, X.H., Feng, S.Y., Chen, X.L. et al. (2015). Minimally invasive image-guided keyhole aspiration of cerebral abscesses. *Int. J. Clin. Exp. Med.* 8: 155–163.
44. Sonneville, R., Ruimy, R., Benzonana, N. et al. (2017). An update on bacterial brain abscess in immunocompetent patients. *Clin. Microbiol. Infect.* 23: 614–620.

5 Herpes Simplex Virus Infections of the CNS

Bette K. Kleinschmidt-DeMasters[1], Catherine (Katy) Keohane[2], and Françoise Gray[3,4]

[1] Department of Pathology, Neurosurgery, and Neurology, University of Colorado School of Medicine, Aurora, CO, USA
[2] Department of Pathology and School of Medicine, University College Cork, Brookfield Health Science Complex, Cork, Ireland
[3] Retired from Department of Pathology, Lariboisière Hospital, APHP, Paris, France
[4] University Paris Diderot (Paris 7), Paris, France

Abbreviations

AIDS	acquired immune deficiency syndrome
CMV	cytomegalovirus
CNS	central nervous system
CSF	cerebrospinal fluid
DRG	dorsal root ganglion/ganglia
EBV	Epstein-Barr virus
HHV	human herpes virus
HSV	herpes simplex virus
HSVE	HSV encephalitis
MRI	magnetic resonance imaging
NMDAR	N-methyl-D-aspartate receptor
PCR	polymerase chain reaction
SEM	skin, eye, mouth
VZV	varicella-zoster virus

Definition

Herpesviruses are large, enveloped, spherical viruses, ranging from 120 to more than 200 nm in diameter. They have a unique four-layered structure: a core containing the large, double-stranded DNA genome is enclosed by an icosapentahedral capsid composed of capsomeres. The capsid is surrounded by an amorphous protein coat called the "tegument." It is encased in a glycoprotein-bearing lipid bilayer envelope [1].

The family Herpesviridae is divided into three subfamilies. Although there are more than 100 known herpesviruses, only 8 are pathogenic to humans and 5 cause pathologically proven productive CNS infections.

The α-herpesviridae are characterized by an extremely short reproductive cycle, rapid destruction of the host cell, and the ability to replicate in a wide variety of host tissues. They characteristically establish latent infection in sensory nerve ganglia. They include:
HSV-1: herpes simplex virus 1/human herpesvirus 1
HSV-2: herpes simplex virus 2/human herpesvirus 2
VZV: varicella-zoster virus/human herpesvirus 3

β-herpesviridae have a long reproductive cycle and restricted host range; they include:
CMV: cytomegalovirus/human herpes virus 5
HHV-6: human herpesvirus 6

Infections of the Central Nervous System: Pathology and Genetics, First Edition. Edited by Fabrice Chrétien, Kum Thong Wong, Leroy R. Sharer, Catherine (Katy) Keohane and Françoise Gray.
© 2020 John Wiley & Sons Ltd. Published 2020 by John Wiley & Sons Ltd.

HHV-7: human herpesvirus 7

γ-herpesviridae have a restricted host range and include:

EBV: Epstein-Barr virus/human herpesvirus 4

HHV-8: human herpesvirus 8

HHV-8 is the causative agent of Kaposi sarcoma. In Zambian individuals positive for human immunodeficiency virus (HIV) with Kaposi sarcoma, infection by HHV-8 has been demonstrated in CNS resident cells, primarily neurons [2]. Rare clinical observations of encephalitis, encephalomyeloradiculitis, or meningomyelitis associated with HHV-7 infection have been reported [3]. A possible association between HHV-6 and multiple sclerosis has been suggested [4]. However, only five herpes viruses have consistently caused pathologically proven CNS infectious damage: HSV-1, HSV-2, VZV, CMV, and EBV.

This chapter will describe infections of the CNS in HSV-1 and HSV-2. VZV and EBV infections are described in Chapter 6 and CMV infection in Chapter 7.

Definition of the disorder, major synonyms, and historical perspective

HSV-1 and HSV-2 produce two major disease patterns: (i) primary and recurrent HSV infections in adults and children, which may be asymptomatic, cause mucocutaneous lesions, or more rarely, keratitis or CNS infections; and (ii) primary neonatal infection acquired perinatally.

Colloquial terms for orolabial herpes infections are "cold sores" or "fever blisters." "Herpetic whitlow" refers to vesicular lesions on the thumb or fingers.

Greeks coined the word "herpes," meaning "to creep or crawl" along the skin. Hippocrates used this term to describe skin lesions, some of which were likely herpetic infections [5]. In the 1920s, the Mathewson commission was one of the earliest reports to suggest HSV caused encephalitis in humans [6]. Goodpasture and others demonstrated that material from herpetic lip and genital lesions produced encephalitis when introduced into the scarified cornea or skin of rabbits [7]. The first pediatric case report of herpes simplex virus encephalitis (HSVE) was published in 1941 [8] and the first adult case in 1944 [9].

Microbiological characteristics

Replication of all herpesviruses is a multistep process. The interaction of the four viral envelope glycoproteins (i.e. gD, gH, gB, and gL) with cell surface receptors is important for cell entry. The tegument protein VP16 is important for replication and activates immediate early gene expression [10]. This is followed by transcription of immediate-early genes, which encode for the regulatory proteins. Expression of immediate-early gene products is followed by the expression of proteins encoded by early and then late genes. Assembly of the viral core and capsid takes place within the nucleus, followed by envelopment at the nuclear membrane and transport out of the nucleus through the endoplasmic reticulum and the Golgi apparatus. Glycosylation of the viral membrane occurs in the Golgi apparatus. Mature virions are transported to the outer membrane of the host cell inside vesicles. Release of progeny virus is accompanied by cell death [1].

All herpes family viruses share the ability to establish latency and reactivation, but only HSV-1, HSV-2, and VZV are neurotropic and establish latency in the dorsal root ganglia (DRG). Latency primarily occurs in the sensory ganglion of the nerve(s) innervating the site of primary infection (i.e. the trigeminal ganglion for HSV-1 and sacral DRG for HSV-2). The virus travels intra-axonally along sensory nerves in a retrograde fashion to access the sensory nerve ganglion. During latency, HSV-1 or HSV-2 genome localizes to the host ganglion neuronal cell nucleus but does not integrate into the host DNA. Rather, it maintains a circular form outside the host DNA but still within the host nucleus ("episomal") and shows only limited gene transcription [10]. Throughout this stage, from when latency is first established until HSV is reactivated, the latency-associated transcript (LAT) locus is the only highly expressed gene. This gene helps to maintain survival of the infected neuron with assistance from noncoding micro-RNAs (mRNAs) [10]. HSV-1 and HSV-2 have lifelong latency.

Recurrent infections are usually the result of the reactivation of virus from a latent state, although a second primary infection with a different HSV viral strain also occurs. If reactivated, the virus is transported via fast anterograde microtubule-associated pathways down the sensory nerve to the distal axon [10], where it can replicate in various types of cells, especially epithelial cells, at the nerve terminus.

Epidemiology: incidence and prevalence, sex, age, geographical distribution, and risk factors

Infection in children and adults

Primary infections from HSV-1 or HSV-2 require intimate person-to-person contact; humans are the sole hosts and no intermediate host is required.

As of January 2017, the World Health Organization (WHO) estimates that, globally an estimated 3.7 billion people younger than age 50 (67%) have HSV-1 infection [11]. HSV-1 infection occurs worldwide and is usually acquired in childhood, with up to 95% of adults in the western world being seropositive. The overwhelming majority of persons with HSV-1 never develop encephalitis, keratitis, or other severe disease manifestation [12].

HSV-2 is principally acquired through sexual activity and, thus, occurs a bit later. It is estimated that 16.2% of all Americans ages 14–49 years have genital herpes [10]. According to WHO, 417 million people ages 15–49 (11%) worldwide have HSV-2 infection [11].

Genital HSV-2 infections show the highest incidence in Africa, followed by the Americas. Incidence increases with age, although the highest numbers of those newly infected are adolescents. More women are infected with HSV-2 than men as a result of more efficient sexual transmission of HSV from men to women. HSV-2 infection increases the risk of acquiring and transmitting HIV infection [11] and treatment of the HSV infection reduces this risk [10].

Although there is >70% homology between the DNA of HSV-1 and HSV-2, infection with one type of HSV does not confer complete immunity for the other.

The percentage of persons infected who go on to develop meningitis or encephalitis caused by HSV-1 and HSV-2 is low. However, within cohorts of patients who have had meningitis or encephalitis, HSV-1 and HSV-2 are the major, but not the most frequent, culprits.

Of 26 429 adult patients with meningitis or encephalitis reviewed in the United States between 2011 and 2014, the most common etiology was enterovirus, followed by "unknown cause," bacterial meningitis, HSV, noninfectious cause, fungi, arboviruses, and other viruses [13]. When a cause could be identified, a large recent German study of adult "aseptic" (i.e. nonbacterial) meningitis or encephalitis cases found the leading viral causes of meningitis were enteroviruses (36%), HSV (15%), and VZV (12%), whereas encephalitis or meningoencephalitis was caused by HSV or VZV (13% each) [14]. Another study of aseptic meningitis showed HSV was the most common identifiable cause in adults, and in children it was enterovirus [15].

Although many studies are small, the quoted annual incidence of HSVE ranges from 2.5–12 cases per million, and mortality from 4–11% for inpatients to 10–14% at one year. Most studies found near-equal gender involvement and similar mean or median age (50–66 years), except in HSVE cases from India (80% male) and Iran (mean age 34.9 years) [16].

Rare documented risk factors for HSVE include previous neurosurgical procedures [17] and full-blown acquired immunodeficiency syndrome (AIDS) [18].

Neonatal infection

According to WHO, neonatal herpes infection is rare, occurring in an estimated 10 per 100 000 births globally. The risk for neonatal herpes is greatest when a mother acquires HSV infection for the first time in late pregnancy. Women with genital herpes before they become pregnant are at low risk of transmitting HSV to their infants [11].

Infection in adults and children

Primary infection

The symptoms of HSV infections in adults and children >6 months of age are dictated by the route of transmission.

HSV-1 is mainly transmitted by oral-to-oral contact with blisters or vesicles ("cold sores"), saliva, and surfaces in or around the mouth of a person with the infection. In most patients, initial infection by HSV-1 involves the oropharyngeal mucosa. In children younger than age 5, primary HSV-1 infection can cause gingivostomatitis, with fever, sore throat, redness and edema of the pharynx, and vesicular or ulcerative lesions of oropharyngeal mucosa. Recurrent labial HSV-1 infections most commonly occur at the vermillion border of the lip. Intraoral lesions as a manifestation of recurrent disease are uncommon in hosts who are immunocompetent but do occur in persons who are immunocompromised [1]. Less commonly, HSV-1 causes herpetic keratitis, the most common infectious cause of blindness in the United States [1].

HSV-2 is almost exclusively sexually transmitted, causing infection in the genital or anal area ("genital herpes"). Primary infection may be associated with fever, malaise, anorexia, and lymphadenopathy; up to 10% of those infected are estimated to develop aseptic meningitis with the primary infection [1]. Although most genital herpes is a result of HSV-2, increasing numbers are due to HSV-1 infection transmitted through oral-genital contact.

Classic HSVE
Etiology
HSVE is the most common, sporadic, and fatal form of encephalitis. Only one-third of patients with HSVE have the disease because of first exposure to HSV (i.e. primary HSV infection). The majority of adult cases occurs in persons already seropositive for HSV at the onset of symptoms. Approximately one-half of adults with HSVE reactivate their latent virus, whereas in others, the isolates suggest that HSVE occurred after reinfection with a different HSV strain [12]. Only 6–10% of patients with HSVE have a history of orolabial herpes [19]. HSVE is mainly the result of HSV-1 and neonatal herpes to HSV-2 infection, but a minor percentage of each of these infections can be produced by the other virus. In recent studies, when subtypes have been established, >90% of HSVE in adults and older children are caused by HSV-1, with 4–6% of HSVE cases caused by HSV-2 [19, 20]. HSV-2 infection has been cited as being more frequent in atypical cases of HSVE, characterized by mild or atypical clinical disease course, absence of focal findings, and slow progression in the absence of antiviral therapy [20, 21].

Clinical features
Patients present with a combination of nonspecific features of encephalitis and focal neurological signs because of involvement of the temporal and frontal lobes (see Chapter 4). Most patients develop fever, headache, and confusion, and frequent neurological signs include dysphasia, hemiparesis, ataxia, and focal seizures. Although the onset may be fulminant, many patients have an influenza-like prodromal illness. Some patients present with insidious personality changes and behavioral abnormalities over several days.

Computed tomography (CT) scans, magnetic resonance imaging (MRI), and electroencephalogram (EEG) show focal abnormalities usually involving one or both temporal lobes (cf. Chapter 4), but the changes are non-specific and may not be present until relatively late.

Cerebrospinal fluid (CSF) examination usually reveals moderate leukocytosis, variable numbers of red cells, and elevated proteins but may be normal in the early stage. Polymerase chain reaction (PCR)-based detection of HSV DNA in the CSF is now the gold standard for diagnosis (sensitivity 96%, specificity 99% [22]) and has supplanted biopsy and serology. False-negative PCR can occur early in the illness, and if the clinical suspicion is high, acyclovir should be continued empirically and repeat CSF HSV PCR obtained within three to seven days [22].

Long-term outcomes for HSVE before the advent of effective antiviral therapy (acyclovir) were poor with a 70% mortality [23]. With treatment, this has decreased significantly, but a favorable outcome requires rapid diagnosis and prompt treatment with acyclovir [24]. However, too few patients that survive return to completely normal neurological and cognitive function [23]. Long-term challenges include memory and language loss, significant changes in employment status, access to correct rehabilitation services, and other social problems [25]. Reactivation of encephalitis after therapy has been reported.

Pathology, including histopathology, electron microscopy, and immunocytochemistry

Acute phase

The macroscopic features in the acute phase are stereotyped and distinctive: there is generalized swelling (Figure 5.1a) and bilateral asymmetric necrotic and hemorrhagic lesions predominantly involving the temporal lobes and limbic regions (i.e. insulae, cingulate gyri, and posterior orbital frontal cortex). The changes vary in intensity from near-normal, to softening with discoloration in the earliest phase (Figure 5.1b), to hemorrhagic necrosis, or frank hematoma.

Microscopically, the earliest lesions can have a limited inflammatory response, the predominant feature being shrinkage and eosinophilia of neurons, capillary dilatation, marked congestion, and petechial hemorrhages (Figure 5.2a) [26]. Inflammation can be scant and, when present, is mostly composed of lymphocytes around vessels in superficial cortex (Figure 5.2b), leptomeninges, [26] or perivascular spaces (Figure 5.2b and c). Neutrophils can be seen in the necrotic tissue, which often involves broad zones (Figure 5.2c), especially by the onset of the second week. Although this can simulate anoxic encephalopathy, the necrotic areas in HSVE are either patchy or very widespread and fail to show laminar necrosis.

Overall, scattered cells (neurons and glia) contain intranuclear inclusion bodies, either classic intranuclear eosinophilic discrete Cowdry A inclusions or more diffuse violaceous inclusions (Figure 5.2d). Immunocytochemistry reveals abundant intranuclear and cytoplasmic viral antigen in many neurons and glial and endothelial cells as the virus egresses the cell before total cell lysis (Figure 5.2e).

At a more advanced stage, the lesions are more characteristic and include foci of hemorrhage and necrosis (Figure 5.3a) with parenchymal infiltration by lymphocytes and macrophages. Severe tissue destruction, gliosis, and cavitation can be found (Figure 5.3b). Mononuclear cells in the leptomeninges, perivascular cuffing, neuronophagia, and diffuse microglial hyperplasia more characteristic of meningoencephalitis are also present (Figure 5.3c). Nuclear inclusions are usually sparse, and the virus is more easily identified by immunohistochemistry. HSV is demonstrable for up to about three weeks after the onset of encephalitis, but the number of immunopositive cells declines considerably after two weeks [26]. Viral antigen is less likely to be demonstrable after treatment with acyclovir. Especially during the first two weeks, electron microscopy (EM) is often successful in revealing HSV nucleocapsid in the nuclei of infected cells. Viral DNA can be detected on paraffin-embedded

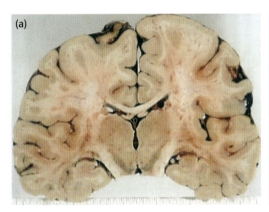
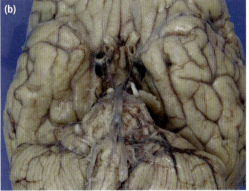

Figure 5.1 Acute herpes simplex virus encephalitis (HSVE), gross examination. (a) Bilateral swelling of cerebral hemispheres slightly more on the right side with discoloration of the white matter and mild accentuation of blood vessels. Acute death (<48 hours) from herpes simplex virus 1 (HSV-1) encephalitis. There is no visible necrosis. Microscopy showed viral inclusions and mild perivascular lymphocytic inflammation. (b) Gross brain specimen of an 82-year-old woman with Alzheimer disease who first experienced new-onset seizures six days prior to demise. She was febrile on admission but was thought to be septic, but HSVE was never suspected; note the swelling and discoloration in the right inferomedial temporal lobe is more prominent than in the left.

Infections of the Central Nervous System

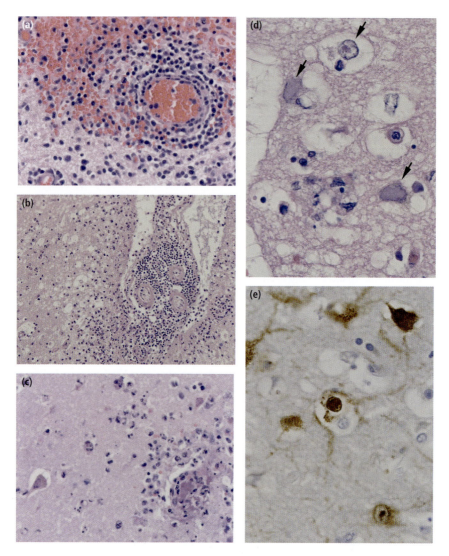

Figure 5.2 Acute herpes simplex virus encephalitis (HSVE), microscopy of earliest lesions. (a) Brain biopsy from a 59-year-old woman who presented with headache, nausea, vomiting, and in whom neuroimaging showed cortical thickening in the medial right temporal lobe without associated enhancement. Glioma was suspected, but biopsy showed intense lymphocytic inflammation and petechial hemorrhages. Hematoxylin and eosin (H&E). (b) Microscopically, the brain from the patient illustrated in Figure 5.1b. shows lymphocytic inflammation in the leptomeninges, with neutrophils predominating in the adjacent necrotic brain parenchyma (H&E). (c) The necrotic parenchyma with neutrophilic reaction contains red and dead neurons, which, without close inspection, could be mistaken for acute anoxic encephalopathy (H&E). (d) Herpes simplex virus (HSV) can infect neurons and all types of glial cells; this image shows a classic "owl's eye" Cowdry A inclusion in the infected cell at left (arrow), which contains a large, discrete, eosinophilic intranuclear viral inclusion and shows clearing/vesicular change in the host nucleus and margination of the host nuclear chromatin to the nuclear membrane. The other two infected cells, middle and right (arrows), have viral particles that completely fill the host cell nucleus, resulting in a violaceous, uniform appearance, albeit still with margination of host chromatin. Without co-immunostaining, it can sometimes be difficult to identify the host cell type (H&E). (e) Immunostaining for HSV in the same patient illustrated in Figure 5.2d parallels the features seen on H&E. Note that the Cowdry A inclusions are immunopositive but so are the host nuclear membrane of the infected cell and often the entire cytoplasm (as in the pyramidal neuron at lower right) as the virus egresses the nucleus where viral assembly occurred (Immunostain for HSV with light hematoxylin counterstain).

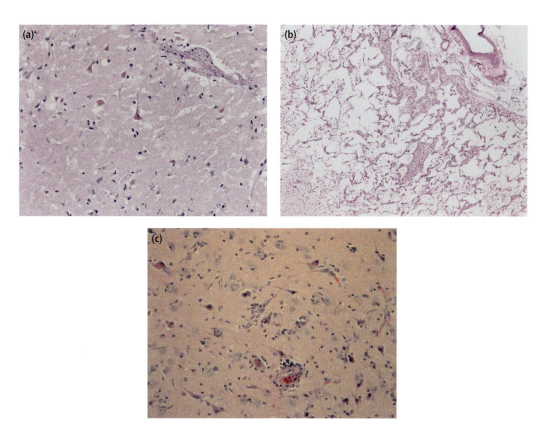

Figure 5.3 Herpes simplex virus encephalitis (HSVE) at a more advanced stage. (a) This 74-year-old man with past medical history of sarcoidosis presented to an outside hospital with acute onset of right arm and leg weakness and right arm twitching. After extensive work up for autoimmune and infectious etiologies, the patient's initial herpes simplex virus (HSV) polymerase chain reaction (PCR) was negative, but a repeat study returned positive herpes simplex virus 1(HSV-1) but negative for herpes simplex virus 2 (HSV-2); he succumbed one month later. Despite the fact that this was well beyond the phase when normally inflammation would have ensued and viral antigen would have been cleared, his brain showed "pseudo-ischemic" features, with near absence of inflammation and extremely widespread virus by immunohistochemistry (hematoxylin and eosin [H&E]). (b) This 48-year-old woman with a seizure disorder after HSVE lived 11 years before demise; note the extensive cavitation of the affected temporal lobe cortex (H&E). (c) Temporo/occipital biopsy in a 29-year-old woman with headache for two weeks, new-onset complex partial seizures, and magnetic resonance imaging (MRI) appearances thought to represent infiltrating neoplasm. Histology showed necrotic areas with macrophages (not illustrated) and adjacent perivascular lymphocytic inflammation, diffuse microglial hyperplasia, and numerous intraneuronal inclusions immunopositive for HSV-1.

or frozen sections by in situ hybridization or PCR amplification [27].

Chronic phase

In patients who are untreated or unsuccessfully treated and die weeks after the onset of the disease, hemorrhagic necrosis will have progressed to cavitation and atrophy with collapse of the affected temporal lobes and yellow and brown discoloration of the surrounding brain parenchyma and overlying meninges.

Microscopically, the affected parenchyma is replaced by cavitated glial scar tissue containing occasional microglial nodules and some residual mononuclear inflammation [26, 27]. The virus is no longer demonstrable by culture, EM, or immunohistochemistry but may be detectable by PCR [27].

Atypical HSVE

HSVE resulting from either HSV-1 or HSV-2 is usually an acute, monophasic illness. Some patients, especially children, can have a relapse within weeks or months after the initial event and in a subset of these, PCR testing in the CSF is negative for virus [28]. It has been recently recognized that these virus-negative relapses are likely the result of an autoimmune response, with N-methyl-D-aspartate receptor (NMDAR) antibodies being detected [29]. NMDAR encephalitis following HSVE may be due to molecular mimicry or an immune response to neuronal damage caused by the initial HSVE [29].

Occasionally, some patients develop non-necrotizing, often noninflammatory atypical forms of HSVE that may involve a site other than the temporal or frontal lobes, usually the brainstem. These forms are often more slowly progressive than classic HSVE with persistence of viral antigen and DNA. Although the likelihood of developing HSVE is probably not increased by immunosuppression, this seems to predispose to atypical forms, as most cases are reported in patients with AIDS [21, 30, 31].

Granulomatous herpes simplex encephalitis

Granulomatous herpes simplex encephalitis is a very rare form of HSVE and has only been reported in children [32]. In most cases, an initial episode of "typical HSVE" has been complicated by the development of intractable seizures [33], progressive neurological deficits, and enlarging regions of abnormality on imaging, in some cases, after an interval of several years. CSF HSV viral DNA load may be low [34]. Neuropathological examination reveals chronic granulomatous inflammation with multinucleated giant cells, foci of necrosis sometimes with a multicystic appearance, [34] and mineralization. Immunohistochemistry to demonstrate the virus in tissue may be negative by the time of biopsy or autopsy, but the virus may be detectable by PCR [34].

Spinal cord disease associated with hsv infection

Both HSV-1 and HSV-2 can cause myelitis and radiculitis, although HSV-2 is more often responsible. Myelitis is a rare complication. The disease may be limited to a few cord segments and followed by complete recovery suggesting a non-necrotizing inflammatory process. Pathological reports are few.

HSV-2 may also cause an ascending necrotizing myelopathy, usually in patients who are immunocompromised. Histology reveals extensive coagulative necrosis of the cord parenchyma and mononuclear inflammation in the leptomeninges and roots. HSV antigen is usually abundant in the cord, and viral particles may be visible on EM [35].

Aseptic meningitis

Aseptic meningitis is a frequent complication of primary genital infection by HSV-2. In addition, HSV-2 DNA can be identified in the CSF of most patients who experience recurrent aseptic meningitis (also known as Mollaret meningitis, recurrent HSV meningitis, or recurrent benign lymphocytic meningitis), with HSV-1 accounting for a small proportion of cases [23, 36].

Neonatal HSVE

Etiology

Neonatal HSVE is acquired in utero, during delivery, or the first four weeks of life and differs in its pathogenesis and clinical and pathological manifestations from the adult disease. One-half to three-quarters of neonatal HSV infections are the result of HSV-2 [37–39]. About 5% of cases are acquired in utero, 85% during vaginal delivery by contact with infected maternal genital lesions, and 10% by contact with infected secretions from the mother or another source during the early postnatal period. Caesarean section is recommended for pregnant women with active genital HSV lesions at time of delivery to decrease the risk of perinatal transmission.

Encephalitis may be one component of a disseminated infection or an isolated manifestation of neonatal HSV infection. During disseminated infection, HSV is thought to enter the CNS hematogenously and be distributed widely throughout the CNS and other organs. In isolated HSVE, the pattern of distribution is often similar to that in adults suggesting a similar intra-axonal mechanism of entry into the brain.

Clinical features

Three main patterns of neonatal HSV infection have been delineated [40]: (i) disseminated disease, with visceral organ involvement (including infection of the brain in two-thirds to three-quarters of patients); (ii) CNS disease (with no other visceral organ involvement but with skin lesions in two-thirds of patients); or (iii) disease limited to the skin, eyes, or mouth (i.e. SEM disease), and the CNS appears unaffected although a small proportion of children have long-term neurological sequelae [1]. Neonatal HSVE is most common in the first month of life. Symptoms are usually non-specific including fever, seizures, poor feeding, and lethargy [37].

PCR-based detection of HSV DNA in the CSF is positive and unlike in children and adults with HSVE, viral DNA can be detected in the serum even in neonates with isolated encephalitis.

A recent study identified three different anatomical patterns of predominant brain involvement by MRI. The inferior frontal and temporal pole area was involved in 38% of neonates, a watershed distribution was present in 46%, and corticospinal tract involvement in 31% [37]. Corticospinal tract involvement was characterized as affecting white matter fibers of the tracts and the pre- and postcentral cortical gyri, with or without involvement of the lateral nucleus of the thalamus [37]. Corticospinal tract involvement was also identified in an independent study of 29 cases [39]. Similar to pediatric and adult HSVE, these areas of involvement were not always symmetrical.

Symptoms may differ between infants infected with HSV-1 and HSV-2. Corey et al. noted that infants with HSV-2 neonatal encephalitis presented with a higher frequency of seizures, greater pleocytosis and protein concentrations in the CSF, and more frequent evidence of structural damage on CT scans of the brain than those with HSV-1 encephalitis [38].

The outcome of neonatal HSV infection depends on the pattern. In SEM disease, mortality is near zero, whereas it is 15% for encephalitis and 60% for disseminated neonatal HSV infection [1]. Long-term sequelae including microcephaly, seizure disorders, ophthalmological defects, cerebral palsy, and mental retardation occur in approximately 60% of survivors, even with therapy, [1] and are usually greater in those surviving HSV-2 than HSV-1 infection [38] and those with MRI involvement of the corticospinal tract [37].

Neuropathology

At gross examination, the brain is usually swollen congested and extensively softened, sometimes with parenchymal or ventricular hemorrhages. Long-term survivors may show microcephaly, ventricular enlargement, hemorrhagic infarct, diffuse porencephalic changes or hydranencephaly, intracranial calcifications, chorioretinitis, and optic atrophy.

Microscopically, at the time of autopsy, the lesions tend not to be restricted to any particular part of the brain and can involve both gray and white matter in the cerebrum (Figure 5.4a), cerebellum, or brainstem. There is necrotizing encephalitis with meningeal and parenchymal infiltration by lymphocytes and macrophages (Figure 5.4b). Some lesions may be hemorrhagic or calcified (Figure 5.4c). Viral inclusions may be found and viral antigen and DNA demonstrated, particularly during the first days of infection.

Genetics and pathogenesis

Although clearly exposure to virus by direct person-to-person contact results in the initial orolabial, genital, or neonatal infection, less is known about why only a few patients develop HSVE despite the nearly ubiquitous exposure and seroconversion in the general population. A number of mutations have been identified that relate to possible alterations in innate immunity and may be associated with increased susceptibility to HSVE, including *TLR3, TRAF3, UNC98B1, TRIF, TBK1, STAT1,* and *NEMO* [12].

Treatment, future perspective, and conclusions

The current standard of care for herpes simplex virus infections requiring treatment is acyclovir. Acyclovir is a DNA replication inhibitor; the drug, 9-(2-hydroxyethoxymethyl) guanine, had a lower toxicity and better efficacy than previously used drugs and was declared the drug of choice in HSV infection by the Food and Drug Administration in 1998. It can also be used to treat herpes in newborns [41].

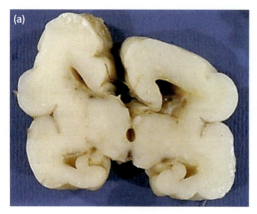
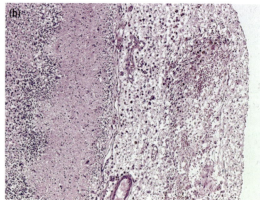
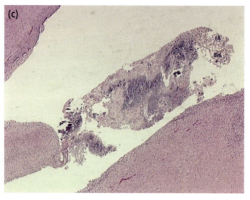

Figure 5.4 Neonatal Herpes simplex virus encephalitis (HSVE). (a) Intrauterine herpes simplex virus 1 (HSV-1) infection. Preterm fetal immature brain showing yellowish discoloration mainly around the ventricular surfaces. (b and c) At microscopy there is necrotizing encephalitis with meningeal and parenchymal infiltration by lymphocytes and macrophages (b) and intraventricular necrotic material with calcification (c) (hematoxylin and eosin [H&E]). Source: Courtesy Professor Homa Adle-Biassette.

The WHO website notes that is it "working to accelerate research to develop new strategies for prevention and control of genital and neonatal HSV-1 and HSV-2 infections. Such research includes the development of HSV vaccines and topical microbicides. Several candidate vaccines and microbicides are currently being studied" [11].

References

1. Whitley, R.J. (1996). Herpesviruses. In: *Medical Microbiology*, 4e (ed. S. Baron), Chapter 68. Galveston (TX): University of Texas Medical Branch at Galveston. https://www.ncbi.nlm.nih.gov/pubmed/21413307.
2. Tso, F.Y., Sawyer, A., and Kwon, E.H. (2017). Kaposi's sarcoma-associated herpesvirus infection of neurons in HIV-positive patients. *J. Infect. Dis.* 215: 1898–1907.
3. Parra, M., Alcala, A., Amoros, C. et al. (2017). Encephalitis associated with human herpesvirus-7 infection in an immunocompetent adult. *Virol. J.* 14: 97.
4. Hogestyn, J.M., Mock, D.J., and Mayer-Proschel, M. (2018). Contributions of neurotropic human herpesviruses herpes simplex virus 1 and human herpesvirus 6 to neurodegenerative disease pathology. *Neural Regen. Res.* 13: 211–221.
5. Roizman, B. and Whitley, R.J. (2001). The nine ages of herpes simplex virus. *Herpes: the journal of the IHMF* 8: 23–27.
6. Commission M (1929). *Epidemic Encephalitis: Etiology, Epidemiology, Treatment; Report of a Survey by the Mathewson Commission*. New York: Columbia university Press.
7. Goodpasture, E.W. (1993). Herpetic infection, with especial reference to involvement of the nervous system. 1929. *Medicine* 72: 125–132.

8. Smith, M.G., Lennette, E.H., and Reames, H.R. (1941). Isolation of the virus of herpes simplex and the demonstration of intranuclear inclusions in a case of acute encephalitis. *Am. J. Pathol.* 17: 55–68.
9. Zarafonetis, C.J. and Smadel, J.E. (1944). Fatal herpes simplex encephalitis in man. *Am. J. Pathol.* 20: 429–445.
10. Steiner, I. and Benninger, F. (2013). Update on herpes virus infections of the nervous system. *Curr. Neurol. Neurosci. Rep.* 13: 414.
11. World Health Organization (WHO). *Herpes simplex virus*. https://www.who.int/news-room/fact-sheets/detail/herpes-simplex-virus (accessed 17 July 2019).
12. Deigendesch, N. and Stenzel, W. (2017). Acute and chronic viral infections. *Handb. Clin. Neurol.* 145: 227–243.
13. Hasbun, R., Rosenthal, N., Balada-Llasat, J.M. et al. (2014). Epidemiology of meningitis and encephalitis in the United States, 2011–2014. *Clin. Infect. Dis.* 65: 359–363.
14. Kaminski, M., Grummel, V., Hoffmann, D. et al. (2017). The spectrum of aseptic central nervous system infections in southern Germany – demographic, clinical and laboratory findings. *Eur. J. Neurol.* 24: 1062–1070.
15. Shukla, B., Aguilera, E.A., Salazar, L. et al. (2017). Aseptic meningitis in adults and children: diagnostic and management challenges. *J. Clin. Virol.* 94: 110–114.
16. Modi, S., Mahajan, A., Dharaiya, D. et al. (2017). Burden of herpes simplex virus encephalitis in the United States. *J. Neurol.* 264: 1204–1208.
17. Jaques, D.A., Bagetakou, S., L'Huillier, A.G. et al. (2016). Herpes simplex encephalitis as a complication of neurosurgical procedures: report of 3 cases and review of the literature. *Virol. J.* 13: 83.
18. Quinnan, G.V. Jr., Masur, H., Rook, A.H. et al. (1984). Herpesvirus infections in the acquired immune deficiency syndrome. *JAMA* 252: 72–77.
19. Skoldenberg, B. (1996). Herpes simplex encephalitis. *Scand. J. Infect. Dis. Suppl.* 100: 8–13.
20. Aurelius, E., Johansson, B., Skoldenberg, B., and Forsgren, M. (1993). Encephalitis in immunocompetent patients due to herpes simplex virus type 1 or 2 as determined by type-specific polymerase chain reaction and antibody assays of cerebrospinal fluid. *J. Med. Virol.* 39: 179–186.
21. Fodor, P.A., Levin, M.J., Weinberg, A. et al. (1998). Atypical herpes simplex virus encephalitis diagnosed by PCR amplification of viral DNA from CSF. *Neurology* 51: 554–559.
22. Bradshaw, M.J. and Venkatesan, A. (2016). Herpes simplex virus-1 encephalitis in adults: pathophysiology, diagnosis and management. *Neurotherapeutics* 13: 493–508.
23. Tyler, K.L. (2004). Herpes simplex virus infections of the central nervous system: encephalitis and meningitis, including Mollaret's. *Herpes* 11 (Suppl 2): 57a–64a.
24. Patoulias, D., Gavriiloglou, G., Kontotasios, K. et al. (2017). HSV-1 encephalitis: high index of clinical suspicion, prompt diagnosis, and early therapeutic intervention are the triptych of success-report of two cases and comprehensive review of the literature. *Case Rep. Med.* 2017: 5320839.
25. Cooper, J., Kierans, C., Defres, S. et al. (2017). Care beyond the hospital ward: understanding the sociomedical trajectory of herpes simplex virus encephalitis. *BMC Health Serv. Res.* 17: 646.
26. Esiri, M.M. (1982). Herpes simplex encephalitis. An immunohistological study of the distribution of viral antigen within the brain. *J. Neurol. Sci.* 54: 209–226.
27. Nicoll, J.A., Maitland, N.J., and Love, S. (1991). Autopsy neuropathological findings in "burnt out" herpes simplex encephalitis and use of the polymerase chain reaction to direct viral DNA. *Neuropathol. Appl. Neurobiol.* 17: 375–382.
28. Hoftberger, R., Armangue, T., Leypoldt, F. et al. (2013). Clinical neuropathology practice guide 4-2013: post-herpes simplex encephalitis: N-methyl-D-aspartate receptor antibodies are part of the problem. *Clin. Neuropathol.* 32: 251–254.
29. Galli, J., Clardy, S.L., and Piquet, A.L. (2017). NMDAR encephalitis following herpes simplex virus encephalitis. *Curr. Infect. Dis. Rep.* 19: 1.
30. Chretien, F., Belec, L., Hilton, D.A. et al. (1996). Herpes simplex virus type 1 encephalitis in acquired immunodeficiency syndrome. *Neuropathol. Appl. Neurobiol.* 22: 394–404.
31. Schiff, D. and Rosenblum, M.K. (1998). Herpes simplex encephalitis (HSE) and the immunocompromised: a clinical and autopsy study of HSE in the settings of cancer and human immunodeficiency virus-type 1 infection. *Hum. Pathol.* 29: 215–222.
32. Love, S., Koch, P., Urbach, H., and Dawson, T.P. (2004). Chronic granulomatous herpes simplex encephalitis in children. *J. Neuropathol. Exp. Neurol.* 63: 1173–1181.
33. Hackney, J.R., Harrison, D.K., Rozzelle, C. et al. (2012). Chronic granulomatous herpes encephalitis in a child with clinically intractable epilepsy. *Case Rep. Pediatr.* 2012: 849812.
34. Schutz, P.W., Fauth, C.T., Al-Rawahi, G.N. et al. (2014). Granulomatous herpes simplex encephalitis in an infant with multicystic encephalopathy: a distinct clinicopathologic entity? *Pediatr. Neurol.* 50: 392–396.

35. Britton, C.B., Mesa-Tejada, R., Fenoglio, C.M. et al. (1985). A new complication of AIDS: thoracic myelitis caused by herpes simplex virus. *Neurology* 35: 1071–1074.
36. Picard, F.J., Dekaban, G.A., Silva, J., and Rice, G.P.A. (1993). Mollaret's meningitis associated with herpes simplex type 2 infection. *Neurology* 43: 1722–1727.
37. Kidokoro, H., de Vries, L.S., Ogawa, C. et al. (2017). Predominant area of brain lesions in neonates with herpes simplex encephalitis. *J. Perinatol.* 37: 1210–1214.
38. Corey, L., Whitley, R.J., Stone, E.F., and Mohan, K. (1988). Difference between herpes simplex virus type 1 and type 2 neonatal encephalitis in neurological outcome. *Lancet* 1: 1–4.
39. Bajaj, M., Mody, S., and Natarajan, G. (2014). Clinical and neuroimaging findings in neonatal herpes simplex virus infection. *J. Pediatr.* 165: 404–407.
40. Kimberlain, D.W. and Whitley, R.J. (2005). Neonatal herpes: what we have learnt. *Semin. Pediatr. Infect. Dis.* 16: 7–16.
41. Mandal, A. (2019). Herpes simplex history. https://www.news-medical.net/health/Herpes-Simplex-History.aspx (accessed 10 October 2018).

6

Varicella-Zoster Virus and Epstein-Barr Virus Infections of the CNS

Catherine (Katy) Keohane[1] and Françoise Gray[2,3]

[1] Department of Pathology and School of Medicine, University College Cork, Brookfield Health Science Complex, Cork, Ireland
[2] Retired from Department of Pathology, Lariboisière Hospital, APHP, Paris, France
[3] University Paris Diderot (Paris 7), Paris, France

Abbreviations

ADEM	acute demyelinating encephalomyelitis
AIDS	acquired immune deficiency syndrome (AIDS)
CMV	cytomegalovirus
CNS	central nervous system
CSF	cerebrospinal fluid
CVS	congenital varicella syndrome
DRG	dorsal root ganglion/ganglia
EBER	EBV-encoded small RNA
EBV	Epstein-Barr virus
HAART	highly active antiretroviral treatment
HHV	human herpes virus
HIV	human immunodeficiency virus
HSV	herpes simplex virus
HZ	herpes zoster
IM	infectious mononucleosis
PCR	polymerase chain reaction
PHN	postherpetic neuralgia
VZV	varicella-zoster virus

Definition

Herpesviruses are large, enveloped, spherical viruses, ranging from 120 to more than 200 nm in diameter. They have a unique four-layered structure: a core containing the large, double-stranded DNA genome is enclosed by an icosapentahedral capsid composed of capsomeres. The capsid is surrounded by an amorphous protein coat called the "tegument." It is encased in a glycoprotein-bearing lipid bilayer envelope [1].

The family Herpesviridae is divided into three subfamilies. Although there are more than 100 known herpesviruses, only 8 are pathogenic to humans and 5 cause pathologically proven productive CNS infections.

The α-herpesviridae are characterized by an extremely short reproductive cycle, rapid destruction of the host cell, and the ability to replicate in a wide variety of host tissues. They characteristically

Infections of the Central Nervous System: Pathology and Genetics, First Edition. Edited by Fabrice Chrétien, Kum Thong Wong, Leroy R. Sharer, Catherine (Katy) Keohane and Françoise Gray.
© 2020 John Wiley & Sons Ltd. Published 2020 by John Wiley & Sons Ltd.

establish latent infection in sensory nerve ganglia. They include:

HSV-1: Herpes simplex virus 1/human herpesvirus 1

HSV-2: Herpes simplex virus 2/human herpesvirus 2

VZV: Varicella-zoster virus/human herpesvirus 3

β-herpesviridae have a long reproductive cycle and restricted host range; they include:

CMV: Cytomegalovirus/human herpes virus 5

HHV-6: Human herpesvirus 6

HHV-7: Human herpesvirus 7

γ-herpesviridae have a very restricted host range and include:

EBV: Epstein–Barr virus/human herpesvirus 4

HHV-8: Human herpesvirus 8

This chapter will describe infections of the CNS by VZV and EBV. HSV-1 and HSV-2 infections are described in Chapter 5 and CMV infection in Chapter 7, respectively.

Infection of the CNS by varicella-zoster virus

Definition, major synonyms, and microbiological characteristics

Varicella-zoster virus (VZV), or human herpes virus 3, produces two distinct cutaneous exanthematous diseases: chickenpox (varicella) and shingles (zoster). The name "varicella" is a diminutive of "variola" (smallpox) because the distribution of both rashes is similar. Unlike smallpox, the course of chickenpox is benign. Zoster derives from the Greek for "girdle," named because of the dermatomal distribution of the rash.

The microbiological characteristics of VZV are highly similar to those of HSV-1 and HSV-2 (see Chapter 5).

Epidemiology

VZV is a ubiquitous, highly infectious, neurotropic, and exclusively human α-herpesvirus. Primary infection leads to acute varicella or "chickenpox," usually from exposure either through direct contact with a skin lesion or via airborne spread from respiratory droplets. After initial infection, VZV establishes lifelong latency in neurons of cranial nerve ganglia, dorsal root ganglia (DRG), and autonomic ganglia along the entire neuroaxis. The infection can reactivate years to decades later as herpes zoster (HZ) or "shingles" [1].

VZV is highly contagious. More than 90% of adults acquire the disease in childhood and become latently infected. In many countries, the majority of children and young adults have been vaccinated. Attenuated VZV in varicella vaccine also becomes latent after childhood vaccination [2].

Primary varicella typically presents with fever, malaise and a vesicular, pruritic, disseminated rash mainly involving the trunk and face. Symptoms usually resolve within 7–10 days. In rare cases, primary varicella leads to more severe disease with visceral invasion. The CNS is involved in about 1 of 1000 cases [3]. Adults and very young children are more likely to develop these complications, which may be life-threatening. Rates of hospitalization and mortality resulting from varicella have dropped since the introduction of routine childhood varicella vaccination [2].

HZ is the result of reactivation of latent ganglionic VZV infection. Nearly all patients with HZ develop vesicular skin lesions in a dermatomal distribution, accompanied by pain, which usually resolves over months but may persist for years (postherpetic neuralgia [PHN]). HZ cannot be transmitted from one individual to another, but spread of the virus from HZ vesicles may lead to the development of varicella in a susceptible host.

The overall annual incidence of HZ in the general population is 1.5–3.0 cases per 1000 persons and is estimated to occur in up to 20% of individuals during their lifetimes. HZ most often affects persons who are older, in whom the annual incidence exceeds 1% [4].

In the United States, ~8% of zoster episodes occur in patients who are immunocompromised [5]. In patients with acquired immunodeficiency syndrome (AIDS), the risk of zoster varies with the stage of human immunodeficiency virus (HIV) infection and treatment, but rates are typically increased many-fold, and episodes can be recurrent and protracted. In the regions most affected by the HIV/AIDS pandemic, zoster in young adults is often a marker of HIV infection.

Clinical features of the neurological complications of VZV infection

Neurological complications of primary infection are uncommon; the most frequent is transient acute cerebellar ataxia [6]. Rarer complications include aseptic meningitis, transverse or ascending myelitis, Guillain-Barré syndrome, CNS vasculitis, and postinfectious acute disseminated encephalomyelitis (see Chapter 26). These complications are generally more common and severe in adults and persons who are immunocompromised [3].

In addition to neuralgia, reactivation of VZV can cause rarer acute neurological complications, including ophthalmic zoster, Ramsay Hunt syndrome, meningoencephalitis, and myelitis.

Since the 1990s, the spectrum of VZV-related CNS disease is recognized as wider than previously thought, particularly in patients with AIDS. Clinicopathological features include leukoencephalitis, ventriculitis, acute meningomyeloradiculitis, or cerebral infarcts [7]. The diagnosis may be difficult when there is no history of HZ rash or if the skin manifestation is remote from the time of neurological signs. Clinical and radiological signs are often nonspecific or misleading. Isolation of the virus or polymerase chain reaction (PCR)-based detection of VZV DNA in the cerebrospinal fluid (CSF) enables early diagnosis and immediate treatment with acyclovir.

Neuropathology

The pathological changes in zoster infection are usually limited to the DRG or to ganglia of a sensory cranial nerve and the nerve root. Changes may extend to the corresponding segment of the spinal cord, with intense lymphocytic inflammation sometimes associated with vasculitis and necrosis. Viral antigen and DNA can be identified in nerve cells, glial cells, Schwann cells, and blood vessels [8].

Most pathological reports of CNS infection by VZV are in patients with AIDS. Several patterns of VZV encephalitis and myeloradiculitis have been described, and all may occur in the same patient:

Bulbar encephalitis or transverse myelitis is the result of viral spread from the trigeminal or corresponding DRG, respectively, and is usually associated with a dermatomal zoster rash. The lesions are usually necrotizing and occasionally hemorrhagic.

Multifocal leukoencephalitis [7, 9] is characterized by multiple well-demarcated, often confluent, round or oval lesions scattered throughout the white matter with a predilection for the gray and white junctions and periventricular regions (Figure 6.1a). Microscopically they have a characteristic targetlike pattern with central necrosis surrounded by a well-demarcated zone of myelin pallor (Figure 6.1b). In recent lesions, the central area shows coagulative necrosis; older lesions are cystic and contain numerous lipid-laden macrophages and residual blood vessels. The peripheral zone shows edema, incomplete necrosis with a few residual myelinated fibers, capillary endothelial swelling, reactive astrocytosis, and microglial proliferation. Inflammation is mild or absent. Cowdry type A eosinophilic inclusion bodies, immunopositive for VZV, are numerous in the peripheral zone and adjacent unaffected parenchyma and can involve all cell types: neurons, glia, endothelial cells, and macrophages (Figure 6.1c and d).

Ventriculitis [10] may be acute or chronic with complete necrosis of the ventricular wall (Figure 6.2a) and marked vasculitis. In developing lesions, the ependymal lining appears irregular and foci of VZV-infected cells protrude into the ventricular lumen (Figure 6.2b).

Leptomeningeal vasculitis or vasculopathy [7] is often associated with meningitis and produces hemorrhagic infarcts in the brain or spinal cord. Various vascular lesions may be observed sometimes in the same brain: acute necrotizing arteritis, granulomatous vasculitis or severe non-inflammatory vasculopathy with marked intimal proliferation, severe stenosis, and occasional focal thrombosis.

Spinal cord involvement may take the form of an extensive hemorrhagic meningomyeloradiculitis with vasculitis (Figure 6.2c) [10].

VZV-related CNS lesions are rare in patients who are immunocompetent, but the two main patterns are bulbar encephalitis or transverse myelitis, with a usually granulomatous vasculitis involving large basal and parenchymal arteries, very similar to primary angiitis of the CNS [3].

Infections of the Central Nervous System

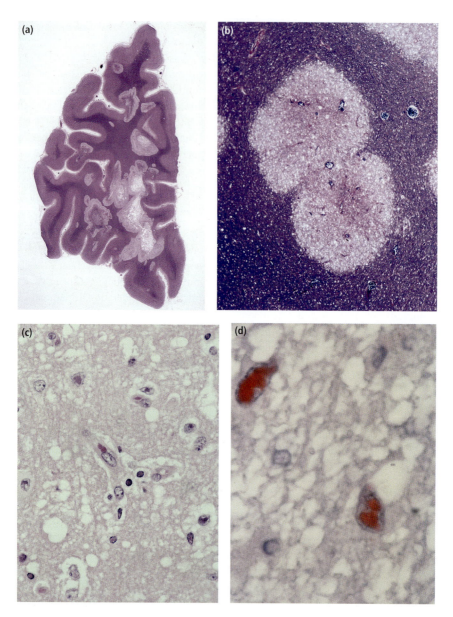

Figure 6.1 Varicella-zoster virus (VZV). Multifocal leukoencephalitis in a patient with acquired immune deficiency syndrome (AIDS). (a) Coronal section of the left frontal lobe. Confluent necrotic foci in the white matter more marked at the cortico-subcortical junction (hematoxylin and eosin [H&E]). (b) Targetlike lesions with central coagulative necrosis surrounded by a well-demarcated zone of myelin pallor (Hematoxylin phloxin-Luxol). (c) In the peripheral edematous zone, numerous cells (i.e. neurons, glia, and endothelial cells) are positively immunostained for VZV. (d) At higher magnification, Cowdry type A intranuclear bodies in astrocytes are positively immunostained for VZV.

In patients with AIDS, acyclovir combined with recovery of immune function due to highly active antiretroviral treatment (HAART) may result in "burnt-out" lesions [11]. These are centrally necrotic, containing foamy macrophages but lack the inflammation, acute astrocytic reaction, viral inclusions, and antigen that are present in active disease (Figure 6.3).

Varicella-Zoster Virus and Epstein-Barr Virus Infections of the CNS Chapter 6

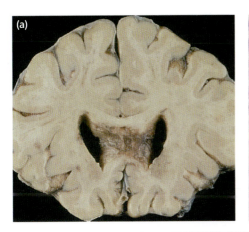
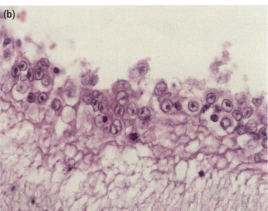
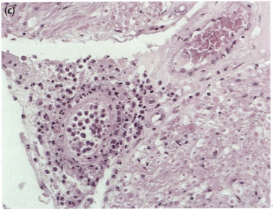

Figure 6.2 Varicella-zoster virus (VZV) ventriculitis and acute meningomyeloradiculitis with vasculitis in a patient with acquired immune deficiency syndrome (AIDS). (a) Coronal section at the level of the genu of corpus callosum. The lining of the lateral ventricles is replaced by an irregular layer of brown necrotic tissue. Source: Courtesy Professor F. Scaravilli. (b) In a more recent case, the ependymal lining appears irregular with foci of VZV-infected cells containing Cowdry type A intranuclear inclusion bodies, protruding into the ventricular lumen (hematoxylin and eosin [H&E]). (c) Acute meningomyeloradiculitis vasculitis in a spinal root with transmural infiltration of the vessel wall by inflammatory cells (H&E).

Pathogenesis

Pathological reports of neurological complications of primary VZV infection are lacking. Because many of the complications may be linked with other mechanisms, it is questionable whether direct CNS infection by the virus plays a role in their genesis.

In contrast, following viral reactivation, productive VZV infection has been demonstrated within all the types of pathology described. These different types likely reflect the various routes of viral spread to the brain or spinal cord from latent ganglionic infection [8].

In focal encephalitis or myelitis, neuropathological findings suggest centripetal neural spread to the brain or spinal cord from VZV trigeminal or spinal ganglionic infection.

In multifocal leukoencephalitis, disseminated lesions (predominantly at the gray and white junctions) are more consistent with hematogenous spread to the brain following viremia.

Periventricular involvement (isolated or in multifocal leukoencephalitis) may also result from hematogenous spread because there are no tight junctions between endothelial cells in the periventricular microvasculature [8].

Infections of the Central Nervous System

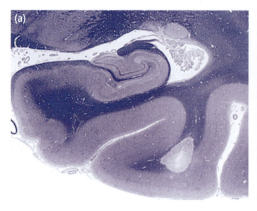 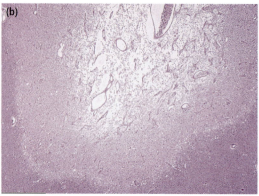

Figure 6.3 "Burnt-out" varicella-zoster virus (VZV) encephalitis in a patient with acquired immune deficiency syndrome (AIDS) treated by high doses of acyclovir and highly active antiretroviral treatment (HAART). (a) Coronal section of the right hemisphere at the level of Ammon's horn. A necrotic subcortical lesion is present in the temporal lobe (Luxol fast blue/cresyl violet). (b) The lesion has a targetoid appearance of VZV leukoencephalitis, the central region consists of loosely arranged blood vessels and scattered macrophages (hematoxylin and eosin [H&E]).

Focal necrotizing vasculitis adjacent to VZV ganglionitis may indicate local spread of infection. However, disseminated necrotizing vasculitis remote from the zoster focus strongly suggests hematogenous spread of infection [8]. Another possibility is seeding of CSF by infected ependymal cells [10] (also suggested for other hemorrhagic meningomyeloradiculitis cases such as CMV-associated with vasculitis and necrotizing ventriculitis [12]).

Neonatal varicella

Etiology

Varicella in pregnancy is unusual because most women of childbearing age are immune. The consequences of varicella infection in utero depend on the stage of gestation. If maternal varicella is acquired during the first two trimesters, the fetus is at risk for congenital varicella syndrome (CVS) with an incidence of <1% [13]. VZV PCR has a poor positive predictive value for fetal disease or disease severity.

Clinical features

CVS is characterized by skin scars, intrauterine growth restriction, seizures, mental retardation, ocular symptoms (i.e. microphthalmia, chorioretinitis, cataracts, Horner syndrome, ptosis, and nystagmus), limb abnormalities (i.e. hypoplasia of bones and muscle, absent digits, talipes), and dysfunction of the autonomic nervous system. The skin scars are usually on the abnormal limb. Affected fetuses are often growth restricted and born prematurely. The prognosis is generally poor. Infant mortality is high, resulting from intractable gastroesophageal reflux, recurrent aspiration pneumonia, and respiratory failure [14].

Pathology

Neuropathological reports are few and mostly old. Necrotic lesions and scars may be seen on gross examination of the cerebral hemispheres; there may be ventricular dilatation or polymicrogyria. The meninges and brain parenchyma show a diffuse chronic inflammatory infiltrate with granulation tissue, microglial nodules, necrosis, and gliosis. There is neuronal loss in spinal cord anterior horns and DRG, and the posterior and lateral columns are shrunken and gliotic [15]. Muscles in affected limbs show denervation atrophy.

Pathogenesis

VZV is a neurotropic virus. Many of the CVS defects are regarded as a direct result of infection in neural cells of the spinal cord and ganglia, with destruction of the plexi during embryogenesis, leading to denervation of the limb bud and subsequent hypoplasia [13]. The cutaneous defects are also likely to reflect VZV infection of sensory nerves.

Treatment and future perspective

Acyclovir is the treatment for VZV infections. It has revolutionized VZV CNS infection and has proved effective even in protracted disease. In some patients positive for HIV, acyclovir-resistant VZV strains have emerged; these can be treated by foscarnet.

Both varicella-zoster immune globulin and acyclovir have been given to mothers with varicella during pregnancy; their efficacy in preventing CVS is unknown, whereas varicella-zoster immune globulin improves the prognosis of perinatal varicella.

Live attenuated VZV vaccines used to prevent varicella and HZ have proven safe and effective for both diseases.

A more concentrated live attenuated vaccine against zoster has been introduced in some countries for individuals who are older and immunocompetent. In trials, this vaccine halved zoster incidence and reduced PHN by two-thirds, but it lacks lifelong protection, and its efficacy is poor in older individuals. It is contraindicated in immunosuppressed groups. A new subunit vaccine (HZ/su) shows extremely high vaccine efficacy (around 90% against zoster and PHN) [16].

Because live vaccines have the potential to reactivate and cause clinical disease, newer inactivated vaccines are being developed.

Infection of the CNS by Epstein–Barr virus

Definition, epidemiology, microbiological characteristics, and genetics

EBV, also called human herpesvirus 4, is a lymphotropic, γ-herpes virus, first identified in lymphoblasts from Burkitt lymphoma [17]. Later, it was recognized to be highly prevalent worldwide. Epidemiological studies indicate more than 90% of the world's population is seropositive for EBV [18]. Primary infection may be associated with the development of infectious mononucleosis (IM) and a combination of latent or low-level productive infection probably causes or contributes to a wide range of lymphocytic, epithelial, and soft-tissue tumors, including primary cerebral lymphomas [3]. EBV has also been associated with diverse non-neoplastic neurological diseases such as Guillain-Barré syndrome or multiple sclerosis, but pathological data are limited.

There is wide geographical variation in the incidence of these complications, perhaps partly because of variations in the EBV genome [18]. The two main genotypes, type 1 and type 2, are distinguished by differences in *EBNA-2* gene, with only 54% homology between them. Types 1 and 2 can be further subdivided into different virus strains. Most genetic variability investigations were based on studying the *LMP-1* oncogene because it has a greater degree of polymorphism than most other EBV genes [19].

EBV is transmitted by intimate contact, particularly via saliva exchange. The virus is usually acquired during childhood or adolescence. Similar to other herpesviruses, following a primary infection, EBV has a latent phase where it infects epithelial cells in oropharyngeal epithelium and salivary glands, then enters circulating B lymphocytes, and persists for life in a latent state in resting memory B cells.

Clinical features

Typically, the primary infection is asymptomatic and occurs during childhood. However, the infection can cause IM, particularly in adults. The predominant findings are fever, debilitating fatigue, pharyngitis, lymphadenopathy, and hepatosplenomegaly. Blood examination reveals lymphocytosis and later, enlarged atypical lymphocytes. Diagnosis is usually made by specific antibody tests. In some cases, EBV DNA has to be identified using Southern blotting, PCR, or in situ hybridization.

Headache is frequent in IM and may be associated with neck stiffness and CSF pleocytosis. EBV DNA and specific antibodies are present in CSF during the acute illness. Rarer complications include polyradiculopathy, transverse myelitis, optic neuritis, and encephalitis. In some cases, the encephalitis probably corresponds to acute demyelinating encephalomyelitis (ADEM). Criteria for the diagnosis of neurological disease associated with primary EBV infection include: lymphocytic

Infections of the Central Nervous System

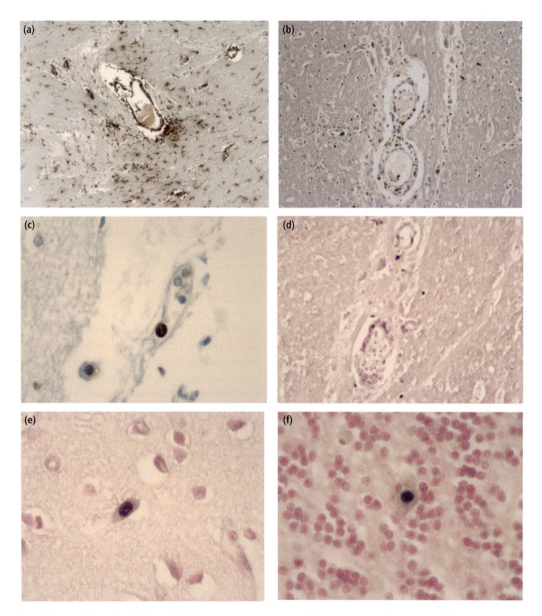

Figure 6.4 Epstein-Barr virus (EBV) encephalitis in an immunocompetent patient. This 48-year-old man was admitted for persistent fever complicated by severe hypotension. He had lymphadenopathy and splenomegaly; there was no overt immunosuppression. EBV DNA was positive. He died rapidly from severe hypoxia associated with acute respiratory distress syndrome. Histology showed that almost all organs, particularly lymph nodes, lungs, spleen, liver, brain, and heart were infiltrated by large atypical lymphoid cells suggestive of infectious mononucleosis (IM). In the brain, the cellular infiltrate was less dense and predominantly involved the leptomeninges and perivascular spaces. They were more marked at the base of the brain and extended into the perineural spaces. Encephalitic changes were restricted to the brainstem and cerebellum. (a) Pons: microglial activation with rod cells more marked in the perivascular region (CD68 immunostaining). (b) Pons: perivascular lymphocyte cuffing with atypical large lymphoid cells within a dilated blood vessel and in the perivascular space (CD79 immunostaining). (c) Brainstem leptomeninges. A large atypical lymphoid cell is present in the lumen of a blood vessel (CD79 immunostaining). (d) Pons same level as Figure 6.4a. Large lymphoid cells are EBV-encoded small RNA (EBER) + (in situ hybridization for EBER). (e, f) EBER+ nerve cells within the pons (e) and the granule cells of the cerebellum (f) (in situ hybridization for EBER).

and monocytic inflammation both in blood and CSF, elevated viral load in serum and CSF, and positive PCR in CSF [20].

A variety of neurological complications from meningitis to hemorrhagic encephalitis have been associated with EBV reactivation and its presence in CSF [3]. These occur mostly (but not exclusively) in immunosuppression.

Neuropathology

There are few neuropathological studies [21–25]. Most cases report mild nonspecific changes, including cerebral or cerebellar edema, sparse petechial hemorrhages in the spinal cord and cerebrum, and mild meningeal and nerve root inflammation [3]. However fatal acute hemorrhagic encephalitis [22] or encephalopathy is also described, particularly in children [21, 24, 25]. We have seen EBV brainstem and cerebellum encephalitis in a patient who was immunocompetent with fatal EBV reactivation (Figure 6.4). There was focal microglial activation (Figure 6.4a) and lymphocytic infiltration of blood vessel walls and parenchyma with frequent atypical lymphoid cells suggestive of IM (Figures 6.4b and c). Lymphocytes, occasional nerve cells, and glial cells were positively labeled by in situ hybridization for EBV-encoded small RNA (EBER) (Figures 6.4d–f).

Treatment

Most cases of EBV-related encephalopathy or encephalitis have been treated with a combination of antiviral agents such as acyclovir, ganciclovir, or foscarnet sometimes in association with corticosteroids and management of raised intracranial pressure or hydrocephalus [25, 26].

References

1. Gilden, D.H., Kleinschmidt-DeMasters, B.K., LaGuardia, J.J. et al. (2000). Neurologic complications of the reactivation of varicella-zoster virus. *N. Engl. J. Med.* 342: 635–645.
2. Pahud, B.A., Glaser, C.A., Dekker, C.L. et al. (2011). Varicella zoster disease of the central nervous system: epidemiological clinical and laboratory features 10 years after the introduction of the varicella vaccine. *J. Infect. Dis.* 203: 316–323.
3. Love, S., Wiley, C.A., and Lucas, S. (2015). Viral infection. In: *Greenfield's Neuropathology*, 9e (eds. S. Love, H. Budka, J.W. Ironside and A. Perry), 1087–1191. CRC Press.
4. Whitley, R.J. (1996). Herpesviruses. In: *Medical Microbiology*, 4e (ed. S. Baron), Chapter 68. Galveston (TX): University of Texas Medical Branch at Galveston. https://www.ncbi.nlm.nih.gov/pubmed/21413307.
5. Yawn, B.P., Saddier, P., Wollan, P.C. et al. (2007). A population-based study of the incidence and complication rates of herpes zoster before zoster vaccine introduction. *Mayo Clin. Proc.* 82: 1341–1349.
6. Connolly, A.M., Dodson, W.E., Prensky, A.L., and Rust, R.S. (1994). Course and outcome of acute cerebellar ataxia. *Ann. Neurol.* 35: 673–679.
7. Gray, F., Belec, L., Lescs, M.C. et al. (1994). Varicella zoster infection of the central nervous system in acquired immune deficiency syndrome. *Brain* 117: 987–999.
8. Schmidbauer, M., Budka, H., Pilz, P. et al. (1992). Presence, distribution and spread of productive varicella zoster virus infection in nervous tissues. *Brain* 115: 383–398.
9. Gray, F., Mohr, M., Rozenberg, F. et al. (1992). Varicella-zoster virus encephalitis in acquired immunodeficiency syndrome: report of four cases. *Neuropathol. Appl. Neurobiol.* 18: 502–514.
10. Chrétien, F., Gray, F., Lescs, M.C. et al. (1993). Acute varicella-zoster virus ventriculitis and meningo-myelo-radiculitis in acquired immunodeficiency syndrome. *Acta Neuropathol.* 86: 659–665.
11. Lorin de la Grandmaison, G., Carlier, R., Chrétien, F. et al. (2005). "Burnt out" varicella-zoster-virus encephalitis in an AIDS patient following treatment by highly active antiretroviral therapy. *Clin. Radiol.* 60: 613–617.
12. Mahieux, F., Gray, F., Fénelon, G. et al. (1989). Acute myeloradiculitis due to cytomegalovirus as the initial manifestation of AIDS. *J. Neurol. Neurosurg. Psychiatry* 52: 270–274.
13. Smith, C.K. and Arvin, A.M. (2009). Varicella in the fetus and newborn. *Semin. Fetal Neonatal Med.* 14: 209–217.
14. Gershon, A. (2001). Chickenpox, measles and mumps. In: *Infectious Diseases of the Fetus and Newborn Infant*, 5e (eds. J. Remington and J. Klein), 683–732. Philadelphia: WB Saunders.
15. Harding, B. and Baumer, J. (1976). Congenital varicella-zoster. A serologically proven case with necrotizing encephalitis and malformation. *Acta Neuropathol.* 76: 311–315.
16. Warren-Gash, C., Forbes, H., and Breuer, J. (2017). Varicella and herpes zoster vaccine development: lessons learned. *Expert Rev. Vaccines* 16: 1191–1201.

17. Epstein, M.A., Achong, B.G., and Barr, Y.M. (1964). Virus particles in in cultured lymphoblasts from Burkitt's lymphoma. *Lancet* 1: 702–703.
18. Tzellos, S. and Farrell, P.J. (2012). Epstein-Barr virus sequence variation-biology and disease. *Pathogens* 1: 156–174.
19. Smatti, M.K., Al-Sadeq, D.W., and Ali, N.H. (2018). Epstein–Barr virus epidemiology, serology, and genetic variability of LMP-1 oncogene among healthy population: an update. *Front. Oncol.* 8: 211.
20. Bathoorn, E., Vlaminckx, B.J., Schoondermark-Stolk, S. et al. (2011). Primary Epstein-Barr virus infection with neurological complications. *Scand. J. Infect. Dis.* 43: 136–144.
21. Sworn, M. and Urich, H. (1970). Acute encephalitis in infectious mononucleosis. *J. Pathol.* 100: 201–205.
22. Francisci, D., Sensini, A., Fratini, D. et al. (2004). Acute fatal necrotizing encephalitis caused by Epstein-Barr in a young adult immunocompetent man. *J. Neurovirol.* 10: 414–417.
23. Ringelstein, E.B., Sobczak, H., Pfeifer, B. et al. (1984). Polyradiculomeningoencephalitis caused by Epstein-Barr virus infection: description of a case with fatal outcome. *Fortschr. Neurol. Psychiatr.* 52: 73–82.
24. Roulet Perez, E., Maeder, P., Cotting, J. et al. (1993). Acute fatal parainfectious cerebellar swelling in two children: a rare or overlooked situation? *Neuropediatrics* 24 (6): 346–351.
25. Biebl, A., Webersinke, C., Traxler, B. et al. (2009). Fatal Epstein-Barr virus infection in a 12-year-old child: an underappreciated neurological complication? *Nat. Clin. Pract. Neurol.* 5: 171–174.
26. Rafailidis, P.I., Mavros, M.N., Kapaskelis, A. et al. (2010). Antiviral treatment for severe EBV infections in apparently immunocompetent patients. *J. Clin. Virol.* 49 (3): 151–157.

7 Cytomegalovirus Infections of the CNS

Homa Adle-Biassette[1,2] and Natacha Teissier[2,3]

[1] Department of Pathology, Lariboisière Hospital, APHP, Paris, France
[2] Paris University, NeuroDiderot, INSERM F-75019, Paris, France
[3] Department of Pediatric Otolaryngology, Robert Debre Hospital, APHP, Paris, France

Abbreviations

AIDS	acquired immunodeficiency syndrome
CID	cytomegalic inclusion disease
CMV	cytomegalovirus
CNS	central nervous system
CSF	cerebrospinal fluid
ELISA	enzyme-linked immunosorbent assay
HAART	highly active antiretroviral treatments
HHV-5	herpesvirus-5
HIV	human immunodeficiency virus
MCMV	murine cytomegalovirus
MGN	microglial nodules
MIE	major IE genes
MRI	magnetic resonance imaging
PML	progressive multifocal leukoencephalopathy
TORCH	Toxoplasmosis, Other agents, Rubella, Cytomegalovirus, and Herpes simplex
US	ultrasound

Definition of the disorder, major synonyms, and historical perspective

Human cytomegalovirus (CMV) or herpesvirus-5 (HHV-5) is a double-stranded DNA virus and is a member of Herpesviridae family and Betaherpesvirinae subfamily.

The disease was formerly known as cytomegalic inclusion disease (CID).

The first description in 1881 (in a stillborn infant) is attributed to Joseph Ribbert, a German pathologist [1]. The term "cytomegalia" was coined by Goodpasture and Talbot in 1921, who described cytoplasmic and intranuclear inclusions in a 2-month-old infant, attributed to a filtrable virus [2]. The virus was later isolated from mouse and human salivary gland in tissue cell cultures [3] and from human skin tissue cultures of a microcephalic infant with an illness resembling CID [4]. With the development of antibody tests, antibodies to CMV could be found in "normal" infants, but significantly higher levels were found in infants who were microcephalic.

Epidemiology: incidence and prevalence, sex, age, geographical distribution, and risk factors

CMV infection is ubiquitous; its seroprevalence depends on socioeconomic and ethnic factors and is close to 100% in emerging countries. Prevalence increases with age: 40% of children acquire the infection in the first decade, whereas more than 80% of patients older than 60 are seropositive. In children, CMV infection is more frequent in low-birth-weight and premature babies [5].

Transmission of CMV can occur (i) by direct contact with infectious body fluids (e.g. urine, saliva, tears); (ii) by maternal genital secretions during delivery, or through breast milk; (iii) sexually; or (iv) via organ transplantation and blood transfusion. CMV can be secreted in body fluids of young children for months. Infection can occur as a primary infection, reinfection, or reactivation of latent virus. Once a person becomes infected, the virus establishes lifelong latency with limited viral gene expression; it may reactivate intermittently [6, 7] in patients who become immunocompromised and is then associated with increased morbidity and mortality. Patients at high risk for serious complications from CMV infection are [8]:
- Fetuses, very-low-birth-weight and premature infants for congenital and perinatal CMV infection,
- People with compromised immune systems (organ and bone marrow transplant and AIDS]- with CD4 count <100) for childhood and adult CMV infection.

Autopsy findings in patients with AIDS before and after the introduction of highly active antiretroviral treatment (HAART) showed that the incidence of systemic CMV infection decreased from 37 to 22%, and that of CMV infection of the CNS from 20 to 11% [9].

Congenital CMV infection involves 0.5–1% of all live births. One-third of mothers with primary CMV infection will infect their baby transplacentally; 10% of their babies will be symptomatic at birth [10]. Maternal age influences the risk of materno-fetal infection, as does contact with toddlers. Young mothers with children in childcare facilities are at high risk of infection because congenitally infected children can shed CMV in saliva and urine for two to four years.

Materno-fetal transmission correlates with viral titers and inversely correlates with antibody titers, especially with neutralizing immunoglobulin G (IgG) of great avidity (see section on Laboratory Tests). CMV binds to IgG for transplacental passage by transcytosis [11]. With high-avidity IgG, the complex is recognized by chorionic villi macrophages, leading to viral destruction. However, with low-avidity IgG, the complex escapes lymphocyte recognition, facilitating fetal infection. Materno-fetal transmission may increase in the presence of a coexisting bacterial or viral infection [12]. In children born to mothers with human immunodeficiency virus (HIV)symptomatic CMV infection occurs in 23.1% of newborns infected with human immunodeficiency virus 1 (HIV-1)compared to 6.7% in neonates uninfected with HIV-1 [13].

Several other factors influence the outcome in congenital CMV infection. The risk of fetal transmission correlates inversely with gestational age [14]. If the infection happens in the six months preceding conception, materno-fetal transmission is still possible but less frequent. The consequences of a primary or a recurrent infection during pregnancy are not the same on the fetus. In primary infection, materno-fetal transmission is estimated at 30–50%, and there is a high risk of embryofetopathy and fetal growth restriction. Even if preconception immunity is present, it is not completely protective: the mother can demonstrate viral reactivation or be reinfected with another CMV serotype, and transplacental infection can still occur leading to embryofetopathy [15].

Microbiological characteristics

The four major components of beta-herpesviruses are the core, the capsid, the tegument, and the envelope. The tegument contains two essential complexes for viral entry (i.e. glycoprotein B and gH–gL dimer) [8] and the majority of virion-associated proteins for disassembly and assembly of the virions during entry and egress, and for regulating the host immune response, such as the lower matrix phosphoprotein of 65 kDa or pp65 (the most abundant tegument protein), and the upper matrix protein (or pp71) [16].

Like other herpesviruses, during productive infection, CMV expresses genes in a temporally controlled cascade, designated immediate-early (IE), early, and late. The major IE genes (MIE) *UL123* and *UL122* (IE1/IE2) play a critical role in subsequent viral gene expression and the efficiency of viral replication. Suppression of IE proteins is thought to contribute to CMV latency, whereas the expression of IE genes is associated with reactivation. Viral IE proteins modulate the host cell environment and stimulate the expression of viral early genes. Viral early genes encode proteins necessary for viral DNA replication. After DNA replication, delayed early and viral late genes are expressed; these encode structural proteins for the virion and permit the assembly and egress of newly formed progeny viral particles. Synthesis of the viral genome occurs in the host cell nucleus.

CMV latency is not a totally quiescent state but is characterized by limited viral gene expression. During latency, *miR-UL112-1* promotes the downregulation of lytic *IE-gene* expression to prevent T-cell recognition of latently infected cells [6].

Clinical features including appropriate investigations

Clinical manifestations
Children and adults
In healthy individuals with a normal immune system, primary infection may be asymptomatic or present as a mononucleosis-like syndrome with symptoms including prolonged fever, rash, headache, myalgia, malaise, and sore throat. Atypical lymphocytosis and jaundice may develop in some patients. Latent infection is usually asymptomatic in those with normal immunity. The significance of CMV detection in adults who are immunocompetent and critically ill is debatable [8]. In patients who are immunocompromised, the clinical manifestations may be localized or disseminated to several organs such as liver, esophagus, colon, and lung, leading to severe end-organ dysfunction.

Symptomatic CMV disease is classified as CMV syndrome or tissue-invasive CMV disease. CMV syndrome is characterized by fever, myelosuppression, and CMV DNA detection in blood. The diagnosis of tissue-invasive disease requires tissue evidence of cytopathic effects and CMV antigens or nucleic acids.

CMV retinitis is a potentially blinding manifestation of CMV infection. It was commonly seen in advanced AIDS in the era before modern combination antiretroviral therapy, but it is also less frequently recognized in patients with immune deficiency from multiple causes [17].

The nervous system is also commonly involved; the spectrum of neurological disorders in patients with AIDS ranges from subacute or acute encephalitis and ventriculoencephalitis, transverse myelitis to lumbar radiculopathy, distal symmetrical polyneuropathy, and mononeuritis multiplex.

CMV CNS disease in HIV/AIDS typically manifests as a progressive encephalopathy or has an acute onset with rapid progression that helps distinguish it from HIV encephalitis or progressive multifocal leukoencephalopathy (PML). Patients with diffuse CMV encephalitis may have fever and present with a dementia-like syndrome with decreased memory, attention, motor, and sensory deficits or ataxia that can be confused with HIV-related dementia. In CMV ventriculoencephalitis, patients have a more aggressive course of neurological deficits, radiculopathy, and nystagmus. Mass lesions manifest as focal deficits.

Peripheral neuropathies may respond to antiviral therapy when started early [18]. Rare case reports describe CMV immune-recovery-vitritis. One case report of CMV infection with multiple small vessel cerebral infarcts has been described in a recipient of HAART, in the setting of early immune reconstitution [19].

Congenital CMV infection
Congenital CMV infection is the most prevalent cause of congenital neurological handicap [15, 20, 21] and after genetic disorders, the second cause of hearing loss. In the United States, it is estimated that 40000 children (0.2–2% of newborns) per year present with congenital CMV infection; 400 are fatal. Five to 10% of infected infants are symptomatic with severe neurological deficits [22]; of these, 10% may have a fatal outcome as a result of severe systemic infection. About 60% of children with symptomatic congenital infection may develop cerebral lesions with neurological sequelae, such as microcephaly, seizures, hypotonia, feeding disorders, as well as chorioretinitis and hearing loss. Others

may present with growth retardation, jaundice, organomegaly, and low platelet count. Eighty-five to 90% of congenital infections are asymptomatic at birth; 5–15% of these infants will later develop clinical sequelae such as mental restriction and sensorineural hearing loss. Severe lesions usually predominate in early gestation.

In congenital infection, the risk of hearing loss is estimated at 9.9% in children who are asymptomatic compared with 32.8% in children who are symptomatic [23]. The mean delay of hearing loss onset is 15 months in children who are symptomatic, and 20 months in children who are asymptomatic.

Imaging studies

Magnetic resonance imaging (MRI) studies usually show a nonspecific increased T2/fluid attenuated inversion recovery (FLAIR) signal in the white matter in CMV encephalitis. Periventricular enhancement may be observed in cases of ventriculitis, and enhancement of cauda equina or meninges can be seen in CMV polyradiculomyelitis. The differential diagnosis includes HIV encephalitis, PML, and primary periventricular CNS lymphoma, which presents with an enhancing mass effect.

Laboratory tests

Laboratory methods for diagnosis of CMV infection include serology, culture, antibody detection, molecular testing, and histopathology.

- In the cerebrospinal fluid (CSF), lymphocytic pleocytosis and, occasionally, low glucose or polymorphonuclear pleocytosis may be present with encephalitis (more often with ventriculoencephalitis than diffuse encephalitis) and polyradiculomyelitis.
- CMV-specific IgG and immunoglobulin M (IgM) antibodies (serology) are usually detected by enzyme-linked immunosorbent assay (ELISA). The presence of CMV IgG indicates that a person was infected with CMV. CMV IgM is produced during primary CMV infection, reactivation of latent infection, or reinfection, including by a different strain. IgM positivity combined with low IgG avidity is an accurate indicator of primary infection within the preceding three to four months. IgG avidity is defined as the strength with which IgG binds to antigenic epitopes and matures gradually during the six months following primary infection [24].
- The first laboratory methods for CMV detection consisted of human fibroblast cultures inoculated with body fluids such as CSF, blood, urine, or saliva, leading to cytopathic effects in tube cell cultures within two days to three weeks. The viral identity is verified by immunofluorescence. The shell-vial assay is more rapid and uses monoclonal antibodies directed against early antigens of replicating CMV. These methods are relatively specific but are poorly sensitive compared to other methods.
- CMV-specific matrix-protein pp65 antigenemia detects antigen in leukocytes during the early phase of CMV replication by immunofluorescence, immunoperoxidase, and other antigen-detection methods. The test gives both a qualitative and quantitative result and correlates closely with viremia and clinical disease severity in immunosuppressed populations.
- Molecular methods to detect or amplify CMV nucleic acids are rapid and sensitive, even at early stage disease before positive serology. Qualitative and quantitative (real-time polymerase chain reaction [PCR]) methods have been developed for the detection of CMV DNA. However, viral DNA may be detected during latent infection and in nonviable viral particles during treatment; therefore, low-level viral load may represent latent viral DNA or subclinical infection. Detecting CMV DNA in the CSF is highly suggestive of CNS disease, although CSF pleocytosis containing latent CMV in CSF leukocytes may produce false-positive results. Compared to CMV DNA, the detection of viral RNA using real-time PCR is more indicative of active CMV infection and replication. RNAs are sensitive to degradation in vitro; thus, the sensitivity of the method is lower compared to the pp65 antigen test and the detection of CMV DNA. Numerous studies emphasize the interassay and interlaboratory variability even using an international reference standard.
- To test the susceptibility of viral isolates to antiviral drugs, genotypic methods provide objective results and are more rapid and sensitive than phenotypic methods [25]. However, phenotypic assays are still required for confirmation of potential new drug-resistant mutations identified by genotyping.
- Histopathological examination remains the gold standard and most clinically relevant test because CMV is a common finding in patients who are immunosuppressed without clinical manifestations. Moreover, tissue-invasive CMV diseases may be observed in the absence of significant viremia.

In numerous countries, CMV infection is not routinely screened during pregnancy. PCR on amniotic fluid is performed in addition to serology in maternal symptomatic disease or when ultrasound is abnormal. Ultrasound (US) abnormalities are observed in about 43.5% of infected fetuses. The main US findings (i.e. hyperechogenic bowel, intrauterine growth restriction, microcephaly, brain calcifications, and cerebral ventriculomegaly) are not specific for CMV infection. However, an anechogenic cavity located at the occipital horn extremity or near the temporal horn may be a helpful sign [26]. These likely correspond to periventricular pseudocysts related to infection and necrosis of ventricular or periventricular regions [27]. The contribution of fetal MRI has also been extensively described.

In neonates, maternal IgG antibodies cross the placenta, whereas IgM does not; therefore, detecting CMV IgM supports a congenital infection. The other standard laboratory test for diagnosing congenital CMV infection is PCR on saliva, usually in combination with urine for confirmation. This avoids false-positive results because mothers who are seropositive shed CMV virus in their breast milk.

Pathology

CMV infection of the CNS in adults and children

Recipients of organ and bone marrow transplants and patients with AIDS with CD4 count <100 are at high risk for CMV. CMV is the most frequent viral infection in the CNS of patients with AIDS, in whom five patterns of lesions are observed [28].

- Isolated inclusion-bearing cells in the CNS or peripheral nervous system.
- Diffuse nodular encephalitis characterized by the presence of dispersed microglial nodules (MGNs) and cytomegalic cells that can be single or found within MGNs. Immunohistochemistry is helpful to demonstrate viral antigens.
- Necrotizing encephalitis (Figures 7.1a, 7.2a–d, 7.3a, b): focal or dispersed necrotic foci containing cytomegalic cells and MGN. Cytomegalic cells are pathognomonic for CMV and may show "owl's eye" inclusions with a characteristic space around the inclusion (Figure 7.2b). Cytomegalic cells may be found outside areas of necrosis (Figures 7.2c, d). Lymphocytic vasculitis (Figures 7.2f), necrotizing vasculitis, and thrombosis are associated lesions.
- Necrotizing ventriculoencephalitis (Figures 7.1b, 7.2e–h): the ventricular wall is necrotic, containing numerous cytomegalic cells. MGNs and macrophages are present and associated with variable density of lymphocytes and may be associated with lymphocytic vasculitis, necrotizing vasculitis, and thrombosis.
- Myeloradiculopathy or mononeuritis multiplex (Figures 7.3b–f) that can be secondary to a ventriculoencephalitis.

These lesions can be associated with other pathogens within the same cell (e.g. CMV plus HIV [28]) or in the same organ (CMV plus PML). They can

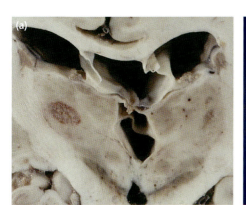 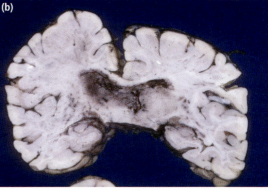

Figure 7.1 Macroscopic appearance (a): Focal parenchymal necrosis: coronal section at the level of red and subthalamic nuclei. Note the presence of multiple necrotic and hemorrhagic lesions in the thalami and in the right caudate nucleus. (b): Ventriculoencephalitis. Coronal section of the hemispheres at the level of the thalami. The corpus callosum, the ventricular wall, and the thalami are necrotic and hemorrhagic.

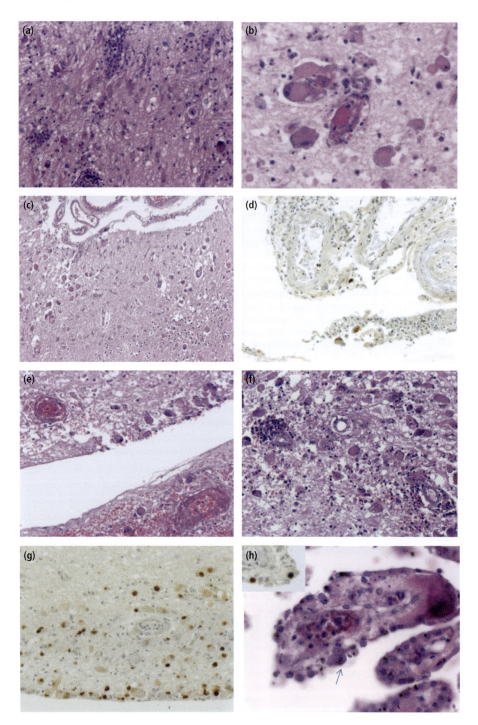

Figure 7.2 Microscopic appearance of the lesions in the cerebral hemispheres. (a) Dispersed cytomegalic cells, microglial nodules (MGN), and lymphocytes. (b) Cytomegalic cells with characteristic intracellular "owl's eye" viral inclusions around a thrombosed vessel. (c) Numerous cytomegalic cells in the cortex, note the lack of MGN. (d) Cytomegalovirus (CMV)-related meningitis, composed of lymphocytes, macrophages, and polymorphonuclear cells; the presence of CMV-infected cells is demonstrated using immunohistochemistry. (e) Ventriculoencephalitis: necrosis of ventricular walls and of the thalamus. Note the denuded ependymal layer replaced by cytomegalic cells. Necrotic and thrombosed vessels are also present. (f) Ventriculoencephalitis: numerous dispersed cytomegalic cells and vasculitis. (g) Ventriculoencephalitis: Immunohistochemical staining showing cytomegalic CMV-positive cells in the ventricular wall and adjacent parenchyma. (h) Ventriculoencephalitis: Cytomegalic cell in the epithelial lining of the choroid plexus (arrow) (inset: immunohistochemistry showing the CMV-positive cells).

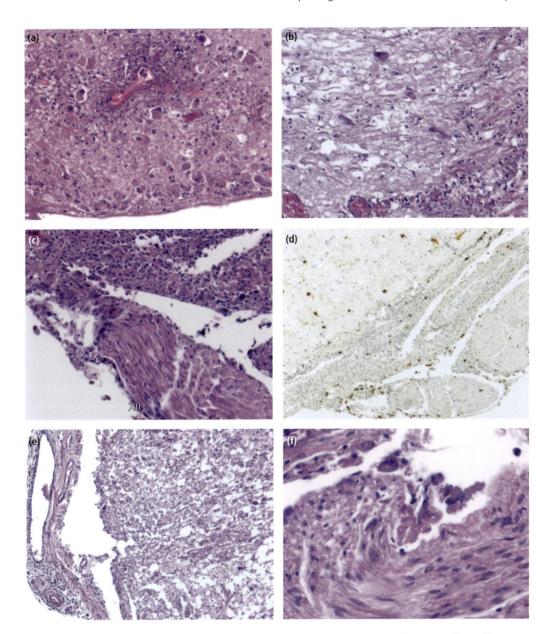

Figure 7.3 Microscopic appearance of the lesions in the brainstem, spinal cord, and peripheral nerves. (a) Necrotic cytomegalovirus (CMV) infection of the medulla, containing dispersed cytomegalic cells and a necrotic vessel surrounded by lymphocytes and macrophages. (b) Infection of the medulla with meningitis and numerous cytomegalic cells in meninges and hypoglossal nerve. (c) Necrosis of the fifth cranial nerve, containing cytomegalic cells and mixed inflammatory infiltrates. (d) Lower magnification of serial section of B immunostained using an anti-CMV antibody showing numerous CMV-positive cells in the medulla, meninges, and hypoglossal nerve. (e–f) meningo-myeloradicultis showing meningitis, necrosis of the spinal cord infiltrated by lymphocytes and macrophages, and numerous cytomegalic cells (e), which are also present in the spinal root (f).

also be associated with other complications of immunosuppression (e.g. other opportunistic infections, tumors, and toxic and metabolic disorders).

Congenital CMV infection

Congenital infection can be caused by *Toxoplasma gondii,* rubella, cytomegalovirus, and herpes simplex virus (TORCH), leading to fetal and neonatal morbidity and mortality. In congenital CMV infection, CNS lesions are usually widespread, involving the hippocampus, olfactory bulb, eyes, and inner ears.

The neuropathology of brain malformations and inner ear lesions related to congenital CMV infection has been extensively reviewed [27, 29]. Lesions include:

- Microcephaly
- Diffuse meningoencephalomyelitis characterized by meningitis, widespread MGNs, and cytomegalic cells that can be isolated or found within MGNs (Figures 7.4c–e). Innate and adaptive immune responses are present but do not react against all CMV-infected cells.
- Cortical abnormalities, consisting of polymicrogyria (Figure 7.4a) associated with areas of dysplastic cortex (Figure 7.5a), atrophy of the cortical plate; neuronal heterotopia (Figure 7.4b), and rupture of the glia limitans (Figure 7.4c, d).
- Microcalcifications or calcifications in the form of nodules or bands (Figures 7.4c, f).
- Hemorrhagic lesions and hemosiderin deposits (Figure 7.4f).
- Necrosis and cellular loss (Figure 7.5b, c), especially in the ventricular and subventricular zones (where progenitors are abundant), and germinolytic cysts (Figures 7.4b, d–f).
- Cochlear and vestibular infections. These are consistently present. Their severity correlates with the CNS lesions [29].

Two main factors influence the neuropathologic outcome: the density of CMV-positive cells and the tropism of CMV for stem and progenitor cells. This suggests that the spectrum of CMV-induced brain abnormalities is caused not only by tissue destruction (likely resulting from both direct cytopathic effects and bystander damage induced by inflammation and microglial activation) but also by the particular vulnerability of stem cells during early brain development.

Pathogenesis

A major site of human cytomegalovirus (HCMV) latency is the CD34+ hematopoietic progenitor cell population in bone marrow, whereas myelomonoytic and dendritic cells appear to play a role in the carriage and reactivation of HCMV in vivo. CMV replicates in virtually all cell types.

CMV infection elicits a series of cell-mediated immune responses initiated by innate microglial cells and macrophages and natural killer (NK) cells, followed by adaptive CD4+ and cytotoxic CD8+ T cells, memory T-cell populations, and B-cell high-avidity neutralizing antibodies [30]. Innate immune defenses against viral infections also involve different programmed cell death pathways [31, 32].

As a countermeasure of all herpesviruses, CMV harbors the largest number of genes dedicated to evading innate and adaptive immunity in the host [8, 33]. Viruses have evolved numerous strategies to interfere with the induction or execution of the host cell death [31]. CMV represents a lifelong challenge to T-cell surveillance and immune dysfunction. Therefore, the virus also needs immune evasion strategies during latency.

For the risk factors and pathogenesis of congenital infection please also refer to the section on Epidemiology and Risk Factors).

Animal models

Studies of murine cytomegalovirus (MCMV) infections of adult mice have served as a model of CMV biology and pathogenesis. MCMV infection of newborn mice has been used as a model of perinatal CMV infection [34].

Treatment, future perspective, and conclusions

The reduction of immunosuppressive therapy is considered whenever possible. Currently, intravenous ganciclovir and oral valganciclovir are the drugs of choice for the treatment of CMV disease [8]. Foscarnet and cidofovir are second-line agents because of their associated toxicities. Recommendations for CMV

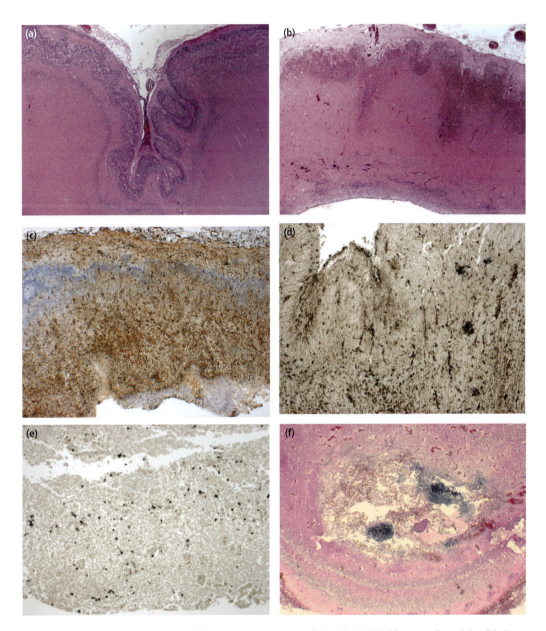

Figure 7.4 Congenital cytomegalovirus (CMV) infection. (a) Polymicrogyria adjacent to a normal cortex (on the right). (b) Microcephaly, dysplastic cortical plate, and loss of germinal cells in the ventricular zone. (c) Vimentin (brown)-Iba1 (black) double labeling in a fetus with microcephaly; note the dysplastic cortical plate, calcifications, loss of germinal cell in the ventricular zone, loss of radial glial cells in the ventricular subventricular zone, disorganized network of radial glial fibers, and paucity of microglial nodules (MGN). (d) vimentin (brown)-Iba1 (black) double labeling in a fetus with microcephaly. MGN are dispersed in the polymicrogyric cortical plate; note the loss of radial glial fibers. (e) CMV (black)-Iba1 (brown) double labeling in the ventricular zone showing abundant cytomegalic CMV-positive cells contrasting with the lack of MGN. (f) Temporal cyst at the rostral part of the temporal horn of the lateral ventricles. The cyst wall is necrotic, hemorrhagic, and sprinkled by calcifications.

Infections of the Central Nervous System

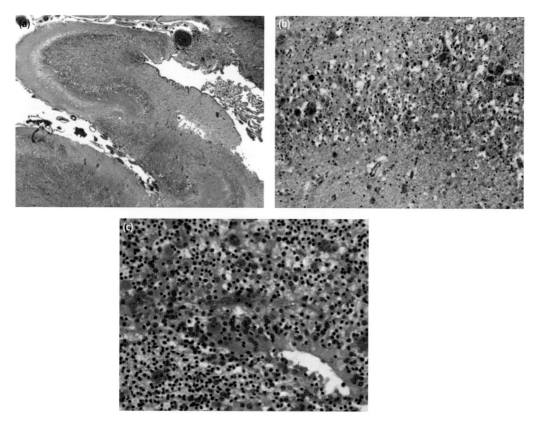

Figure 7.5 Congenital cytomegalovirus (CMV) infection. (a) Dysplastic hippocampi. (b) Necrosis and neuronal loss in the pyramidal layer of the Ammon's horn containing numerous cytomegalic cells. (c) Infection of the olfactory bulb; the ventricular zone is necrotic and surrounded by cytomegalic cells.

management in recipients of solid organ transplants, those with congenital infections, [35] and neonates have been proposed [36].

References

1. Dudgeon, J.A. (1971). Cytomegalovirus infection. *Arch. Dis. Child.* 46: 581–583.
2. Goodpasture, E.W. and Talbot, F.B. (1921). Concerning the nature of 'protozoan-like' cells in certain lesions of infancy. *Am. J. Dis. Child.* 21: 415–425.
3. Stern, H. (1968). Isolation of cytomegalovirus and clinical manifestations of infection at different ages. *BMJ* 1: 665–669.
4. Weller, T.H., Macauley, J.C., Craig, J.M. et al. (1957). Isolation of intranuclear inclusion producing agents from infants with illnesses resembling cytomegalic inclusion disease. *Proc. Soc. Ex. Biol. Med.* 94: 4–12.
5. Cheeran, M.C., Lokensgard, J.R., and Schleiss, M.R. (2009). Neuropathogenesis of congenital cytomegalovirus infection: disease mechanisms and prospects for intervention. *Clin. Microbiol. Rev.* 22: 99–126, Table of Contents.
6. Lau, B.E., Poole, E., Van Damme, L. et al. (2016). Human cytomegalovirus miR-UL112-1 promotes the down-regulation of viral immediate early-gene expression during latency to prevent T-cell recognition of latently infected cells. *J. Gen. Virol.* 97: 2387–2398.
7. Jackson, S.E., Redeker, A., Arens, R. et al. (2017). CMV immune evasion and manipulation of the immune system with aging. *Geroscience* 39: 273–291.

8. Griffiths, P., Baraniak, I., and Reeves, M. (2015). The pathogenesis of human cytomegalovirus. *J. Pathol.* 235: 288–297.
9. Jellinger, K.A., Setinek, U., Drlicek, M. et al. (2000). Neuropathology and general autopsy findings in AIDS during the last 15 years. *Acta Neuropathol.* 100: 213–220.
10. Fowler, K.B., Stagno, S., and Pass, R.F. (2003). Maternal immunity and prevention of congenital cytomegalovirus infection. *JAMA* 289: 1008–1011.
11. Maidji, E., McDonagh, S., Genbacev, O. et al. (2006). Maternal antibodies enhance or prevent cytomegalovirus infection in the placenta by neonatal fc receptor-mediated transcytosis. *Am. J. Pathol.* 168: 1210–1226.
12. Pereira, L., Maidji, E., McDonagh, S. et al. (2003). Human cytomegalovirus transmission from the uterus to the placenta correlates with the presence of pathogenic bacteria and maternal immunity. *J. Virol.* 77: 13301–13314.
13. Guibert, G., Warszawski, J., Le Chenadec, J. et al. (2009). Decreased risk of congenital cytomegalovirus infection in children born to HIV-1-infected mothers in the era of highly active antiretroviral therapy. *Clin. Infect. Dis.* 48: 1516–1525.
14. Pass, R.F., Fowler, K.B., Boppana, S.B. et al. (2006). Congenital cytomegalovirus infection following first trimester maternal infection: symptoms at birth and outcome. *J. Clin. Virol.* 35: 216–220.
15. Kenneson, A. and Cannon, M.J. (2007). Review and meta-analysis of the epidemiology of congenital cytomegalovirus (CMV) infection. *Rev. Med. Virol.* 17: 253–276.
16. Kalejta, R.F. (2008). Tegument proteins of human cytomegalovirus. *Microbiol. Mol. Biol. Rev.* 72: 249–265, table of contents.
17. Port, A.D., Orlin, A., Kiss, S. et al. (2017). Cytomegalovirus Retinitis: A Review. *J. Ocul. Pharmacol. Ther.* 33: 224–234.
18. Centner, C.M., Bateman, K.J., and Heckmann, J.M. (2013). Manifestations of HIV infection in the peripheral nervous system. *Lancet Neurol.* 12: 295–309.
19. Anderson, A.M., Fountain, J.A., Green, S.B. et al. (2010). Human immunodeficiency virus-associated cytomegalovirus infection with multiple small vessel cerebral infarcts in the setting of early immune reconstitution. *J. Neuro-Oncol.* 16: 179–184.
20. Cannon, M.J. and Pellett, P.E. (2005). Risk of congenital cytomegalovirus infection. *Clin. Infect. Dis.* 40: 1701–1702; author reply 1702-3.
21. Cannon, M.J., Schmid, D.S., and Hyde, T.B. (2010). Review of cytomegalovirus seroprevalence and demographic characteristics associated with infection. *Rev. Med. Virol.* 20: 202–213.
22. Boppana, S.B., Fowler, K.B., Britt, W.J. et al. (1999). Symptomatic congenital cytomegalovirus infection in infants born to mothers with preexisting immunity to cytomegalovirus. *Pediatrics* 104 (1 Pt 1): 55–60.
23. Goderis, J., Keymeulen, A., Smets, K. et al. (2016). Hearing in children with congenital cytomegalovirus infection: results of a longitudinal study. *J. Pediatr.* 172: 110–115 e112.
24. Prince, H.E. and Lape-Nixon, M. (2014). Role of cytomegalovirus (CMV) IgG avidity testing in diagnosing primary CMV infection during pregnancy. *Clin. Vaccine Immunol.* 21: 1377–1384.
25. Lurain, N.S. and Chou, S. (2010). Antiviral drug resistance of human cytomegalovirus. *Clin. Microbiol. Rev.* 23: 689–712.
26. Picone, O., Teissier, N., Cordier, A.G. et al. (2014). Detailed in utero ultrasound description of 30 cases of congenital cytomegalovirus infection. *Prenat. Diagn.* 34: 518–524.
27. Teissier, N., Fallet-Bianco, C., Delezoide, A.L. et al. (2014). Cytomegalovirus-induced brain malformations in fetuses. *J. Neuropathol. Exp. Neurol.* 73: 143–158.
28. Scaravilli, F. and Gray, F. (1993). Opportunistic infections. In: *Atlas of the Neuropathology of HIV Infection*, 1e (ed. F. Gray), 49–120. Oxford: Oxford Science Publications.
29. Teissier, N., Delezoide, A.L., Mas, A.E. et al. (2011). Inner ear lesions in congenital cytomegalovirus infection of human fetuses. *Acta Neuropathol.* 122: 763–774.
30. Klenerman, P. and Oxenius, A. (2016). T cell responses to cytomegalovirus. *Nat. Rev. Immunol.* 16: 367–377.
31. Brune, W. and Andoniou, C.E. (2017). Die another day: inhibition of cell death pathways by cytomegalovirus. *Viruses* 9 (9): E249.
32. Jorgensen, I., Rayamajhi, M., and Miao, E.A. (2017). Programmed cell death as a defence against infection. *Nat. Rev. Immunol.* 17: 151–164.
33. Gardner, T.J. and Tortorella, D. (2016). Virion glycoprotein-mediated immune evasion by human cytomegalovirus: a sticky virus makes a slick getaway. *Microbiol. Mol. Biol. Rev.* 80: 663–677.
34. Cekinovic, D. and LisnicVJ, J.S. (2014). Rodent models of congenital cytomegalovirus infection. *Methods Mol. Biol.* 1119: 289–310.

35. Torre-Cisneros, J., Aguado, J.M., Caston, J.J. et al. (2016). Management of cytomegalovirus infection in solid organ transplant recipients: SET/GESITRA-SEIMC/REIPI recommendations. *Transplant. Rev. (Orlando)* 30: 119–143.

36. Rawlinson, W.D., Boppana, S.B., Fowler, K.B. et al. (2017). Congenital cytomegalovirus infection in pregnancy and the neonate: consensus recommendations for prevention, diagnosis, and therapy. *Lancet Infect. Dis.* 17: e177–e188.

8 Adenovirus Meningoencephalitis

Harry V. Vinters[1] and Xinhai R. Zhang[2]

[1] Department of Pathology and Laboratory Medicine (Neuropathology) and Neurology, David Geffen School of Medicine UCLA and Ronald Reagan UCLA Medical Center, Los Angeles, CA, USA
[2] Department of Pathology, RUSH University Medical Center, Chicago, IL, USA

Abbreviations

ADV	adenovirus
ADVE	adenovirus encephalitis
AIDS	acquired immune deficiency syndrome
CMV	cytomegalovirus
CNS	central nervous system
CSF	Cerebrospinal fluid
DNA	deoxyribonucleic acid
EEG	electroencephalogram
HIV	human immunodeficiency virus
HSC	Hospital for Sick Children
HSV	herpes simplex virus
IL-1	interleukin-1
MRI	magnetic resonance imaging
PCR	polymerase chain reaction
WBC	white blood cells

Introduction

Adenovirus (ADV) is a medium-sized nonenveloped virus with an icosahedral nucleocapsid containing double-stranded DNA. It was first isolated from adenoid tissue in the early 1950s, hence, the derivation of its name. An excellent review within recent years has placed ADV in the context of *all* microbial pathogens that may cause acute encephalitis (i.e. bacteria, viruses, rickettsiae, etc.) and discusses the proof required to detect a confirmed, probable, or possible etiologic agent in a given case [1].

ADV is a common cause of febrile respiratory illness (i.e. bronchitis, croup), gastrointestinal infection, and conjunctivitis. Although systemic ADV infection can impact neurologic function or dysfunction, direct infection of the CNS by the virus is quite rare. A recent authoritative review of ADV associated with CNS dysfunction presents minimal details of neuropathologic features of adenovirus encephalitis (ADVE), probably because they are so rarely described [2]. This study from the Hospital for Sick Children (HSC) in Toronto, Canada, included data from the HSC Encephalitis Registry (1996–2016) and Microbiology Database (2000–2016) as well as the world literature. Their pooled analysis included 48 children who were immunocompetent, 38 from the literature and 10 from the HSC. Eighteen of 48 (38%) affected children either died or suffered permanent neurologic sequelae; predictors of poor long-term outcome included younger age, coagulopathy, serotype 2 virus, absence of meningismus, and (especially) the presence of seizures. The spectrum of neurologic disease was extremely variable, ranging from mild

Infections of the Central Nervous System: Pathology and Genetics, First Edition. Edited by Fabrice Chrétien, Kum Thong Wong, Leroy R. Sharer, Catherine (Katy) Keohane and Françoise Gray.
© 2020 John Wiley & Sons Ltd. Published 2020 by John Wiley & Sons Ltd.

aseptic meningitis and reversible encephalopathy to acute necrotizing encephalitis [2]. In the HSC study, which includes a thorough literature review, median age of affected children was two years, and 40% were female. Of 48 subjects, the large majority (30/48) fully recovered, whereas 18 manifested severe postinfection disability or death.

Epidemiology

This chapter summarizes what is known about the rare phenomenon of CNS ADV infection resulting in meningoencephalitis or "pure" ADVE. In the broader context of viral encephalitides, ADVE is much less frequent than those resulting from herpes simplex virus (HSV), cytomegalovirus (CMV), human immunodeficiency virus (HIV), or enteroviruses, to name only four common pathogens (discussed in Chapters 5, 7, 22, and 23, respectively). The relative frequency of ADVE varies substantially with (i) subject age, (ii) the region of the world in which a given epidemiologic or public health study has been carried out, and (iii) the epoch of time when the investigation occurred. A two-year surveillance study of encephalitis from Finland, extending over the years 1993–1994 that looked at more than 791 000 children, concluded that the microbial diagnosis was ADV in 5% of cases [3]. An investigation from the late 1990s in China found 9 children with severe ADV infection [4]. Their mean age was 22 months (range 5–50 months) and all presented with respiratory tract infections; 6 had hepatitis, 3 encephalitis, and 3 conjunctivitis. Only 1 child died from disease, but more than half had long-term pulmonary complications.

Using molecular analysis, a population-based study of 110+ cerebrospinal fluid (CSF) samples obtained between 2012 and 2015 from patients with encephalitis in Warsaw, Poland, found a viral agent in almost 43% of samples, most commonly HSV and enterovirus [5]. Not a single case of ADV was encountered in this survey. An Italian study of CSF samples from the same time period, focusing on older subjects (65 years or older), found that 35.4% of "positives" showed HSV, 23.1% had evidence of enteroviruses, but not a single sample showed a "footprint" of ADV infection [6]. By contrast, a study from India looking at children with acute encephalitis syndrome found ADV was the second-most common virus encountered, seen in almost 11% of subjects (vs. HSV-1 in 31.5%) [7]. Schwartz et al. [2] also emphasized the regional and geographic variability of ADV CNS infection, noting that ADV was implicated in 5% of children with encephalitis examined in Finland [3] and 3.3% of similar young subjects in Taiwan. They make the point that the majority of ADV infections are almost certainly self-limited because only a small percentage of those affected are hospitalized or seen in emergency departments. Thus, studies from large academic centers likely overestimate the incidence of ADV-related neurologic problems.

Clinical and neuroimaging features

As one would suspect, both the clinical manifestations and neuroimaging features of ADVE are quite variable. Clinical manifestations may include seizures, raised intracranial pressure, irritability, and severe headache with or without vomiting. Seizures appear to be the strongest predictor of poor clinical outcome. Focal neurologic deficits may be determined by the region(s) of brain involved. Electroencephalograms (EEGs) may show focal slowing. Computed tomography (CT) scans and magnetic resonance imaging (MRI) may be normal or show ischemic change with or without features of a necrotizing encephalitis or demyelination. Obviously, such findings may also be attributed, at least in part, to systemic hypoxia-ischemia secondary to severe pulmonary disease (common and often a defining feature in ADV infection) rather than ADVE itself. CSF findings show a modest increase in white blood cells (WBCs); in at least one small study, CSF WBC counts ranged up to 1019 mm^3, and in three of four patients were predominantly polymorphonuclear leukocytes (in one subject with lymphocytic leukemia they were 100% lymphocytes). CSF protein is variably increased but rarely above 340 mg/dl, and glucose is normal or low normal [8, 9]. Surprisingly, most infants and children with ADV-associated CNS disease, including those with encephalitis, CSF pleocytosis, and MRI abnormalities, have no detectable ADV in their CSF.

Diagnostic considerations

Molecular diagnostics of CSF and other fluids, with an emphasis on searching for viral pathogens, is a rapidly evolving field. Older publications [8] stress the value of looking for characteristic cytopathic effects of putative viral isolates in cell culture. This is laborious and has a significant subjective component. Electron microscopic examination of tissue samples and stool could be rewarding but is also very labor intensive. Direct fluorescent antibody staining can be performed using fluorophore-labeled anti-ADV monoclonal antibody. In the current era, virus isolation is rarely attempted or necessary and has been supplanted by polymerase chain reaction (PCR)-based technology, often using commercial kits [2] available from companies such as Altona Diagnostics or biotech giant Luminex. Multiplex PCR platforms have been developed that enable simultaneous screening for multiple viral pathogens (including ADV) in a single specimen [10]. Metagenomic sequencing can be used to screen for multiple viruses and has a fairly rapid turnaround time [11]. This method directly sequences all of the DNA in a sample at once and is described as being highly sensitive with "nearly unlimited coverage of pathogen detection compared with conventional culture-dependent clinical microbiology and nucleic acid amplification tests."

Neuropathology

Most reports of ADVE are based on single case reports or rarely a larger series of patients, in whom the diagnosis was confirmed by CSF studies, including PCR or sometimes viral culture [2, 9]. Brain biopsy is rarely carried out, and autopsies are infrequent because it is rarely fatal. The rare necropsies performed on subjects with ADVE are especially valuable, but their neuropathologic findings cannot necessarily be extrapolated to a larger population. One detailed study of ADVE in a recipient of a bone marrow transplant [12] showed an externally unremarkable brain but with significant abnormalities on sectioning and microscopy: symmetrical softenings and hemorrhagic lesions were noted in the inferomedial temporal cortex and amygdaloid nuclei, hypothalamus, and septum pellucidum. Symmetrical hemorrhagic lesions were seen in the inferior colliculi, perivascular and parenchymal lymphocytes were prominent, and characteristic neuronal intranuclear inclusions were present. Characteristic viral particles were confirmed by dramatic published electron micrographs.

We have described an unfortunate 4-year-old child with acquired immune deficiency syndrome (AIDS) who developed encephalitis two months prior to death, in the context of disseminated ADV affecting many organs including pancreas and adrenals [13]. ADV was cultured from the CSF. At autopsy the brain showed complete sloughing of the cerebral ependymal lining with marked gliosis and edema of the periventricular white matter (Figure 8.1). Cells with large, "smudged" intranuclear inclusions, consistent with ADV inclusions, were identified in subependymal regions of the brain. In situ hybridization confirmed ADV DNA in many periventricular cells. ADV may be localized to neurons, with surprisingly sparse inflammation in the surrounding brain parenchyma (Figure 8.2). However, in its extreme (thankfully rare) form, meningoencephalitis secondary to ADV may mimic severe bacterial sepsis [14]. Serotypes 7 and 2 appear to be most strongly associated with CNS morbidity and mortality, but the numbers available are small. ADV is frequently used as a vector to introduce "gene therapy" into gliomas, which may eventually become associated with a unique ADV-related brain pathology in this neuro-oncologic context [15].

Pathogenesis and animal models

The pathogenesis of ADVE is not well understood. One of the "mysteries" is that there may be significant brain injury, manifest as neuronal loss and even necrosis, in the absence of detectable virus within the CNS [2]. This suggests a "parainfectious pathogenesis." A potentially toxic effect of the ADV "penton antigen" or component of the viral capsid antigen observed to be toxic to cultured cells has been suggested. An immunopathologic mechanism resulting from antigen–antibody complexes

Infections of the Central Nervous System

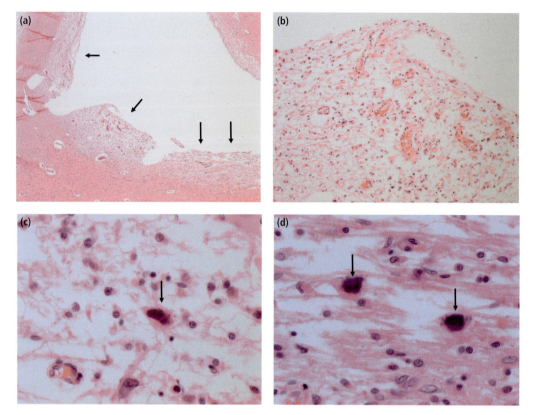

Figure 8.1 A case of adenovirus encephalitis (ADVE) in a child with acquired immunodeficiency syndrome (AIDS). There was extensive loss of ependymal lining throughout the ventricular system (a, arrows hematoxylin and eosin [H&E] × 2), and "subependymal" astrocytosis and edema (b H&E × 10). Enlarged cells in the periventricular region showed "smudged" hyperchromatic nuclei with effacement of the normal nuclear architecture and morphology (c, d arrows H&E ×40). Adenovirus (ADV) was proven by in situ hybridization studies. (Source: For details, see reference 13 by Anders et al.)

in the circulation has been postulated. Infiltrating T lymphocytes in the brain may be mediators of ADV-related brain injury.

In mouse models, some ADV strains show greater neurotropism than others. In murine models, varying degrees of encephalomyelitis can be induced depending on the mouse strain mouse used. For example, one study showed a fatal hemorrhagic encephalomyelitis may eventuate in adult C57BL/6 but *not* in BALB/c mice [16]. Newborn and suckling mice develop a fulminant encephalomyelitis characterized by infectious virus and viral lesions in many organs. In the adult mice with ADVE, symptoms of CNS disease included tremors, seizures, ataxia, and paralysis. By light microscopy, affected brains showed petechial hemorrhages, edema, neovascularization, and mild inflammatory changes in the spinal cord and brain. Ultrastructure of affected tissues showed activated microglia and swollen astrocytic endfeet, suggesting blood-brain barrier (BBB) dysfunction [16]. The most abundant viral mRNA was found in the CNS. In other experiments, a protective role has been implicated for interleukin-1 (IL-1) in the course of murine ADV type 1-induced encephalitis [17]. In the absence of IL-1 signaling, the investigators noted an increase in the transcription of interferon-stimulated genes. Further experimental studies are likely to shed light on important pathogenetic mechanisms in ADVE.

Adenovirus Meningoencephalitis Chapter 8

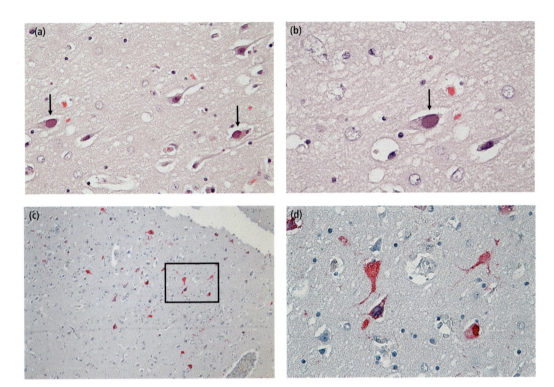

Figure 8.2 Adenovirus encephalitis (ADVE). Note the minimal inflammation within cortex. (a and b) Arrows indicate characteristic nuclear inclusions, substantially different than the Cowdry type A intranuclear inclusions seen in cytomegalovirus infection. Panel b (hematoxylin and eosin [H&E] × 40) shows a magnified view of the inclusion highlighted at left (a, H&E × 63). Panels c and d show a section stained with primary antibody to adenovirus (ADV) antigen. Note prominent neuronal cytoplasmic staining. Region highlighted by the rectangle in (c, immunohistochemistry [IHC] × 10) is shown at magnified view in (d, IHC × 40). (Source: Micrographs courtesy of Dr. Wun-Ju Shieh of the Centers for Disease Control in Atlanta, Georgia.)

Treatment and future directions

Because most medical centers (possibly apart from pediatric hospitals) encounter so few cases of ADVE, clinical trials aimed at optimizing therapy for this rare entity are difficult to carry out. Treatment is usually supportive and individualized, depending on the severity of the CNS infection. Pathologists must be vigilant for undiagnosed cases that come to brain biopsy or autopsy because they may be highly illuminating.

Acknowledgments

Kazu Williams and Dr. Marcia Cornford (Harbor-UCLA Medical Center) assisted with preparation of the micrographs. Authors are especially grateful to Dr. Wun-Ju Shieh of the Centers for Disease Control in Atlanta, Georgia, who provided the case illustrated in Figure 8.2.

References

1. Granerod, J., Cunningham, R., Zuckerman, M. et al. (2010). Causality in acute encephalitis: defining aetiologies. *Epidemiol. Infect.* 138: 783–800.
2. Schwartz, K.L., Richardson, S.E., MacGregor, D. et al. (2019). Adenovirus-associated central nervous system disease in children. *J. Pediatr.* 205: 130–137.
3. Koskiniemi, M., Korppi, M., Mustonen, K. et al. (1997). Epidemiology of encephalitis in children. A prospective multicentre study. *Eur. J. Pediatr.* 156: 541–545.

4. Chuang, Y., Chiu, C.H., Wong, K.S. et al. (2003). Severe adenovirus infection in children. *J. Microbiol. Immunol. Infect.* 36: 37–40.
5. Popiel, M., Perlejewski, K., Bednarska, A. et al. (2017). Viral etiologies in adult patients with encephalitis in Poland: a prospective single center study. *PLoS One* 12: e0178481.
6. Parisi, S.G., Basso, M., Del Vecchio, C. et al. (2016). Viral infections of the central nervous system in elderly patients: a retrospective study. *Int. J. Infect. Dis.* 44: 8–10.
7. Kumar, R., Kumar, P., Singh, M.K. et al. (2018). Epidemiological profile of acute viral encephalitis. *Indian J. Pediatr.* 85: 358–363.
8. Kelsey, D.S. (1978). Adenovirus meningoencephalitis. *Pediatrics* 61: 291–293.
9. Landry, M.L. and Hsiung, G.D. (1988). Adenovirus associated meningoencephalitis in a healthy adult. *Ann. Neurol.* 23: 627–628.
10. Pham, N.T., Ushijima, H., Thongprachum, A. et al. (2017). Multiplex PCR for the detection of 10 viruses causing encephalitis/encephalopathy and its application to clinical samples collected from Japanese children with suspected viral. *Clin. Lab.* 63: 91–100.
11. Fang, X., Xu, M., Fang, Q. et al. (2018). Real-time utilization of metagenomics sequencing in the diagnosis and treatment monitoring of an invasive adenovirus B55 infection and subsequent herpes simplex virus encephalitis in an immunocompetent young adult. *Open Forum Infect. Dis.* 16 (5): ofy114.
12. Davis, D., Henslee, P.J., and Markesbery, W.R. (1988). Fatal adenovirus meningoencephalitis in a bone marrow transplant patient. *Ann. Neurol.* 23: 385–389.
13. Anders, K.H., Park, C.S., Cornford, M.E., and Vinters, H.V. (1990-91). Adenovirus encephalitis and widespread ependymitis in a child with AIDS. *Pediatr. Neurosurg.* 16: 316–320.
14. Reyes-Andrade, J., Sanchez-Cespedes, J., Olbrich, P. et al. (2014). Meningoencephalitis due to adenovirus in a healthy infant mimicking severe bacterial sepsis. *Pediatr. Infect. Dis. J.* 33: 416–419.
15. Castro, M.G., Candolfi, M., Wilson, T.J. et al. (2014). Adenoviral vector-mediated gene therapy for gliomas: coming of age. *Expert. Opin. Biol. Ther.* 14: 1241–1257.
16. Guida, J.D., Fejer, G., Pirofski, L.-A. et al. (1995). Mouse adenovirus type 1 causes a fatal hemorrhagic encephalomyelitis in adult C57BL/6 but not BALB/c mice. *J. Virol.* 69: 7674–7681.
17. Castro-Jorge, L.A., Pretto, C.D., Smith, A.B. et al. (2017). A protective role for interleukin-1 signaling during mouse adenovirus type 1-induced encephalitis. *J. Virol.* 91: e02106–e02116.

9 Polyomavirus Infections of the CNS

Susan Morgello
Department of Pathology, Neurology, and Neuroscience, Icahn School of Medicine, Mount Sinai, New York, NY, USA

Abbreviations

AAN	American Academy of Neurology
AIDS	Acquired immunodeficiency syndrome
BBB	blood-brain barrier
BKV (also BKPyV)	BK virus
cART	combination antiretroviral therapy
CNS	central nervous system
CSF	cerebrospinal fluid
CT	computerized tomography
DMT	disease modifying therapy
EM	electron microscopy
FLAIR	fluid-attenuated inversion recovery
GCE	gray matter encephalopathy
GCN	granule cell neuronopathy
HIV	human immunodeficiency virus
IRIS	immune reconstitution inflammatory syndrome
JCV (also JCPyV)	John Cunningham virus
JCVE	JC virus encephalopathy
LT-Ag	large T antigen
MME	meningitis/meningoencephalitis
MRI	magnetic resonance imaging
MS	multiple sclerosis
NCCR	noncoding control region
PCR	polymerase chain reaction
PML	progressive multifocal leukoencephalopathy
Sm t-Ag	small t antigen
SV40	Simian virus 40

CNS disorders caused by polyomaviridae: history and syndromes

In 1958, Astrom, Mancall, and Richardson described three patients with hematopoietic neoplasia who developed subacute, relentlessly progressive neurologic disorders resulting in death [1]. Autopsy neuropathology was characterized by disseminated, perivascular, and coalescing regions of demyelination, bizarre glial pleomorphism, and oligodendrocytes with enlarged, deeply basophilic nuclei [1]. Additional patients with progressive multifocal leukoencephalopathy (PML) were reported in 1961, and an "uncharacterized" virus, in the setting of immunocompromise, was hypothesized to be involved in pathogenesis [2]. In 1965,

---

Infections of the Central Nervous System: Pathology and Genetics, First Edition. Edited by Fabrice Chrétien, Kum Thong Wong, Leroy R. Sharer, Catherine (Katy) Keohane and Françoise Gray.
© 2020 John Wiley & Sons Ltd. Published 2020 by John Wiley & Sons Ltd.

Zu Rhein and Chou demonstrated viral particles in glial nuclei by electron microscopy (EM), suggesting that the disorder resulted from cytocidal effects of virions on oligodendroglia [3]. In 1971, Padgett and colleagues isolated polyomavirus from brain tissue of a patient with PML [4], and the existence of a subacute, overwhelmingly fatal, virally induced demyelinating disorder was established.

Over ensuing decades there was uncertainty regarding which particular viral species constituted the etiologic agent of PML, and with revisions in taxonomy, a distinct family was established for polyomaviridae (papova viruses were split into polyoma and papilloma; John Cunningham virus [JCV] became JCPyV but will be abbreviated by its older acronym JCV herein) [5]. The uncertainty persisted partly because of the strong protein-genetic homology (approximately 70%) among betapolyomaviridae JCV, BK virus (BKV), and Simian virus 40 (SV40), and the fact that all could be detected in human tissues and tumors [6–8]. It is now clear that PML is a JCV-related neuropathology, although rare individuals with BKV-related CNS demyelination are reported [9]. The spectrum of polyoma-related CNS disorders has expanded, both with regard to clinicopathologic entities and individuals at risk. Although PML is by far the most common CNS pathology with JCV, granule cell neuronopathy (GCN), gray matter encephalopathy (GCE), and meningitis and meningoencephalitis (MME) are now recognized [10]. With improving sensitivity and specificity of molecular diagnostics, detection of BKV-associated meningoencephalitis is more frequent [11]. Finally, our understanding is evolving of those at risk for CNS polyomavirus infection and how immunity and its therapeutic modulation contribute to viral pathogenesis. With each medical era, new types of immunosuppression provide insights into the mechanisms by which these highly prevalent viruses transform from commensal to injurious agents.

Microbiological and genetic characteristics of polyomaviridae

Polyomaviridae are small, nonenveloped, double-stranded, covalently linked circular DNA viruses; JCV, the etiologic agent of PML, is 5130 base pairs in size (JCV structure, function, and life cycle are reviewed in [12]) (Figure 9.1). Circular JCV DNA is packaged into a 40- to 45-nm icosahedral virion by a capsid composed of three structural proteins, VP1, VP2, and VP3; VP1 forms the outer shell, and VP2 and VP3 are located in the inner layer. The virus contains a bidirectional regulatory region, which allows transcription of early regulatory genes (small t and large T antigens, and smaller T′ proteins) in one direction and structural capsid proteins VP1, VP2, and VP3 as well as a late regulatory agnoprotein in the other direction. There is significant homology among JCV, BKV, and SV40 in coding regions, but large divergence in the regulatory region; this noncoding control region (NCCR) is a critical determinant of cellular tropism, virulence, and clinical disease.

Although this chapter focuses on CNS infections, it is important to note that all polyomaviridae

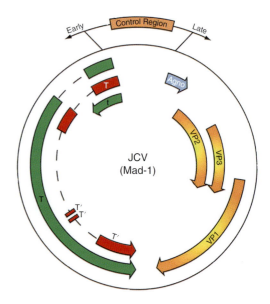

Figure 9.1 Diagram of a prototype John Cunningham virus (JCV) genome. The Mad-1 strain was the first virus isolated from a patient with progressive multifocal leukoencephalopathy (PML). It is a 5130 base pair DNA circle; a noncoding control region (NCCR) contains regulatory elements that allow transcription in two directions; early gene products (i.e. large and small t antigens and T′ proteins) in one direction and late gene products (i.e. VP1, VP2, VP3, and agnoprotein) in another.

express large T (LT-Ag) and small t (Sm t-Ag) antigens; these are well-documented oncogenes, capable of inactivating tumor suppressors pRb, p130, p53, and protein phosphatase 2A, and interacting with many other cell-signaling molecules [7, 13]. JCV, BKV, and SV40 are oncogenic in cell culture and animal models, experimentally induce brain tumors, and have been demonstrated to varying degrees in human brain tumor tissues [7]. However, there is no definitive evidence that polyomaviruses contribute to human brain tumor formation [13]. It is difficult to document a specific causal association because the ubiquity of these viruses contrasts with the rarity of both primary brain tumors and CNS infections.

Epidemiology, risk factors

It is estimated that up to 80% of adults are infected with JCV and BKV, based on seroepidemiology [14]. Acquisition of serum antibodies begins in childhood, more rapidly for BKV than JCV, with 80% and 50% seropositivity by the second decade, respectively [14]. The portal of primary infection is unclear. JCV can be detected in tonsil of adults and children but is rarely present in oropharyngeal secretions [15]. In contrast, asymptomatic shedding in urine has been observed in 50% of adults, and abundant JCV has been detected in urban sewage, likely a result of urinary excretion [15]. There are no animal hosts; there is no evidence to support vertical transmission.

After primary infection, JCV and BKV establish latency, capable of reactivation in the setting of immunocompromise. Up to 44% of transplant recipients demonstrated urinary excretion in early studies; prior to availability of combination antiretroviral therapy (cART), JCV in circulating peripheral blood mononuclear cells could be found in almost 40% of individuals with human immunodeficiency virus (HIV), and 90% of those with biopsy-proven PML [14, 16]. The ubiquity of these viruses is in remarkable contrast to the much lower frequency of PML. The greatest population incidence was in individuals with HIV before the cART era; it was estimated that 4% of those with the acquired immunodeficiency syndrome (AIDS) would develop PML [17]. Other immunosuppressed populations have a lower frequency: for those receiving natalizumab, a biological agent used to treat autoimmune disorders, the incidence of PML is variably estimated at 3.85 per 1000 patients or 1 per 1000 patient-treatment years; a similar incidence is seen in solid-organ transplantation [18, 19].

CNS polyomavirus infections are opportunistic. Most individuals with PML have immune compromise or dysregulation as a result of a disease process or disease-modifying therapy (DMT); depending on the medical era, the spectrum of predisposing conditions varies [20]. Individuals at risk were identified in the era of burgeoning cancer chemo and radiation therapies, particularly with hematopoietic neoplasms; in the decades of immunosuppression with solid organ, and later, stem-cell and bone-marrow transplantation; and during the HIV epidemic prior to effective cART. More recently, PML occurred unexpectedly in individuals with autoimmune disorders receiving therapy with natalizumab, a selective adhesion molecule antagonist that targets α4 integrin, blocking translocation of activated leukocytes across the blood-brain barrier (BBB). Initially, natalizumab-associated PML was observed in patients with multiple sclerosis (MS), but it was later identified in a wider spectrum of disorders. This experience, and the observation that other DMTs also increase risks for PML, led to developing criteria to stratify DMT PML risk [20]. This is important for therapeutic management but also influences the frequency of PML signs and symptoms that vary with underlying predisposing conditions (noted in a recent American Academy of Neurology [AAN] consensus statement for PML diagnostic criteria [21]).

Clinical features and diagnosis

Because PML lesions are typically bilateral, multifocal, and progressive, a variety of clinical phenomena may be observed. Disease onset is subacute but requires attention to accurate history; it is not uncommon for patients with PML to be mistakenly classified as having sustained strokes. Neurologic

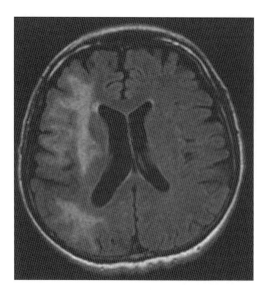

Figure 9.2 Magnetic resonance imaging (MRI) of a patient with progressive multifocal leukoencephalopathy (PML) displays nonenhancing T2 signal abnormality in the hemispheric white matter without mass effect. The lesion is extensively subcortical without ventricular predilection. (Source: Image courtesy of Dr. Jessica Robinson-Papp.)

findings are typically diffuse but asymmetric, commonly including behavioral and cognitive abnormalities, motor weakness, gait dysfunction, speech and language disturbances, visual field deficits, and incoordination [21]. Sensory loss, seizures, diplopia, and headache are less frequent [21]. Optic nerve or peripheral nerves disease does not occur, and clinical myelopathy has not been reported, albeit cerebral involvement might mask spinal symptoms. Without immune reconstitution, the disease usually progresses to death less than a year after presentation [2].

On neuroimaging, PML lesions do not have mass effect, are hypodense on computed tomography (CT), and hypointense on T1-weighted and hyperintense on T2-weighted and fluid-attenuated inversion recovery (FLAIR) magnetic resonance imaging (MRI) (Figure 9.2). Classically in the white matter, lesions occur in supra- and infratentorial regions and, in early disease, may be small and focal, mimicking cerebral small vessel disease [22]. Lesions can be deep or superficial; in subcortical arcuate fibers, a "scalloped" appearance impinging into cortex can be seen [21]. At clinical presentation, 42% of lesions are unilobar, 19% multilobar, and 35% widespread [22]. In classical PML, lesions do not enhance, but up to 15% of cases may show faint, peripheral contrast enhancement, thought to indicate inflammation [21]. "Inflammatory PML," defined by this enhancement, is also a function of the predisposing risk; in natalizumab-associated PML, contrast enhancement is present in up to 40% of patients [22], and is also a feature of PML-associated immune reconstitution inflammatory syndrome (IRIS). Typically, restoring immune function improves PML prognosis. With immune reconstitution, long-term survival may be realized with or without persistent neurologic deficits. In a series of cART-treated HIV-PML, clinical improvement was seen in 17%, partial improvement in 46%, and stable deficits in 37%; on MRI, leukomalacia secondary to white matter destruction in regions with prior PML was identified [23]. With PML-IRIS, individuals whose immune status is improving display paradoxical worsening of neurologic symptoms as immunity "overshoots" and becomes destructive to the brain. It has been suggested that PML-IRIS can be radiographically distinguished from "inflammatory PML" by the presence of swelling, with higher frequency of perilesional edema [22].

A clinical variant of JCV infection selectively involves the posterior fossa with cerebellar atrophy and subacute onset of cerebellar signs such as ataxia, dysmetria, and dysarthria [10]. On MRI, cerebellar atrophy and posterior fossa white matter abnormalities may be seen, particularly in pons and middle cerebellar peduncles, a manifestation of JCV-induced GCN. Another variant is JCV meningitis, in which patients present with signs of meningeal irritation [10]. JCV encephalitis (JCVE), in which lesions are restricted to gray matter regions of cerebral hemispheres is very rare [10]. Finally, BKV encephalitis and meningoencephalitis are described in a handful of case reports, but because no validated standards for diagnosis exist, it is difficult to identify a clinical syndrome, although most reported presentations have been non-focal [9, 24].

Cerebrospinal fluid (CSF) analysis is critical to the diagnosis of polyoma-related CNS disease. Cell counts are typically low (reflecting immunocompromise) and proteins elevated [21]. Highly specific and sensitive demonstration of JCV (or BKV) DNA in

Polyomavirus Infections of the CNS Chapter 9

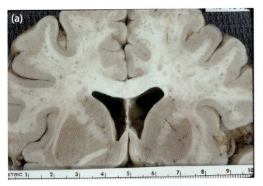
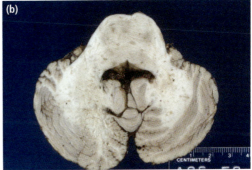
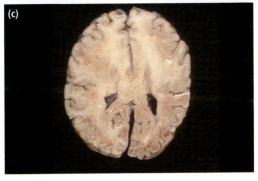

Figure 9.3 Macroscopic appearance of progressive multifocal leukoencephalopathy (PML). (a). The earliest lesions of PML are small, multifocal regions of gray discoloration in the white matter, as seen in this coronal section through the cerebral hemispheres. (Source: Image courtesy of Dr. David E. Wolfe.) (b). As the lesions continue to grow and mature, demyelination becomes more extensive and imparts a "moth eaten" appearance to white matter. This can be seen in the left cerebellar hemisphere in this semihorizontal section. Other lesions are apparent in pons and right cerebellar hemisphere; it is typical to see lesions of differing ages. (c). Eventually, large, contracted plaques may come to occupy large regions of white matter, as seen in this semihorizontal section through cerebral hemispheres. Note the subcortical predilection of lesions. (Source: Image courtesy of Dr. Hilda Laufer.)

CSF can be made by polymerase chain reaction (PCR); if positive in the setting of a compatible clinical presentation, a definitive diagnosis of PML can be made without biopsy [21]. In the absence of clinical findings, caution must be exercised because low viral copy numbers can sometimes be found in individuals without CNS infection who have systemic reactivation [21]. Accordingly, brain biopsy remains a gold standard for diagnosis.

Neuropathology

PML

Lesions of PML range in size from microscopic perivascular zones of acute infection, to small regions of parenchymal discoloration, to larger foci of demyelination imparting a "moth-eaten" appearance to white matter, to coalescent plaques that may be virtually holo-lobar or holo-hemispheric [2, 25] (Figure 9.3). Demyelinating foci can be found in supra- and infratentorial locations, with a predilection for subcortical regions in cerebral hemispheres and cerebellum and cerebellar peduncles in posterior fossa. Spinal cord involvement is rare [26]. Lesion distribution is helpful in distinguishing PML from MS; MS displays prominent involvement of the optic nerves and plaques are often periventricular, whereas PML spares optic nerves and lacks periventricular predilection. In patients with prolonged survival, remote lesions are well demarcated and focally cystic, with a combination of features resembling plaques and infarcts, corresponding to parenchymal destruction seen on

Infections of the Central Nervous System

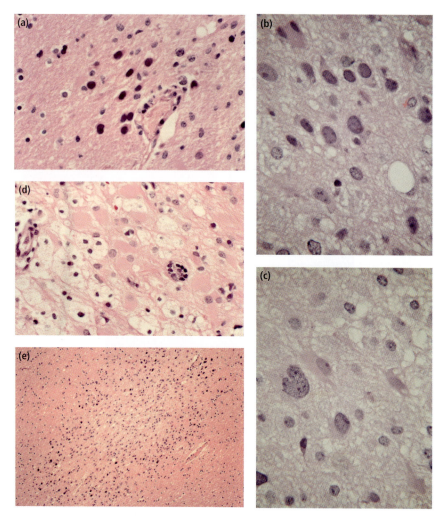

Figure 9.4 Microscopic appearance of progressive multifocal leukoencephalopathy (PML). (a) Enlarged oligodendroglial nuclei with deeply basophilic viral inclusions, adjacent to a small blood vessel in hemispheric white matter. These inclusions are characteristic of PML. (b) Viral inclusions may sometimes have a more amphophilic hue; characteristic nuclear enlargement is still present. (c) Glial atypia is pronounced in PML, as seen with this astrocyte that has an irregular nuclear contour and multiple nucleoli. Out of context, cells like these may be mistaken for neoplasm. (d) Demyelination occurs with oligodendroglial cell death, and lipid-laden macrophages become prominent, as seen in this micrograph. (e) In contrast, earlier lesions of PML demonstrate a spreading ring of oligodendroglial inclusions surrounding central zones of myelin pallor and vacuolization.

MRI. Cystic peripherally located remote lesions in cerebral hemispheres can be distinguished from infarcts by relative sparing of the cortical ribbon.

Microscopically, PML is characterized by the triad of enlarged oligodendroglial nuclei with viral inclusions, bizarrely pleomorphic astrocytes, and variable stages of demyelination with lipid-laden macrophages (Figure 9.4). Oligodendroglial inclusions are "hazy," diffusely fill the enlarged nucleus, and are amphophilic to deeply basophilic. On EM, numerous round to polygonal and occasionally filamentous intranuclear virions measuring up to 45 nm in diameter are seen. Pleomorphic astrocytes are enlarged, with hyperchromatic nuclei, irregular nuclear contours, and

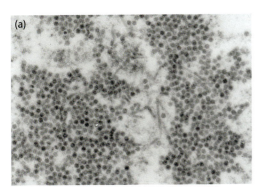 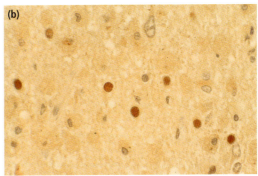

Figure 9.5 Special techniques in assessing polyomavirus pathologies. (a) Electron microscopy (EM) can be used to visualize John Cunningham virus (JCV) in the nuclei of infected glia. Here, polygonal, round, and occasionally filamentous virions measuring 40 nm in diameter are seen in an oligodendroglial nucleus. (Source: EM courtesy of Dr. Hilda Laufer.) (b) Immunohistochemistry for polyomavirus large T antigen highlights viral infection of oligodendroglia (diaminobenzidene chromogen).

sometimes multilobation or multinucleation [25]. It is critical to recognize these cells in the context of PML, because in isolation, they may be mistaken for neoplasm. Both cell types sustain JCV infection; in the case of oligodendroglia, productively and with eventual cell death; in the case of astrocytes, with resultant atypia, but only infrequent intranuclear virions identified on EM (Figure 9.5a). Infection in both cell types can be confirmed by immunohistochemistry; a commercially available antibody to LT-Ag is often used in clinical practice but cannot distinguish JCV from BKV because of extensive viral homology (Figure 9.5b).

The earliest lesions of PML consist of infected oligodendroglia in perivascular locations accompanied by white matter pallor; as lesions age and spread, increasing numbers of bizarre astrocytes, myelin destruction, and lipid-laden macrophages occur, until confluent zones of demyelination are produced with numerous macrophages. If there is long-term survival, cystic lesions with peripheral pallor and gliosis are seen; in our experience, there is sometimes minimal evidence of continued viral replication with occasional inclusion-bearing oligodendroglia. In subacute progressive disease, it is common to encounter lesions of variable maturation because continuous viremia results in parenchymal seeding over time.

JCV-Associated gray matter pathologies

Although PML has a devastating effect on white matter, it also commonly involves gray matter [25] (Figure 9.6). In cerebral cortex and deep gray matter, PML cytopathology is glial, and pyramidal neurons are histologically intact, but in cerebellum, a distinct gray matter neuropathology occurs. The earliest descriptions of PML noted focal destruction of the granule cell layer, with or without contiguous white matter demyelination, with sparing of Purkinje cell neurons, and with peripherally located, enlarged granule cell nuclei [2, 25]. In the absence of supratentorial white matter PML, and clinically manifesting as a cerebellar syndrome, this pathology is the hallmark of JCV-associated GCN [10]. Immunohistochemistry for LT-Ag demonstrates infection of granule cells. Distinction from classical PML is supported by association of GCN with JCV molecular variants carrying deletions in VP1 [10]. JCVE is a rarer gray matter variant, in which infection of pyramidal neurons and astrocytes of cerebral cortex characterizes initial disease presentation [10]. Morphologically, both neurons and cortical glia display atypia. An unusual feature is the lack of VP1 expression in many neurons with abundant immunohistochemical detection of LT-Ag, suggesting the neuronal infection is abortive. VP1 deletions found in GCN are not identified in JCVE.

Infections of the Central Nervous System

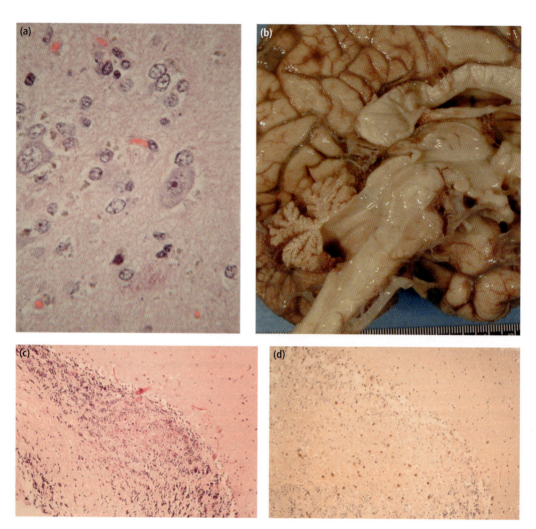

Figure 9.6 Gray matter manifestations of John Cunningham virus (JCV). (a) When progressive multifocal leukoencephalopathy (PML) involves gray matter regions, neurons appear histologically intact, while surrounding glia demonstrate atypia, as seen in this section of cerebral cortex. (b) In the cerebellum, granule cell neurons may be preferentially infected, resulting in the JCV variant granule cell neuronopathy (GCN). Grossly, remarkable atrophy of the cerebellum and pons are seen, as demonstrated in this midsagittal section. (c) Microscopically, infected granule cell neurons display nuclear enlargement. (d) Immunohistochemistry demonstrates large T antigen in the infected granule cells; there has been a reduction in their numbers because of neuronal cell death, but Purkinje neurons remain intact.

JCV-Associated inflammatory pathologies

Since the early descriptions of PML, mononuclear inflammatory infiltrates were occasionally described; these are usually perivascular, extend into parenchyma, and are T-cell predominant, mixed infiltrates with variable plasma cell components [27]. The number of oligodendroglial inclusions is generally inversely proportional to the extent of inflammation, reflecting the underlying immune competence. Longer survival correlates with inflammation [27]. The most severe inflammatory pathology is characteristic of PML-IRIS. With PML-IRIS, predominantly CD8 T-cell mixed inflammatory infiltrates extend beyond recognizable PML, in a nonspecific pattern of perivenous encephalitis [28].

Another inflammatory variant is JCV-associated MME, in which productive infection of choroid plexus epithelium, arachnoid, and elongated cells in subarachnoid space and meningeal arteries can be demonstrated, with variable involvement of underlying brain parenchyma [10].

BKV-Associated pathologies

Published accounts of neuropathology are rare, but it appears BKV can induce the full spectrum of lesions seen with JCV [9]. Foci of white matter demyelination with oligodendroglial inclusions; pyramidal neuron infection with paucity of VP1 expression, and MME have all been described [9, 24].

Molecular biology and pathogenesis

The elucidation of JCV life cycle and PML pathogenesis has depended on in vitro systems and direct analysis of human biospecimens in health and disease [18]. JCV uses sialic acid residues to infect cells and requires the serotonin receptor 5HT-2a for glial cell entry. After receptor binding, JCV enters the cell by clathrin-dependent endocytosis, traffics from endosomes to endoplasmic reticulum, and then through the cytosol into the nucleus [12, 18]. Replication and transcription are tightly controlled, and cell-type and species specific; this specificity is dependent on the hypervariable NCCR, which contains the origin of replication (ORI), promoter, and enhancer elements [18]. After early gene transcription, LT-Ag, the host cell DNA polymerase, and a variety of host proteins participate in JCV DNA replication. Late gene transcription occurs after replication is initiated, enabling virion assembly [12, 18].

JCV has been detected in a variety of cells and tissues, including (but not limited to): B cells in brain, tonsils, lymphoid organs, peripheral blood and bone marrow; tonsillar stromal cells; hematopoietic progenitor cells; glial cells; and renal epithelium [12, 18]. Currently, the favored model of pathogenesis entails immunosuppression-induced reactivation in kidney; migration from kidney into brain via B-cell lymphocyte trafficking across the BBB; and then infection of glial elements [12]. Alternatively, some have suggested disease initiation from latent sites in bone marrow or brain [18]. Regardless of the model, one of the mysteries of pathogenesis is why polyoma-associated CNS disease is so rare when infections are so prevalent.

Part of this mystery has been solved by elucidating molecular alterations enabling CNS infection. Viruses recovered from PML lesions, or prototype viruses, show marked divergence in the NCCR when compared to species from kidney and urine, or archetype viruses. The Mad-1 strain of JCV, the original sequence isolated from a patient with PML at the University of Wisconsin–Madison, is a prototype virus and contains a 98 base pair tandem repeat in the NCCR, a common motif in PML viruses thought to be important for CNS expression [12, 18]. In contrast, archetype viruses, lacking the duplication, are rarely associated with PML lesions. B cells contain both archetype and prototype viruses, raising the possibility that NCCR rearrangements conferring brain tropism and neurovirulence occur in this cell compartment, favoring a model of systemic viral activation leading to mutations that cross the BBB and initiate infection [12, 18].

Animal models

Attempts to create a model of JCV-induced demyelination have failed, partly because of species- and cell-type–specific restrictions for JCV replication [18]. Many attempts to establish infection by injecting animals or creating transgenic models with JCV have resulted in primary brain tumors [29]. A PML-like disease in immunosuppressed rhesus monkeys is seen with SV40, and JCV T-ag transgenic mice with dysmyelination have been created but are not models of PML. Intracerebral JCV injection of neonatally immuno- and myelin-deficient mice (Rag2–/– Mbp shi/shi mice) with engrafted human glial progenitor cells results in demyelination, but because of apoptosis and not productive oligodendroglial infection [29]. To date, animal models with JCV-induced PML pathology do not exist.

Treatments and future perspectives

Currently, there are no effective antiviral therapies demonstrated in clinical trials for PML, although individual case reports describe treatment response

[30]. Treatments include nucleotide and nucleoside analogs such as cidofovir and cytarabine to interfere with viral DNA synthesis and serotonin receptor 5-HT2a antagonists such as mirtazapine to inhibit JCV cell entry. The best therapy for PML is reversal of the underlying immunodeficiency. If PML-IRIS develops, paradoxical treatment with suppressive corticosteroids is indicated [30].

Unfortunately, reversing immunodeficiency is sometimes not feasible. For transplant recipients, graft survival may be jeopardized, and cancer-related immunodeficiency may not give recourse to immune reconstitution. Current research is focused on development of novel antivirals and strategies for immunization and adoptive transfer of ex vivo generated JCV-specific T cells [30].

Although PML remains a serious malady with significant morbidity and mortality, advances in our understanding of pathogenesis and increasing sophistication in manipulating immunity will continue to transform a once inexorably fatal condition into one compatible with prolonged survival.

References

1. Astrom, K.E., Mancall, E.L., and Richardson, E.P. (1958). Progressive multifocal leukoencephalopathy: a hitherto unrecognized complication of chronic lymphatic leukemia and Hodgkin's disease. *Brain* 81: 93–111.
2. Richardson, D.P. (1961). Progressive multifocal leukoencephalopathy. *New Engl. J. Med.* 265 (17): 815–823.
3. Zu Rhein, G.M. and Chou, S.M. (1965). Particles resembling papova viruses in human cerebral demyelinating disease. *Science* 148: 1477–1479.
4. Padgett, B.L., Zu Rhein, G.M., Walker, D.L. et al. (1971). Cultivation of papova-like virus from human brain with progressive multifocal leukoencephalopathy. *Lancet* 1: 1257–1260.
5. Polyomaviridae Study Group of the International Committee on Taxonomy of Viruses, Calvignac-Spencer, A., Feltkamp, M.C. et al. (2016). A taxonomy update for the family Polyomaviridae. *Arch. Virol.* 161: 1739–1750.
6. Vilchez, R.A. and Kusne, S. (2006). Molecular and clinical perspectives of polyomaviruses: emerging evidence of importance in non-kidney transplant populations. *Liver Transpl.* 12: 1457–1463.
7. White, M.K., Gordon, J., Reiss, K. et al. (2005). Human polyomaviruses and brain tumors. *Brain Res. Rev.* 50: 69–85.
8. Frisque, R.J., Bream, G.L., and Cannella, M.T. (1984). Human polyomavirus JC virus genome. *J. Virol.* 51 (2): 458–469.
9. Darbinyan, A., Major, E.O., Morgello, S. et al. (2016). BK virus encephalopathy and sclerosing vasculopathy in a patient with hypohidrotic ectodermal dysplasia and immunodeficiency. *Acta Neuropathol. Commun.* 4: 73.
10. Miskin, D.P. and Koralnik, I.J. (2015). Novel syndromes associated with JC virus infection of neurons and meningeal cells: no longer a gray area. *Curr. Opin. Neurol.* 28: 288–294.
11. Hirsch, H.H. and Steiger, J. (2003). Polyomavirus BK. *Lancet Infect. Dis.* 3: 611–623.
12. White, M.K. and Safak, M. (2016). Molecular biology of JC virus and the human demyelinating disease, progressive multifocal leukoencephalopathy. In: *Neurotropic Viral Infections, Volume Two: Neurotropic Retroviruses, DNA Viruses, Immunity and Transmission*, 2e (ed. C.S. Reiss), 75–110. Switzerland: Springer International Publishing.
13. Moens, U., Rasheed, K., Abdulsalam, I., and Sveinbjornsson, B. (2015). The role of Merkel cell polyomavirus and other human polyomaviruses in emerging hallmarks of cancer. *Viruses* 7: 1871–1901.
14. Walker, D.L. and Padgett, B.L. (1983). The epidemiology of human polyomaviruses. In: *Polyomaviruses and Human Neurological Diseases* (eds. J.L. Sever and D.L. Madden), 99–106. New York: Alan R Liss.
15. Matos, A., Duque, V., Luxo, C. et al. (2012). Individuals infected with JC polyomavirus do not present detectable JC virus DNA in oropharyngeal fluids. *J. Gen. Virol.* 93: 692–697.
16. Tornatore, C., Berger, J.R., Houff, S.A. et al. (1992). Detection of JC virus DNA in peripheral lymphocytes from patients with and without progressive multifocal leukoencephalopathy. *Ann. Neurol.* 31: 454–462.
17. Chaisson, R.E. and Griffin, D.E. (1990). Progressive multifocal leukoencephalopathy in AIDS. *JAMA* 264 (1): 79–82.
18. Ferenczy, M.W., Marshall, L.J., Nelson, C.D.S. et al. (2012). Molecular biology, epidemiology, and pathogenesis of progressive multifocal leukoencephalopathy, the JC virus-induced demyelinating disease of the human brain. *Clin. Microbiol. Rev.* 25: 471–506.
19. Mateen, F.J., Muralidharan, R., Carone, M. et al. (2011). Progressive multifocal leukoencephalopathy

20. Berger, J.R. (2017). Classifying PML risk with disease modifying therapies. *Mult. Scler. Relat. Dis.* 12: 59–63.
21. Berger, J.R., Aksamit, A.J., Clifford, D.B. et al. (2013). PML diagnostic criteria. Consensus statement from the AAN Neuroinfectious disease section. *Neurology* 80: 1430–1438.
22. Wattjes, M.P., Richert, N.D., Killestein, J. et al. (2013). The chameleon of neuroinflammation: magnetic resonance imaging characteristics of natalizumab-associated progressive multifocal leukoencephalopathy. *Mult. Scler.* 19: 1826–1840.
23. Lima, M.A., Bernal-Cano, F., Clifford, D.B. et al. (2010). Clinical outcome of long-term survivors of progressive multifocal leukoencephalopathy. *J. Neurol. Neurosurg. Psychiatry* 81: 1288–1291.
24. Bourlon, C., Alamoudi, S., Kumar, D. et al. (2017). A short tale of blood, kidney and brain: BK virus encephalitis in an allogeneic stem cell transplant recipient. *Bone Marrow Transplant.* 52: 907–909.
25. Richardson, E.P. Jr. and deWebster, H.F. (1983). Progressive multifocal leukoencephalopathy: its pathological features. In: *Polyomaviruses and Human Neurological Diseases* (eds. J.L. Sever and D.L. Madden), 191–203. New York: Alan R Liss.
26. Bernal-Cano, F., Joseph, J.T., and Koralnik, I.J. (2007). Spinal cord lesions of progressive multifocal leukoencephalopathy in an acquired immunodeficiency syndrome patient. *J. Neurovirol.* 13: 474–476.
27. Hair, L.S., Nuovo, G., Power, J.M. et al. (1992). Progressive multifocal leukoencephalopathy in patients with human immunodeficiency virus. *Hum. Pathol.* 23: 663–667.
28. Vendrely, A., Bienvenu, B., Gasnault, J. et al. (2005). Fulminant inflammatory leukoencephalopathy associated with HAART-induced immune restoration in AIDS-related progressive multifocal leukoencephalopathy. *Acta Neuropathol.* 109: 449–455.
29. White, M.K., Gordon, J., Berger, J.R., and Khalili, K. (2015). Animal models for progressive multifocal leukoencephalopathy. *J. Cell. Physiol.* 230: 2869–2874.
30. Pavlovic, D., Patera, A.C., Nyberg, F. et al. (2015). Progressive multifocal leukoencephalopathy: current treatment options and future perspectives. *Ther. Adv. Neurol. Disord.* 8: 255–273.

10 Measles Virus Infection of the CNS

Catherine (Katy) Keohane[1], Leroy R. Sharer[2], and Françoise Gray[3,4]

[1] Department of Pathology and School of Medicine, University College Cork, Brookfield Health Science Complex, Cork, Ireland
[2] Division of Neuropathology, Department of Pathology, Immunology, and Laboratory Medicine, Rutgers New Jersey Medical School and University Hospital, Newark, NJ, USA
[3] Retired from Department of Pathology, Lariboisière Hospital, APHP, Paris, France
[4] University Paris Diderot (Paris 7), Paris, France

Abbreviations

ADEM	acute disseminated encephalomyelitis
CNS	central nervous system
CSF	cerebrospinal fluid
EEG	electroencephalogram
HIV	human immunodeficiency virus
MIBE	measles inclusion body encephalitis
MV	measles virus
NIAID	National Institute of Allergy and Infectious Diseases
NK-1	neurokinin-1
PVRL4	poliovirus receptor-related 4 protein
RNA	ribonucleic acid
PCR	Polymerase chain reaction
SLAM	signaling lymphocytes-activation molecule
SNPs	single nucleotide polymorphisms
SSLE	subacute sclerosing leucoencephalitis
SSPE	subacute sclerosing panencephalitis
WHO	World Health Organization

Introduction

Measles is characterized by high fever, conjunctivitis, and a maculopapular rash. The measles virus (MV) is a highly contagious human pathogen [1]. Effective live vaccines have greatly reduced its morbidity and mortality, but measles is still prevalent in certain developing countries [2]. It causes acute and subacute infections.

Infection is acquired when viral-laden fomites, usually from coughs or sneezes, infect conjunctival or respiratory cells, followed by viral replication and viremia. Fever and upper respiratory tract symptoms appear 10–14 days following initial infection. A morbilliform skin rash appears a few days later. Recovery is the normal outcome.

Acute measles may involve the CNS in two ways: as aseptic meningitis, which has a benign outcome, or as acute disseminated encephalomyelitis (ADEM) or postinfectious encephalitis (cf. Chapter 26), which occurs in 1 in 1000 cases of measles infection and 1 in 2 000 000 following measles vaccination [3]. Neurological sequelae may be severe in 25% of cases, and death rate was 1 per 10 000 reported cases of measles infection [4].

MV infection also causes two rare subacute encephalitides: subacute sclerosing panencephalitis (SSPE) and immunosuppressive measles inclusion body encephalitis (MIBE).

Infections of the Central Nervous System: Pathology and Genetics, First Edition. Edited by Fabrice Chrétien, Kum Thong Wong, Leroy R. Sharer, Catherine (Katy) Keohane and Françoise Gray.
© 2020 John Wiley & Sons Ltd. Published 2020 by John Wiley & Sons Ltd.

Microbiological characteristics of MV

MV is a pleomorphic enveloped virus of the genus *Morbillivirus* in the Paramyxovirus family. The virus particles may be spherical or filamentous, 100–300 nm in diameter and up to 1000 nm in length. The nucleocapsid contains single-stranded, antisense RNA that is complexed with the nucleocapsid protein (N) and two other proteins: large protein (L) and phosphoprotein (P), which together confer RNA-dependent RNA polymerase activity. The matrix protein (M) is present on the inner aspect of the surrounding envelope, and the hemagglutinin (H) and fusion (F) proteins are on the outer aspect. Neutralizing antibodies are produced to both (H) and (F) proteins, and cell surface glycoproteins and give lifelong immunity. The matrix protein (M) is important for viral assembly [5].

CD46 (membrane cofactor protein) was the first identified MV receptor but serves this function for laboratory-adapted strains only and probably not in vivo. Signaling lymphocyte-activation molecule (SLAM), expressed by T and B lymphocytes, macrophages, dendritic cells, and thymocytes, is an established receptor for MV in vivo but is not expressed by respiratory tract epithelial cells, endothelial cells, or neurons, which are nonetheless also infected by the virus. Poliovirus receptor-related 4 (PVRL4) protein (nectin 4) may serve as the MV receptor for epithelial cells and the substance P receptor, neurokinin-1 (NK-1) as the viral receptor for neurons [for review, see 6].

Upon binding to the virus, F protein initiates fusion of the envelope with the cell membrane, leading to release of the nucleocapsid into the cytoplasm. There, the RNA is transcribed to produce multiple copies of viral proteins, before a positive-sense RNA genomic intermediate is synthesized, which acts as a template for the synthesis of new genomes. The nucleocapsids are assembled in large numbers in the cytoplasm and also accumulate within the nucleus. The H and F proteins are transported to, and incorporated in, the cell membrane. The M protein is needed for association of the nucleocapsid with the envelope proteins at the cell surface and for subsequent budding of the virus through the modified cytoplasmic membrane to form a mature virion. M protein is also an inhibitory regulator of MV ribonucleic transcriptional activity. In addition to their role in viral budding, the H and F proteins mediate local fusion of adjacent cells [6].

Epidemiology and genetics

MV is highly contagious. Humans and primates are the hosts, but only human-to-human infection occurs. Infection by MV remains one of the leading causes of death among young children worldwide [7]. In 2014, MV caused 114 900 deaths globally, mostly in children age <5 years in Asia and Africa. Infants and young children are particularly at risk; in outbreaks 40% of cases occur in children younger than 16 months [8]. Successful vaccination programs using live attenuated virus have been instituted in many countries. However, in some countries measles has re-emerged following unproven concerns about complications of the triple vaccine [9, 10], and the United States had more cases in 2014 than in any year since 1996 [11], attributed to declining herd immunity. A significant number of cases occur in previously vaccinated people [12, 13].

Single nucleotide polymorphisms (SNPs) in candidate immune response genes, in addition to *HLA* alleles, explain approximately 30% of the interindividual variability in measles-specific humoral immune response and suggest tight genetic control over measles vaccine-induced immunity. Genetic variants modulating cell surface viral receptors and related molecules also play a role [14]; these include *SLAM, CD 46, CD209/DC-SIGN* as well as cytokine and cytokine receptor genes *IL2, IL1, ILI2B, IL4RA, IL12RB1, IL7R, IL6, TNFA*, antiviral effector and innate immunity genes and innate genes *TLR2, TLR3, TLR4, TLR5, TLR6, TLR7, TLR8, MyD88, MD2, MAP3K7, IKBKE, TICAM1, NFKBIA, IRAK2, TRIM5, DDX58/RIG-I, OAS1, ADAR, MX2, OAS3, VISA,* vitamin A *RARA, RARB, RARG* and vitamin D *RXRA* receptor genes and *HLA* genes [14, 15]. For detailed discussion see [15].

Subacute sclerosing panencephalitis

Definition of the disorder, major synonyms, and historical perspective

SSPE is a rare, subacute or chronic, slowly progressive fatal inflammatory disease of the CNS caused by persistent aberrant MV infection. One early report by Dawson in 1933 [16] described it as "inclusion body encephalitis" in a child who died after several years of slow deterioration that ended in a vegetative state. Dawson identified intranuclear eosinophilic inclusion bodies, reminiscent of viral inclusions. A cause was not identified. In 1945, in Antwerp, van Bogaert [17] described a child with a similar history; the white matter pathology showed sclerosing lesions, which van Bogaert called "subacute sclerosing leucoencephalitis" (SSLE). Clinicians began to identify these cases as "Dawson's encephalitis." Their clinical course was similar and they all died. Their brains showed both inclusion bodies and diffuse sclerosing lesions involving white and gray matter. Ultimately the common name, SSPE, first suggested by Greenfield [18], became accepted.

Epidemiology

SSPE occurs 5–10 years after initial MV infection. Some cases occur post vaccination. Global incidence is one case per million population per year [19]. Vaccination reduces the risk 10-20-fold [20]. The annual incidence of SSPE has declined steadily in countries with measles vaccination programs and is typically below 0.05 per million population, but it remains higher at more than 20 per million in countries with poor measles control [21].

Estimates of the risk vary from 4 to 11 per 100 000 patients with measles [21]. For unknown reasons, the male-to-female ratio is approximately 2 : 1 [22]. There is a 16-fold increased risk in children whose primary infection occurs at younger than two years of age compared with >5 years.

Pathogenesis and genetics

Despite occasional reports [23], proof of direct CNS infection in acute measles is lacking, although electroencephalogram (EEG) abnormalities and cerebrospinal fluid (CSF) lymphocytosis suggest that the virus accesses the CNS.

Key factors in the pathogenesis of SSPE are thought to be (i) an inadequate cellular immune response allowing virus to persist within infected cells and (ii) hypermutation of particular regions of the viral genome that encode the M, H, and F proteins, with subsequent clonal expansion of mutated virus within the brain [6]. Sequence analysis of MV genomes in SSPE shows mutations throughout the genome. Infected neurons and oligodendroglia contain mutated viral genome and truncated genome with deletions. These mutations result in (i) absence of the matrix protein M on the inner aspect of the envelope, (ii) alteration of the hemagglutinin protein H, responsible for binding to the cell surface receptor, and (iii) alteration of the fusion protein F. The virus is unable to bud to the exterior but cell-to-cell transfer is possible, so virus spreads within the brain by local cell fusion. By this manner of spread, MV evades the immune system, which produces high titers of antibodies to viral proteins other than the M protein. The strong humoral immune response provides a continuing selective pressure that favors expansion of the mutated virus. An immature cellular immune system in early life, combined with the presence of circulating maternal antibodies to MV during the first months of life, may similarly promote the emergence of mutant clones and contribute to the increased risk of SSPE that follows infection at a very early age.

Demyelination may be a result of viral or cytokine-induced oligodendroglial or myelin damage or other immune response against oligodendrocytes or myelin [24].

Clinical presentation

Onset of SSPE is usually between 5 and 15 years but the range extends from 1 to 35 years. Most patients have a history of measles usually at an early age (before two years in about half of cases) [22]. Rarely, SSPE occurs during infancy as a complication of maternal infection shortly before delivery [25]. The average interval from measles to SSPE is seven years [22], but in cases complicating maternal infection, the latent period is reduced to a few months [25], and in older-onset cases, the interval may be as long as 22 years [26].

Classically, the disease has four stages [27].
- The first stage is characterized by insidious development of intellectual impairment and behavioral abnormalities. At least half of patients develop visual disturbances because of macular chorioretinitis (which may be the earliest manifestation).
- After about one to two months, most patients enter the second stage lasting two to three months, during which intellectual decline accelerates and episodic motor disturbances become prominent. Patients often show repetitive symmetrical myoclonic jerks every 5–10 seconds, associated with characteristic changes on electroencephalogram (EEG).
- During the third stage, which usually lasts one to four months, patients become uncommunicative and develop various combinations of ataxia, spasticity, choreoathetosis, and dystonia with gradual disappearance of myoclonus. Drop attacks may occur.
- The fourth and final stage may last for months to years during which stupor, mutism, and autonomic disturbances occur, with coma finally leading to death.

The disease progression is very variable. Median survival is 1.8 years, but death may occur within months or disease may progress only intermittently with survival for more than 10 years. Some patients experience periods of clinical improvement or stabilization that can last several years [28]. Short fulminant cases are also described, most often in familial cases suggesting genetic susceptibility [29].

Characteristic slow waves are found on EEG. MV antibody titer is increased in CSF as compared to serum (normal ratio 1 : 200). Measles RNA can be identified in fresh-frozen biopsy or postmortem brain tissue by immunofluorescence using monoclonal antibody to the anti-nucleocapsid protein (N) and can be detected by sequencing the real-time polymerase chain reaction (PCR) amplicon from fresh-frozen brain.

Neuropathology

Autopsied brain may be macroscopically normal or, in prolonged survival, show atrophy. The lesions involve both gray and white matter. In the gray matter, the cortex is predominantly affected, but involvement of the basal ganglia, mainly the thalamus, is frequent, and there may be extension to the brainstem. The white matter is demyelinated, gli-

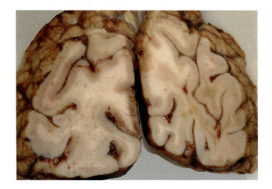

Figure 10.1 Subacute sclerosing panencephalitis (SSPE) macroscopic appearance. The occipital white matter is pale and gliotic bilaterally.

otic and may be thin and atrophic in prolonged cases (Figure 10.1 and 10.2).

Microscopic examination shows the features of subacute encephalitis. There is neuronal loss, occasional neuronophagia, and astrocytic and microglial reaction. Inclusion bodies may be found in neuronal and glial, mainly oligodendroglial, nuclei (Figure 10.3). Immunocytochemistry for measles antigen enables infected cells to be easily seen (Figure 10.4a) and can be used to identify the MV strain genotype, which can be helpful in supporting a vaccine or nonvaccine origin [30]. In situ hybridization for MV using a radiolabeled probe may also demonstrate the virus (Figure 10.4b). Inclusion bodies can be scarce and are better detected by immunohistochemistry. Inflammatory cells may be scanty but leptomeningeal, perivascular, and parenchymal inflammatory infiltrates including lymphocytes and macrophages are found in both gray and white matter. In late cases, there may be considerable neuronal loss with atrophy of the cortex and basal ganglia, associated with severe gliosis. Tau-positive neurofibrillary tangles of the Alzheimer type have been reported.

Measles inclusion body encephalitis

Definition of the disorder and major synonyms

This subacute type of measles encephalitis develops within months of the initial systemic infection in patients with depressed cell-mediated immunity,

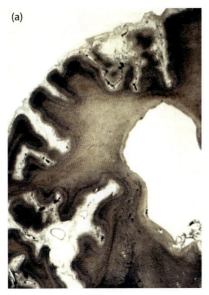 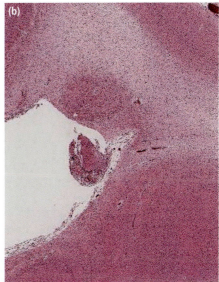

Figure 10.2 Subacute sclerosing panencephalitis (SSPE) lesions of the white matter. (a) Whole mount section showing marked loss of deep myelin, Loyez stain. (b) Occipital white matter loss (hematoxylin and eosin [H&E] × 40).

especially those with congenital or acquired T-lymphocyte deficiency, including patients with human immunodeficiency virus (HIV), and cancer, and undergoing chemotherapy. Several names have been used for this condition: "acute measles encephalitis associated with immunosuppression," "subacute measles virus encephalitis," or "measles inclusion-body encephalitis" (MIBE).

Epidemiology
Most affected patients are children with leukemia or lymphoma or other causes of immunosuppression [31]. In patients with the acquired immune deficiency syndrome (AIDS), similar changes have been reported after measles vaccination [32]. Very rarely, MIBE has been reported in patients who are immunocompetent. In one such case, a vaccine strain of measles was responsible [33].

Pathogenesis
The relatively few detailed serological and molecular genetic studies conducted in MIBE suggest that viral clones present in the CNS have undergone mutations of the genomic sequences encoding the M, H, and F proteins, resulting in their restricted or abnormal expression, similar to SSPE [34].

The mechanisms of persistence and spread of the virus are probably the same in MIBE and SSPE but, because of impaired cell mediated immunity in MIBE, the disease course is usually more rapid, viral inclusions are more abundant, and lymphocytic inflammation is milder or absent [6].

Clinical features
Following initial usually good clinical recovery from the acute illness, seizures, confusion, altered consciousness, and visual defects develop one to seven months post infection. There may be epilepsia partialis continua. The disease progresses to coma and in most cases, death within a few weeks of onset. A few patients have survived but have severe neurological dysfunction. EEG changes are non-specific. CSF is generally normal.

Neuropathology
The diagnosis is made only on pathological examination.

Gross examination of the brain is usually normal but may show focal softening and discoloration of the white matter.

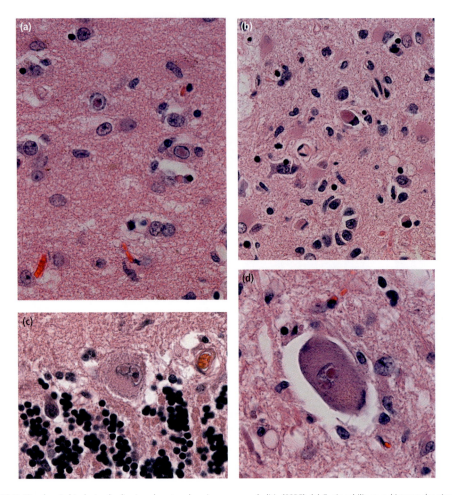

Figure 10.3 Measles viral inclusion bodies in subacute sclerosing panencephalitis (SSPE). (a) Eosinophilic round intranuclear inclusions. (b) Cytoplasmic inclusions probably in astrocytes. Astrocytic hyperplasia and hypertrophy are also evident. (c) Inclusions in a Purkinje cell (d) and in a hypoglossal nucleus neuron.

Microscopically, there may be extensive zones of necrosis of gray and white matter. The lesions may be focal or widespread throughout the brain; involvement of the spinal cord has been found in children with AIDS. The diagnostic feature is the presence of eosinophilic inclusion bodies that are readily seen on routine stains (Figure 10.5) [35] but can also be demonstrated by immunohistochemistry and electron microscopy. These are mostly intranuclear and involve neurons more than astrocytes and oligodendrocytes. Cytoplasmic inclusions may also be found. Occasionally, virus-containing multinucleated giant cells, which can occur in the lung in acute MV infection, may be found. Reactive astrocytes, inflammatory infiltrates, and microglia may be very scanty, or absent, and the inclusions may be missed.

Animal models

Although animals are not natural reservoirs for measles infection, hamsters, rats, and mice, both genetically modified and not, have been used to study the effects of MV on the CNS [36]. The identification of the human receptors for measles CD46 and CD150 (SLAM) has facilitated the study of measles pathogenesis in humanized mice for

Measles Virus Infection of the CNS **Chapter 10**

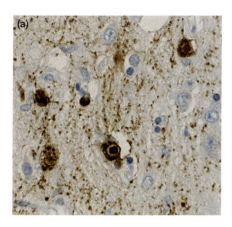
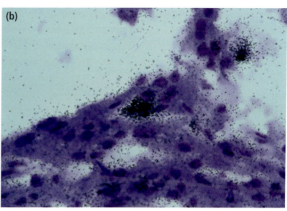

Figure 10.4 Subacute sclerosing panencephalitis (SSPE). (a) Immunocytochemistry shows strongly positive uptake within the intranuclear inclusions. DAB × 200. (b) In situ hybridization for measles virus (MV) in a case of SSPE using a radiolabeled probe × 200. Source: *Courtesy Dr. Peter Dowling, at Rutgers New Jersey Medical School.*

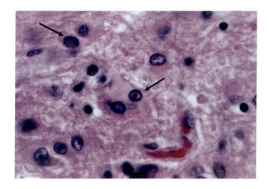

Figure 10.5 Measles inclusion body encephalitis (MIBE) in a boy, age 2½ years, with acquired immunodeficiency syndrome (AIDS; mother was an intravenous drug user) with measles myelitis. The child also had vacuolar myelopathy [35]. Large intranuclear inclusions (arrows). There is almost no inflammatory response. (hematoxylin and eosin [H&E] × 400).

analysis of virus-host interactions and immune responses for viral clearance [37]. For detailed animal models see [37].

Treatment

There is no specific antiviral treatment for MV, but most patients recover from the acute illness without sequelae. Vaccination is effective and safe in the overwhelming majority of children but, unfortunately, is not globally available. In general, measles vaccination is contraindicated in children who are immunosuppressed, except those with HIV infection because their morbidity and mortality from natural measles is very high [2]. Current vaccination programs, although successful, have been insufficient to induce herd immunity in the population because of (i) higher rates of primary and secondary vaccine failure in clinical practice versus that seen in clinical trials; (ii) the inability to guarantee a minimum of two doses of vaccine to every individual in the population, including subgroups in which vaccination is contraindicated; (iii) cost; (iv) cold-chain requirements, and (v) variations in immune responses because of genetic variations [15]. For these reasons, some have advocated development of a third-generation measles vaccine based on "vaccinomics" [15, 38]. Vaccinomics integrates immunogenomics and immunogenetics with systems biology and immune profiling [38].

SSPE and MIBE are usually fatal, and treatments consist of controlling seizures and supportive and palliative care. The nucleoside analogue ribavirin was used successfully to treat MIBE in a four-year-old girl with leukemia [39]. Turner et al. [40] reported two children who received a single dose of measles, mumps, and rubella vaccine in the first year of life, developed MIBE after kidney transplantation but partially recovered neurologically, which the authors attributed to a combination of prior vaccination, reduced immunosuppressive therapy, and treatment with intravenous immunoglobulin and ribavirin.

References

1. Griffin, D. (2013). Measles virus. In: *Fields virology*, 6e (eds. D. Knipe, P. Howley, J. Cohen, et al.), 1042–1069. Philadelphia, PA: Lippincott Williams & Wilkins.
2. Coughlin, M.M., Beck, A.S., Bankamp, B., and Rota, P.A. (2017). Perspective on global measles epidemiology and control and the role of novel vaccination strategies. *Viruses* 9: 11.
3. Centers for Disease Control (1981). Measles encephalitis -United States, 1962-79. *MMWR* 30: 362–364.
4. Centers for Disease Control (1998). Measles mumps and rubella-vaccine use and strategies for elimination of measles rubella and congenital rubella syndrome and control of mumps; recommendations of the advisory committee on immunisation practices (ACIP). *MMWR* 47: 1–57.
5. Maldonado, Y.A. (2003). Rubeola virus (measles and subacute sclerosing panencephalitis). In: *Principles and Practice of Pediatric Infectious Diseases*, 2e (eds. S.S. Long, L.K. Pickering and C.G. Prober), 1148–1155. Philadelphia: Churchill Livingstone.
6. Love, S., Wiley, C.A., and Lucas, S. (2015). Viral infection. In: *Greenfield's Neuropathology*, 9e (eds. S. Love, H. Budka, J.W. Ironside and A. Perry), 1144–1147. CRC Press.
7. Moss, W.J. and Griffin, D.E. (2012). Measles. *Lancet* 379: 153–164.
8. Mason, W.H., Ross, L.A., Lanson, J., and Wright, H.T. Jr. (1993). Epidemic measles in the postvaccine era: evaluation of epidemiology, clinical presentation and complications of suspected measles in hospitalized children. *Pediatr. Infect. Dis. J.* 12: 42–48.
9. McBrien, J., Murphy, J., Gill, D. et al. (2003). Measles outbreak in Dublin, 2000. *Pediatr. Infect. Dis. J.* 22: 580–584.
10. Katz, S.L. and Hinman, A.R. (2004). Summary and conclusions: measles elimination meeting, 16 to 17 march 2000. *J. Infect. Dis.* 189 (Suppl 1): S43–S47.
11. Orenstein, W. and Seib, K. (2014). Mounting a good offense against measles. *N. Engl. J. Med.* 371: 1661–1663.
12. Seward, J.F. and Orenstein, W.A. (2012). Editorial commentary: a rare event: a measles outbreak in a population with high 2-dose measles vaccine coverage. *Clin. Infect. Dis.* 55: 403–405.
13. De Serres, G., Boulianne, N., Defay, F. et al. (2012). Higher risk of measles when the first dose of a 2-dose schedule of measles vaccine is given at 12-14 months versus 15 months of age. *Clin. Infect. Dis.* 55: 394–402.
14. Tan, P.L., Jacobson, R.M., Poland, G.A. et al. (2001). Twin studies of immunogenicity – determining the genetic contribution to vaccine failure. *Vaccine* 19 (17–19): 2434–2439.
15. Haralambieva, I.H., Ovsyannikova, I.G., Shane Pankratz, V. et al. (2013). The genetic basis for interindividual immune response variation to measles vaccine: new understanding and new vaccine approaches. *Expert Rev. Vaccines* 12: 57–70.
16. Dawson, J.R. Jr. (1933). Cellular inclusions in cerebral lesions of lethargic encephalitis. *Am. J. Pathol.* 9: 7–15.
17. van Bogaert, L. (1945). Une leucoencéphalite sclérosante subaiguë. *J. Neurol. Neurosurg. Psychiatry* 8: 101–120.
18. Greenfield, J.G. (1950). Encephalitis and encephalomyelitis in England and Wales during the last decade. *Brain* 73: 141–166.
19. Dimova, P. and Bojinova, V. (2000). Subacute sclerosing panencephalitis with atypical onset. Clinical computed tomographic and magnetic imaging correlations. *Child. Neurol.* 15: 258–260.
20. Farrington, C.P. (1991). Subacute sclerosing panencephalitis in England and Wales transient effects and risk estimates. *Stat. Med.* 10: 1733–1744.
21. Campbell, H., Andrews, N., Brown, K.E., and Miller, E. (2007). Review of the effect of measles vaccination on the epidemiology of SSPE. *Int. J. Epidemiol.* 36 (6): 1334–1348.
22. Modlin, J.F., Halsey, N.A., Eddins, D.L. et al. (1979). Epidemiology of subacute sclerosing panencephalitis. *J. Pediatr.* 94: 231–236.
23. Ter Meulen, V., Muller, D., Kackell, Y., and Katz, M. (1972). Isolation of infectious measles virus in measles encephalitis. *Lancet* 2: 1172–1175.
24. Stohlman, S.A. and Hinton, D.R. (2001). Viral induced demyelination. *Brain Pathol.* 11: 92–96.
25. Dasopolou, M. and Covanis, A. (2004). Subacute sclerosing panencephalitis after intrauterine infection. *Acta Paediatr.* 93: 1251–1253.
26. Singer, C., Lang, A.E., and Suchowersky, O. (1997). Adult onset subacute sclerosing panencephalitis: case report and review of the literature. *Mov. Disord.* 12: 342–353.

27. Jabbour, J.T., Garcia, J.H., Lemmi, H. et al. (1969). Subacute sclerosing panencephalitis: a multidisciplinary study of eight cases. *JAMA* 207: 2248–2254.
28. Cobb, W.A., Marshall, J., and Scaravilli, F. (1984). Long survival in subacute sclerosing panencephalitis. *J. Neurol. Neurosurg. Psychiatry* 47: 176–183.
29. Sharma, V., Gupta, V.B., and Eisenhut, M. (2008). Familial subacute sclerosing panencephalitis. *Pediatr. Neurol.* 3: 215–217.
30. Wight, C., Jin, L., Nelson, S.C. et al. (2003). An autopsy-proven case of fulminant subacute sclerosing panencephalitis. *Neuropathol. Appl. Neurobiol.* 29: 312–320.
31. Aicardi, J., Goutieres, F., Arsenio-Nusnes, M.L., and Lebon, P. (1977). Acute measles encephalitis in children with immunosuppression. *Pediatrics* 59: 232–239.
32. Budka, H., Urbanits, S., Liberski, P.P. et al. (1996). Subacute measles virus encephalitis a new and fatal opportunistic infection in a patient with AIDS. *Neurology* 46: 586–587.
33. Bitnun, A., Shannon, P., Durward, A. et al. (1999). Measles inclusion-body encephalitis caused by the vaccine strain of measles virus. *Clin. Infect. Dis.* 29: 855–861.
34. Suryanaryana, K., Baczko, K., ter Meulen, V., and Wagner, R.R. (1994). Transcription inhibition and other properties of matrix proteins expressed by M genes cloned from measles virus and diseased human brain tissue. *J. Virol.* 68: 1532–1543.
35. Sharer, L.R., Dowling, P.C., Michaels, J. et al. (1990). Spinal cord disease in children with HIV-1 infection: a combined molecular biological and neuropathological study. *Neuropathol. Appl. Neurobiol.* 16: 317–331.
36. Reuter, D. and Schneider-Schaulies, J. (2010). Measles virus infection of the CNS: human disease, animal models and approaches to therapy. *Med. Microbiol. Immunol.* 199: 261–271.
37. Sellin, C.I. and Horvat, B. (2009). Current animal models: transgenic animal models for the study of measles pathogenesis. In: *Measles. Current Topics in Microbiology and Immunology* (eds. D.E. Griffin and O. MBA), 330. Springer Verlag Heidelberg.
38. Poland, G.A., Ovsyannikova, I.G., Kennedy, R.B. et al. (2011). Vaccinomics and a new paradigm for the development of preventive vaccines against viral infections. *OMICS* 15: 625–663.
39. Mustafa, M.M., Weitman, S.D., Winick, N.J. et al. (1993). Subacute measles encephalitis in the young immunocompromised host: report of 2 cases diagnosed by polymerase chain rection and treated with ribavirin and review of literature. *Clin. Infect. Dis.* 16: 654–660.
40. Turner, A., Jeyaratnam, D., Haworth, F. et al. (2006). Measles –associated encephalopathy in children with renal transplant. *Am. J. Transplant.* 6: 1459–1465.

11 Rubella Virus

Bette K. Kleinschmidt-DeMasters

Department of Pathology, Neurosurgery, and Neurology, University of Colorado School of Medicine, Aurora, CO, USA

Abbreviations

ADEM	Acute disseminated encephalomyelitis
CRS	Congenital rubella syndrome
CSF	Cerebrospinal fluid
GBS	Guillain-Barré syndrome
MMR	Measles, mumps, rubella
MMRV	Measles, mumps, rubella, varicella
RT-PCR	Reverse transcriptase-polymerase chain reaction testing
RV	Rubella virus
SSPE	Subacute sclerosisng panencephalitis

Definition of the disorder, major synonyms, and historical perspective

Rubella is often known among laypersons as "German" or "3-day" measles. The original name for the exanthematous childhood disease was the German term, *Rötheln*. Henry Veale described 30 cases in 1866 and felt that "Rötheln is harsh and foreign to our ears. Rubeola notha and Roseola idiopathica are too long for general use and certainly are expressive of conclusions which are yet to be proved. I therefore venture to propose Rubella as a substitute for Rötheln" [1]. It has been referred to as rubella (Latin, "little red") ever since [2]. A viral etiology was suspected before, but not confirmed until, 1962 [2]. The notion of the benign nature of rubella infection was shattered in 1941 when Norman Gregg, an ophthalmologist, described its association with devastating consequences in infants infected in the early weeks of pregnancy [1].

Rubella virus (RV) causes four different clinical disorders: (i) an acquired, generally benign, self-limiting postnatal infection that usually occurs in children and causes fever and rash; (ii) rubella encephalitis, a complication of the acquired infection seen in <0.1% of patients; (iii) congenital rubella syndrome (CRS) in infants born to mothers affected by acquired viral infection during the first trimester and manifesting microcephaly, cataracts, and hearing loss; and (iv) very rare progressive rubella panencephalitis, a disorder causing neurological deterioration that can follow a decade or more after either acquired postnatal infection or CRS.

Microbiological characteristics

RV is a single-stranded, positive-sense enveloped RNA virus of the Togaviridae family. No arthropod or tick vector is required for transmission: human-to-human transmission is via respiratory droplets that infect cells in the upper respiratory tract. The virus then spreads locally in lymphoid tissues before being hematogenously disseminated throughout the body [2]. Viral production in the

Infections of the Central Nervous System: Pathology and Genetics, First Edition. Edited by Fabrice Chrétien, Kum Thong Wong, Leroy R. Sharer, Catherine (Katy) Keohane and Françoise Gray.
© 2020 John Wiley & Sons Ltd. Published 2020 by John Wiley & Sons Ltd.

upper respiratory tract parallels the development of craniocervical lymphadenopathy, which is the key clinical finding. In women who are pregnant, maternal viremia results in the infection of the placenta and the fetus.

The RV virion is small and encodes three structural proteins, the C1 coat protein and two envelope glycoproteins, E1 and E2, as well as two nonstructural proteins [2, 3]. RV enters cells through receptor-mediated endocytosis [2]. A 700+ nucleotide region in the E1 glycoprotein is the site for genotyping different strains of RV; genotyping can be critical for detecting whether strains of virus during epidemics are already circulating, based on previous genotyping data, or newly introduced [4].

Epidemiology: incidence and prevalence, sex, age, geographical distribution, and risk factors

Before the advent of effective vaccine coverage, epidemics typically occurred at six- to nine-year intervals [2] and still maintain this pattern in parts of the world where vaccination is not routine, such as Ethiopia [5]. Because rubella-caused rash, fever, and lymphadenopathy is almost always mild and without sequelae, the main reason for effective vaccination is to reduce CRS. Vaccination programs in countries with broad coverage of at-risk populations with either measles, mumps, and rubella (MMR) or measles, mumps, rubella, with varicella (MMRV) vaccines, given at 12–15 months of age with second dose before kindergarten or first-grade school entry, has hugely reduced disease burden because of the high rate of seroconversion (>95%) [2].

However, outbreaks continue to be reported, largely due to suboptimal or absent vaccination programs in some countries, including Japan [6, 7], Tunisia [8, 9], China [10], Romania [4], and Poland [11]. An outbreak in Japan in 2012–2013 caused acute infection in more than 15 000 persons, most of whom were young adult males who had not received vaccination in childhood and also resulted in 43 cases of CRS [7].

Vaccination challenges still remain in Europe in that 1708 cases of rubella were reported in 28 countries in the European region from 1 July 2015 to 30 June 2016 [12]. The highest incidence was in Poland, where 1553 cases were reported, followed by 91 cases in Germany. As a result of circulating rubella, CRS still occurs in the European Union, with 7–23 cases reported annually. Travel to areas where infection is endemic can also result in infection in unvaccinated persons [13, 14].

Clinical features

Major symptoms
Exanthem-producing febrile acute infection
Most acquired postnatal, exanthem-producing infections in children are mild to minimally symptomatic, with some studies suggesting that up to 40% of children with rubella infection do not develop clinical disease; more severe disease tends to occur in adults [2]. In unvaccinated populations, acute rubella infection is usually seen in school-age children [10, 15].

Patients are contagious for two weeks, one week prior and one week after onset of rash [2]. In almost all patients, infection or vaccination yields lifelong immunity. In rare instances, recurrent infection occurs but is generally asymptomatic, devoid of viremia, and only detectable by laboratory testing [2].

Clinically evident acquired rubella infection produces a lymphadenopathy, "the absence of which should raise suspicion of alternative diagnoses" [2]. The lymphadenopathy characteristically involves the posterior auricular, posterior cervical, and suboccipital lymph nodes [15] and may persist for weeks [2].

The rubella rash is erythematous, maculopapular (Figure 11.1), and less severe than that seen with measles [15]. It begins on the face, spreads to the trunk, and disappears over three to five days. Low-grade fever, inflammation of nasal mucosal membranes, and conjunctivitis are variable [15].

Encephalitis
Neurologic complications of rubella include encephalitis, aseptic meningitis, myelitis, or Guillain-Barré syndrome (GBS). These complications, usually appearing within six days of the rash, consist of headache, vomiting, somnolence, and seizures in cases of encephalitis. Overall, less than 0.1% of rubella cases are associated with neurologic complications. [15]

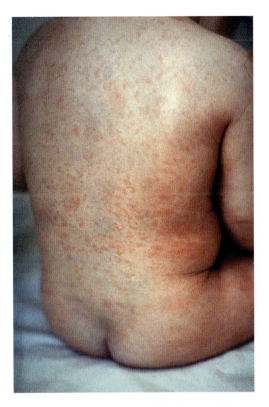

Figure 11.1 Acquired, postnatal rubella infection rash. (Source: Center for Disease Control website, with permission.)

To put the low incidence of rubella encephalitis into perspective, in a recent study investigating the etiology of acute viral meningitis and encephalitis in Chinese children [16], rubella was the cause of 2.2% of proven encephalitis and 3.3% of proven meningitis cases, far less frequent than neurological complications of enterovirus or herpesvirus [17]. The 2011–2012 outbreak in Tunisia reported a higher incidence of encephalitis [8]. Childhood rubella encephalitis was associated with at least one episode of seizures (95%), maculopapular rash (81%), status epilepticus (76%), and death in 2/21 children (9.5%, median age nine years) [9]. Survivors, fortunately, had no neurological sequelae six months after discharge from the intensive care unit[9].

Reports of fulminant and fatal encephalitis associated with a vaccine strain of rubella virus, with disease onset 10 days after vaccination, are exceedingly rare [17]. The occasional patient with rubella-associated Guillain-Barré syndrome manifests symmetrical weakness with hyporeflexia.

Unlike encephalitis, complications in non-CNS organs are not rare, especially in rubella occurring in young adults. In the Japanese 2012–2013 outbreak mostly affecting young adults, sequelae included arthralgia/arthritis (19.4%), thrombocytopenic purpura (0.5%), and hepatic dysfunction (0.3%) compared with encephalitis (0.1%) [6].

CRS

Hallmark clinical features of CRS are cataracts, sensorineural hearing loss, and congenital heart disease, consisting of patent ductus arteriosus or septal defects. Although these features are the hallmarks, rubella virus can infect many tissues, causing intrauterine growth retardation, microphthalmia, chorioretinitis, hepatosplenomegaly, hepatitis, 'blueberry muffin' rash, interstitial pneumonitis, osteopathy, or thrombocytopenia [15]. One study found that rubella defects occurred in all infants infected before the 11th gestational week (principally congenital heart disease and deafness) and in 35% of those infected at 13–16 weeks (deafness alone). No defects attributable to rubella were found in 63 children infected after 16 weeks [18].

Progressive rubella panencephalitis

The rarest clinical manifestation of rubella infection, progressive rubella panencephalitis, can occur as a late sequela of CRS or acute rubella infection [3]. Spasticity, ataxia, intellectual deterioration, and seizures show onset in the second decade [19]. The neurodegenerative disorder shows more

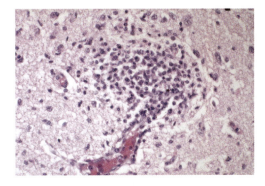

Figure 11.2 Encephalitis associated with acute rubella infection occurs in <0.1% of persons in most outbreaks and can show microglial clusters in brain tissue. (Source: From the collection of the late Dr. Sydney Schochet.)

Infections of the Central Nervous System

cerebellar symptomatology than measles-associated subacute sclerosing panencephalitis [20].

Laboratory testing

A definite clinical diagnosis of acquired rubella infection based on rash features is not possible because overlap exists with other childhood rash-producing disorders, especially measles. Laboratory confirmation of acquired rubella infection depends on measurement of serum titers of rubella-specific immunoglobulin M (IgM) and immunoglobulin G (IgG), with a single positive IgM sample or a fourfold increase in titer between acute and convalescent serum samples (i.e. two to three weeks apart) [2]. Isolation of virus from throat swabs, urine, or synovial fluid is usually not performed, and reverse transcriptase-polymerase chain reaction (RT-PCR) testing may be superior to viral isolation.

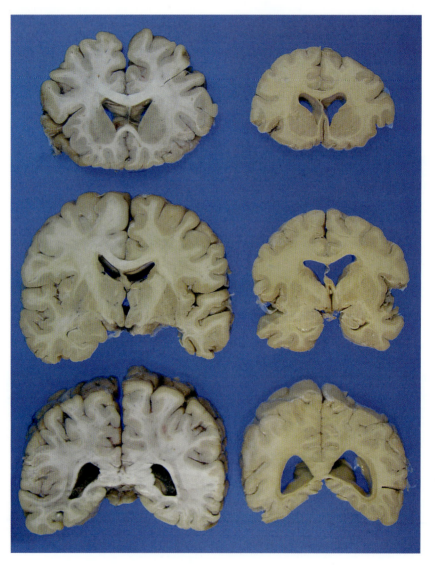

Figure 11.3 Congenital rubella syndrome (CRS): Microcephaly. Microcephalic brain on the right from a woman, conceived during the last US pandemic 1963–1965, and who had severe developmental delay and cataracts, was mute, deaf, and blind, and died at 41 years of age. At autopsy her brain weighed 870 g (right); compared with a 1350-g brain from a normal 76-year-old man (left). Note the absence of malformations.

Rubella Virus **Chapter 11**

Acute rubella encephalitis is confirmed by rubella IgM in the appropriate clinical setting of neurological symptoms [2].

Progressive rubella panencephalitis diagnosis is based on the clinical syndrome in combination with cerebrospinal fluid (CSF) analysis; neuroimaging studies show global cerebral and specifically cerebellar volume loss [2]. CSF may show mild lymphocytic pleocytosis, elevated total protein related to elevations in immunoglobulin, and even oligoclonal bands [2].

Pathology

Acute rubella encephalitis shows neuronal degeneration, absence of demyelination, petechial hemorrhages, sometimes relatively minimal inflammation, and few microglial nodules (Figure 11.2) [2].

Progressive rubella panencephalitis is described as showing perivascular lymphocytes and plasma cells most prominent in white matter, along with

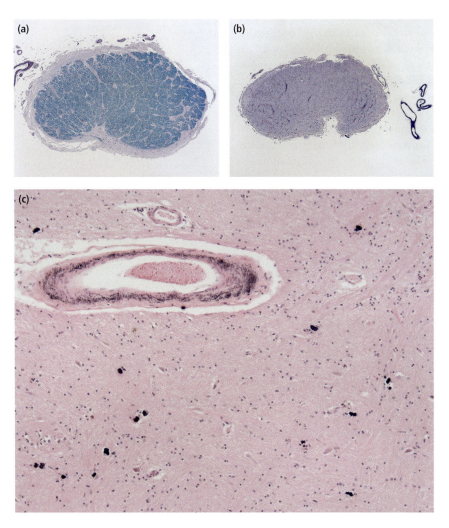

Figure 11.4 Congenital rubella syndrome (CRS): Microscopy. Same patient as Figure 11.3, she likely also showed unilateral pigmentary retinopathy in addition to cataracts, as evidenced by the unilateral optic nerve atrophy and total myelin loss. (b) (Luxol fast blue-periodic acid Schiff) compared to the normal unaffected nerve (a). She also showed the classic mineralization of small vessels and basophilic mineral deposits in basal ganglia (c).

neuronal loss, microglial nodules, and gliosis. Unlike subacute sclerosing panencephalitis (SSPE) caused by measles, there is minimal gray matter involvement, no viral neuronal inclusions, and more cerebellar involvement [2].

CRS causes microcephaly, usually unassociated with other malformations (Figure 11.3). Microscopically, extensive damage to cerebral blood vessels is seen, especially in cerebrum, particularly smaller arterial and venous branches of leptomeninges and those supplying the centrum ovale and deep gray matter (striatum, thalamus) [20, 21]. Infants show destruction of vessel walls and replacement by deposits of amorphous granular material. Death at a later time period results in extensive vascular dystrophic mineralization (Figure 11.4c). Optic atrophy or pigmentary retinitis can result in severe optic nerve atrophy or myelin loss (Figure 11.4a and b).

Recent immunohistochemical studies demonstrated RV antigens in the outer granular layer of the cerebellum [4] and in the ciliary body which could play an important role in cataractogenesis [22].

Genetic and pathogenesis

There is no well-described genetic explanation as to why only certain infected individuals develop rubella encephalitis or progressive rubella panencephalitis.

The pathogenesis of acute rubella encephalitis is thought to be direct infection by virus, with neuronal degeneration but no demyelination, the latter distinguishing it from postinfectious or acute disseminated encephalomyelitis (ADEM).

Progressive rubella panencephalitis may be because of immune complex deposition [23], although one of the original studies also suggested CNS viral replication in vascular endothelium [24].

The pathogenesis of CRS is due to rubella virus-induced cell-cycle arrest, apoptosis, and cytoskeletal and mitochondrial changes [25, 26]. These data correlate well with the major CNS feature of CRS, microcephaly.

Treatment, future perspective, and conclusions

Given the mildness of almost all cases of acquired rubella infection, only control of fever, or arthralgias if they occur, is necessary. Prevention of all forms of rubella infection, especially CRS, is through vaccination coverage. Large-scale monitoring programs and initiatives such as the World Health Assembly Global Vaccine Action Plan and the World Health Organization plan to eliminate measles and, in some regions also rubella, by 2020 [27] are already seeing results.

References

1. Forbes, J.A. (1969). Rubella: historical aspects. *Am. J. Dis. Child.* 118: 5–11.
2. Tyor, W. and Harrison, T. (2014). Mumps and rubella. *Handb. Clin. Neurol.*: 591–600.
3. Frey, T.K. (1994). Molecular biology of rubella virus. *Adv. Virus Res.* 44: 69–160.
4. Lazar, M., Perelygina, L., Martines, R. et al. (2015). Immunolocalization and distribution of rubella antigen in fatal congenital rubella syndrome. *EBioMedicine* 3: 86–92.
5. Getahun, M., Beyene, B., Gallagher, K. et al. (2016). Epidemiology of rubella virus cases in the pre-vaccination era of Ethiopia, 2009–2015. *BMC Public Health* 16: 1168.
6. Sugishita, Y., Shimatani, N., Katow, S. et al. (2015). Epidemiological characteristics of rubella and congenital rubella syndrome in the 2012–2013 epidemics in Tokyo, Japan. *Jpn. J. Infect. Dis.* 68: 159–165.
7. Ugiie, M., Nabae, K., and Shobayashi, T. (2014). Rubella outbreak in Japan. *Lancet* 383: 1460–1461.
8. Messedi, E., Fki-Berrajah, L., Gargouri, S. et al. (2014). Clinical epidemiological and molecular aspects of rubella outbreak with high number of neurological cases, Tunisia 2011–2012. *J. Clin. Virol.* 61: 248–254.
9. Chaari, A., Bahloul, M., Berrajah, L. et al. (2014). Childhood rubella encephalitis: diagnosis, management, and outcome. *J. Child Neurol.* 29: 49–53.
10. Chang, C., Ma, H., Liang, W. et al. (2017). Rubella outbreak and outbreak management in a school setting, China, 2014. *Hum. Vaccin. Immunother.* 13: 772–775.

11. Abramczuk, E., Częścik, A., Pancer, K., and Gut (2016). Problem of rubella in Poland after compensatory outbreak in 2013. *Przegl. Epidemiol.* 70: 549–554.
12. Bianco, V., Spera, A.M., Simeone, D. et al. (2017). An update on epidemiology of congenital rubella syndrome: how far from the World Health Organization goals. *Minerva Med.* 108: 483–485.
13. Hadano, Y. and Honda, J. (2017). Adult rubella in a returned traveler. *Intern. Med.* 56: 2085.
14. Hyle, E.P., Rao, S.R., Jentes, E.S. et al. (2017). Missed opportunities for measles, mumps, rubella vaccination among departing U.S. adult travelers receiving pretravel health consultations. *Ann. Intern. Med.* 167: 77–84.
15. Bale, J.F. Jr. (2014). Measles, mumps, rubella, and human parvovirus B19 infections and neurologic disease. *Handb. Clin. Neurol.* 121: 1345–1353.
16. Ai, J., Xie, Z., Liu, G. et al. Etiology and prognosis of acute viral encephalitis and meningitis in Chinese children: a multicentre prospective study. *BMC Infect. Dis.* 17: 494.
17. Gualberto, F.A., de Oliveira, M.I., Alves, V.A. et al. (2013). Fulminant encephalitis associated with a vaccine strain of rubella virus. *J. Clin. Virol.* 58: 737–740.
18. Miller, E., Cradock-Watson, J.E., and Pollock, T.M. (1982). Consequences of confirmed maternal rubella at successive stages of pregnancy. *Lancet* 2: 781–784.
19. Townsend, J.J., Baringer, J.R., Wolinsky, J.S. et al. (1975). Progressive rubella panencephalitis. Late onset after congenital rubella. *N. Engl. J. Med.* 292: 990–993.
20. Rorke, L.B. and Spiro, A.J. (1967). Cerebral lesions in congenital rubella syndrome. *J. Pediatr.* 70: 243–255.
21. Rorke, L.B. and Spiro, A.J. (1967). Cerebral lesions associated with congenital rubella syndrome. *J. Neuropathol. Exp. Neurol.* 26: 115–117.
22. Nguyen, T.V., Pham, V.H., and Abe, K. (2015). Pathogenesis of congenital rubella virus infection in human fetuses. Viral infection in the ciliary body could play an important role in cataractogenesis. *EBioMedicine* 2: 59–63.
23. Wolinsky, J.S., Waxham, M.N., Hess, J.L. et al. (1982). Immunochemical features of a case of progressive rubella panencephalitis. *Clin. Exp. Immunol.* 48: 359–366.
24. Townsend, J.J., Wolinsky, J.S., and Baringer, J.R. (1976). The neuropathology of progressive rubella panencephalitis of late onset. *Brain* 99: 81–90.
25. Atreya, C.D., Mohan, K.V., and Kulkarni, S. (2004). Rubella virus and birth defects: molecular insights into the viral teratogenesis at the cellular level. *Birth Defects Res. A Clin. Mol. Teratol.* 70: 431–437.
26. Lee, J.Y. and Bowden, D.S. (2000). Rubella virus replication and links to teratogenicity. *Clin. Microbiol. Rev.* 13: 571–575.
27. Datta, S.S., O'Connor, P.M., Jankovic, D. et al. (2018). Progress and challenges in measles and rubella elimination in the WHO European region. *Vaccine* 36: 5408–5415.

12 Henipavirus Encephalitis

Kum Thong Wong[1] and Kien Chai Ong[2]

[1] Department of Pathology, Faculty of Medicine, University of Malaya, Kuala Lumpur, Malaysia
[2] Department of Biomedical Science, Faculty of Medicine, University of Malaya, Kuala Lumpur, Malaysia

Abbreviations

CNS   central nervous system
HeV   Hendra virus
MRI   magnetic resonance imaging
NiV   Nipah virus

Definition of the disorders, major synonyms, and historical perspective

Hendra virus (HeV) was discovered in 1994 after an outbreak in horses and humans in Australia [1]. It was named after the town of Hendra in Queensland, Australia, near where the first outbreak occurred. A few years later in 1999, Nipah virus (NiV) was first isolated after outbreaks in pigs and humans in Malaysia from 1998 to 1999 [2]. The virus was named after the Sungai Nipah Village (or Nipah River Village) in the state of Negri Sembilan, Malaysia. Because both viruses have now been classified under the *Henipavirus* genus, the term "henipavirus encephalitis" has been used to include both HeV and NiV infections because they share similar features.

Microbiological characteristics

The *Henipavirus* genus (family Paramyxoviridae; subfamily Paramxyxovirinae) was originally created for HeV and NiV [3]. Henipaviruses are enveloped, pleomorphic virions averaging about 500 nm (range: 40–1900 nm) and contain typical paramyxoviral "herringbone" nucleocapsids. The unusually large (>18 000 nucleotides), negative-sense, single-stranded RNA viral genomes comprise six genes encoding for the nucleocapsid, phosphoprotein, matrix protein, fusion glycoprotein (F), attachment glycoprotein (G), and the large polymerase (Figure 12.1). The G protein enables attachment to host cell Ephrin B2 or B3 receptors, leading to F protein fusion, and viral entry into cells.

Epidemiology: Incidence and prevalence, sex, age, geographical distribution, and risk factors

A total of 7 human HeV infections with four fatalities have been reported so far, with no cases reported outside Australia [4]. In Malaysia, there were likely

---

Infections of the Central Nervous System: Pathology and Genetics, First Edition. Edited by Fabrice Chrétien,
Kum Thong Wong, Leroy R. Sharer, Catherine (Katy) Keohane and Françoise Gray.
© 2020 John Wiley & Sons Ltd. Published 2020 by John Wiley & Sons Ltd.

Infections of the Central Nervous System

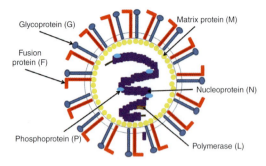

Figure 12.1 Diagrammatic representation of the henipavirus virion with an outer, plasma-membrane–derived envelope through which the viral G and F glycoproteins protrude. The matrix protein is found under the envelope. The central core consists of the nucleocapsid, viral RNA, phosphoprotein, and polymerase. Source: Reproduced from [3] with permission from John Wiley & Sons.

more than 350 human NiV infections, including at least 265 cases of acute NiV encephalitis with 105 fatalities [5]. NiV outbreaks in Bangladesh and India (Bengal) were reported from 2001 onward, probably involving more than 250 people with a higher fatality rate of about 70%. In 2014, 17 people were believed to be infected by NiV in the Philippines [6]. Another outbreak was reported in India (Kerala) in 2018, involving at least 18 people.

The natural host of henipaviruses is the bat, mainly from the *Pteropus* genus (fruit bat or flying fox). Human henipavirus infection may occur in three main ways: direct bat-to-human, bat-to-intermediate host-to-human, and human-to-human transmissions.

The best evidence for direct bat-to-human transmission occurred in Bangladesh where humans were infected by drinking raw date palm sap contaminated by bats infected with NiV [5].

The most common transmission is probably via intermediate hosts from contaminated animal urine and oronasal secretions, either by direct contact or airborne exposure. Human HeV infections in Australia were strongly linked to exposure to horses who were infected. In NiV outbreaks in Malaysia and Singapore, pigs were the main intermediate host, whereas other infected domestic animals, like dogs, may play a minor role. In Bangladesh, domestic animals like goats and cows have been implicated; in the Philippines, horses were thought to be involved in NiV transmission [3].

Human-to-human transmission of infection was firmly established in the NiV outbreaks in Bangladesh and India, in patient contacts including healthcare workers [5]. Human-to-human HeV transmission has not been documented so far.

Clinical features

The incubation period of henipavirus infections ranges from a few days to about three weeks. Milder manifestations include fever, nonspecific influenza-like illness, lethargy, myalgia, and headache [7, 8]. Although acute henipavirus encephalitis is the most serious complication, it is likely that many infections may remain asymptomatic or only result in mild symptoms. Much less is known about acute HeV encephalitis than acute NiV encephalitis, but in general, the clinical manifestations are probably similar. Acute HeV encephalitis is characterized by drowsiness, confusion, ataxia, ptosis, and seizures. One patient with pneumonitis and chest radiograph showing diffuse alveolar shadowing [8] had autopsy evidence of acute encephalitis, which was not clinically apparent [9].

In addition to milder manifestations, acute NiV encephalitis presents with reduced consciousness, areflexia or hyporeflexia, hypotonia, pin-point pupils with variable reactivity, tachycardia, hypertension, and abnormal doll's eye reflex. Segmental myoclonus involving the diaphragm, limbs, neck, and face, if present, may be unique to acute NiV encephalitis. Meningism, generalized tonic–clonic convulsions, nystagmus, and cerebellar signs are also observed.

Magnetic resonance imaging (MRI) in acute henipavirus encephalitis showed multiple, disseminated, generally small discrete hyperintense lesions mainly in the cerebral cortex and subcortical and deep white matter [4].

Mortality in acute henipavirus encephalitis ranged from about 40 to 70% [3]. A slight majority of surviving patients from Malaysia had no long-term sequelae [7], but others may develop neurological and neuropsychiatric sequelae and gait or movement disorders [10]. Fatal intracerebral hemorrhage is a rare complication. Probably less than 10% of survivors of acute NiV infection

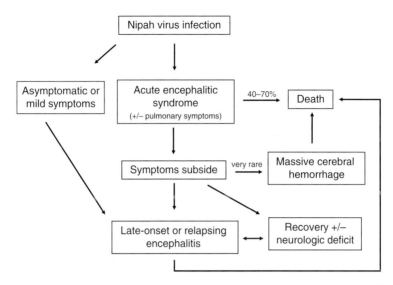

Figure 12.2 Flowchart showing possible clinical syndromes, complications, sequelae, and outcomes after acute Nipah infection. +/-, with or without. Source: Reproduced from [12] with permission from Springer Nature.

(asymptomatic, mild infection, or acute encephalitis) develop relapsing encephalitis occurring weeks to years after exposure to virus [11, 12] (Figure 12.2). So far, there has been only 1 case of relapsing HeV encephalitis [13], whereas about 20 relapsing NiV encephalitis cases have been reported. Brain MRI in relapsing henipavirus encephalitis shows more extensive and confluent hyperintense cortical lesions. Virus could not be cultured from cerebrospinal fluid (CSF), nasotracheal secretions, urine, and brain tissue in NiV-relapsing encephalitis [11].

Detection of anti-henipavirus antibodies by enzyme-linked immunosorbent assay (ELISA) and specific polymerase chain reaction (PCR)-based methods and sequencing to identify henipaviruses are now more widely available for outbreak investigations and diagnosis in animals and humans [14]. In human NiV infection, immunoglobulin M (IgM) seroconversion occurred by two weeks and immunoglobulin G (IgG) seroconversion by about four weeks, persisting for at least three months and several years, respectively [15]. Specific IgM or IgG have also been detected in human HeV infections [16]. Serum neutralization tests that use live viruses as the gold standard to confirm henipavirus infection require biosafety level-4 facilities and so may not be possible in most laboratories. A sensitive surrogate assay using pseudo-typed vesicular stomatitis virus bearing the NiV F and G proteins has been used for henipavirus infections [17].

Pathology of human henipavirus infection

Based on findings in 3 autopsies of HeV and more than 30 autopsies of NiV infections, the pathology of acute HeV and NiV infections appears to be similar [18]. Blood vessels are a major viral target as reflected in the systemic, disseminated small vessel vasculopathy, including varying degrees of endothelial infection or ulceration, vasculitis (Figure 12.3a and g) and vasculitis-induced thrombosis or occlusion (Figure 12.3a) in the CNS, lung, kidney, and other major organs. Thrombosis or occlusion is often associated with parenchymal ischemia or microinfarction (Figure 12.3d) [19]. In some cases, endothelial multinucleated syncytia (Figure 12.3b), a unique feature of henipavirus infection, can be detected (in about 25% of acute NiV infection). Viral antigens/RNA and nucleocapsids have been detected in vascular endothelium, multinucleated giant cells, and smooth muscle.

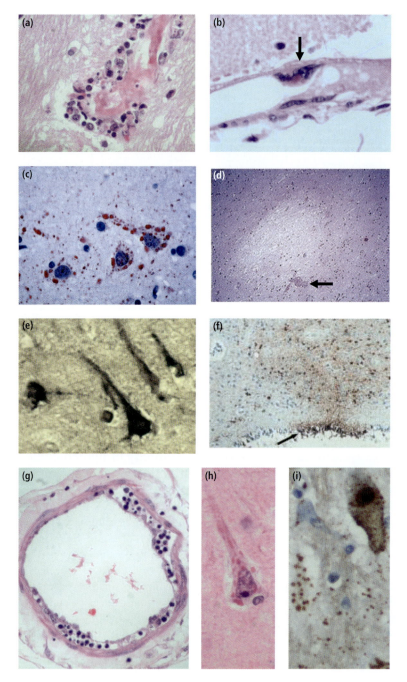

Figure 12.3 Pathology of henipavirus infection: Vasculopathy in Nipah virus encephalitis showing vasculitis, thrombosis (a), and endothelial multinucleated syncytia with viral inclusion (b, arrow). There are numerous Nipah viral inclusions and antigens within neurons (c), especially around necrotic plaques (d). Necrotic plaques may also have evidence of adjacent vascular thrombo-occlusion (d, arrow). Vasculitis in Hendra encephalitis may manifest as mild endotheliitis (g). Hendra viral inclusions (h), antigens (f, i), and RNA (e) can be demonstrated in neurons. Viral antigens in a necrotic plaque and adjacent ependymal lining (f, arrow). Hematoxylin and eosin stain (a, b, d, g, h). Immunohistochemistry with new fuchsin (c) and DAB (f, i) chromogens, hematoxylin counterstain. In situ hybridization with nitro blue tetrazolium/5-bromo-4-cholor-3-indolyl phosphate (NBT/BCIP) substrate, and hematoxylin counterstain. Original magnification: ×40 (a–i). Source: Figure a reproduced from [24] with permission from Springer Nature; Figures c, d reproduced from [19] with permission from Elsevier; Figures e, f, g, h, i reproduced from [9] with permission from John Wiley and Son.

Vasculopathy in the CNS is probably the most severe and frequently found adjacent to discrete necrotic or more subtle vacuolar, plaque-like lesions (Figure 12.3d and f).

Paramyxoviral-type, eosinophilic cytoplasmic (Figure 12.3h) and nuclear inclusions may be found in some neurons in the vicinity of these lesions or around vasculopathy. Antigens/RNA can be readily demonstrated in these neurons or much more rarely, in glial cells (Figure 12.3c, e, f, and i). As such, the plaque-like lesions are probably the combined effects of microinfarction and neuronal infection, although "pure" plaque-like, infected neurons without microinfarction can be found as well. White matter necrotic lesions probably represent "pure" microinfarcts because glial cells are far less susceptible to infection. Neuronophagia, microglial nodule formation, foamy macrophages, perivascular cuffing, and meningitis can also be found. The dual pathogenic mechanisms of vasculopathy and parenchymal cell infection occurring in the CNS and other major organs may be unique to acute henipavirus infection [19].

The pathological features of relapsing henipavirus encephalitis were based on one HeV and two NiV autopsies [9, 11, 18]. Again, relapsing HeV and NiV encephalitides appear similar, but the pathology is confined only to the CNS. Extensive, geographical parenchymal necrosis, edema, and inflammation are found mainly in neuronal areas where there is also prominent perivascular cuffing, severe neuronal loss, reactive gliosis, and neovascularization. Viral inclusions, antigens, RNA, and nucleocapsids can be demonstrated mainly in surviving neurons (Figure 12.4). Severe meningitis was found in many areas. Notably, the vasculopathy seen in acute henipavirus encephalitis is absent, and blood vessels are negative for antigens or RNA. The presence of viral inclusions, nucleocapsids, antigens, and RNA confirmed that relapsing henipavirus encephalitis represents a recurrent infection, rather than postinfectious encephalitis [11]. The absence of vasculopathy and extra-CNS organ involvement suggests reactivation of latent viral foci within the CNS after the acute phase and not CNS reinfection by viremia.

Clinically and pathologically, relapsing henipavirus encephalitis appears to share some similarities to subacute sclerosing panencephalitis, but unlike this entity, so far, viral mutations have not been implicated in relapsing NiV encephalitis [20]. The risk factors for relapsing henipavirus encephalitis are unknown. Viral immunosuppression, well known in measles, has not been reported but may be one possible predisposing factor for relapsing henipavirus encephalitis.

Animal models and pathogenesis

There is a wide range of susceptible animals that can be naturally and experimentally infected,

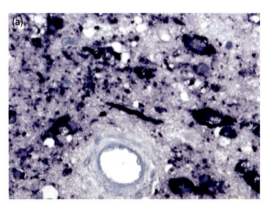
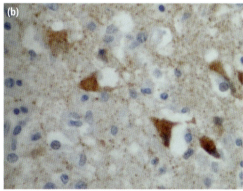

Figure 12.4 Viral antigens in relapsing encephalitis: (a) Viral RNA within neurons in relapsing Nipah encephalitis. Note that the blood vessel shows no evidence of vasculopathy. (b) Viral antigens within neurons in relapsing Hendra encephalitis. Source: Reproduced from [18] with permission from Springer Nature.

including the definitive host (bat), known intermediate hosts (i.e. horse, pig, dog), and other experimental animal models (i.e. mouse, hamster, cat, guinea pig, ferret, chicken embryo, African green monkey, and squirrel monkey) [21]. Overall, these animal studies have contributed much to our understanding of henipavirus pathogenesis, confirming human autopsy findings that the acute infection is a disseminated, multiorgan disease caused by the dual pathogenic mechanisms of vasculopathy and parenchymal cell infection.

Apart from hematogenous spread into the CNS via viremia and damaged blood vessel or blood-brain barrier (BBB), some animal models have demonstrated neuroinvasion via infected nasal mucosa and olfactory bulb [22, 23]. So far, there has been no evidence for this in humans [24]. In experimentally infected hamsters, HeV and NiV infections did not appear to demonstrate very significant differences [25].

The viral determinants that contribute to NiV and HeV pathogenesis remain poorly understood. Recently, NiV V and W proteins were demonstrated to play an important role in pathogenesis and disease outcomes in a ferret model [26]. However, the specific pathogenetic mechanisms involving these proteins are still unknown. Reverse genetics demonstrate that the genetic determinants of viral budding and fusogenic properties of NiV and HeV are different [27].

Treatment, future perspective, and conclusions

To date, there are no approved vaccines or therapeutic agents for human henipavirus infection. In animal models, ribavirin or ribavirin and chloroquine combinations are ineffective against the infection. Other drugs have been suggested as having possible anti-henipavirus effects [28].

Passive immunization strategies using cross-reacting, henipavirus-specific antibodies raised against F and G viral proteins have been found to be effective in animal models [28]. Two patients with acute HeV infection empirically treated with these antibodies apparently showed no adverse side effects, but the antiviral effectiveness could not be verified. Many new vaccine candidates for active immunization have been developed and tested, using different approaches including live recombinant vaccines, subunit vaccines, and virus-like particles that mainly express henipavirus F or G proteins [21]. One of the recombinant subunit vaccines that contained the HeV G glycoprotein has now been licensed for use by the equine industry in Australia.

Because of their worldwide distribution and extensive flying range, pteropid bats, in particular, are potentially highly effective in virus dissemination [29]. Future henipavirus outbreaks following spillover events in new areas or countries are probably inevitable, as shown by the recent outbreaks in the Philippines and India (Kerala) and the seroconversion in some Africans involved with butchering bats for bushmeat [30]. The concept of One Health that integrates activities and contributions of international scientists, ecologists, veterinarians, health professionals, politicians, and other stakeholders may be needed to minimized future outbreaks of bat-borne zoonoses [31].

References

1. Field, H.E. (2016). Hendra virus ecology and transmission. *Curr. Opin. Virol.* 16: 120–125.
2. Chua, K.B., Bellini, W.J., Rota, P.A. et al. (2000). Nipah virus: a recently emergent deadly paramyxovirus. *Science* 288: 1432–1435.
3. Ong, K.C. and Wong, K.T. (2015). Henipavirus encephalitis: recent developments and advances. *Brain Pathol.* 25: 605–613.
4. Mahalingam, S., Herrero, L.J., Playford, E.G. et al. (2012). Hendra virus: an emerging paramyxovirus in Australia. *Lancet Infect. Dis.* 12: 799–807.
5. Clayton, B.A. (2017). Nipah virus: transmission of a zoonotic paramyxovirus. *Curr. Opin. Virol.* 22: 97–104.
6. Ching, P.K., de los Reyes, V.C., Sucaldito, M.N. et al. (2015). Outbreak of Henipavirus infection, Philippines, 2014. *Emerg. Infect. Dis.* 21: 328–331.
7. Goh, K.J., Tan, C.T., Chew, N.K. et al. (2000). Clinical features of Nipah virus encephalitis among pig farmers in Malaysia. *N. Engl. J. Med.* 342: 1229–1235.
8. Playford, E.G., McCall, B., Smith, G. et al. (2010). Human Hendra virus encephalitis associated with

equine outbreak, Australia, 2008. *Emerg. Infect. Dis.* 16: 219–223.
9. Wong, K.T., Robertson, T., Ong, B.B. et al. (2009). Human Hendra virus infection causes acute and relapsing encephalitis. *Neuropathol. Appl. Neurobiol.* 35: 296–305.
10. Sejvar, J.J., Hossain, J., Saha, S.K. et al. (2007). Long term neurological and functional outcome in Nipah virus infection. *Ann. Neurol.* 62: 235–242.
11. Tan, C.T., Goh, K.J., Wong, K.T. et al. (2002). Relapsed and late-onset Nipah encephalitis. *Ann. Neurol.* 51: 703–708.
12. Wong, K.T., Shieh, W.J., Zaki, W.R. et al. (2002). Nipah virus infection, an emerging paramyxoviral zoonosis. *Springer Semin. Immunopathol.* 24: 215–218.
13. O'Sullivan, J.D., Allworth, A.M., Paterson, D.L. et al. (1997). Fatal encephalitis due to novel paramyxovirus transmitted from horses. *Lancet* 349: 93–95.
14. Wang, L.F. and Daniels, P. (2012). Diagnosis of henipavirus infection: current capabilities and future directions. *Curr. Top. Microbiol. Immunol.* 359: 179–196.
15. Ramasundram, V., Tan, C.T., Chua, K.B. et al. (2000). Kinetics of IgM and IgG seroconversion in Nipah virus infection. *Neurol. J. Southeast Asia* 5: 23–28.
16. Selvey, L.A., Wells, R.M., McCormack, J.G. et al. (1995). Infection of humans and horses by a newly described morbillivirus. *Med. J. Aust.* 162: 642–645.
17. Kaku, Y., Noguchi, A., Marsh, G.A. et al. (2012). Second generation of pseudotype-based serum neutralization assay for Nipah virus antibodies: sensitive and high-throughput analysis utilizing secreted alkaline phosphatase. *J. Virol. Methods* 179: 226–232.
18. Wong, K.T. (2010). Emerging epidemic viral encephalitides with a special focus on henipavirus. *Acta Neuropathol.* 120: 317–335.
19. Wong, K.T., Shieh, W.J., Kumar, S. et al. (2002). Nipah virus infection: pathology and pathogenesis of an emerging paramyxoviral zoonosis. *Am. J. Pathol.* 161: 2153–2167.
20. Wong, K.T. (2010). Nipah and Hendra viruses: recent advances in pathogenesis. *Future Virol.* 5: 129–131.
21. Broder, C.C., Weir, D.L., and Reid, P.A. (2016). Hendra virus and Nipah virus animal vaccines. *Vaccine* 34: 3525–3534.
22. Munster, V.J., Prescott, J.B., Bushmaker, T. et al. (2012). Rapid Nipah virus entry into the central nervous system of hamsters via the olfactory route. *Sci. Rep.* 2: 736.
23. Weingartl, H., Czub, S., Copps, J. et al. (2005). Invasion of the central nervous system in a porcine host by Nipah virus. *J. Virol.* 79: 7528–7534.
24. Wong, K.T. and Tan, C.T. (2012). Clinical and pathological manifestations of human henipavirus infection. *Curr. Top. Microbiol. Immunol.* 24: 2269–2272.
25. Rockx, B., Brining, D., Kramer, J. et al. (2011). Clinical outcome of henipavirus infection in hamsters is determined by the route and dose of infection. *J. Virol.* 85: 7658–7671.
26. Satterfield, B.A., Cross, C.W., Fenton, K.A. et al. (2015). The immunomodulating V and W proteins of Nipah virus determine disease course. *Nat. Commun.* 6: 7483.
27. Yun, T., Park, A., Hill, T.E. et al. (2015). Efficient reverse genetics reveals genetic determinants of budding and fusogenic differences between Nipah and Hendra viruses and enables real-time monitoring of viral spread in small animal models of henipavirus infection. *J. Virol.* 89: 1242–1253.
28. Broder, C.C., Xu, K., Nikolov, D.B. et al. (2013). A treatment for and vaccine against the deadly Hendra and Nipah viruses. *Antivir. Res.* 100: 8–13.
29. Halpin, K., Hyatt, A.D., Fogarty, R. et al. (2011). Pteropid bats are confirmed as the reservoir hosts of henipaviruses: a comprehensive experimental study of virus transmission. *Am. J. Trop. Med. Hyg.* 85: 946–951.
30. Pernet, O., Schneider, B.S., Beaty, S.M. et al. (2014). Evidence of henipavirus spillover into human populations in Africa. *Nat. Commun.* 5: 5342.
31. Smith, I. and Wang, L.F. (2013). Bats and their virome: an important source of emerging viruses capable of infection humans. *Curr. Opin. Virol.* 3: 84–91.

13 Rabies

Guilherme Dias de Melo[1], Perrine Parize[1], Grégory Jouvion[2], Laurent Dacheux[1], Fabrice Chrétien[2,3,4], and Hervé Bourhy[1]

[1] Lyssavirus Epidemiology and Neuropathology Unit, French National Reference Centre for Rabies, WHO Collaborating Centre for Reference and Research on Rabies, Pasteur Institute, Paris, France
[2] Experimental Neuropathology Unit, Pasteur Institute, Paris, France
[3] Paris University, Paris, France
[4] Department of Neuropathology, Sainte Anne Hospital, Paris, France

Abbreviations

ARAV	Aravan lyssavirus
ABLV	Australian bat lyssavirus
BBLV	Bokeloh bat lyssavirus
CSF	cerebrospinal fluid
CT scan	computed tomography scan
DUVV	Duvenhage lyssavirus
EBLV-1	European bat 1 lyssavirus
EBLV-2	European bat 2 lyssavirus
GBLV	Gannoruwa bat lyssavirus
HE	hematoxylin and eosin
IKOV	Ikoma lyssavirus
IRKV	Irkut lyssavirus
KBLV	Kotalahti bat lyssavirus
KHUV	Khujand lyssavirus
LBV	Lagos bat lyssavirus
LLEBV	Lleida bat lyssavirus
MOKV	Mokola lyssavirus
PEP	Postexposure prophylaxis
RABV	Rabies lyssavirus
RNA	ribonucleic acid
RNP	Ribonucleoprotein
RT-PCR	reverse transcription-polymerase chain reaction
SHIBV	Shimoni bat lyssavirus
TWBLV	Taiwan bat lyssavirus
WCBV	West Caucasian bat lyssavirus

Introduction, microbiological characteristics, and historical perspective

Rabies is an almost invariably fatal zoonotic disease caused by lyssaviruses (family Rhabdoviridae). It is characterized by an acute encephalomyelitis that can present as classic "furious" or "paralytic" rabies. Lyssaviruses are neurotropic viruses transmitted from animals (dogs and other carnivores, bats, etc.) to humans by bites, scratches, licking of broken skin, and contact of infectious material with the mucosae [1].

There are currently 16 officially recognized different species of lyssavirus. These species comprise

---

Infections of the Central Nervous System: Pathology and Genetics, First Edition. Edited by Fabrice Chrétien, Kum Thong Wong, Leroy R. Sharer, Catherine (Katy) Keohane and Françoise Gray.
© 2020 John Wiley & Sons Ltd. Published 2020 by John Wiley & Sons Ltd.

the following viruses: rabies lyssavirus (RABV), Lagos bat lyssavirus (LBV), Mokola lyssavirus (MOKV), Duvenhage lyssavirus (DUVV), European bat 1 lyssavirus (EBLV-1), European bat 2 lyssavirus (EBLV-2), Australian bat lyssavirus (ABLV), Aravan lyssavirus (ARAV), Khujand lyssavirus (KHUV), Irkut lyssavirus (IRKV), West Caucasian bat lyssavirus (WCBV), Shimoni bat lyssavirus (SHIBV), Ikoma lyssavirus (IKOV), Bokeloh bat lyssavirus (BBLV), Lleida bat lyssavirus (LLEBV), and Gannoruwa bat lyssavirus (GBLV) [2]. A further two putative bat lyssaviruses await classification: Taiwan bat lyssavirus (TWBLV) and Kotalahti bat lyssavirus (KBLV).

Lyssaviruses are enveloped viruses whose genome consists of an unsegmented single-stranded negative RNA. The electron-microscopic appearance of lyssaviruses are classically compared to "bullets." Their average length is 180 nm (130–250 nm) with a mean diameter of 75 nm (60–110 nm). The genome, about 12 kb, consists of a leader sequence, five genes encoding the five viral proteins (nucleoprotein N, phosphoprotein P, matrix protein M, glycoprotein G, and L polymerase) and a trailer sequence. N protein is associated with the viral genome to form the ribonucleoprotein (RNP) of helical structure. The P and L proteins interact with this ribonucleoprotein to form the viral nucleocapsid. The G protein is found in the form of trimeric spicules inserted on the surface of the viral envelope. It is responsible for inducing the production of neutralizing antibodies and stimulating T lymphocytes. After self-assembly, the M protein lines up on the internal surface of the viral envelope, forming a bridge between the envelope and the RNP complex [1].

On 6 July 1885, when Louis Pasteur began immunizing little Joseph Meister at the Ecole Normale in Paris, France (Figure 13.1), rabies became the second human disease (after smallpox) preventable by vaccination. However, rabies is still a neglected disease in many developing countries. Once the first signs of rabies encephalitis manifest, there is no cure and the mortality rate is around 100%. The neuropathogenic mechanisms leading to death in patients infected with rabies are still unknown.

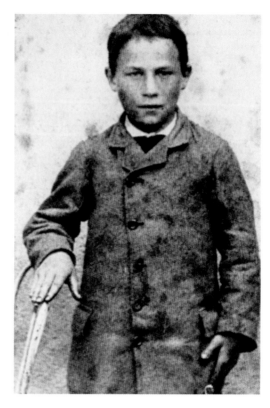

Figure 13.1 Joseph Meister in 1885, the first human to receive Louis Pasteur's live attenuated rabies vaccine on 6 July 1885 (Pasteur Institute-Musée Pasteur).

Epidemiology

All mammals are susceptible to rabies, but only a few species are important reservoirs for the disease (dogs, some other carnivores, and bats).

Human-to-human transmission of rabies is exceptional and almost exclusively reported in the setting of tissue and solid-organ transplantation.

Dogs are responsible for up to 99% of human deaths. Mass vaccination campaigns targeting dogs or wild carnivores constitute the principal strategy for rabies control both in animals and humans.

North America, Western Europe, Australia, Japan, and a few other countries are currently free of dog rabies and dog-transmitted human rabies (except from imported dogs) (Figure 13.2).

Endemicity of dog rabies and dog-transmitted human rabies, 2016
Endémicité de la rage canine et de la rage humaine à transmission canine, 2016

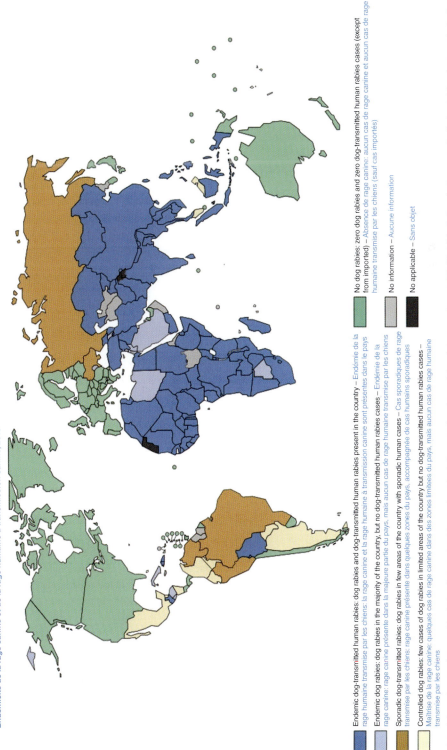

Figure 13.2 Endemicity of dog rabies and dog-transmitted human rabies, 2016 (Source: from World Health Organization (WHO) Endemicity of dog rabies and dog-transmitted human rabies, 2016. www.who.int/rabies).

A very small number of human cases are transmitted by terrestrial wildlife including foxes, wolves, jackals, racoons, skunks, or mongooses, depending on the continent.

Bats are responsible for several human cases annually in the Americas where chiropteras can be infected by RABV. In the rest of the world, bats are regularly infected by non-RABV lyssaviruses and rarely transmit to humans.

Rabies is 100% preventable by early postexposure management including meticulous washing, flushing and disinfection of all wounds and postexposure prophylaxis (PEP) with vaccines and, if required, anti-rabies immunoglobulins [3]. However, rabies is still responsible for an estimated 59 000 human deaths every year worldwide, with approximately 40% of cases in children age <15 years. Human cases occur largely in Asia and Africa, where control measures in dogs are not implemented and PEP is hardly available for the majority of the population [4].

Pathogenesis

In humans

Rabies can be transmitted to humans by bites, scratches, or direct exposure of mucosal surfaces to saliva from an infected animal or by transplantation of organs or tissues from a donor infected with rabies. The virus travels by retrograde axonal transport to the spinal cord, along either the dorsal root (sensory neuron) or the ventral root (motor neuron) probably depending on the site and depth of the virus inoculation [5].

Dog RABV predominantly infects the motor endplates at the site of inoculation. It attaches to myocytes though its glycoprotein (G-protein) and replicates in muscle, entering motor fibers using postsynaptic nicotinic acetylcholine receptors [6]. Virus spreads rapidly toward the CNS (between 5 and 100 mm/d) exclusively by retrograde axonal and transneuronal transport (centripetal propagation), including dorsal root ganglia connected to the infected motoneurons, hitchhiking along axonal vesicles [6, 7]. They can travel by binding to receptors other than nicotinic acetylcholine receptors, such as neural cell adhesion molecule (CD56) and low-affinity nerve growth factor receptor (NTR75). Other receptors such as glycans, heparan sulfate, and metabotropic glutamate receptor subtype-2 have also been identified recently [8, 9]. Conversely, some bat RABV variants can also infect and multiply in epithelial cells and fibroblasts, even at low temperatures (34°C). Accordingly, lesions caused by an infected bat, even minor skin scratches, constitute higher risks of infection [6], and clinical presentation may vary from that because of exposure to nonflying animals [5].

More slowly, RABV also spreads anterogradely in axons (centrifugal propagation) toward all innervated organs, including salivary glands, skin, hair follicles, and heart, via passive diffusion. This is an ineffective distance-dependent route. Within the CNS, RABV spreads by trans-synaptic diffusion and deregulates neurotransmitters such as serotonin, gamma aminobutyric acid (GABA), and muscarinic acetylcholine. The blood-brain barrier is not affected, limiting access of immune mediators into the CNS. RABV regulates its growth rate in a manner that preserves the integrity of the neuronal network and evades the immune system. Expression of low levels of G protein is a key factor preventing neuronal apoptosis, thereby assuring brain invasion [7, 10].

The incubation period of human rabies varies from a few days to several years, with an average of two to three months. This variation probably relates to the infective dose more than wound location. Nevertheless, bites on the head, neck, and hands have the highest risk and fastest incubation period, mainly because of the rich innervation and reduced distance from the CNS [6, 10]. During incubation, RABV probably remains at low replicating levels in muscle at the infection site before entering the motor pathway. This low-replicating rate has been associated with the presence of microRNAs that can interfere with viral protein expression [10]. On the other hand, short incubation periods are usually related to high titers of inocula, where RABV can directly infect motor endplates, or penetrating nerve injury, when the virus is inoculated directly into motor axons. By the time of onset of clinical signs, RABV has disseminated widely throughout the CNS [1, 10].

Clinically, rabies manifests as either furious or paralytic. The pathophysiology underlying these different forms is still not elucidated. Virus variants, wound location, previous vaccination, incubation period, and virus localization in the brain have all been linked with the different clinical forms, but none of these hypotheses has been validated. The furious form may be related to a higher viral load in the brain and to more CNS-infected areas. High levels of T cells and inflammatory mediators are present in the paralytic form, associated with reduced centrifugal spread and loss of axonal integrity. Accordingly, furious rabies seems to be virus-mediated, whereas inflammation and demyelination seem to be characteristic of the paralytic form [6, 10].

Animal models

Although all mammals are susceptible to infection, a few animal models have been used to study rabies pathogenesis using different inoculation routes to reproduce the long incubation period and high mortality rate [5, 6]. Mice are widely used but are not strictly comparable to human rabies because sensory neurons may also be infected by RABV giving an additional entry route to the CNS. Nonhuman primates, rats, and guinea pigs seem to be better models to mimic human rabies pathogenesis because RABV exclusively invades the CNS via neuromuscular junctions and motor pathway in these animals [6, 10].

Due to the species-specific characteristics of RABV infection, and for ethical reasons, initial broad studies are usually performed in rodents. They are flexible models, allowing the use of different inoculation doses and routes with shorter incubation periods. Nonhuman primates are then preferable for final studies to be more applicable to humans and to corroborate the findings in rodents.

Clinical features and diagnosis

Clinical diagnosis

Rabies is an acute encephalitis that can manifest clinically as either the encephalitic furious form (two-thirds of cases) or the paralytic "dumb" form (one-third of cases) [6, 10]. Rare atypical forms can be observed in patients exposed to bats. The primary diagnosis of rabies relies on the clinical presentation and history of exposure to a suspect rabid animal or RABV, however a history of exposure may be lacking. Inconsistent nonspecific prodromes (e.g. flulike symptoms, neuropathic pain at the site of bite) can precede the onset of neurological symptoms.

Furious rabies is characterized by phobic spasms (i.e. hydrophobia or aerophobia), spontaneous inspiratory spasms, fluctuating alteration in consciousness (i.e. hyperactivity, anxiety, altered attention span), and signs of autonomic dysfunction (i.e. hypersalivation, excessive sweating, priapism, pupil abnormalities, tachycardia, and hypotension). Phobic spasms are pathognomonic and frequent in patients with encephalitic rabies but may not be observed at all stages of the disease.

The paralytic form is more difficult to identify and can be misdiagnosed as Guillain-Barré syndrome. The features include ascending paralysis with intact sensory function and frequent facial diparesis. Phobic spams can be observed in up to 50% of paralytic forms. The evolution of rabies is characterized by neurologic dysfunction progressing to coma and death. On average, death occurs 7 and 11 days after the onset of symptoms in the encephalitic and paralytic forms, respectively.

Cerebrospinal fluid (CSF) can show meningitis or be normal. Other routine biological tests are nonspecific. Brain computed tomography (CT) scan is nearly always normal, but magnetic resonance imaging (MRI) can show abnormal signals in the gray matter (i.e. thalamus, pons, caudate and putamen of basal ganglia, midbrain nuclei) [11].

The differential diagnosis of rabies mainly includes viral encephalitides (i.e. arboviruses, enteroviruses, herpesvirus), neurological manifestations of malaria, Guillain-Barré syndrome, and tetanus.

Laboratory diagnosis

The best method for *intra-vitam* (antemortem) diagnosis of human rabies is examination of a skin biopsy from a richly innervated zone (e.g. the base of the neck in an area rich in hair follicles) [12–14]. The virus is regularly found in nerve cells surrounding the base of hair follicles. The biopsy can be performed by a dermatologist using a biopsy punch-type instrument (4 mm diameter). Saliva is the second-best sample. Sequential samples must be collected directly or, failing that, by swabbing (at least three to six hours apart between each sample) [15]. The intermittent excretion of the virus in saliva

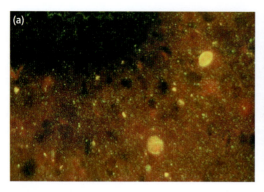 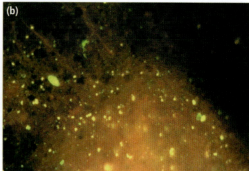

Figure 13.3 Detection of rabies antigens on two human cerebral samples (a and b) by direct immunofluorescence. Inclusions of rabies virus (RABV) nucleocapsids are represented by green dots of various sizes present in the cytoplasm of infected cells (400×).

necessitates at least three samples. CSF and serum can also be examined, although their diagnostic sensitivity is lower at the beginning of infection [12–14]. Detection of viral RNAs on samples is by real-time reverse transcriptase-polymerase chain reaction (RT-PCR) or by conventional RT-PCR [12, 15, 16]. For each positive case, subsequent genotyping is essential to determine the viral species, geographical origin, animal species to which the isolate is preferentially adapted, and to highlight new variants.

At postmortem, the diagnosis is made on cerebral biopsies (i.e. cerebral cortex, hippocampus, or cerebellum) or, failing that, on a skin biopsy (as described previously). Rapid techniques for collecting occipital or retro-orbital brain samples have been described. All these biological samples must be collected in a dry tube, stored immediately at −20 °C and shipped frozen to ensure maximum integrity.

Rabies antigens can be detected on postmortem brain tissue from hippocampus, medulla oblongata, cerebral cortex, or cerebellum by direct immunofluorescence, representing the reference method, along with the direct rapid immunohistochemical test (Figure 13.3). It is very fast (less than two hours) and performed on touch preparations or smears (previously fixed with acetone). Mono- or polyclonal anti-nucleocapsid antibodies linked to fluorescein enable detection of all the different lyssavirus species, depending on the spectrum of detection of the selected reagent. Diagnosis can be completed by isolation of RABV on cell culture (murine neuroblastoma type cells). This is rapid (< 24 h) and very sensitive, provided the virus has retained its infectivity. Viral inclusions in cell cytoplasm are revealed by direct immunofluorescence as previously described.

Pathology, including histopathology and immunocytochemistry

Although rabies is a severe fatal disease, macroscopic lesions in the CNS are mild or absent. Histology, using hematoxylin and eosin (H&E) staining, reveals an encephalomyelitis, classically characterized by: (i) mononuclear cell infiltrates of lymphocytes, plasma cells, and macrophages; (ii) perivascular lymphocyte cuffs; (iii) glial nodules; and (iv) Negri bodies (Figure 13.4 a–e) [17]. Negri bodies are intracytoplasmic round or oval acidophilic inclusions measuring from 0.25 to 27 μm. They consist of aggregates of nucleocapsids and are detected in neuronal cytoplasm in the brainstem, hippocampus, cerebellum, and several other brain regions. Negri bodies are not observed in all infected cases, and so cannot be considered as the only diagnostic criteria for rabies [18].

Other lesions including meningitis, degeneration or necrosis of ganglion cells, neuronophagia, thrombosis, hemorrhages, and vacuolation of neurons and neuropil have been reported [7, 19].

Lesions are also detectable in the peripheral nerves and spinal cord. Inflammation is more severe in the midbrain and medulla.

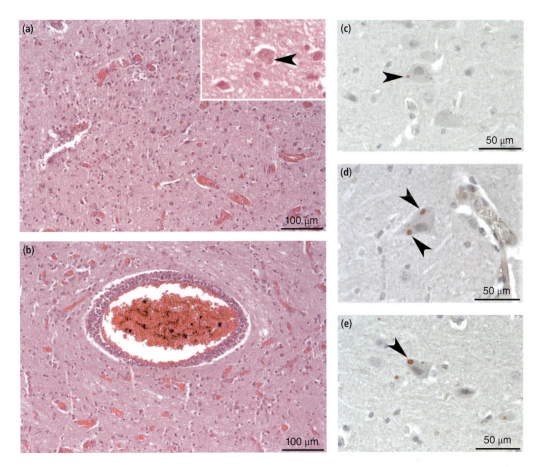

Figure 13.4 Pathology of rabies, human infection. (a) Mild inflammatory lesions in the brain, characterized by multifocal gliosis, mononuclear cell infiltrates, and vacuolation of the neuropil, with rare Negri bodies (inset, black arrowhead) detected in the cytoplasm of neurons. (b) Perivascular lymphocyte cuffs can be observed (hematoxylin and eosin [H&E] staining). (c–e) Immunohistochemistry against specific Ag of rabies virus (RABV) is helpful in detecting infected neurons (black arrowheads).

Immunohistochemistry against RABV antigens is important for diagnosis because histological lesions are clearly non-specific (Figure 13.3).

For all rabies tissue investigations and postmortem examination, appropriate precautions must be taken to protect staff, and safety guidelines and protocols should be followed, such as those that can be found at the Centers for Disease Control and Prevention website.

Treatment and future perspective

Rabies is 100% preventable by early postexposure management, including meticulous washing, flushing and disinfection of all wounds, and PEP, including vaccines, and, if required, anti-rabies immunoglobulins [3, 20]. After the onset of clinical symptoms, the outcome is nearly always fatal. There are only a few reports of survival in patients who were not vaccinated; most had been exposed to bats. Their survival is most probably attributed to the combination of a virus poorly adapted to humans and an exceptional immune response of the host.

Unfortunately, to date, there is no effective validated therapy for the management of rabies [21, 22]. Confirmation of the diagnosis is a priority, both to ensure a curable differential diagnosis is not missed and to institute PEP in others potentially exposed to the same rabid animal.

The management of rabies cases relies mostly on symptom relief and palliative care to alleviate suffering for patients and their families [23]. The patients should be managed in a quiet room and physical restraint avoided. Healthcare workers must take precautions to avoid droplet, transdermal, or mucosal exposure to infectious fluids (i.e. saliva and tears). To alleviate the sensation of thirst, spastic signs, and anxiety, treatment can include rehydration, anxiolysis, and analgesia. Parenteral or intrarectal routes are recommended in patients suffering from hydrophobia. More aggressive treatment could be provided in patients who are young, immunocompetent, and exposed to bats, especially if they have a history of pre-exposure prophylaxis or PEP.

Several therapeutic approaches are currently under investigation in vitro and in animal models and may enable viral eradication and clinical cure in rabies cases in the future.

Conclusion

More than 130 years after Louis Pasteur's first vaccine protocol, rabies is still responsible for about 59 000 deaths annually. Further understanding of rabies neuropathogenesis and pathophysiology is needed to develop potential therapies for patients infected with rabies. However, progresses in prevention of infection in humans and dogs is the most promising way to reach the goal of zero human deaths resulting from dog rabies by 2030.

References

1. Fooks, A.R., Banyard, A.C. et al. (2014). Current status of rabies and prospects for elimination. *Lancet* 384: 1389–1399.
2. Virus Taxonomy (2017). Release (2017) International Committee on Taxonomy of Viruses. http://www.ictvonline.org/virustaxonomy.asp (accessed 31 December 2017).
3. World Health Organization (WHO) (2018). *WHO Expert Consultation on Rabies*. Third report. 1012. Geneva: World Health Organization.
4. Hampson, K., Coudeville, L., Lembo, T. et al. (2015). Estimating the global burden of endemic canine rabies. *PLoS Negl. Trop. Dis.* 9: e0003709.
5. Begeman, L., GeurtsvanKessel, C., Finke, S. et al. (2018). Comparative pathogenesis of rabies in bats and carnivores, and implications for spillover to humans. *Lancet Infect. Dis.* 18: e147–e159.
6. Ugolini, G. and Hemachudha, T. (2018). Rabies: changing prophylaxis and new insights in pathophysiology. *Curr. Opin. Infect. Dis.* 31: 93–101.
7. Singh, R., Singh, K.P., Cherian, S. et al. (2017). Rabies – epidemiology, pathogenesis, public health concerns and advances in diagnosis and control: a comprehensive review. *Vet. Q.* 37: 212–251.
8. Wang, J., Wang, Z., Liu, R. et al. (2018). Metabotropic glutamate receptor subtype 2 is a cellular receptor for rabies virus. *PLoS Pathog.* 14: e1007189.
9. Sasaki, M., Anindita, P.D., Ito, N. et al. (2018). The role of Heparan Sulfate proteoglycans as an attachment factor for rabies virus entry and infection. *J. Infect. Dis.* 217: 1740–1749.
10. Hemachudha, T., Ugolini, G., Wacharapluesadee, S. et al. (2013). Human rabies: neuropathogenesis, diagnosis, and management. *Lancet Neurol.* 12: 498–513.
11. Laothamatas, J., Hemachudha, T., Mitrabhakdi, E. et al. (2003). MR imaging in human rabies. *AJNR Am. J. Neuroradiol.* 24: 1102–1109.
12. Dacheux, L., Larrous, F., Lavenir, R. et al. (2016). Dual combined real-time reverse transcription polymerase chain reaction assay for the diagnosis of lyssavirus infection. *PLoS Negl. Trop. Dis.* 10: e0004812.
13. Dacheux, L., Wacharapluesadee, S., Hemachudha, T. et al. (2010). More accurate insight into the incidence of human rabies in developing countries through validated laboratory techniques. *PLoS Negl. Trop. Dis.* 4: e765.
14. Duong, V., Tarantola, A., Ong, S. et al. (2016). Laboratory diagnostics in dog-mediated rabies: an overview of performance and a proposed strategy for various settings. *Int. J. Infect. Dis.* 46: 107–114.
15. Dacheux, L., Reynes, J.M., Buchy, P. et al. (2008). A reliable diagnosis of human rabies based on analysis of skin biopsy specimens. *Clin. Infect. Dis.* 47: 1410–1417.
16. Hayman, D.T., Banyard, A.C., Wakeley, P.R. et al. (2011). A universal real-time assay for the detection of lyssaviruses. *J. Virol. Methods* 177: 87–93.
17. Adle-Biassette, H., Bourhy, H., Gisselbrecht, M. et al. (1996). Rabies encephalitis in a patient with AIDS: a clinicopathological study. *Acta Neuropathol.* 92: 415–420.
18. Caicedo, Y., Paez, A., Kuzmin, I. et al. (2015). Virology, immunology and pathology of human

rabies during treatment. *Pediatr. Infect. Dis. J.* 34: 520–528.
19. Pathak, S., Horton, D.L., Lucas, S. et al. (2014). Diagnosis, management and post-mortem findings of a human case of rabies imported into the United Kingdom from India: a case report. *Virol. J.* 11: 63.
20. WHO (2018). Rabies vaccines: WHO position paper, April 2018 – recommendations. *Vaccine* 36: 5500–5503.
21. Zeiler, F.A. and Jackson, A.C. (2016). Critical appraisal of the Milwaukee protocol for rabies: this failed approach should be abandoned. *Can. J. Neurol. Sci.* 43: 44–51.
22. Rogée, S., Larrous, F., Jochmans, D. et al. (2019). Pyrimethamine inhibits rabies virus replication in vitro. *Antiviral. Res.* 161: 1–9. https://doi.org/10.1016/j.antiviral.2018.10.016.
23. Tarantola, A., Crabol, Y., Mahendra, B.J. et al. (2016). Caring for patients with rabies in developing countries – the neglected importance of palliative care. *Tropical Med. Int. Health* 21: 564–567.

14 Flaviviruses 1: General Introduction and Tick-Borne Encephalitis

Herbert Budka

Institute of Neurology, Medical University of Vienna, Vienna, Austria

Abbreviations

ADE	antibody-dependent enhancement
BBB	blood-brain barrier
BSL3	biosafety level 3
C	capsid protein
DALYs	disability-adjusted life years
DENV	dengue virus
DHF	dengue hemorrhagic fever
DSS	dengue shock syndrome
DTV	deer tick virus
E	envelope protein
ELISA	enzyme-linked immunosorbent assay
ER	endoplasmic reticulum
FV	flavivirus
GrB	granzyme B
H&E	hematoxylin and eosin
HIT	hemagglutination inhibition test
I	*Ixodes* spp.
IFA	immunofluorescence assay
IFN	interferon
Ig	immunoglobulin
IHC	immunohistochemistry
JE	Japanese encephalitis
JEV	Japanese encephalitis virus
M	membrane (protein)
MBFV	mosquito-borne flavivirus
MIA	microsphere immunoassay
NS	nonstructural (proteins)
OHFV	Omsk Hemorrhagic Fever virus
POWV	Powassan virus
pr	precursor (peptide)
prM	precursor of membrane (protein)
PRNT/micro-VNT	plaque reduction neutralization/micro-virus neutralization tests
SHA	slowly sedimenting hemagglutinin (non-infectious subviral particle)
SLEV	St. Louis encephalitis virus
TBE	tick-borne encephalitis
TBEV	tick-borne encephalitis virus
TBEV-Eu	tick-borne encephalitis virus, European subtype
TBEV-FE	tick-borne encephalitis virus, Far East subtype

Infections of the Central Nervous System: Pathology and Genetics, First Edition. Edited by Fabrice Chrétien, Kum Thong Wong, Leroy R. Sharer, Catherine (Katy) Keohane and Françoise Gray.
© 2020 John Wiley & Sons Ltd. Published 2020 by John Wiley & Sons Ltd.

TBEV-Sib	tick-borne encephalitis virus, Siberian subtype
TBFV	tick-borne flavivirus
WNV	West Nile virus
YF	yellow fever
YFV	Yellow Fever virus
ZIKV	Zika virus

Flaviviruses: general introduction

Significance, classification, and historical perspective

Flaviviruses (FVs) are among the most important infectious agents worldwide, with dengue virus (DENV) and Japanese encephalitis virus (JEV) identified as global research priorities [1]. FVs distribute to roughly half of the planet's landmasses (Figure 14.1a). The present classification system distinguishes the family Flaviviridae, the subjacent genus *Flavivirus,* which contains more than 70 species of viruses (see abbreviations and Figure 14.2b for the more relevant ones), and finally specific virus subtypes [2]. FVs may be separated according to their vectors as tick-borne viruses and a rather heterogeneous group transmitted by mosquitoes *(Aedes* or *Culex)* [2, 3] (Figure 14.2b). Recognition of arthropod vectors resulted in the former compilation of arthropod borne viruses (arboviruses) that encompassed FVs (originally group B arboviruses) as well as toga-, bunya-, and reoviruses. A timeline of historical landmarks of FV research is given in Figure 14.1b [2].

Genetics and microbiological characteristics of FVs

FVs are single positive-stranded RNA viruses with a genome of about 11 000 nucleotides that has a single, open reading frame encoding a large polypeptide (Figure 14.2a, upper graph). Processing of the polypeptide is co- and post-translationally performed by the virus as well as host proteases (Figure 14.2a, center). Structural proteins comprise the capsid (C), pre-M (prM), and envelope (E) proteins; prM is cleaved by furin into the precursor (pr) fragment and the membrane (M) protein [6]. In addition, there are 7 nonstructural (NS) proteins (NS1, 2A, 2B, 3, 4A, 4B and 5) (Figure 14.2a, center). These 10 distinct viral proteins localize to the endoplasmic reticulum (ER) membrane (Figure 14.2a, bottom). The E protein is responsible for both receptor binding and membrane fusion and, thus, decisive for virus entry into the cell [6]. Because of its essential function, the E protein is the main target of FV neutralizing antibodies [6].

The genetic relatedness of FV species clusters into vector-specific groups (Figure 14.2b).

The structure of FV particles is depicted in Figure 14.3a and b. Morphogenesis starts by budding at ER membranes and results first in immature particles. Further details are explained in the legend of Figure 14.3a and b [6–8].

The cellular cycle of FVs (Figure 14.3c) starts with binding of the virus to cell receptors; identification of specific receptors for FVs has remained a major gap of knowledge. Further steps are explained in the legend of Figure 14.3c [6, 7].

Epidemiology

Globally, the most important FV is DENV that is endemic in (sub)tropical areas (Figure 14.1a) where about 2.5 billion people live; yearly, it causes about 50–100 million infections, 500 000 cases of dengue hemorrhagic fever (DHF) and 20 000 deaths due to dengue shock syndrome (DSS) [6]. The vast DENV distribution overlaps with endemic areas of yellow fever (YF; estimated 20 000 annual cases) and Japanese encephalitis (JE; estimated 50 000 annual cases) [6]. In contrast, the three strains of tick-borne encephalitis virus (TBEV) locate to a broad strip in temperate latitudes of Eurasia (Figure 14.1a). West Nile virus (WNV), DENV, and TBEV are described as of high risk for impact of climate change in Europe, with severe consequences to society [9].

The host range and epidemiology of FVs is strongly determined by the distribution of their vectors. *Culex*-transmitted viruses are neurotropic, with frequent meningoencephalitis, and circulate among birds, whereas *Aedes*-transmitted viruses affect primates and usually cause hemorrhagic fevers [3]. Simultaneous outbreaks (such as presently in the Americas with DENV, Zika virus [ZIKV] and chikungunya virus) may result from

Flaviviruses 1: General Introduction and Tick-Borne Encephalitis **Chapter 14**

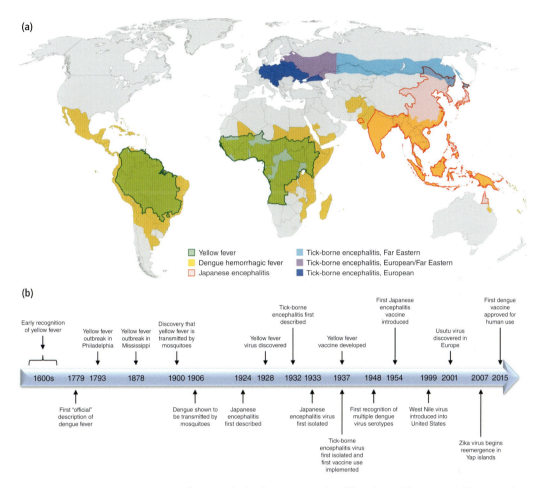

Figure 14.1 (a) Global distribution of major flaviviruses (FVs). Information was adapted from data and figures provided by Centers for Disease Control and Prevention (CDC) and World Health Organization (WHO) websites. (b). A timeline of historical highlights of FV research. Source: (a and b) are figures 1 and 2 in [2], with kind permission.

several FVs transmitted by the same vector or one FV transmitted by different vectors [10].

Mosquito-borne flaviviruses (MBFVs) and tick-borne flaviviruses (TBFVs) circulate between arthropod vectors and vertebrate hosts, frequently without any damaging effect on the host [11]. The transmission and amplification cycle of MBFVs is depicted in Figure 14.4a. In contrast to MBFVs, the transmission cycle of TBFVs (Figure 14.4b) is more complex. Ticks are persistently infected when feeding on a viremic host and transmit the virus between all developmental stages (i.e. larvae, nymphs, adults including transovarial transmission), and by cofeeding with adjacent biting ticks on a nonviremic host [12]. The primary reservoirs are mostly rodents but also infected birds, the latter capable of long-distance travel. If milk-producing animals are infected and viremic, alimentary infection via unpasteurized milk and dairy products can occur [11]. For evaluation of patients, epidemiological data should include history of exposure, vaccination status, and history of tick or mosquito bites [13]. Some evidence for FV persistence in humans is emerging by use of polymerase chain reaction (PCR) and isolation of infectious virus, although the site of persistence is still disputed [11].

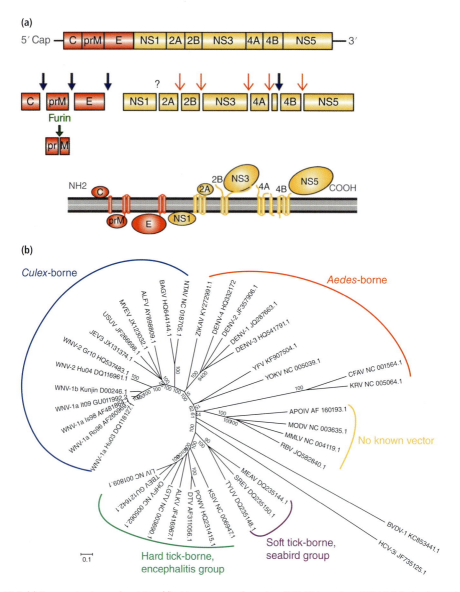

Figure 14.2 (a) Genome structure and proteins of flaviviruses (FVs). Upper graph shows the coding regions of the genome, in the center are the cleaved products after processing of the polypeptide, and below the location of viral proteins in relation to the endoplasmic reticulum (ER) membrane (cytoplasm is above, ER lumen below). Structural proteins are in red; nonstructural proteins in green. Cleavage sites by host proteases are marked by blue arrows; those by virus proteases by red arrows. Source: Modified by Prof. F. X. Heinz, Vienna, from figure 38.2 in [5], with kind permission. (b) Genetic relatedness of FVs, evaluated using genetic alignments of complete genomic sequences. GenBank accession numbers are given next to the name of each virus. Clockwise from upper left: WNV, West Nile virus; JEV, Japanese encephalitis virus; USUV, Usutu virus; MVEV, Murray Valley encephalitis virus; ALFV, Alfuy virus; BAGV, Bagaza virus; NTAV, Ntaya virus; ZIKAV, Zika virus; DENV, Dengue virus; YFV, Yellow fever virus; YOKV, Yokose virus; CFAV, Cell Fusing Agent virus; KRV, Kamiti River virus; APOIV, Apoi virus; MODV, Modoc virus; MMLV, Montana Myotis Leukoencephalitis virus; SREV, Saumarez Reef virus; TYUV, Tyuleniy virus; KSIV, Karshi virus; POWV, Powassan virus; DTV, deer tick virus; ALKV, Alkhurma virus; LGTV, Langat virus; OHFV, Omsk Hemorrhagic Fever virus; TBEV, tick-borne encephalitis virus; LIV, louping ill virus. Two outgroups were used, HCV for Hepatitis C virus (*Hepacivirus* genus, Flaviviridae family) and BVDV for Bovine Viral Diarrhea virus (*Pestivirus* genus, Flaviviridae family). FVs and WNV strains isolated in Europe are underlined. The phylogenetic tree was constructed using neighbor-joining with Jukes–Cantor parameter distances (scale bar) in MEGA, version 5.2 [4]. A bootstrapped confidence interval (1000 replicates) and a confidence probability value based on the standard error test were also calculated using MEGA. Source: From [5], with kind permission.

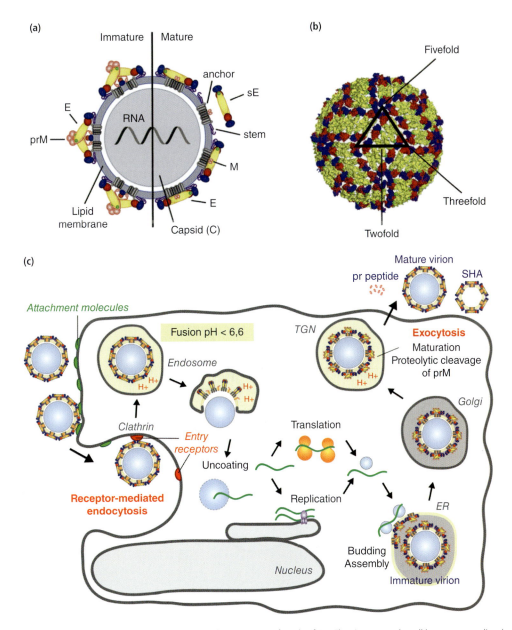

Figure 14.3 (a and b) Flaviviruses (FVs) structure. (a) Schematic representation of an FV particle. Left: immature virion; right: mature virion. The unstructured spherical capsid contains the positive-stranded genomic RNA and multiple copies of the capsid protein C. Immature virions are covered by spiky complexes of 60 trimers of precursor of membrane-envelope (prM-E) heterodimers. The proteolytic cleavage of prM results in the reorganization of the E proteins and the formation of smooth-surfaced particles covered with 90 E dimers. sF, soluble form of E that lacks the membrane anchor and an adjacent sequence element called "stem"; M, Membrane-associated cleavage product of prM. (b) Herringbone-like arrangement of 90 E protein dimers at the virion surface as determined by cryo-electron microscopy (PDB 14KR). The triangle indicates two-, three-, and fivefold symmetry axes. Source: These are figures 1a and b in [6] with kind permission. (c) Life cycle of FVs. The virus enters the cell by receptor-mediated endocytosis. The acid pH of endosomes induces structural changes in E that mediate fusion of viral and endosomal membranes with release of the nucleocapsid into the cytoplasm. After uncoating, the genome is translated and replicated. The assembly of new viral particles locates to the endoplasmic reticulum (ER), leading first to immature, prM-containing particles that are transported via cell exocytosis. In the trans-Golgi network (TGN), the acid pH cause conformational changes on the viral surface where the precursor (pr) peptide is cleaved but still associated with the E protein. Only after the virus has left the cell, the pr peptide is released and mature infectious particles develop. SHA, slowly sedimenting hemagglutinin (noninfectious subviral particle). Source: Modified by Prof. F. X. Heinz, Vienna, from figure 38.3a in [7], with kind permission.

Infections of the Central Nervous System

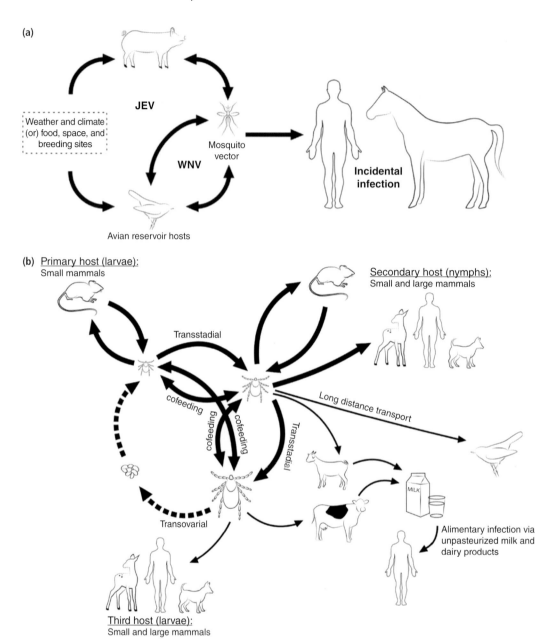

Figure 14.4 (a) Schematic representation of a mosquito-borne flavivirus (MBFV) amplification and transmission cycle. West Nile virus (WNV) is cycled between the mosquito and avian hosts that play an amplification and maintenance role. Swine are important amplifying hosts for Japanese encephalitis virus (JEV), and mosquitoes that acquire blood meals on infected pigs can become infected and transmit the virus. Similar to tick-borne flaviviruses (TBFVs), MBFV infection in humans and large animals, such as horses, is accidental. Source: This is figure 2 in [11], with kind permission. (b) FV maintenance and transmission cycle in ticks and vertebrate hosts. Ticks are crucial for viral persistence because they remain infected once they acquire viral infection. Infected ticks are capable of transmitting TBFVs to other ticks when they feed in close proximity on the same animal, as well as to the different stages of the tick life cycle. TBFVs persist also in a cycle between small mammals (e.g. rodents) and the ticks that feed on them. Large mammals and humans tend to be incidental, dead-end hosts. Source: This is figure 1 in [11], with kind permission.

Sexual transmission has been recently described for ZIKV but not (yet) for other FVs [2]. Mother-to-child transmission was also discovered for ZIKV, whereas similar data are available only for WNV, and transmission by breastfeeding has been established for some FVs [2].

Clinical features

Human infection by encephalitogenic FVs usually follows a biphasic course [11], as will be detailed for tick-borne encephalitis (TBE). A first flulike phase features arthralgia, headache, discomfort, and fatigue. In the second phase, neurologic symptoms range from mild meningism to severe encephalitis. Survivors of encephalitis may have severe neurological defects because of neural tissue destruction or virus persistence, which has been shown for WNV, JEV, and TBEV [11].

Clinical FV diagnostics mostly rely on serology using immunoglobulin G (IgG) and immunoglobulin M (IgM) immunoassays [6]. They usually detect immunodominant epitopes on the E or NS1 proteins. In general, broad serological cross-reactivity exists among FVs and is used to define 10 serocomplexes [3]. Some E epitopes, however, can be virus specific. The detection methodology includes plaque reduction neutralization/micro-virus neutralization tests (PRNT/micro-VNT), hemagglutination inhibition tests (HITs), immunofluorescence assays (IFA), enzyme-linked immunosorbent assay (ELISA), and microsphere immunoassays (MIA) [3]. Although ELISAs are the preferred screening tests because of their affordability, rapidity, reproducibility, and sensitivity, the specificity of many tests is a concern [3]. A risk of cross-reactivity exists in particular where several FVs are circulating in a population. The titer of antibodies does not always correlate with clinical outcome, and knowledge of the epidemiological background is important when interpreting serological results [3, 13].

Nucleic acid detection by PCR is specific but may not be helpful when, at the height of clinical symptoms but at the end of viremia, the virus titer may drop to undetectable levels [6].

Pathology

Fortunately, many viral infections, including those by FVs, run a favorable course of aseptic meningitis or mild meningoencephalitis and only exceptionally involve the neuropathologist for diagnosis [14]. Neuropathological experience usually concerns fatal cases. The neuropathology of FV encephalitis is not specifically distinguishable between virus types [15]; it features all major elements of the encephalitic syndrome spectrum, with disseminated microglial nodules, gliosis, perivascular lymphomononuclear cuffing, and variable neuronal damage ranging from disseminated neuronophagia to larger necroses (edematous-necrolytic areas). Human cases with neuropathology have been reported in encephalitis by Powassan virus (POWV) [16], deer tick virus [17], St. Louis encephalitis virus (SLEV) [18, 19], JEV [20, 21], WNV [22, 23], Sao Paulo virus [24], and TBEV [14, 25–30]. Because of the relatively nonspecific morphology, virologic examination or molecular analysis is required for an etiologic diagnosis [14, 25]. However, some detailed topographical mapping of inflammatory lesions was recommended (e.g. for distinction of JE from encephalitis resulting from enterovirus 17) [21].

Arguably, the techniques of immunocytochemistry (ICC), in situ hybridization (ISH), and PCR had one of the most profound diagnostic impacts in neuropathology of viral infections; when done appropriately with adequate controls and tissue selection, they provide an etiologic diagnosis with high sensitivity and specificity [14] However, in JE the viral antigen is progressively cleared in patients who survive six days or more [20]. Neurons in normal-appearing regions and neuronophagias were JEV-antigen positive, as were antigenic masses in the center of so-called acellular plaques, whereas glial or vascular endothelial cells were not labeled [31]. In 11/13 brains, the topographic distribution of JEV was regarded as explaining the evolution of post-JE sequelae [32].

Collectively, the neuropathology of human FV encephalitides such as JE and fatal human and animal WNV infection [20, 22, 23, 33, 34], along with our and other studies on TBE [26, 30, 35], suggests an important immunopathological component in FV encephalitogenesis. The role of T-cell–mediated immunity still awaits full clarification [2].

Animal models and pathogenesis

Several animal models have been developed for various FVs, in particular WNV, SLEV, JEV, TBEV, louping ill virus (LIV), and POWV, mostly using mice and hamsters, but occasionally also monkeys [11]. However, most models are poorly representative of the human disease [2]. Depending on virus and strain, mouse models of encephalitogenic FVs are usually monophasic and lethal within one to two weeks; on the other hand, primate models mostly do not develop disease after peripheral inoculation [2]. In a comparison among three FV species, intravenously infected mice suggested different entry routes to the CNS with a neural route via the enteric nervous system for tick-borne encephalitis virus-Far Eastern (TBEV-FE), and a hematogenous or lymphogenous pathway for JEV and WNV, with individual variability in the latter [36]. For JEV and WNV, complex ways of neuroinvasion were suggested, including blood-brain barrier (BBB) impairment by systemic inflammatory cytokines and axonal transport including olfactory pathways [37, 38]. A four amino-acid sequence in the NS5 protein was described as a determinant of neurovirulence in mice infected by chimeric TBEV and Omsk hemorrhagic fever virus (OHFV) [39]. In nonhuman primates infected with various FVs, the time course, composition, and magnitude of cellular inflammatory responses in the CNS are significantly different, again suggesting the type and level of immune responses as determinants of the outcome [40].

Treatment and prophylaxis

Unfortunately no specific antiviral treatment has been developed for FV infections; thus, supportive care is the only therapeutic option [2]. Major obstacles to effective therapies are (i) the need for early diagnosis during viremia, (ii) the lack of viremia at the height of symptoms, (iii) the seeding to tissues including the CNS, and (iv) the host immune response [2]. However, preclinical studies have identified microRNAs capable of inhibiting FV replication [41, 42].

Although FVs can be well targeted by vaccines in principle [6], few human vaccines have been developed against TBEV (inactivated vaccine), JEV (live and inactivated), and yellow fever virus (YFV; live attenuated). Vaccines against widespread WNV and DENV are lacking or insufficiently effective [3] (see also Chapter 15).

Cross-protection in individuals who are vaccinated may become important, and efforts are underway to exploit this using chimeric vaccines [3, 6]. There is a potential risk of antibody-dependent enhancement (ADE; i.e. an adverse boost of second, antigenically related infections by the presence of cross-reacting antibodies from a primary infection, which has been observed in consecutive infections with different DENV serotypes [3]). These concerns about immunopathogenesis are one reason why vaccines against DENV have not appeared on the market [6]. It is unclear whether this complication may emerge with natural infection by other FVs [3].

TBE

Significance, definition, and historical perspective

TBEV is medically a most important pathogen for Eurasia and responsible for more than 10 000 severe infections requiring hospitalization annually [3, 43], including 3000 in Europe [44]. In number of cases it is second to JE among neurotropic FVs [44]. TBE has been recognized by the World Health Organization (WHO) as an international public health problem and has been amply covered in the scientific literature, including a recent dedicated book [45].

TBE became a notifiable disease in the European Union in 2012 [46]; the definition by the European Center for Disease Prevention and Control (ECDC) requires clinical symptoms of CNS infection plus microbiological confirmation of the infection, usually by detection of specific IgG and IgM immunoglobulins [43].

Molecular data indicate that TBEV originated from Western Siberia about 3100 years ago and reached central Europe some 2000 years ago [12]. Some Scandinavian church records suggest a description of a TBE-like disease already in the eighteenth century [44], but the clinical entity of TBE was first reported in 1931 in Austria [47]. TBEV was first isolated in 1937 in Siberia by a Soviet team [44] led by Lev A. Zilber. Working under difficult conditions in the Taiga, they also clarified the transmission of TBEV by ticks [12];

several scientists including Zilber were later victims of persecution under Joseph Stalin and were incarcerated in Gulag camps [48].

Genetics and microbiological characteristics

TBEV occurs as three major subtypes, the European (TBEV-Eu) in central and eastern Europe transmitted by the tick *Ixodes ricinus*, the Siberian (TBEV-Sib) in eastern Europe and western Siberia, and the Far Eastern (TBEV-FE) in eastern Siberia, China, Japan, and surrounding areas—the latter two both transmitted mainly by *Ixodes persulcatus* [44]. Recently two supposedly new strains have been reported in eastern Siberia; further subtypes will possibly be found in the future [12].

The amino-acid sequence varies, within a subtype up to 2% [44]. There are considerable genetic differences between eastern and western strains, with 16.8–16.9% of nucleotide and 6.9–7.2% of amino-acid substitutions [12].

TBEV structural proteins were found to determine the efficiency of nonviremic transmission, whereas NS proteins determine cytotoxicity [49]. The virus is present in the tick's salivary glands, and a skin attachment of only 15 minutes is sufficient for transmission [11]. In addition to the usual transmission by tick bite and occasional alimentary infections by contaminated milk, exceptional TBE cases have been described after slaughter of likely viremic goats, by blood transfusion, breastfeeding, and laboratory investigations [13, 44].

Epidemiology

Prevalence studies found 0.1–5% of *I. ricinus* infected in Europe, whereas in Russia up to 40% of *I. persulcatus* may be infected [11, 13]. Tick activity starts in spring and lasts until November in central Europe, with two peaks in early and late summer [44], resulting in the name *Frühsommermeningoenzephalitis* (FSME; meaning "early summer meningoencephalitis") for TBE in German-speaking countries. In endemic areas, outdoor work and leisure activities are the main risk factors; males are mainly infected [44]. In some areas of Siberia, the Far East, and China, *I. persulcatus* is not the predominant tick species, and transmission has been attributed to *Dermacentor reticulatus, Dermacentor silvarum, Haemaphysalis concinna,* and *Haemaphysalis ovatus* [13]. The geographical distribution of TBE foci is largely driven by ecological factors and the presence of transmitting ticks [50].

One clinical case was estimated to occur for every 100 persons bitten by ticks in endemic areas, a calculation well in accordance with the 1.4% TBE rate in people knowingly bitten by ticks [13]. Seroconversion without prominent disease is common [44]. Seroprevalence rates in Europe for TBEV range from 1 to 20%, whereas Russia has much higher rates (30–100%) [44]. The past two decades experienced both an expansion of endemic foci in Europe, as well as regional increases of cases [44]. The average increase of TBE in 10 European countries was 311% between the periods 1974–1983 and 1994–2003 [51]. Part of the increase is speculated to be the result of climate change [13, 44], but human behavior and improved diagnostics are also possibilities [43]. The notable exception is Austria, where successful vaccination coverage (up to 88%) since 1981 resulted in a significant decline from the highest number of hospitalized cases per country formerly to the present about one-tenth of cases [13, 44].

TBE is endemic in 27 countries in Europe and in Asia [13]. Between 1990 and 2009, a total of 163 937 clinical TBE cases were registered in 20 European countries [13]. A map of the distribution of TBEV in Europe is given in Figure 14.5. Russia has by far the most cases and the highest TBE incidence (cases per 100 000 per year); other countries in Europe with high rates (2005–2009) were Slovenia (14.07), Estonia (11.10), Lithuania (10.59), Latvia (8.76), the Czech Republic (7.02), Switzerland (2.15), Sweden (1.99), Slovakia (1.16), Austria (0.94), Poland (0.66), Hungary (0.60), Germany (0.44), and Finland (0.39) [13]. In heavily affected Slovenia, the annual burden of TBE was estimated as 10.95 disability-adjusted life years (DALYs) per 100 000, with a higher burden in children [52]. Most recently, a detailed country-wise epidemiological report was published and also includes national recommendations for vaccination [43]. Occasional coinfection with *Borrellia burgdorferi* has been described [53].

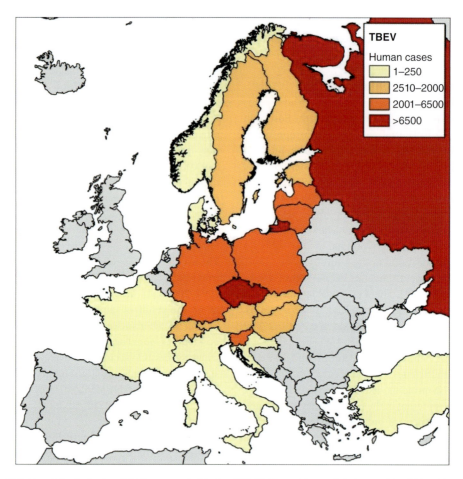

Figure 14.5 Map of the distribution of tick borne encephalitis virus (TBEV) in Europe. Human clinical cases with reliable epidemiological information are aggregated across a 10-year period (2000–2009) and the numbers of cases by country are indicated. Source: Data are from table 1 in [13]. This is Fig. 2b in [3], with kind permission.

Clinical features

Incubation time after a tick bite has a median of 8 days (range 4–28 days); however, a tick bite can occur unnoticed in up to one-third of cases [44]. The typical biphasic clinical course is seen in 72–87%, with a first viremic stage (median 5 days), featuring fever (99%), fatigue (63%), general malaise (62%), and headache and body pain (52%), accompanied by leuko- and thrombocytopenia and some elevated serum transaminases [44]. A lag phase of about 7 days is followed by the second stage, featuring neurological symptoms ranging from mild meningitis to severe encephalitis in about half of all cases, with or without spinal involvement. Seizures develop rarely, but impairment of consciousness is seen in about one-third of cases [44]. Myelitis, preferentially affecting spinal anterior horns, may result in a flaccid, poliomyelitis-like syndrome that mainly involves the upper body parts and occasionally requires ventilatory support. In Germany, 5% of cases need assisted ventilation, and 12% require intensive care [44]. Motor cranial nerves may be affected as well as vestibular and auditory functions. Involvement of the brainstem can lead to respiratory and cardiac failure, with a case fatality rate ranging up to 1.4% [44]. Rarer clinical presentations are an isolated bulbar syndrome and myeloradiculitis with severe back and limb pain and sensory impairment [44]. Increasing age has been shown as a major risk factor for severe morbidity, arguing for preferential vaccination of this population group [44]. In contrast, severe disease is rare in children younger than three years of age [44].

TBEV-IgM and -IgG are usually detectable in serum when the first neurological symptoms develop in the second phase of disease. These Igs are found in the cerebrospinal fluid (CSF) several days later, until day 10 [44], and the CSF-to-serum index is increased [13]. Specific serodiagnosis uses immunoassays for E or prM proteins from purified viruses or viruslike particles that require biosafety level-3 (BSL3) laboratories. The widely used HIT needs a rise in antibody titer for disease diagnosis [44]. Reverse transcription- polymerase chain reaction (RT-PCR) is able to detect virus in the first disease stage but rarely later [44]. CSF investigations show moderate pleocytosis with polymorphs initially and later lymphomononuclear cells that exhibit signs of considerable activation. Magnetic resonance imaging (MRI) and electroencephalogram (EEG) show nonspecific abnormalities in 18 and 77%, respectively [44].

TBEV infection frequently shows long-term morbidity, occasionally including a progressive type of encephalitis [11], mostly with subtypes other than TBEV-Eu [44]. Virus persistence has been described by isolation of viable virus and, somewhat less useful, persisting IgM antibodies in serum and CSF [11]. Some residual symptoms after 6–12 months were described in 26–46% of TBEV-Eu cases, and moderate to severe impairment of quality of life was reported in 30% [44]. If sequelae persist longer than one year, the prognosis for recovery is poor [44].

TBEV-FE may not feature the biphasic course [54] and was described as causing more severe disease than other TBEV subtypes, reportedly with fatality rates of 20–40% [44]. However, many of these grievous data are historic, and Russian publications describe chronic and progressive forms in particular with TBEV-Sib [44].

Pathology

Autopsy in human fatal cases of TBE macroscopically shows the brain with mild to severe hyperemia of parenchyma and leptomeninges, diffuse swelling, and petechial hemorrhages in the cerebrum, brainstem, and spinal cord [26]. The histopathology of TBE has been aptly described in the older literature (e.g. in [27]) as multinodular and patchy polioencephalitis with meningeal involvement. It is the prototype of the classical neuropathological triad of encephalitis: (i) parenchymal damage, (ii) reactive astro- and microgliosis, and (iii) inflammatory cellular infiltration (Figure 14.6) [14, 28]. Edematous changes with vacuolation of neuropil and of white matter are observed in all cases [26]. It was argued that every neuroviral infection usually features a fingerprint signature of selective vulnerability in the nervous system in terms of regional and cellular tropism; for neurotropic FVs in general, and for TBE in particular, there is moderate regional selectivity (preference of brainstem, cerebellum, and spinal cord, Figure 14.6a–e) and high cellular specificity, with viral tropism mainly for neurons (Figure 14.6d and f) [14].

Historically, neuropathology served as an important differential diagnostic tool when molecular diagnoses were not yet available; then, the prominent affection of cerebellar cortex in TBE (Figure 14.6c, d, and f) was used for distinction from acute poliovirus infection [27]. Inflammatory changes are widespread and accentuated in anterior horns (Figure 14.6a), brainstem (Figure 14.6b and e), cerebellum (Figure 14.6c, d, and f, and basal ganglia [29]. Neuronophagia is seen in cases with short clinical duration; in cases with longer disease duration, there is pronounced gliosis and neuronal loss. The midbrain shows predominant involvement of substantia nigra with loss of pigmented neurons. In the cerebellum, neuronophagia of Purkinje cells (Figure 14.6f), gliosis in molecular layer, and Bergmann gliosis (Figure 14.6c) are commonly observed. The maximum inflammatory changes are seen at 10 days [26].

In one detailed immunohistological study on the presence of TBEV antigen, immunoreactivity was widespread and mainly found in large neurons [26]. Numerous labeled neurons appeared morphologically intact, which might suggest that direct neuronotoxicity by viral proteins is not prominent [30]. Positive cases had a maximal disease duration of 35 days. The peak distribution of immunolabeled structures was found between 6 and 13 days.

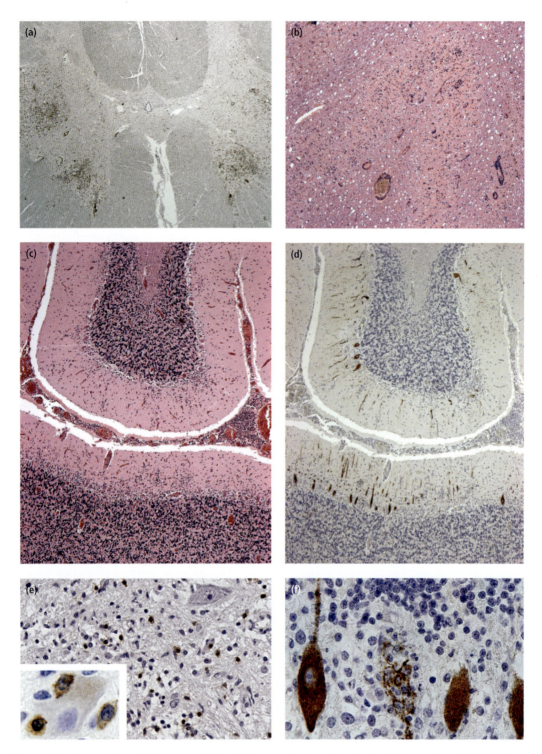

Figure 14.6 Neuropathology of tick-borne encephalitis (TBE). (a) Prominent inflammatory infiltration by microglia and macrophages of spinal gray matter. Immunohistochemistry (IHC) for CD 68, ×20. (b) Prominent inflammatory changes in inferior olives with perivascular cuffing, gliosis and neuronal loss. Hematoxylin and eosin (H&E), ×40. (c and d) Prominent inflammatory changes in cerebellar cortex with Purkinje cell reduction, gliosis of molecular layer, meningeal infiltration (c), and TBEV antigen in remaining Purkinje cell somata and their apical dendrites (d). ×40, (c) H&E and (d) IHC for TBEV [26]. (e) Diffuse parenchymal infiltration in brainstem by cytotoxic T cells, some of which attach to neurons (insert). IHC for CD 8, ×200, insert ×600. (f) TBEV antigen in Purkinje cells and central neuronophagia. IHC for TBEV [26].

Glial, ependymal, choroidal, or endothelial cells were not immunolabeled, and neither were meningeal structures, peripheral nerve, or blood cells. Inflammatory changes and TBEV antigen showed similar predilection sites, but inverse intensities: areas with prominent inflammatory infiltrates and marked neuronal damage contained only few antigen-positive neuronal processes or immunolabeled neuronophagia (Figure 14.6f). In contrast, strongly decorated intact neurons typically were not (yet) accompanied by prominent inflammatory infiltrates [26]. This suggests a time sequence of events, starting with viral production and cytopathogenicity, followed by emerging inflammation. Fas ligand was only occasionally found, and signs of neuronal apoptosis by anti-caspase 3 immunohistochemistry, terminal deoxynucleotidyl transferase dUTP nick end labeling (TUNEL) method, or morphology were not found, indicating that apoptosis is not the main mechanism of neuronal cell death in human cases of fatal TBE [30].

Immunohistochemical characterization of inflammatory infiltrates showed predominance of cytotoxic T cells (Figure 14.6e) and of macrophages or microglia (Figure 14.6a), and only few B cells. Anti-CD3 showed scattered T cells in the parenchyma. B cells were more frequently observed in the perivascular compartment [30]. CD4- and CD8-expressing cells were present in approximately equal amounts. Up to 45% of anti-CD8-immunoreactive cells were found in close contact with neurons (Fig. 14.6e inset), including TBEV-immunoreactive cellular structures, in almost all cases [26]. There was also granzyme B (GrB) expression in parenchymal T cells and occasional deposits of membrane attack complex (MAC, C5b9) in the cytoplasm of single neurons [30]. TBEV-antigen-positive neurons were closely associated with GrB-expressing lymphocytes, showing that cytotoxic T cells contribute to neuronal damage in human TBE [30]. In summary, these findings in fatal human TBE emphasize immunologic mechanisms as major players in nerve cell destruction and suggest a complex inflammatory process that involves multiple closely interrelated elements of the cellular and humoral immune systems [26, 30].

By electron microscopy (EM), TBEV virions are small enveloped spherical structures of about 50 nm diameter, first visualized in human TBE brain by Mazlo and Szanto [55].

Pathogenesis

For TBEV pathogenesis, the first barrier to infection is the skin, which is overcome by the tick bite, followed by initial local replication. The second barrier is the innate and adaptive immune response; if this is overcome, spread to peripheral organs and viremia occurs [56]. The third barrier is the virus entry to the CNS, which is mostly considered hematogenous [44]. However, in contrast to WNV, neuroinvasion has not been well studied for TBEV [56]. After entry to the CNS, the virus replicates in neurons. Recently, transcriptomics of infected neural cells in vitro identified a wide panel of proinflammatory genes and noncoding RNAs [57]. Host innate cellular responses include autophagy and apoptosis, type I interferon (IFN) response, and stimulation of the complement pathway, as well as the antiviral response by natural killer (NK) and antigen-presenting cells, finally followed by adaptive humoral and cellular immune responses [56].

Animal models and pathogenesis

Mouse models have allowed insight into host and TBEV genetic factors that are responsible for outcome of the infection [56]. These include systemic inflammatory and stress responses contributing to a fatal course [58] and also suggest a neural route to the CNS [36]. Infection of mice has confirmed data from human studies that CD8 cells determine immune pathogenesis [35]. Nonhuman primates inoculated with TBEV develop a disease similar to mild TBE and may also develop a chronic infection [2]. Among TBEV subtypes, TBEV-FE has high neurovirulence in animal studies including primates, and TBEV-Sib may cause persistent infections; however, the molecular underpinnings of TBEV neuropathogenicity and variations between subtypes still await clarification [44].

In natural infections of dogs [59] and a monkey kept in an outdoor park in Germany [51], features similar to human TBE and TBEV-antigen-containing neurons were described at necropsy.

Treatment, prevention, and conclusions

Like with other FVs, there is no specific treatment for TBE; the use of steroids is not recommended, nor is hyperimmune IgG for postexposure prophylaxis [44].

TBEV infection can be prevented effectively by vaccination. In Russia and China, vaccines are based on TBEV-FE [54], whereas against TBEV-Eu, two very similar vaccines are licensed: one against the Neudörfl strain (FSME-Immun®) and the other against the K23 strain (Encepur®) [44]. For FSME-Immun, a protection rate of more than 95% was calculated from the significant decrease of cases in Austria [44]. Vaccination is generally recommended for persons inhabiting, working in, or visiting endemic regions who might become exposed to ticks [13].

In conclusion, the past two decades have seen tremendous progress in our knowledge about FV in general, and TBEV in particular. At the end of this chapter on TBE in a book on genetics and neuropathology of infections, it is gratifying to assert that neuropathology has contributed significantly to our understanding of this fascinating disease.

References

1. John, C.C., Carabin, H., Montano, S.M. et al. (2015). Global research priorities for infections that affect the nervous system. *Nature* 527: S178–S186.
2. Holbrook, M.R. (2017). Historical perspectives on flavivirus research. *Viruses* 9: E97.
3. Beck, C., Jimenez-Clavero, A.M., Leblond, A. et al. (2013). Flaviviruses in Europe: complex circulation patterns and their consequences for the diagnosis and control of West Nile disease. *International Journal of Environmental Research and Public Health* 10: 6049–6083.
4. Tamura, K., Peterson, D., Peterson, N. et al. (2011). MEGA5: molecular evolutionary genetics analysis using maximum likelihood, evolutionary distance, and maximum parsimony methods. *Mol Biol Evol* 28: 2731–2739.
5. Beck, C. (2017). Nouvelles stratégies diagnostiques et thérapeutiques contre les flavivirus neurotropes en médecine vétérinaire [doctoral dissertation]. Paris: Université Paris-Sud.
6. Heinz, F.X. and Stiasny, K. (2012). Flaviviruses and their antigenic structure. *Journal of Clinical Virology* 55: 289–295.
7. Heinz, F.X. and Stasny, K. (2009). Flaviviren: Grundlagen. In: *Medizinische Virologie. Grundlagen, Diagnostik, Prävention und Therapie viraler Erkrankungen, 2., komplett überarbeitete und erweiterte Auflage* (eds. H.W. Doerr and W. Gerlich), 380–386. Stuttgart: Thieme.
8. Rey, F.A., Heinz, F.X., Mandl, C. et al. (1995). The envelope glycoprotein from tick-borne encephalitis virus at 2 Å resolution. *Nature* 375: 291–298.
9. Lindgren, E., Andersson, Y., Suk, J.E. et al. (2012). Monitoring EU emerging infectious disease risk due to climate change. *Science* 336: 418–419.
10. Valderrama, A., Díaz, Y., and López-Vergès, S. (2017). Interaction of flavivirus with their mosquito vectors and their impact on the human health in the Americas. *Biochemical and Biophysical Research Communications* 492: 541–547.
11. Mlera, L., Melik, W., and Bloom, M.E. (2014). The role of viral persistence in flavivirus biology. *Pathogens and Disease* 71: 137–163.
12. Kahl, O., Pogodina, V.V., Poponnikova, T. et al. (2017). TBE Milestones. In: *TBE-The Book* (eds. G. Dobler, W. Erber and H.J. Schmitt). Singapore: Global Health Press https://id-ea.org/tbe/chapter-1-tbe-milestones.
13. Süss, J. (2011). Tick-borne encephalitis 2010: epidemiology, risk areas, and virus strains in Europe and Asia – an overview. *Ticks and Tick-borne Diseases* 2: 2–15.
14. Budka, H. (1997). Viral infections. In: *Neuropathology – The Diagnostic Approach* (eds. J.H. Garcia, H. Budka, P.E. Mc Keever, et al.), 353–391. St Louis: Mosby.
15. Haymaker, W. (1961). Mosquito-borne encephalitides. In: *Encephalitides* (eds. L. van Bogaert, J. Radermecker, J. Hozay and A. Lowenthal), 38–56. Amsterdam: Elsevier.
16. Gholam, B.I., Puksa, S., and Provias, J.P. (1999). Powassan encephalitis: a case report with neuropathology and literature review. *CMAJ: Canadian Medical Association Journal* 161: 1419–1422.
17. Tavakoli, N.P., Wang, H., Dupuis, M. et al. (2009). Fatal case of deer tick virus encephalitis. *N Engl J Med* 360: 2099–2107.
18. Leech, R.W. and Harris, J.C. (1977). The neuropathology of Western equine and St. Louis encephalitis: a review of the 1975 North Dakota epidemic. *J Neuropathol Exp Neurol* 36: 611.
19. Reyes, M.G., Gardner, J.J., Poland, J.D., and Monath, T.P. (1981). St Louis encephalitis. Quantitative histologic

20. Johnson, R.T., Burke, D.S., Elwell, M. et al. (1985). Japanese encephalitis: immunocytochemical studies of viral antigen and inflammatory cells in fatal cases. *Ann Neurol* 18: 567–573.
21. Wong, K.T., Ng, K.Y., Ong, K.C. et al. (2012). Enterovirus 71 encephalomyelitis and Japanese encephalitis can be distinguished by topographic distribution of inflammation and specific intraneuronal detection of viral antigen and RNA. *Neuropathology and Applied Neurobiology* 38: 443–453.
22. Sampson, B.A. and Armbrustmacher, V. (2001). West Nile encephalitis: the neuropathology of four fatalities. *Ann N Y Acad Sci* 951: 172–178.
23. Guarner, J., Shieh, W.-J., Hunter, S. et al. (2004). Clinicopathologic study and laboratory diagnosis of 23 cases with West Nile virus encephalomyelitis. *Human Pathology* 35: 983–990.
24. Rosemberg, S. (1980). Neuropathology of S. Paulo south coast epidemic encephalitis (Rocio flavivirus). *J Neurol Sci* 45: 1–12. issn: 0022-0510x.
25. Tomazic, J., Poljak, M., Popovic, P. et al. (1997). Tick-borne encephalitis: possibly a fatal disease in its acute stage. PCR amplification of TBE RNA from postmortem brain tissue. *Infection* 25: 41–43.
26. Gelpi, E., Preusser, M., Garzuly, F. et al. (2005). Visualization of central European tick-borne encephalitis infection in fatal human cases. *J Neuropathol Exp Neurol* 64: 506–512.
27. Seitelberger, F. and Jellinger, K. (1966). Neuropathologie der Zeckenencephalitis (mit Vergleichsuntersuchung der Arbo-Virus-Encephalitiden und der Poliomyelitis) [Neuropathology of tick-borne encephalitis (with comparative studies of arbovirus encephalitides and poliomyelitis)]. *Neuropatologia Polska.* 4: 366–400.
28. Spatz, H. (1930). Encephalitis. In: *Handbuch der Geisteskrankheiten* (ed. O. Bumke), 157. Berlin: Springer.
29. Love, S., Wiley, C.A., and Lucas, S. (2015). Viral infections. In: *Greenfield's Neuropathology*, 9e (eds. S. Love, H. Budka, J.W. Ironside and A. Perry), 1087–1091. Boca Raton – London – New York: CRC Press.
30. Gelpi, E., Preusser, M., Laggner, U. et al. (2006). Inflammatory response in human tick-borne encephalitis: analysis of postmortem brain tissue. *Journal of NeuroVirology* 12: 322–327.
31. Iwasaki, Y., Zhao, J.X., Yamamoto, T., and Konno, H. (1986). Immunohistochemical demonstration of viral antigens in Japanese encephalitis. *Acta Neuropathol* 70: 79–81.
32. Desai, A., Shankar, S.K., Ravi, V. et al. (1995). Japanese encephalitis virus antigen in the human brain and its topographic distribution. *Acta Neuropathol* 89: 368–373.
33. Wang, Y., Lobigs, M., Lee, E., and Mullbacher, A. (2003). CD8+ T cells mediate recovery and immunopathology in West Nile virus encephalitis. *J Virol* 77: 13323–13334.
34. Liu, Y., Blanden, R.V., and Mullbacher, A. (1989). Identification of cytolytic lymphocytes in West Nile virus-infected murine central nervous system. *The Journal of General Virology* 70: 565–573.
35. Růžek, D., Salát, J., Palus, M. et al. (2009). CD8+ T-cells mediate immunopathology in tick-borne encephalitis. *Virology* 384: 1–6.
36. Nagata, N., Iwata-Yoshikawa, N., Hayasaka, D. et al. (2015). The pathogenesis of 3 neurotropic flaviviruses in a mouse model depends on the route of neuroinvasion after viremia. *Journal of Neuropathology & Experimental Neurology* 74: 250–260.
37. Neal, J.W. (2014). Flaviviruses are neurotropic, but how do they invade the CNS? *Journal of Infection* 69: 203–215.
38. Taylor, M.P. and Enquist, L.W. (2015). Axonal spread of neuroinvasive viral infections. *Trends in Microbiology* 23: 283–288.
39. Yoshii, K., Sunden, Y., Yokozawa, K. et al. (2014). A critical determinant of neurological disease associated with highly pathogenic tick-borne flavivirus in mice. *Journal of Virology* 88: 5406–5420.
40. Maximova, O.A., Faucette, L.J., Ward, J.M. et al. (2009). Cellular inflammatory response to flaviviruses in the central nervous system of a primate host. *Journal of Histochemistry & Cytochemistry* 57: 973–989.
41. Smith, J.L., Jeng, S., Mc Weeney, S.K., and Hirsch, A.J. (2017). A MicroRNA screen identifies the Wnt signaling pathway as a regulator of the interferon response during flavivirus infection. *Journal of Virology* 91: e02388–e02316.
42. Teterina, N.L., Maximova, O.A., Kenney, H. et al. (2016). MicroRNA-based control of tick-borne flavivirus neuropathogenesis: challenges and perspectives. *Antiviral Research* 127: 57–67.
43. Erber, W., Schmitt, H.-J., and Vuković Janković, T. (2017). Epidemiology by country – an overview. In: *TBE-The Book* (eds. G. Dobler, W. Erber and H.J. Schmitt). Singapore: Global Health Press https://id-ea.org/tbe/chapter-4-pathogenesis-of-TBE-with-a-focus-on-molecular-mechanisms.
44. Lindquist, L. and Vapalahti, O. (2008). Tick-borne encephalitis. *The Lancet* 371: 1861–1871.

45. Dobler, G., Erber, W., and Schmitt, H.J. (eds.) (2017). *TBE-The Book*. Singapore: Global Health Press.
46. Amato-Gauci, A.J. and Zeller, H. (2012). Tick-borne encephalitis joins the diseases under surveillance in the European Union. *Eurosurveillance* 17: 20299.
47. Schneider, H. (1931). Über epidemische akute "Meningitis serosa". *Wien Klin Wochenschr* 44: 350–352.
48. Zlobin, V.I., Pogodina, V.V., and Kahl, O. (2017). A brief history of the discovery of tick-borne encephalitis virus in the late 1930s (based on reminiscences of members of the expeditions, their colleagues, and relatives). *Ticks and Tick-borne Diseases* 8: 813–820.
49. Khasnatinov, M.A., Tuplin, A., Gritsun, D.J. et al. (2016). Tick-borne encephalitis virus structural proteins are the primary viral determinants of non-viraemic transmission between ticks whereas non-structural proteins affect cytotoxicity. *PLOS ONE* 11: e0158105.
50. Sun, R.-X., Lai, S.-J., Yang, Y. et al. (2017). Mapping the distribution of tick-borne encephalitis in mainland China. *Ticks and Tick-borne Diseases* 8: 631–639.
51. Süss, J., Gelpi, E., Klaus, C. et al. (2007). Tickborne encephalitis in naturally exposed monkey (*Macaca sylvanus*). *Emerging Infectious Diseases* 13: 905–907.
52. Fafangel, M., Cassini, A., Colzani, E. et al. (2017). Estimating the annual burden of tick-borne encephalitis to inform vaccination policy, Slovenia, 2009 to 2013. *Euro surveillance: bulletin Europeen sur les maladies transmissibles = European communicable disease bulletin* 2017: 22.
53. Oksi, J., Viljanen, M.K., Kalimo, H. et al. (1993). Fatal encephalitis caused by concomitant infection with tick-borne encephalitis virus and *Borrelia burgdorferi*. *Clin Infect Dis* 16: 392–396.
54. Xing, Y., Schmitt, H.-J., Arguedas, A., and Yang, J. (2017). Tick-borne encephalitis in China: a review of epidemiology and vaccines. *Vaccine* 35: 1227–1237.
55. Mazlo, M. and Szanto, J. (1978). Morphological demonstration of the virus of tick-borne encephalitis in the human brain. *Acta Neuropathol* 43: 251–253.
56. Kröger, A.Ö. and Överby, A.K. (2017). Pathogenesis of TBE with a focus on molecular mechanisms. In: *TBE-The Book* (eds. G. Dobler, W. Erber and H.J. Schmitt). Singapore: Global Health Press https://id-ea.org/tbe/chapter-4-pathogenesis-of-TBE-with-a-focus-on-molecular-mechanisms.
57. Selinger, M., Wilkie, G.S., Tong, L. et al. (2017). Analysis of tick-borne encephalitis virus-induced host responses in human cells of neuronal origin and interferon-mediated protection. *Journal of General Virology* 98: 2043–2060.
58. Hayasaka, D., Nagata, N., Fujii, Y. et al. (2009). Mortality following peripheral infection with tick-borne encephalitis virus results from a combination of central nervous system pathology, systemic inflammatory and stress responses. *Virology* 390: 139–150.
59. Weissenböck, H., Suchy, A., and Holzmann, H. (1998). Tick-borne encephalitis in dogs: neuropathological findings and distribution of antigen. *Acta Neuropathol* 95: 361–366.

15

Flaviviruses 2: West Nile, St. Louis Encephalitis, Murray Valley Encephalitis, Yellow Fever, and Dengue

Edward S. Johnson[1] and Juan M. Bilbao[2]

[1] Department of Laboratory Medicine and Pathology, University of Alberta, Edmonton, Alberta, Canada
[2] Department of Pathology, University of Toronto, Toronto, Ontario, Canada

Abbreviations

AFP	acute flaccid paralysis
BBB	blood-brain barrier
CCR5	CC-chemokine receptor 5
CNS	central nervous system
CSF	cerebrospinal fluid
CT	computed tomography
DCSIGN	dendritic cell-specific ICAM-3 grabbing non-integrin
DENV	dengue virus
DF	dengue fever
DHF	dengue hemorrhagic fever
DSS	dengue shock syndrome
E protein	envelope protein
ELISA	enzyme-linked immunosorbent assay
FLAIR	fluid attenuation inversion recovery
HLA	human leukocyte antigen
IHC	immunohistochemistry
INF-γ	interferon γ
IRF-3	interferon regulatory factor-3
ISH	in situ hybridization
M protein	membrane protein
MBL	Mannose-binding lectin
MHC	major histocompatibility complex
MICB	MHC class1 polypeptide-related sequence B
MRI	magnetic resonance imaging
MVEV	Murray Valley encephalitis virus
NHP	nonhuman primates
NS1	nonstructural protein 1
NS3	nonstructural protein 3
NS5	nonstructural protein 5
OAS-1	$2'$-$5'$ oligoadenylate synthetase-1
PLCE 1	phospholipase C, epsilon 1
RT-PCR	reverse transcriptase-polymerase chain reaction
SLEV	St. Louis encephalitis virus
TNF-α	tumor necrosis factor alpha
VDR	vitamin D receptor
VEGF	vascular endothelial growth factor
WNF	West Nile fever
WNND	West Nile neuroinvasive disease
WNV	West Nile virus
YFV	Yellow fever virus

Infections of the Central Nervous System: Pathology and Genetics, First Edition. Edited by Fabrice Chrétien, Kum Thong Wong, Leroy R. Sharer, Catherine (Katy) Keohane and Françoise Gray.
© 2020 John Wiley & Sons Ltd. Published 2020 by John Wiley & Sons Ltd.

Introduction

In addition to their mosquito vector–enzootic vertebrate host cycle of transmission and replication, West Nile virus (WNV), St. Louis encephalitis virus (SLEV), Murray Valley encephalitis (MVEV), yellow fever virus (YFV), and dengue virus (DENV) share many other features. Each virus group is usually comprised of serotype strains or lineages that have variations in virological properties, including virulence, some epidemiologic features that overlap, and a common pathogenic mechanism of infection and dissemination in the host. However, other aspects differ, most notably in the pattern of human infection: WNV, SLEV, and MVEV are neurotropic, whereas YFV and DENV are viscerotropic. Similarities among these five viruses permit discussion as a group; differences separate sections for each.

Epidemiology

Geographic distribution

The geographic distribution of these viruses extends worldwide throughout the tropical and subtropical zones (latitudes 35° N to 35° S) with variable incursions into temperate zones [1–5] (Table 15.1). The exceptions are SLEV and MVEV, which have regional distributions. SLEV tends to be restricted to the Western Hemisphere, predominantly in the continental United States and southern Canada. MVEV is endemic to Western Australia, Northern Territory, Papua New Guinea, and Irian Jaya with periodic epidemic spread into southeastern Australia (1951, 1956, 1974, 1981) [2, 3]. Environmental conditions that promote enhancement of the transmitting mosquito-vector population predicate the geographic distribution of each virus and optimally include hot humid weather, intermittent rain, and dry spells. Where these conditions are seasonal (late spring through early autumn), the virus can persist in a reservoir of "overwintering" adult mosquitoes or via vertical transmission into deposited eggs to await hatching in the next seasonal cycle [1, 2, 4].

Burden of human disease

The human diseases associated with these viruses constitute major burdens of illness. WNV is the most recent to achieve global dissemination. Following its initial isolation in the West Nile district of Uganda in 1937, its spread has progressed over decades into the Middle East, Russia, and Europe. After being introduced via the New York epidemic of 1999, it has had an accelerated distribution through North, Central, and South Americas [1, 2, 5]. For the period of 1999–2007 in the United States, the Center for Disease Control and Prevention (CDC) reported an average annual incidence of 0.439 cases per 100 000 per year. During this time WNV displaced SLEV, once the most common neuroinvasive arboviral infection, from an average annual incidence of 0.019 cases to 0.007 cases per 100 000 per year [6]. However, yellow fever and dengue are a greater burden. Notwithstanding problems in data collection, yellow fever has an estimated annual incidence of 200 000 cases per year, including 30 000 deaths, whereas that for dengue is 25–100 million cases per year, of which 25 000 have severe disease [1, 2]. Both diseases are in resurgence because of climate changes, increased urbanization with crowding, introduction of displaced infected immigrants and refugees, unchecked vector populations because of inadequate control measures, and lapses of vaccination protocols or absence of vaccine.

Vectors and hosts

In the course of their phylogenic evolution, these five flaviviruses have partitioned into two groups as denoted by the genus of transmitting vector, differences in the principal amplifying vertebrate hosts, and the patterns of human infection [1, 2]. For WNV, SLEV, and MVEV, the vector is the *Culex* mosquito, the enzootic hosts passeriform or columbiform birds (WNV, SLEV) or ardeid water birds (MVEV), and human infection manifests as meningoencephalomyelitis (Tables 15.1 and 15.2). The corollary for YFV and DENV is the *Aedes* mosquito, man and nonhuman primates (NHP), and hemorrhagic fevers. The species of each genus of mosquito are adapted to specific local habitats, which can influence the characteristics of the transmission cycle. As an example, species of *Aedes*

Table 15.1 Epidemiology of WNV, SLEV, MVEV, YFV, and DENV Infections.

Flavivirus	Number of Serotypes/ Lineages	Geographical Distribution	Mosquito Vector	Amplifying Enzootic Hosts	Other Hosts
WNV	4	Africa Middle East Europe Russia Continental United States Canada Asia[a] Australia[b] Central America Caribbean South America	*Culex* spp.[c]	Passeriform birds[d]	Man Horses Other vertebrate spp. (>30)
SLEV	7	Continental United States[e] Canada[f] Caribbean Central and South America	*Culex* spp.[c]	Passeriform birds[d] Columbiform birds[g]	Man Horses
MVEV	1	Australia[h] Papua New Guinea Irian Jaya	*Culex annulirostris*	Ardeid water birds[i]	Man Horses
YFV	1	Sub-Saharan Africa South America (Tropical)	*Aedes aegypti* and other *Aedes* spp.[j] *Haemagogus* spp.[k] *Sabethes* spp.[k]	Man NHPs	
DENV	4	Africa Asia[l] Australia[m] Central America Caribbean South America	*Aedes aegypti* and other *Aedes* spp.[n]	Man NHPs	

[a] Iran and Indian subcontinent.
[b] Kunjin virus subtype of WNV.
[c] *Culex pipiens, Culex tarsalis, Culex quinquefasciatus, Culex restuans, Culex salinarius, Culex stigmatosoma.*
[d] Passeriform birds: jays, blackbirds, crows, finches, and sparrows.
[e] Except New England States and South Carolina.
[f] Ontario and Manitoba.
[g] Columbiform birds: pigeons and doves.
[h] Western Australia, New Territory, and southeastern Australia (infrequent).
[i] Ardeid birds: herons and egrets.
[j] African forest/savanna vectors: *Aedes africanus, Aedes furcifer, Aedes vittatus, Aedes luteocephalus.*
[k] South American forest vectors.
[l] South Asia, Southeast Asia, and Western Pacific.
[m] Queensland.
[n] *Aedes albopictus, Aedes polynesienis, Aedes scutellaris.*
DENV, Dengue Virus; MVEV, Murray Valley Encephalitis Virus; NHPs, nonhuman primates; SLEV, St. Louis Encephalitis Virus; WNV, West Nile Virus; YFV, Yellow Fever Virus.
Sources: Pierson and Diamond [1]; Thomas et al. [2]; Knox et al. [3]; Reisen [4]; Murgue et al. [5].

Table 15.2 Clinical Features of WNV, SLEV, MVEV, YFV, and DENV Infections.

Flavivirus	Patient Risk Factors	Incubation Period	Clinical Illness	Anatomical Sites	Overall Mortality	Sequelae
WNV	Age > 50 years Male sex HIV infection Immunosuppression SNPs: OAS-1, IRF-3, MX1 genes chemokine receptor CCR5	2–4 days	Meningitis (30–40%) Encephalitis (50–60%) AFP (5–10%)	Brain: brainstem> cerebellum> subcortical gray> cerebral cortex Spinal cord Eye	4–14%	Fatigue/headache Neurodefects: cognition memory motor movement Weakness/paralysis
SLEV	Age > 60 years Male sex HIV infection Immunosuppression	5–15 days	Meningitis Encephalitis	Brain: brainstem> thalamus> cerebellum> basal ganglia/ cerebral cortex Spinal cord	5–20%	Fatigue/headache Memory difficulty Emotional disorder Tremor Unsteadiness Weakness
MVEV	Age – childhood Male sex	1–4 weeks	Encephalitis	Brain: thalamus> brainstem> cerebellum> basal ganglia/ cerebral cortex Spinal cord	15–30%	Neurodefects: cognition movement Emotional disorder Weakness/paralysis
YFV	Age > 40 years Male sex	3–6 days	Yellow fever: Period of Intoxication	Liver Immune system Kidney Heart Capillary bed	20–50%	Fatigue/weakness Secondary infection
DENV	**Secondary** infection: heterologous DENV strain **Primary** infection: infant of immune mother SNPs: HLA, MICB, PLCE1, VDR, DCSIGN, MBL genes	2–7 days	DHF: **thrombocytopenia** DSS	Liver Immune system Capillary bed	1–50%	Fatigue Secondary infection

AFP, acute flaccid paralysis; DCSIGN, dendritic cell-specific ICAM-3 grabbing non-integrin; DENV, dengue virus; DHF, dengue hemorrhagic fever; DSS, dengue shock syndrome; HIV, human immunodeficiency virus; HLA, human leukocyte antigen; IRF-3, interferon regulatory factor-3; MBL, mannose-binding lectin; MICB, Major histocompatibility complex (MHC) Class I polypeptide-related sequence B; MVEV, Murray Valley encephalitis virus; OAS-1, 2'-5 oligoadenylate synthetase-1; PLCE1, phospholipase C, epsilon 1; SLEV, St. Louis encephalitis virus; SNPs, single nucleotide polymorphisms; VDR, vitamin D receptor; WNV, West Nile virus; YFV, Yellow Fever virus.

Incubation period: Refers to period from inoculation of virus to onset of initial nonspecific symptoms; may remit or progress to severe disease.

Overall mortality: Refers to aggregate mortality. For WNV, SLEV, and YFV mortality is higher in patients who are older and those with comorbidity factors; WNV mortality is also higher in patients with encephalitis and AFP. For DENV DHF/DSS, mortality is associated with availability of supportive care measures; if present, approximately 1%.

Capillary bed: Refers to increased capillary permeability in terminal stage with plasma leakage causing pleural and abdominal effusions.

Sources: Pierson and Diamond [1]; Thomas et al. [2]; Knox et al. [3]; Kleinschmidt-De Masters and Becham [8]; Stephens [11]; Khor et al. [12]; Bigham et al. [13].

mosquitoes restricted to savanna–forest habitats in Africa and the corresponding *Haemagogus* and *Sabethes* species in the forested regions of South America principally transmit YFV to monkey populations (jungle or sylvatic cycle), with human exposure uncommon because of the paucity of people. In urban areas, the preferred locale for *Aedes aegypti*, human infection can be high because of population density [7]. Infection of nonenzootic hosts (e.g. man with WNV, SLEV, and MVEV) can restrict virus transmission because these hosts usually do not generate or sustain a level of viremia sufficient to infect a new cohort of feeding mosquitoes (dead-end hosts). Infection may be endemic or epidemic, contingent upon the vector population and the proportion of susceptible unexposed hosts.

Risk factors and genetics

Key factors that predispose to severe forms of infection associated with these viruses are listed in Table 15.2. The higher risk in men is ascribed to their predominance in outdoor occupations, with a greater probability of unprotected exposure to feeding mosquitoes. Iatrogenic transmission of WNV by transfusion of blood products or solid-organ transplantation is documented; the risk for neuroinvasive disease in transplant recipients increases by 40–70% [8]. Screening of individual blood samples and donors of solid organs by WNV nucleic acid testing has almost eliminated this risk for blood products, although not for solid organs because of possible latent viral persistence in the organ tissues. WNV can also be transmitted transplacentally or via lactation from an infected mother [2]. More recent is the documentation of transmission of SLEV by transfused blood products in patients undergoing transplants [9, 10]. Whether similar means of transmission can occur with MVEV, YFV, and DENV has not currently been investigated. Age older than 40 years poses a major risk for severe forms of WNV, SLEV, and YFV infection because of senescent waning of effective immune responses. Immunosuppression by whatever cause is a significant factor for both the severity of infection and systemic dissemination of WNV [8]. Immunological factors also affect the progression of dengue into severe illness, whereby a secondary infection by a different DENV serotype can augment the risk 10-fold due to triggering aberrant immune responses that facilitate rather than protect against disease [1]. Several recent genetic studies have identified single nucleotide polymorphisms in human leukocyte antigen (HLA) and major histocompatibility complex (MHC) class1 polypeptide-related sequence B (MICB) genes as well as non-HLA genes (e.g. phospholipase C, epsilon 1 [PLCE1], vitamin D receptor [VDR], Fcg receptor II, dendritic cell-specific ICAM-3 grabbing non-integrin [DCSIGN], and mannose-binding lectin [MBL]), which influence the risk for severe dengue [11, 12]. Similar studies have noted polymorphisms in the interferon regulatory factor-3 (IRF 3), MX1, and OAS-1 genes, involved in type 1 interferon (IFN) signaling, and chemokine receptor CCR5 that are associated with susceptibility for WNV infection and risk for neuroinvasion, respectively [2, 13].

Clinical features

Shared symptoms and signs

All five infections have a similar spectrum of human disease: asymptomatic infection, overt self-limited constitutional malaise, and severe forms of illness specific to each virus [1–3]. The proportion of people experiencing an asymptomatic infection is difficult to estimate because of under-reporting, but seems to range from 50 to 80%. The same problem applies to gauging the proportion of self-limited illness, to which descriptive names are appended: West Nile fever (WNF–WNV), period of infection (YFV), and dengue fever (DF–DENV). For all viruses, the incubation period after inoculation is approximately two weeks (Table 15.2). Onset of illness is abrupt with a core constellation of symptoms: high fever, headache, fatigue, retro-orbital pain, and myalgia. In addition, there may be symptoms of upper respiratory or gastrointestinal tract infection or back pain sometimes accompanied by bone and joint pain (DENV).

Specific signs include:
- Rash, usually maculopapular (i.e. WNV, DENV, SLEV, MVEV),
- Bradycardia (i.e. YFV, DENV), and
- Cutaneous petechiae and minor mucosal bleeding due to thrombocytopenia (DENV).

Malaise lasts a week or less, representing the period of viremia when the patient is infectious and potentially able to transmit the virus. Though often remitting spontaneously, it can prompt hospitalization or progress to severe illness.

Disease-specific symptoms and signs
West Nile Neuroinvasive Disease
Development of West Nile neuroinvasive disease (WNND), often preceded by a prodrome resembling WNF, occurs in <1% of people infected with WNV. However, the risk is greater in patients with predisposing factors (listed in Table 15.2) and comorbidities of hypertension and diabetes mellitus [2, 8]. Three clinical syndromes are described, which can manifest separately or overlap (Table 15.2) [2, 8, 14]. In addition to customary symptoms and signs, tremor and myoclonus can accompany WNV meningitis. Clinical features of encephalitis mirror the neuroanatomical sites involved with Parkinsonism, cranial nerve palsies (commonly facial nerve), ataxia, and cerebellar signs noted in conjunction with altered consciousness. Severe generalized weakness is a distinctive symptom in 50% of patients. Acute flaccid paralysis (AFP), resulting from spinal cord involvement, is characterized by asymmetrical weakness of one or more limbs with, or without, associated bowel and/or bladder dysfunction (one-third of patients) or paresthesias. Respiratory failure can ensue, requiring assisted ventilation. Ophthalmic disease can occur independently, is self-limited, and manifests as optic neuritis, chorioretinitis, uveitis, retinal vasculitis, and hemorrhage. Neurological recovery is marred by sequelae in 70–75% of patients (listed in Table 15.2), which can be long term (40% at eight years) [8].

St. Louis encephalitis
Neuroinvasive disease with SLEV is heralded by a prodrome as described. The proportion of patients with meningitis, encephalitis, and myelitis is similar to WNND, as are the symptoms and signs and topographical distribution of disease (Table 15.2) [2]. Although less aggressive than WNV, patients aged >60 years have greater risk for encephalitis, morbidity, and mortality. Sequelae occur in 30–50% of survivors and parallel WNND [1].

Murray valley encephalitis
The onset of encephalitis is preceded by a prodrome of two to five days duration in 1 in 150 to 1 in 1000 patients infected with MVE [3]. However, it is unknown how many patients with this nonspecific syndrome remit without encephalitis. Neurological illness, resembling WNND, commences with alterations in consciousness progressing to coma or, in children, seizures. Four clinical scenarios are described: relentless progression to death, flaccid paralysis due to spinal cord disease, brainstem involvement with cranial nerve palsies and tremor, and remitting encephalitis with complete recovery (40%) [3, 15]. Case mortality is 15–30%, and long-term sequelae (similar to WNND and St. Louis encephalitis) occur in 30–50% of survivors [2, 3]. Outcomes appear worse with flaccid paralysis and in persons who are young and those who are elderly [3].

Yellow fever
An estimated 15% of people infected with yellow fever proceed, after a short remission, from the period of infection into the period of intoxication heralded by relapse of fever and prostration. As a multisystem disease, major clinical features [1, 2, 7] are:
- Moderate to severe icteric hepatitis,
- Hemorrhagic diathesis (i.e. gastrointestinal bleeding, oozing from gums and puncture sites, cutaneous petechiae, and purpura),
- Acute tubular necrosis with renal failure and metabolic acidosis,
- Cardiac arrhythmias, enlargement, and failure, and
- Hypotension and terminal shock.

Neurological complications of confusion, seizures, and coma may occur as secondary manifestations. Mortality is high with death in 7–10 days; convalescence is prolonged with risk of bacterial infections.

Dengue
The severe forms of dengue, dengue hemorrhagic fever (DHF) and dengue shock syndrome (DSS), occur in approximately 2–4% of infections and are more often associated with reinfection by a second heterologous serotype [2, 16]. Following an illness

resembling DF, there is a transition into DHF. The major pathophysiologic feature is an increase in capillary permeability with plasma leakage into pleural and abdominal cavities [1, 2, 17]. Fever abates before this critical phase, during which there is hemoconcentration and ensuing hypotension. It lasts 24–48 hours and can rapidly shift into terminal shock (i.e. DSS) with multiorgan failure. The other denoting feature is a hemorrhagic diathesis, heralded by thrombocytopenia, with petechial and gastrointestinal bleeding. A concurrent hepatitis can occur. Mortality is high unless there is supportive clinical treatment, including fluid replacement. Duration of illness is 7–10 days, followed by a short convalescence that in adults can be prolonged by fatigue and bradycardia.

A variety of associated neurological disorders has been documented in clinical reports, summarized in a recent comprehensive review [18]. The estimated incidence of these complications is 0.5–5.4% of laboratory-confirmed infections, although outliers have posted higher percentages. Dengue encephalopathy and encephalitis comprise the majority in patients with either primary or secondary infection. These disorders are more likely associated with DHF than DF and share the clinical features of altered consciousness (confusion to coma) and onset of seizures. Focal neurologic signs are more often associated with cases designated as encephalitis. Nonetheless, the distinction between encephalopathy and encephalitis remains poorly delineated as a result of incomplete or inconsistent diagnostic criteria applied among the case series. Cerebrospinal fluid (CSF) analyses, including laboratory diagnostic tests for DENV, have not helped because of infrequent testing and discordance with the clinical setting or, in fatal cases, the absence of inflammation on neuropathologic examination. Stroke, particularly hemorrhagic, has been confirmed in the convalescent phase in a population-based cohort study. Patients with dengue had an incidence of 5.33 versus 3.72 per 1000 per person years in controls; the risk was 2.49 higher in the first two months [19]. Immune-mediated syndromes and neuromuscular complications have been described and the most common neuro-ophthalmologic complications are dengue maculopathy and retinal vasculopathy.

Neuro-imaging

In West Nile encephalitis, magnetic resonance imaging (MRI) studies are more sensitive than computed tomography (CT) in detecting lesions in 40–70% of patients; lesions usually appear a week after onset of illness [14]. On T2-weighted windows and fluid attenuation inversion recovery (FLAIR), the lesions are hyperintense and distributed as listed in Table 15.2 with a predilection for the thalamus, substantia nigra, and anterior horns of the spinal cord; abnormalities can occur in the subcortical white matter. Lesions in the periventricular regions, leptomeninges, and spinal roots may enhance with gadolinium. In Murray Valley encephalitis, MRI demonstrates a bilateral pattern of similar abnormalities in the thalamus, temporal lobes, red nucleus, and spinal cord [3]. Although invaluable in providing a timely preliminary diagnosis, because of overlap with WNND and Japanese encephalitis, these findings are not conclusive. CT imaging is less sensitive, showing changes in severe disease. Neuroimaging findings in St. Louis encephalitis have not been well-studied, but non-enhancing T2-weighted hyperintense lesions in the substantia nigra on MRI have been emphasized [2]. CT and MRI findings in dengue encephalopathy and encephalitis are not well-documented. When described, cerebral edema is the most common abnormality, then "encephalitis-like" changes (not specified), T2/FLAIR focal hyperintense signals, and rarely, intracranial hemorrhage [18].

Laboratory findings

All five viral diseases have a common profile of clinical laboratory abnormalities; what differs between each is the extent. Hematological findings, early in illness, include a leukocytosis that shifts to a leukopenia [1, 2, 14], and except for SLEV/MVEV infections, thrombocytopenia, which is more severe in yellow fever and dengue. In the latter two infections, there are additional coagulation defects [7, 17]. Corresponding to the DSS phase of dengue, the hematocrit can increase ≥20% [17]. Serum aspartate and alanine aminotransferase levels are increased, variable, and mild for WNV and SLEV infections, but marked in dengue and yellow fever. Direct bilirubin level is similarly elevated, more in yellow fever in which bilirubin and transaminase levels parallel the severity of hepatic disease [7]. Other biochemical abnormalities include an increase in creatine kinase and hyponatremia because of inappropriate antidiuretic hormone syndrome. In yellow fever, renal impairment is characterized by albuminuria and three - to eight-fold increase in serum creatinine [7].

The CSF in West Nile, St. Louis, and Murray Valley meningoencephalitis reveals a mild to moderate increase in protein paralleled by a pleocytosis, usually lymphocytic [2, 3, 15]. When undertaken in yellow fever and dengue, the findings are often normal; if abnormal, the protein content is elevated. In dengue, a pleocytosis may be present, but lacks correlation with the CSF protein or patient's clinical status [18]. In all diseases, glucose content is normal.

Shared findings are observed in electrophysiologic tests. Except for yellow fever, electroencephalography often is abnormal, commonly showing diffuse slowing. Focal seizure activity and periodic lateralized epileptiform discharges are also noted in West Nile and St. Louis encephalitis [2, 14]. Electromyography and nerve conduction velocity studies in WNV infection further reveal features of denervation, motor axonal neuropathy, or demyelinating sensorimotor neuropathy [2, 14]. In yellow fever, electrocardiography may disclose ST–T wave abnormalities, extrasystoles, and bradycardia [7].

Serologic studies are the mainstay of diagnosis [2, 7, 14, 17]. The most applicable are antibody capture enzyme-linked immunosorbent assays (ELISA) for detecting flaviviral-specific immunoglobulin M (IgM) antibodies in the serum by days 7–10, and later for immunoglobulin G (IgG) titers. CSF serology in neurotropic infections can detect IgM antibodies earlier, reflecting intrathecal synthesis and neuroinvasion. If IgM antibodies are present in CSF and serum, CSF and serum antibody ratios assist in excluding the possibility of CSF contamination because of breakdown of the blood-brain barrier (BBB). Persistence of serum IgM antibodies varies among viruses: 60 days or less for YFV and DENV, 9 months for SLEV, and 16 months for WNV. In monitoring IgG titers, acute and convalescent sera must be tested to demonstrate a four-fold or more rise for diagnostic confirmation. The more recent introduction of viral antigen detection by ELISA for the E/M antigen and nonstructural protein 1 (NS1) protein confers high specificity but not necessarily sensitivity [7, 17]. Cross-reactivity with heterologous flaviviral antibodies can occur, notably with MVEV [2, 3]; where additional testing is required, greater specificity can be attained using other ELISA formats (e.g. competitive-epitope-blocking), hemagglutination tests, and neutralization tests (plaque reduction neutralization). A variety of molecular platforms is available using reverse transcriptase-polymerase chain reaction (RT- PCR) techniques for viral detection in early viremia in serum and, with less sensitivity, CSF [7, 14, 17]. This methodology is most applicable to screening blood products for WNV and diagnosing delayed or attenuated seroconversion in patients who are immunocompromised [2, 14]. Viral isolation from serum or CSF has a low diagnostic yield but is more suitable for biopsy or autopsy tissue. Different isolation systems are available: intracerebral inoculation of suckling mice, C6/36 or AP61 mosquito cell cultures, and various mammalian cell culture lines (Vero, LLCMK2, and BHK21) [2, 7, 17].

Pathology

WNND

Other than cerebral edema, there are no notable macroscopic findings. Microscopic examination [1, 8, 14], however, discloses features of meningoencephalitis or myelitis: microglial nodules, associated neuronophagia, patchy neuronal loss, and lymphocytic infiltrates. Lymphocytes in the parenchyma are predominantly CD8 T cells and in perivascular cuffs are a mixture of CD4 T and CD20 B lymphocytes (Figure 15.1). Necrosis is uncommon and inflammation varies in intensity. Inflammation is preferentially distributed in gray matter (Table 15.2): substantia nigra and hypoglossal motor nucleus in the brainstem, dentate nucleus and molecular and Purkinje cell layers in the cerebellum (Figure 15.1c), thalamus in the cerebrum, and anterior horns in the spinal cord. Spinal and cranial nerve roots and dorsal root and sympathetic ganglia are less known sites. In patients who are immunocompromised, lesions are more widely

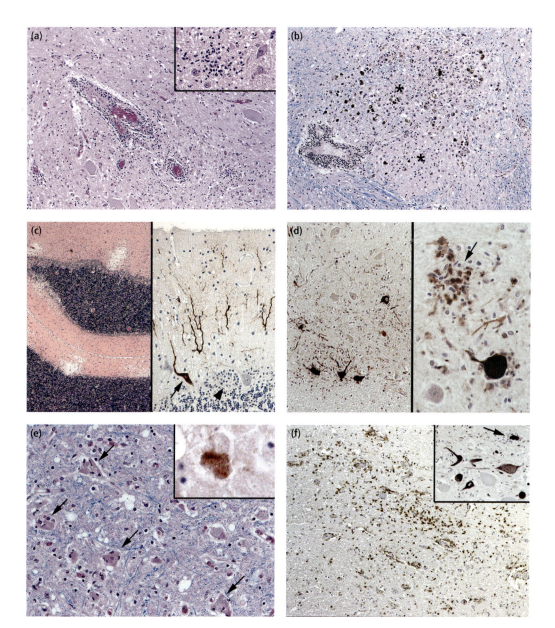

Figure 15.1 Histopathological features of West Nile Virus (WNV) encephalitis. (a) Thalamus: Perivascular chronic inflammatory cell infiltrates track into neuropil. Insert shows a microglial nodule. (b) Substantia nigra: Marked patchy loss of pigmented neurons (asterisk) with chronic inflammatory cells scantily scattered in neuropil but densely cuffing a parenchymal blood vessel. (c) Cerebellum, cortex: Left panel, multifocal rarefaction of the molecular layer due to Purkinje cell injury. Right panel, immunohistochemical demonstration of WNV antigen in Purkinje cell and dendrite (arrow) and nearby dendritic processes but not in cells of the granule cell layer. A microglial nodule (arrowhead) is adjacent to an uninfected Purkinje cell. (d) Cerebellum, dentate nucleus: Left panel, presence of WNV antigen in perikarya and processes of a row of neurons bordering a cluster of uninfected neurons. Right panel, degenerating neuron and its process, diffusely labeled with WNV antigen, is undergoing neuronophagia. In a nearby microglial nodule (arrow), many macrophages contain presumably phagocytized viral antigen. (e) Hypoglossal motor nucleus: Scant parenchymal infiltrate accompanies several neurons (arrows) surrounded by microglia engaged in early neuronophagia; insert shows perikaryal localization of WNV antigen in a neuron. (f) Spinal cord, anterior horn: Leukocyte common antigen (LCA)-labeled lymphocytes are dispersed throughout the neuropil and cuff blood vessels in association with labeled viral infection of neurons, as shown in insert. One neuron is being phagocytozed (arrow). (a), (b), (c) Left panel, and (e) Luxol fast blue – hematoxylin and eosin (H&E); (a) insert, H&E; (c) Right panel, (d) Left and right panels, (e) insert, (f) insert WNV antigen immunohistochemistry; (f) leukocyte common antigen (LCA) immunohistochemistry.

distributed and severe and include hemorrhagic necrosis without vasculitis. Immunohistochemistry (IHC) for WNV antigen (E or NS1 proteins) provides diagnostic confirmation. Usually, only a few neurons are labeled, in perikarya or axons. Nonetheless, IHC is cited to be confirmatory in approximately half of cases examined. In rare instances, electron microscopy (EM) has been useful, demonstrating clusters of 42–50 nm enveloped spherical viral particles within cytoplasmic vesicles.

Inflammation in visceral organs has been documented [8, 14]. Heart, kidney, pancreas, and skeletal muscle are commonly reported sites, whereas WNV antigen, in the absence of inflammation, has been detected in other tissues (i.e. lung, skin, gastrointestinal, and genitourinary tracts). Visceral infection tends to be limited to patients who are immunocompromised.

St. Louis encephalitis

The neuropathology findings and distribution of lesions in SLEV meningoencephalitis are similar to WNND (Table 15.2). There is notable involvement of substantia nigra. Viral antigens in neurons can be demonstrated by immunofluorescence [20], but EM remains a standby.

Murray valley encephalitis

Macroscopic findings are usually absent but, in severe chronic cases, punctate, nondescript rarefactive changes can be noted in the thalamus [21, 22], and the cerebellum may be atrophied [21]. The distribution and microscopic features of lesions are similar to WNND and SLEV [21, 22]. Of note is the brunt borne by the thalamus and, to lesser extent, cerebellum and brainstem. By IHC and in situ hybridization (ISH) techniques, MVEV antigen and RNA (nonstructural protein 5 (NS5) gene) are identified within neurons, single or clusters, in some, but not all, foci of inflammation [22].

Yellow fever

Neuropathology descriptions in yellow fever are scarce. In an oft-cited early study of 20 cases, the most common findings were cerebral edema and perivascular hemorrhages [23]. Although there were no pathognomonic features of encephalitis, half the cases showed slight perivascular cuffs of chronic inflammatory cells. In a single reported fatality in a three-year-old girl who died as a complication of immunization with live attenuated YFV–17D vaccine, perivascular mononuclear infiltrates in the medulla and cerebral cortex were recorded, consistent with acute viral encephalitis [24].

A current update on the neuropathology changes associated with YFV infection was presented at the 95th Annual Meeting of the American Association of Neuropathologists (June 6–9, 2019) in Atlanta, Georgia [25]. In this report, the autopsy findings in the brains of 38 patients who succumbed during the 2017–2018 epidemic in the Sao Paulo district of Brazil were presented. Clinical diagnosis of yellow fever was confirmed in all patients by RT-PCR laboratory testing. The most common macroscopic finding was focal hemorrhage, whereas that on microscopy was hypoxic–ischemic neuronal injury. A few cases showed perivascular hemorrhage or lymphomononuclear inflammatory cell cuffing. In seven brains, scant parenchymal inflammatory cell infiltrates were observed, sparingly, with rare CD8 cells identified along with CD68-labeled microglia. However, neither the presence of microglial nodules nor YFV proteins, as assayed by IHC, was detected. These patients died of acute liver failure, in none of their brains was Alzheimer type II change noted in the astrocytic nuclei. In conclusion, these findings were interpreted as nonspecific in significance, being referable to the patients' systemic illness and not that of encephalitis, thereby corroborating reported findings in the archival literature.

Yellow fever is principally a viscerotropic disease [1, 2, 7]. The major organs afflicted are listed in Table 15.2. In the liver, midzonal necrosis associated with eosinophilic degeneration of hepatocytes (with Councilman bodies) and Kupffer cells is present, accompanied by hepatocyte microvesicular fatty change. Notwithstanding Kupffer cell hyperplasia, inflammation is negligible. These features have been interpreted as consistent with apoptosis and are similarly observed in the renal tubular epithelium and cardiac muscle, including the conduction system. In all these tissues, YFV antigen and viral RNA has been identified by IHC and ISH. There is marked depletion of lymphocytes in spleen and lymphoid tissue in conjunction with the presence of large mononuclear and histiocytic cells.

Widespread hemorrhages are common. Indirect injury to capillaries causing the plasma leakage of the terminal shock syndrome is implied by pulmonary edema and pleural and abdominal effusions.

Dengue

Neuropathological descriptions, whether encephalopathy or encephalitis is clinically associated, are limited and vary in number of cases, completeness of examination, and documentation. The most common findings mentioned are cerebral edema, focal subarachnoid and perivascular hemorrhages, and changes in keeping with ischemia [26, 27]. Notwithstanding rare claims of encephalitis in abbreviated reports [18], inflammatory cells are usually not noted or are present as variable perivascular cuffs that may track into the neural parenchyma [28]. Perivenous cerebral white matter demyelination has been documented in one case [28]. Attempts to identify and localize DENV in brain tissue employing a variety of techniques (isolation, RT-PCR, IHC, and ISH) have yielded conflicting results. The crux has been distinguishing between localization because of uptake by cells of inactive viral particles, viral antigens (E and NS1 proteins), or RNA secreted into the extracellular spaces, and identifying cells that contain replicating virus (e.g. as assessed by the cell-restricted marker nonstructural protein 3 (NS3)). Monocytes and macrophages are consistently identified with viral markers, with a few claims of localization in neurons, astrocytes, microglia, and endothelial cells [1, 29]. Thus, the issue of neuroinvasion by DENV awaits further resolution.

General pathology findings in dengue [26, 27] parallel those in yellow fever (Table 15.2). The difference is severity of lesions. Hepatocyte degeneration in the liver is more variable and Councilman bodies are less common. In the immune system, germinal centers with marked apoptotic lymphocyte depletion contain amorphous eosinophilic deposits comprising complement components, immunoglobulins, and viral E and NS1 proteins. Kidneys may demonstrate minor degenerative changes in tubular epithelium. The most common findings are perivascular multifocal hemorrhages in all tissues and combinations of pleural, pericardial, and abdominal effusions, correlating with the thrombocytopenia, coagulopathy, and increased vascular permeability of DHF/DSS. Other than endothelial swelling, there are no morphologic features of injury to the capillary bed, although apoptosis has been debated. Viral identification and localization by IHC and ISH have consistently demonstrated DENV antigens or RNA in hepatocytes and monocytes and macrophages [27], but viral presence in Kupffer cells and endothelial cells is more contested.

Pathogenesis

Common pathogenic principles

Inherent to the pathogenesis of these flaviviral infections are the principles of viral inoculation, amplification of viral replication in lymphoid tissues and the reticuloendothelial system, and viremia with clearance due to immune response or infection of targeted tissues. The steps entailed are outlined in Box 15.1. The remaining discussion focuses on infection of targeted tissues.

WNV, SLEV, and MVEV neuropathogenesis

Neuroinvasion of the CNS by WNV, SLEV, and MVEV follows the initial phase of infection and viremia. Despite numerous investigative studies with WNV, the mechanisms of viral entry and infectivity remain poorly understood. However, the following viral factors are recognized as important:
- E protein molecular determinants;
- Nonstructural protein mediated evasion of antiviral actions of IFN;
- Generation of quasi-species to elude neutralization by antibodies.

The latter two factors conspire to promote a high viremic load and prolong the duration of viremia, thereby increasing the risk for neuroinvasion. Reciprocally, the coordinated effectiveness of the host innate and adaptive immune response is crucial to clear the viremia. An important innate reaction is the augmented secretion of proinflammatory cytokines, notably tumor necrosis factor alpha (TNF-α) and other IFNs, as mediated by toll-like-receptors (TLRs)-3, -7, and -8 [30]. Nonetheless, high levels of TNF-α may speculatively have a counterproductive action by increasing the permeability of the BBB to facilitate passive diffusion transit of

> **Box 15.1 Common Pathogenic Steps in Flaviviral Infection**
>
> 1. **Mosquito Dermal Inoculation:**
>   - Local immunosuppression of innate immune response by injected mosquito salivary proteins.
>   - Virion uptake by Langerhans dendritic cells and keratinocytes.
> 2. **Virion Transport–Regional Lymph Nodes:**
>   - Migration of dendritic cells.
>   - Transit of free virions in afferent lymph drainage from extracellular tissue spaces.
> 3. **Regional Lymph Nodes:**
>   - Virus replication and amplification in monocytes and macrophages.
>   - Initiation of innate and adaptive immune responses.
>   - Efferent lymphatic drainage of virus bearing monocytes and macrophages and free virions into blood circulation.
> 4. **Primary Viremia:**
>   - Dissemination of virus to secondary lymphoid tissues, Kupffer cells, and bone marrow.
>   - Further viral amplification in tissues and release.
> 5. **Secondary Viremia:**
>   - Augmented viral load in blood.
>   - Clearance:
>   - Emergence of neutralizing IgM antibodies.
>   - Innate immune responses (compliment activation, natural killer (NK) and T-helper (Th) cell activation, cytokine production).
>   - Targeted tissue uptake.
> 6. **Infection of Targeted Organs – Viral Tropism:**
>   - Cell to cell spread and direct damage by virus-induced apoptosis.
>   - Immune response and secondary tissue damage.

blood-borne virions into the CNS [31]. Other proposed mechanisms include transendothelial transport, either by infection or endocytic vesicular trafficking; passage of infected monocytes into the CNS ("Trojan horse" model); and transneural routes, either by retrograde axonal transport along motor neurons or via infected olfactory neuroepithelium transneuronally to the olfactory bulb, in addition to other means. Neurovirulence properties are important for infectivity and spread in the target cell population, the neuron, but how remains unclear. Neuronal death is known to be induced by apoptosis via caspase-3 or noncaspase proteases and possibly cytolysis from excessive virion budding [31]. The regulation of IFN (and other cytokines) and the role of T cells are critical to the control of viral spread and clearance [30]. However, overactive CD8 T cells can cause cytotoxic neuronal injury. Experimental rodent and NHP models have further demonstrated inadequate clearance perpetuates viral persistence and B- and T-cell immune responses in the CNS [1, 31].

Yellow fever

Based on studies in humans and NHP, early infection of several target organs occurs during the primary viremia, aided by viral evasion and downregulation of the host innate immunity, possibly by differential expression of associated genes [7, 32]. Infection of cardiac muscle and hepatocytes coincides with the secondary viremia, which precedes the onset of terminal liver failure. Reduced hepatic synthesis of coagulation factors leads to bleeding diathesis, to which platelet dysfunction and disseminated intravascular coagulopathy may be contributing factors. Renal failure is similarly late, but the roles of direct viral injury, hypotension, and shock remain to be determined. As for the terminal capillary leak syndrome with ensuing shock, a "cytokine storm" of pro- and anti-inflammatory cytokines has been proposed [7], analogous to that in sepsis, although YFV infection of endothelial cells cannot be excluded. Unlike murine models, YFV is not neurotropic in man or NHP. The exception is young infants who develop the rare complication of encephalitis following vaccination or consumption of breast milk from recently vaccinated lactating mothers [7].

Dengue

Disease severity in dengue is contingent upon virulence of infecting serotypes, reinfection by a heterologous DENV serotype, and the repertoire of host immune responses initiated, which can be modified by inherent genetic polymorphisms (Table 15.2). Primary infection by a DENV serotype usually does not progress beyond DF. However, if hematogenous viral load is exceedingly high, the immune reaction effete, or an infant of a previously immune mother is infected, primary infection can transgress to DHF/DSS, with DENV 2 and DENV 3 serotypes having greater virulence [1, 33]. More often DHF/DSS ensues after secondary infection with a heterologous serotype that unleashes a variety of poorly understood interrelated immune mechanisms to propagate facets of the disease. One facet is to augment infection by amplifying viral load through the phenomenon of antibody-dependent enhancement. Incomplete neutralization of the heterologous serotype by pre-existent anti- DENV IgG antibodies forms immune complexes that are selectively taken up via Fcγ receptors on monocytes and macrophages, facilitating viral replication and release from these cells [33]. In addition to compounding suppression of antiviral responses, other immune reactions [34] are proposed: excessive production of pro- and anti- inflammatory cytokines (TNF-α, interleukins [ILs], and INF γ) initiated by heterologous DENV antigen preferentially activating cross-reactive memory T cells; compliment activation; and release of other pro-inflammatory soluble factors (e.g. secretion of DENV NS1 protein and platelet-activating factor). Another possible facet of these interacting mechanisms is the characteristic hemorrhagic diathesis speculatively entailing binding, dysfunction, and shortened survival of platelets; activation of various clotting factors; and generation of a consumptive coagulopathy. A further proposed facet is the plasma leak syndrome, which appears to be a transient physiologic disruption of endothelial permeability in the pleural and abdominal capillary beds. A "cytokine storm" mediated by cross-reactive T-cell responses and complement activation has been proffered as the genesis, along with other possible factors (e.g. upregulation of vascular endothelial growth factor [VEGF]) [2, 33, 34].

Animal models

A diverse range of animals (i.e. mosquitoes, wide varieties of birds, horses, squirrels, and domestic animals) has been employed to study epidemiologic aspects of modes of viral transmission and potential hosts in specific environmental settings [1]. For analysis of factors referable to pathogenesis, patterns of virus dissemination in different hosts, and the testing of various candidate vaccines and antiviral agents, conventionally available laboratory animals are the most applicable. These models are summarized in Table 15.3 and discussed in further detail in cited references [1, 35, 36].

Treatment and vaccines

Treatment

Other than general medical supportive measures, there is no specific therapy for these five flaviviral infections. However, special aspects of each disease require attention:
- WNV/SLEV/MVEV encephalomyelitis: seizure control, assisted ventilation as necessary, and adjustments in immunosuppression for transplant recipients [2, 3, 8, 14]
- Yellow fever: management of hepatic and renal failure, bleeding diathesis, and blood pressure [2, 7]
- Dengue: monitoring stage of disease for parenteral fluid intervention [2, 17].

Prevention of secondary infections is uniform. No guidelines for antiviral therapies exist. Experimental animal studies and random clinical case reports suggest amelioration of WNV, SLEV, and YFV infections with IFN-α [1, 2, 9, 10], but validation by clinical trials is awaited. A similar caveat applies to treatments with immune gamma globulin and monoclonal antibodies for WNV infection [1, 2].

Vaccines

The live attenuated vaccine YF–17D for yellow fever, the only one licensed, confers long-lasting immunity that exceeds 10 years in 95% of recipients [2, 7]. Rare severe adverse events [1, 2, 7] include anaphylactic reactions, YF-associated neurologic disease, and YF-associated viscerotropic disease. The most salient associated neurologic disease is the risk of non-fatal meningoencephalitis in infants ≤6 months of age, for which vaccination is contraindicated. The majority of other contraindications and precautions

Table 15.3 Conventional Animal Models for WNV, SLEV, YFV, and DENV Infections.

Flavivirus	Model	Route	Pattern of Infection	Applications	Limitations
WNV	NHP:				
	Rhesus macaque	ID	Asymptomatic/mild illness (WNF)	Vaccines/antivirals	No encephalitis; expense
	Baboon	ID	Mild illness (WNF)	Vaccines/antivirals	No encephalitis; expense
	Rhesus macaque	IC	Encephalitis[a]	Neuropathogenesis	Relevance[b]
	Golden Hamster	IN, IP, O	Encephalitis[a] Kidney[a]	Pathogenesis Immune responses Vaccines/antivirals	Mortality
	Mice:				
	Wild Type	A, ID, Sc	Range: asymptomatic/ WNF/WNND	Pathogenesis	Small animal size
	Immunodeficient Genetically modified			Neuro-invasion Immune responses Host genetic factors	Short course of disease Relevance[b]
SLEV	NHP:				
	Rhesus macaque	IC	Encephalitis[a]	Pathogenesis Protective immunity[d]	Sc inoculation: no encephalitis
	Golden Hamster	A, IN, IP, Sc	Encephalitis Viscera[c]	Neuro-invasion routes Pathogenesis Viral persistence	
	Mice:				
	Wild Type	A, IC, IP, Sc	Encephalitis Viscera[c]	Pathogenesis Immune responses Viral virulence Antiviral cytokines	
YFV	NHP:				
	Rhesus macaque/ Cynomolgus monkey	Sc	Liver/Kidney/Immune system	Pathogenesis Viral virulence	Severity of illness No biphasic pattern
	Golden Hamster	IP	Liver/Immune system	Pathogenesis Protective immunity[d] Viral virulence	Needs virus adaptation No kidney infection
	Mice:				
	Wild Type	IC, IN, IP	Encephalitis	Viral virulence Vaccines/antivirals	Needs virus adaptation No visceral disease Age-dependent infection
	IFN-SD[e]	Sc	Liver/Immune system	Pathogenesis Immune responses	Relevance[b]
DENV	NHP:				
	Chimpanzee	ID, Sc	Asymptomatic/mild overt disease	Immune responses[h]	Reliability of infection
	Rhesus macaque	Sc		Vaccines	Expense
	Mice:				
	Wild Type	ID, IP, IV	No infection/some features of DF	Immune responses[h]	Needs virus adaptation
		IC	Encephalitis	Vaccines	Relevance[b]
	IFN-SD[e]	IP, IV	Features of DHF Encephalitis (variable)[g]	Pathogenesis Immune responses[h] Antivirals	Variable expression Relevance[b]
	Chimeras[f]	ID, IP, Sc	Features of DF Encephalitis	Pathogenesis Vaccines/antivirals	Incomplete disease Relevance[b]

(Continued)

Table 15.3 (Continued)

^a Infection persists for several months.
^b Pattern of infection does not mimic that in humans because of type of animal model, preparation of viral inoculum, or route of administration.
^c Lungs, kidney, and spleen.
^d Effect of prior immunization with either varying virulent strains for SLEV studies, or heterologous flaviviruses for YFV studies.
^e IFN-SD mice: mouse strains lacking IFN-α/β and γ receptors or IFN-α/β receptor.
^f SCID or nonobese diabetic (NON)/SCID mouse strains engrafted with human tumor cell lines or human CD34+ progenitor stem cells, respectively.
^g Influencing factors include inoculum dosage and class of deficient interferon receptor in mouse model.
^h Refers to immune responses following primary infection, sequential heterologous DENV strain infection, or simulated secondary infection by previous passive transfer of anti-DENV monoclonal antibodies to induce ADE.

A, aerosol; ADE, antibody-dependent enhancement; DENV, dengue virus; DF, dengue fever; DHF, dengue hemorrhagic fever; IC, intracranial; ID, intradermal; IFN-α/β, interferon alpha/beta; IFN-SD, interferon signaling deficient; IN, intranasal; IP, intraperitoneal; IV, intravenous; NHP, Nonhuman primates; O, oral; Sc, subcutaneous; SCID, severe combined immunodeficient; SLEV, St. Louis Encephalitis virus; WNF, West Nile fever; WNV, West Nile virus; WNND, West Nile neuroinvasive disease; WT, wild type; YFV, Yellow Fever Virus.

Sources: Pierson and Diamond [1]; Clark et al. [35]; Zompi and Harris [36].

refer to disturbances in immune status. For the other flaviviruses, chimeric vaccines are in development that combine the nonstructural gene backbone of YF-17D with the heterologous premembrane and envelope genes of WNV [1, 2] or the four serotypes of DENV [1, 16, 17], the tetravalent vaccine of which (*Dengavaxia*) is in clinical trials [2] and licensed recently for certain populations. Other chimeric vaccines in progress employ a DENV 2 or DENV 4 backbone for WNV [2], or a DENV 2 backbone for combination with the other three serotypes [16, 17]. Additional research approaches for flaviviral vaccines include use of viral vectors (poxvirus, adenovirus, and measles), DNA vaccines, and utilization of inactivated whole virus for formulation of yellow fever and dengue vaccines [1].

Acknowledgments

The authors wish to thank Dr. Leroy R. Sharer, Professor of Pathology (Neuropathology), New Jersey Medical School, Rutgers, The State University of New Jersey for his review and comments on the manuscript. They also are grateful to the adroit assistance provided by Mr. Tom Turner, Pathology Photography, Department of Laboratory Medicine and Pathology, University of Alberta for assembling the montage for Figure 15.1.

References

1. Pierson, T.C. and Diamond, M.S. (2013). Chapter 26: Flaviviruses. In: *Field's Virology*, 6e (eds. D.M. Knipe and P.M. Howley), 748–794. Philadelphia, PA: Lippincott Williams and Wilkins.
2. Thomas, S.J., Endy, T.P., Rothman, A.L., and Barrett, A.D. (2015). Flaviviruses (dengue, yellow fever, Japanese encephalitis, West Nile encephalitis, St. Louis encephalitis, tick-borne encephalitis, Kyasanur Forest disease, Alkhurma hemorrhagic fever, Zika). In: *Mandell, Douglas, and Bennett's Principles and Practice of Infectious Diseases*, 8e (eds. J.E. Bennett, R. Dolin, M.J. Blaser, et al.), 1881–1903. Philadelphia, PA: Elsevier/Saunders.
3. Knox, J., Cowan, R.C., Doyle, J.S. et al. (2012). Murray Valley encephalitis: a review of clinical features, diagnosis and treatment. *Med. J. Aust.* 196: 322–326.
4. Reisen, W.K. (2003). Epidemiology of St. Louis encephalitis virus. *Adv. Virus Res.* 61: 139–183.
5. Murgure, B., Zeller, H., and Deubel, V. (2002). The ecology and epidemiology of West Nile virus in Africa, Europe, and Asia. *Curr. Top. Microbiol.* 267: 195–221.
6. Reimann, C.A., Hayes, E.B., DiGuiseppi, C. et al. (2008). Epidemiology of neuroinvasive arboviral disease in the United States, 1999–2007. *Am. J. Trop. Med. Hyg.* 76: 974–979.
7. Monath, T.P., Gershman, M., Staples, J.E., and Barrett, A.D. (2013). Chapter 38: Yellow fever vaccine. In: *Vaccines*, 6e (eds. S.A. Plotkin, W. Orenstein and P.A. Offit), 870–968. Philadelphia, PA: Saunders.

8. Kleinschmidt-De Masters, B.K. and Beckham, J.D. (2015). West Nile virus encephalitis 16 years later. *Brain Pathol.* 25: 625–633.
9. Hartmann, C.A., Vikran, H.R., Seville, M.T. et al. (2017). Neuroinvasive St. Louis encephalitis virus infection in solid organ transplant recipients. *Am. J. Transplant.* 17: 2200–2206.
10. Venkat, H., Adams, L., Sunenshine, R. et al. (2017). St. Louis encephalitis virus possibly transmitted through blood transfusion – Arizona, 2015. *Transfusion* 57: 2987–2994.
11. Stephens, H.A.F. (2010). HLA and other gene associations with dengue disease severity. *Curr. Top. Microbiol. Immunol.* 338: 99–114.
12. Khor, C.C., Chau, T.N.B.C., Pang, J. et al. (2011). Gene-wide association study identifies susceptibility loci for dengue shock syndrome at MICB and PLCE1. *Nat. Genet.* 43: 1139–1141.
13. Bigham, A.W., Buckingham, K.J., Hussain, S. et al. (2011). Host genetic risk factors for West Nile virus infection and disease progression. *PLoS One* 6: e24745.
14. Guyre, K.A. (2009). West Nile virus infections. *J. Neuropathol. Exp. Neurol.* 68: 1053–1060.
15. Burrow, J.N.C., Whelan, P.I., Kilburn, C.J. et al. (1998). Australian encephalitis in the Northern Territory: clinical and epidemiological features, 1987 – 1996. *Aust. NZ J. Med.* 28: 590–596.
16. Halstead, S.B. and Thomas, S.J. (2013). Chapter 44: Dengue vaccine. In: *Vaccines*, 6e (eds. S.A. Plotkin, W. Orenstein and P.A. Offit), 1043–1051. Philadelphia, PA: Saunders.
17. WHO/TDR (2009). *Dengue: Guidelines for Diagnosis, Treatment, Prevention and Control: New Edition*. Geneva: World Health Organization.
18. Carod-Artal, F.J., Wichmann, O., Farrar, J., and Gascon, J. (2013). Neurological complications of dengue virus infection. *Lancet Neurol.* 12: 906–919.
19. Li, H.-M., Huang, Y.-K., Su, Y.-C., and Kao, C.-H. (2018). Risk of stroke in patients with dengue fever: a population-based cohort study. *CMAJ* 190: E285–E290.
20. Reyes, M.G., Gardner, J.J., Poland, J.D., and Monath, T.P. (1981). St. Louis encephalitis. Quantitative histologic and immunofluorescent studies. *Arch. Neurol.* 38: 329–334.
21. Robertson, E.G. (1952). Murray Valley encephalitis: pathological aspects. *Med. J. Aust.* 1: 107–110.
22. Fu, T.L., Ong, K.C., Tran, Y.D. et al. (2016). Viral neurotropism is important in the pathogenesis of Murray Valley encephalitis. *Neuropathol. Appl. Neurobiol.* 42: 307–310.
23. Stevenson, L.D. (1939). Pathologic changes in the nervous system in yellow fever. *Arch. Pathol.* 27: 249–266.
24. Anonymous (1966). Fatal viral encephalitis following 17D yellow fever vaccine inoculation. *JAMA* 198: 203–204.
25. Frassetto, F. and Rosemberg, S. (2019). Neuropathological alterations in cases of yellow fever submitted to autopsy. *J. Neuropathol. Exp. Neurol.* 78: 528.
26. Bhamarapravati, N., Tuchina, P., and Boonyapaknavik, V. (1967). Pathology of Thailand haemorrhagic fever: a study of 100 autopsy cases. *Ann. Trop. Med. Parasitol.* 61: 500–501.
27. Aye, K.S., Charngkaew, K., Win, N. et al. (2014). Pathologic highlights of dengue hemorrhagic fever in 13 autopsy cases from Myanmar. *Hum. Pathol.* 45: 1221–1233.
28. Chimelli, L., Dumas Hahn, M., Barretto Netto, M. et al. (1990). Dengue: neuropathological findings in 5 fatal cases from Brazil. *Clin. Neuropathol.* 9: 157–162.
29. Balsitis, S.J., Coloma, J., Castro, G. et al. (2009). Tropism of dengue virus in mice and humans defined by viral nonstructural protein 3-specific immunostaining. *Am. J. Trop. Med. Hyg.* 80: 416–424.
30. Suthar, M.S., Diamond, M.S., and Gale, M. (2013). West Nile infection and immunity. *Nat. Rev. Microbiol.* 11: 115–128.
31. Cho, H. and Diamond, M.S. (2012). Immune responses to West Nile virus infection in the central nervous system. *Viruses* 4: 3812–3820.
32. Engelmann, F., Josset, L., Girke, T. et al. (2014). Pathophysiologic and transcriptomic analyses of viscerotropic yellow fever in a rhesus macaque model. *PLoS Negl. Trop. Dis.* 8: e3295.
33. Martina, B.E.E., Koraka, P., and Osterhaus, A.D.M.E. (2009). Dengue virus pathogenesis: an integrated view. *Clin. Microbiol. Rev.* 27: 564–581.
34. Malavige, G.N. and Ogg, G.S. (2017). Pathogenesis of vascular leak in dengue virus infection. *Immunology* 151: 261–269.
35. Clark, D.C., Brault, A.C., and Hunsperger, E. (2012). The contribution of rodent models to the pathological assessment of flaviviral infections of the central nervous system. *Arch. Virol.* 157: 1423–1440.
36. Zompi, S. and Harris, E. (2012). Animal models of dengue virus infection. *Viruses* 4: 62–82.

16 Flaviviruses 3: Zika Virus Infection of the CNS

Leila Chimelli[1,2]

[1] Laboratory of Neuropathology and Molecular Genetics, State Brain Institute Paulo Niemeyer, Rio de Janeiro, Brazil
[2] Federal University of Rio de Janeiro (UFRJ), Rio de Janeiro, Brazil

Abbreviations

CNS   central nervous system
iPSCs induced pluripotent stem cells
NPCs neural progenitor cells
ZIKV Zika virus

Definition of the disorder and historical perspective

Zika virus (ZIKV) infection is caused by a virus belonging to the Flaviviridae family, genus *Flavivirus*, and is transmitted by mosquitoes of the genus *Aedes*. It was initially isolated in 1947 from the serum of a sentinel rhesus macaque in the Zika forest, Uganda, Africa, and remained neglected until human Zika infection was reported in Micronesia (2007) and French Polynesia (2013). A widespread epidemic of ZIKV infection became apparent in 2015 in South and Central America and was linked to development of congenital malformations leading to a Public Health Emergency of International Concern [1–4].

ZIKV infection during pregnancy has been reported to cause severe cerebral changes in the fetus, initially demonstrated by neuroimaging [5, 6] and then in fetal and neonatal postmortem material [7–12].

Clinical features, including appropriate investigations

Symptoms include mild fever, arthralgia, rash, headache, and myalgia, but frequently infection may be asymptomatic. More severe sequelae of ZIKV infection in adults include Guillain-Barré syndrome, acute myelitis, and meningoencephalitis.

A major concern associated with ZIKV infection is the increased incidence of microcephaly in infants born to mothers who are infected. In addition, other malformations including ventriculomegaly, cerebellar hypoplasia, and fetal akinesia deformation sequence (arthrogryposis) are associated with congenital ZIKV infection. Calcification detected with cerebral ultrasound is an early hallmark [13].

Pathology

The main changes are calcifications and microcephaly, but ventriculomegaly associated with normal or large head circumference, hypoplasia of cerebral tracts, and disturbances of neuronal migration also occur. Calcification is especially noticeable at the

Infections of the Central Nervous System: Pathology and Genetics, First Edition. Edited by Fabrice Chrétien, Kum Thong Wong, Leroy R. Sharer, Catherine (Katy) Keohane and Françoise Gray.
© 2020 John Wiley & Sons Ltd. Published 2020 by John Wiley & Sons Ltd.

Infections of the Central Nervous System

gray and white matter junctions, in the basal ganglia, and thalamus. There are few individual case reports or small series of postmortem studies of the CNS in congenital ZIKV infection [7–11].

Chimelli et al. [12] reported the largest neuropathological study involving 10 cases, including three stillborn and seven neonates (i.e. six born at term and four premature between 32 and 36 weeks of gestation) who survived from 15 minutes to 37 hours. Most mothers had ZIKV symptoms in the first trimester of gestation, and most babies had arthrogryposis.

Macroscopic findings

The meninges are transparent, congested, or focally thickened.

Three patterns can be observed. One pattern shows severe ventriculomegaly as a result of midbrain damage with aqueduct stenosis or atresia (Figure 16.1a and b). The ventriculomegaly is usually asymmetric, especially in the occipital lobes where the parenchyma is very thin with agyria, sometimes acquiring a cystic appearance with abundant cerebrospinal fluid.

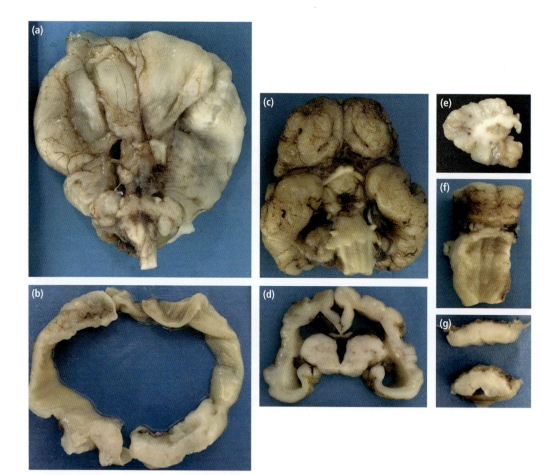

Figure 16.1 Macroscopic appearance (a) Brain from a baby with hydrocephalus and (c), another brain from a baby with microcephaly. Both are seen from the base. The surfaces are smooth or have shallow sulci and show calcification (yellow areas in c). Coronal sections show very thin (b) or slightly thicker parenchyma (d). At the base, the flattened thalami are seen in (b) and simplified hippocampi can be recognized in (d). One cerebellar hemisphere (e) shows irregular or smooth surface, the fourth ventricle is dilated (f). and the basis pontis and pyramids are flat (g).

In the second pattern, the brains are small and associated with mild to moderate (ex-vacuo) ventriculomegaly (Figure 16.1c and d). In these cases, the cranial bones may overlap or be fused and the occipital bones are prominent. The brain surface shows shallow sulci or agyria, sometimes with a cobblestone appearance. In these cases, the aqueduct is patent or even dilated, as is the fourth ventricle (Figure 16.1f).

In both types and in both patterns, the hippocampus is frequently not well identified and may be vertically oriented or malformed (Figure 16.1d). The corpus callosum is either absent (particularly when there is severe hydrocephalus, Figure 16.1b) or very thin (Figure 16.1d). Basal ganglia and thalami are small, malformed, or not well recognized (Figure 16.1d). There is cerebellar hypoplasia with an irregular or smooth cortical surface (Figure 16.1e), and the fourth ventricle is enlarged (Figure 16.1f). The brainstem is frequently small, particularly the basis pontis, which is flat, and the pyramids may not be detectable (Figure 16.1g). Calcifications are easily seen in the cortical mantle, at the junctions between gray and white matter, in deep gray nuclei, and in the brainstem, especially in cases with severe ventriculomegaly, when the midbrain is distorted and the aqueduct is not visible, a characteristic of the first pattern. The spinal cord is usually thin and dorsal root ganglia are normal.

The third pattern, observed in one baby infected at 28 weeks gestation with normal-sized head and ventricles, is a well-formed brain with mild calcification in the deep hemispheric white matter.

Histopathological findings

Diffuse severe brain damage, with extensive destruction and calcifications, is seen mainly at the gray and white matter junctions, and there are occasional perivascular cuffs of CD8+ T-lymphocytes, microglial nodules, and reactive gliosis [9, 12].

In cases with severe ventriculomegaly, the cerebral parenchyma is very thin, sometimes consisting only of remnants of germinal matrix and leptomeninges (Figure 16.2a). Disturbance of neuronal migration is common in both cerebral (Figure 16.2b) and cerebellar hemispheres and in the brainstem and includes polymicrogyria, meningeal glioneuronal heterotopia (Figure 16.2c and d), and cerebellar cortical dysplasia. Large and irregular clusters of immature cells are usually seen along the ventricular surface and toward the cortex, sometimes intermingled with fine or coarse calcification at various levels of the cerebral parenchyma (Figure 16.2e). Apoptotic bodies are occasionally observed along the ependymal surface and in some remnants of the germinal matrix.

There is also Wallerian degeneration and axonal spheroids in deep gray nuclei and the brainstem, associated with coarse and filamentous calcification, gliosis, and aqueduct stenosis or atresia (particularly in cases with marked ventriculomegaly).

The cerebellum frequently shows cortical dysplasia and mature or immature neuronal heterotopias.

The spinal cord is abnormally shaped due to absence of, or very small, cortico-spinal tracts (Figure 16.3a and b), and motor nerve cell degeneration and loss (Figure 16.3c and b), gliosis and calcification, which explain the arthrogryposis. Ventral roots are abnormally thinner than the dorsal ones (Figure 16.3b), whereas the dorsal columns, dorsal nerve roots, and ganglia are preserved and myelinated.

In situ hybridization for ZIKV in the CNS may demonstrate viral RNA in the meninges, occasionally in the neocortex and the germinal matrix, the latter only when the interval between infection and birth is short.

When infection occurs late in gestation the brain damage is mild, suggesting that the timing of infection during pregnancy is one of the most relevant risk factors for development of congenital ZIKV syndrome.

Genetics and pathogenesis

Sequence analysis defined two main viral strains, the African and the Asian. The Asian strain thrived in the Americas and was reported to underlie congenital malformations [2]. The study of ZIKV biology has greatly benefited from the use of induced pluripotent stem cells (iPSCs), which quickly confirmed that the

Infections of the Central Nervous System

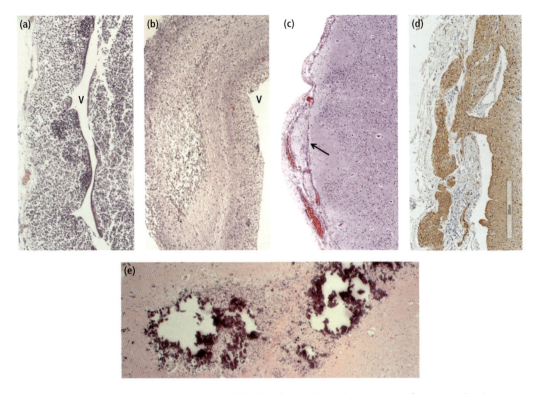

Figure 16.2 Histopathology of the cerebral hemispheres. (a) Section of cerebral hemispheres consisting of immature cells only, continuous between the leptomeninges on the left and ventricular surface (v); (b) disorganized migrating cells over a smooth cortical surface; the lateral ventricle (V) is on the right; (c) polymicrogyria and glioneuronal meningeal heterotopia (arrow); (d) better shown with glial fibrillary acidic protein (GFAP) (d) disclosing glial tissue within the leptomeninges. (e) Extensive hemispheric calcification can be seen.

virus could lead to cell death in neural progenitor cells (NPCs) [14]. Infection of NPCs, neurons and glia (including radial glia and glia limitans), leads to a severe reduction in mature cell numbers and to migration disorders. The AXL receptor in NPCs may be a target for ZIKV in the developing nervous system [15]. A single serine to aspargnine substitution (Ser139→Asn139 [S139N]) in ZIKV polyprotein was reported as increasing ZIKV infectivity in both human and mouse NPCs, leading to more severe microcephaly and higher mortality rates in mice [16]. Evolutionary analysis indicated that the substitution arose before the 2013 outbreak in French Polynesia and had been stably maintained during subsequent spread to the Americas. This functional adaption makes ZIKV more virulent to human NPCs, thus contributing to the increased incidence of microcephaly in recent ZIKV epidemics [16].

Treatment, future perspective, and conclusions

Although great efforts are being made to prevent and treat the consequences of the ZIKV epidemic, particularly the neurodevelopmental disorders, there are many avenues for future research to improve the situation for families and children.

A multidisciplinary approach to treatment is critical for the best clinical outcome, but interventions are likely to vary between countries where demographics, access to health services, and social culture all differ.

Improved sanitation is of utmost importance to avoid the proliferation of mosquitoes and the spread of the infection.

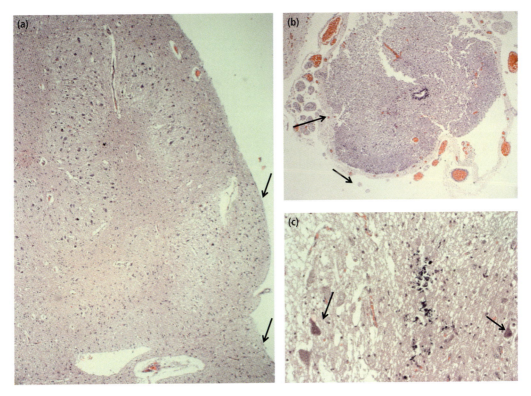

Figure 16.3 Histopathology of brainstem and spinal cord (a) Section at the level of the medulla showing flat pyramids (arrows). Part of the olives can be recognized on both sides; (b) spinal cord with small (undetected) corticospinal tract (long arrow), thin anterior roots (short arrow), compared to the dorsal roots. (c) Detail of the anterior horn showing few remaining motor neurons (arrows) and calcifications in the neuropil.

References

1. Kindhauser, M.K., Allen, T., Frank, V. et al. (2016). Zika: the origin and spread of a mosquito-borne virus. *Bull. World Health Organ.* 94: 675–686.
2. Wang, L., Valderramos, S.G., Wu, A. et al. (2016). From mosquitos to humans: genetic evolution of Zika virus. *Cell Host and Microbe* 19: 561–565.
3. Dasti, J.I. (2016). Zika virus infections: an overview of current scenario. *Asian Pac. J. Trop. Med.* 9: 621–625.
4. Ramos da Silva, S. and Gao, S.J. (2016). Zika virus: an update on epidemiology, pathology, molecular biology, and animal model. *J. Med. Virol.* 88: 1291–1296.
5. Oliveira Melo, A.S., Malinger, G., Ximenes, R. et al. (2016). Zika virus intrauterine infection causes fetal brain abnormality and microcephaly: tip of the iceberg? *Ultrasound Obstet. Gynecol.* 47: 6–7.
6. de Oliveira-Szejnfeld, S., Levine, D., Melo, A.S. et al. (2016). Congenital brain abnormalities and Zika virus: what the radiologist can expect to see? *Radiology* 281: 203–218.
7. Mlakar, J., Korva, M., Tul, N. et al. (2016). Zika virus associated with microcephaly. *N. Engl. J. Med.* 374: 951–958.
8. Acosta-Reyes, J., Navarro, E., Herrera, M.J. et al. (2017). Severe neurologic disorders in 2 fetuses with Zika virus infection, Colombia. *Emerg. Infect. Dis.* 23: 982–984.
9. Sousa, A.Q., Cavalcante, D.I.M., Franco, L.M. et al. (2017). Postmortem findings for 7 neonates with congenital Zika virus infection. *Emerg. Infect. Dis.* 23: 1164–1167.
10. Martines, R.B., Bhatnagar, J., de Oliveira Ramos, A.M. et al. (2016). Pathology of congenital Zika syndrome in Brazil: a case series. *Lancet* 388: 898–904.
11. Driggers, R.W., Ho, C.-Y., Korhonen, E.M. et al. (2016). Zika virus infection with prolonged maternal

viremia and fetal brain abnormalities. *N. Engl. J. Med.* 374: 2142–2151.
12. Chimelli, L., Melo, A.S.O., Avvad-Portari, E. et al. (2017). The spectrum of neuropathological changes associated with congenital Zika virus infection. *Acta Neuropathol.* 133: 983–999.
13. Araujo, A.Q.C., Silva, M.T.T., and Araujo, A.P.Q.C. (2016). Zika virus-associated neurological disorders: a review. *Brain* 139: 2122–2130.
14. Souza, B.S., Sampaio, G.L., Pereira, C.S. et al. (2016). Zika virus infection induces mitosis abnormalities and apoptotic cell death of human neural progenitor cells. *Sci. Rep.* 6: 39775.
15. Nowakowski, T.J., Pollen, A.A., Lullo, E.D. et al. (2016). Expression analysis highlights AXL as a candidate Zika virus entry receptor in neural stem cells. *Cell Stem Cell* 18: 591–596.
16. Yuan, L., Xing-Yao Huang, X.Y., Liu, Z.U. et al. (2017). A single mutation in the prM protein of Zika virus contributes to fetal microcephaly. *Science* 358: 933–936.

17 Flaviviruses 4: Japanese Encephalitis

Shankar Krishna Susarla[1], Anita Mahadevan[1], Bishan Radotra[2], Masaki Takao[3], and Kum Thong Wong[4]

[1] Department of Neuropathology, National Institute of Mental Health and Neurosciences (NIMHANS), Bangalore, India
[2] Department of Histopathology, Postgraduate Institute of Medical Education and Research, Chandigarh, India
[3] Department of Neurology, Saitama International Medical Center, Saitama Medical University, Hidaka, Japan
[4] Department of Pathology, Faculty of Medicine, University of Malaya, Kuala Lumpur, Malaysia

Abbreviations

BBB	blood-brain barrier
CNS	central nervous system
CSF	cerebrospinal fluid
CT	computed tomography
EEG	electroencephalogram
HSP	heat shock protein
IFN	interferon
IL-6	interleukin 6
JE	Japanese encephalitis
JEV	Japanese encephalitis virus
MCP1	monocyte chemotactic protein 1
MRI	magnetic resonance imaging
NO	nitric oxide
PCR	polymerase chain reaction
RIG	retinoic acid inducible gene
RNA	ribonucleic acid
SPECT	single photon emission computed tomography
TLR	toll-like receptor
TNF-α	tumor necrosis factor alpha

Definition of the disorder, major synonyms, and historical perspective

Japanese encephalitis (JE) is the most prevalent mosquito-borne arboviral infection in India, China, Korea, Thailand, Japan, and Indonesia. The first case of JE was reported from Japan in 1871 [1], followed by the first autopsy reports of three cases from Okayama, Japan, in 1912 by Katsurada (in Japanese). Because the encephalitis outbreaks occurred during summer, the disease was termed "encephalitis epidemica B" or "Japanese B encephalitis" to differentiate it from "encephalitis lethargica" that occurs in winter. In 1943, Hayashi successfully produced experimental encephalitis by inoculating the virus into monkeys [2]. The current incidence has fallen to less than 10 per year in Japan as a result of a successful vaccination program.

Infections of the Central Nervous System: Pathology and Genetics, First Edition. Edited by Fabrice Chrétien, Kum Thong Wong, Leroy R. Sharer, Catherine (Katy) Keohane and Françoise Gray.
© 2020 John Wiley & Sons Ltd. Published 2020 by John Wiley & Sons Ltd.

Microbiological characteristics

Japanese encephalitis virus (JEV), belonging to the family of Flaviviridae, is an icosahedral RNA virus, 40–60 nm in size. The virion comprises capsid protein, matrix protein (M), envelope protein (E), and five nonstructural proteins (NS_1, NS_2, NS_3, NS_4, and NS_5). Of these, the envelope E protein plays a critical role in attachment to cells. "Heat shock" protein, HSP-70, is the putative receptor for JEV, identified on cells of neural lineage (Neuro2A cells) [3]. The virulence of the infecting virus is also modulated by mutations in the E gene. A mutation that changes amino acid 720 (L-S) reduces its virulence [4].

Epidemiology

JE is an important CNS viral infection in Asia, West Pacific countries, and Northern Australia. According to a recent World Health Organization (WHO) report, about 68 000 severe clinical cases occur every year [5]. However, the incidence may be even higher because many cases remain undiagnosed and unconfirmed in the Indian subcontinent. The disease occurs in both epidemic and endemic forms [6]. The epidemic form is typically seasonal and is known to occur in countries such as Bangladesh, China, India, Nepal, North and South Korea, Pakistan, and Taiwan. The endemic form occurs sporadically throughout the year particularly in Australia, Cambodia, Indonesia, Malaysia, Myanmar, Philippines, and Sri Lanka. As a result of implementation of vaccination programs in countries such as Japan and Australia, the number of cases in these countries is restricted to a few per year. Both India and China, with large populations, contribute about 95% of JE cases, and the estimated JE incidence in India is still 15 per 100 000.

Although JE can occur in all age groups, children younger than 15 years of age are commonly affected because adults are already immune to the disease. Males are more often affected than females. The disease is fatal in up to 30% cases, and nearly 30–50% survivors develop long-term neurological or neuropsychiatric sequelae.

JE predominantly occurs in rural or agricultural areas, which are often associated with rice farming. Most cases are observed between May and October, with a peak incidence during rainy seasons. This is perhaps related to relentless breeding of mosquitoes during the rainy season because the main vector for JE virus transmission is the *Culex* species mosquito. The enzootic life cycle of the virus is maintained by its transmission to the vertebrate hosts. Bats as well as nesting ardeid birds, such as herons and egrets found in the inland waterways and coastal land, act as virus reservoirs.

Pigs act as amplifier hosts in whom the virus can aggressively replicate, causing significant viremia. The virus can also be further transmitted between pigs through highly infectious oronasal secretions rather than through mosquitoes [7]. For this reason, the virus persists during winter, when the mosquito population is very low. Humans are dead-end hosts because low viral loads in their blood do not allow further spread through mosquitoes; thus, the disease cannot be transmitted among people.

The factors influencing virulence include the age of onset, prior immune sensitization in endemic zones by cross-reacting viruses, and the dose of the inoculum. In endemic areas, children exposed to JEV or other cross-reacting viruses have low mortality because prior exposure to JEV or related viruses confers protection.

Clinical features

Children are the most frequently affected by JE. Symptoms develop 5–15 days after the bite of an infected mosquito. The clinical course of the disease has three phases: the early prodromal, acute encephalitic, and convalescent phases. In the early prodromal phase, the patient manifests fever, headache, nausea, vomiting, chills, and anorexia, lasting 6–24 hours. At this stage, spontaneous recovery is known. During the encephalitic phase, patients manifest convulsions, altered sensorium, behavioral changes, motor paralysis, movement disorders, and delirium. In some patients, status epilepticus is not unusual as a presenting symptom on a background of fever. A variety of movement disorders is common in the late encephalitic phase, including coarse tremors, choreoathetosis, dystonia, and parkinsonism. Although the symptoms of raised intracranial pressure are overt, papilledema is rare. The encephalitic phase usually lasts for a week but may be prolonged following other associated complications [8]. JEV may cause poliomyelitis-like symptoms, especially noted in Vietnamese children. The onset of weakness in children is more rapid and asymmetrical, reflecting damage to the anterior horn cells.

The predictors of poor clinical outcome in JE include: (a) young age, (b) coinfection of CNS by parasitic diseases like cysticercosis and visceral larva migrans [9], (c) presence of immunecomplexes or autoantibodies to myelin basic protein or neurofilament, and (d) raised levels of tumor necrosis factor alpha (TNF-α) in cerebrospinal fluid (CSF) [10, 11]. TNF-α levels in serum and CSF in JE are prognostic indicators of fatal outcomes [12].

Mortality in JE cases usually occurs within the first seven days following the onset of symptoms. Cerebral edema, neuronal damage, and acute pulmonary edema are responsible for early deaths. One-third of patients succumb during the acute phase of illness. Among those who survive, more than half are left with residual neurological deficits, intellectual disability, learning disabilities, and movement disorders. JE acquired during the first and second trimesters of pregnancy can lead to spontaneous abortion or intrauterine fetal death. Recurrence of symptoms has been observed in some children, nearly a year after the acute encephalitic phase, and latent virus can be recovered from the peripheral blood mononuclear cells. Persistence of immunoglobulin M (IgM) antibody and viral antigen can be found in CSF for prolonged periods in 5% of children. Immunological and virological evidence for JEV persistence in human nervous system is well documented, which could account for the long-term clinical sequelae such as behavioral and learning difficulties, postencephalitic parkinsonism, and motor neuron disease, depending on the anatomical localization of viral antigens [13].

In endemic areas, acute encephalitic features strongly suggest a diagnosis of JE. Cerebral malaria, Reye syndrome, acute pyogenic meningitis, and acute tuberculous meningitis in children should be differentiated from JE. Lymphocytic pleocytosis in CSF is common to all, but the lymphocytosis in CSF rapidly decreases in JE, unlike in the other viral infections. Other viral infections like West Nile encephalitis can closely resemble JE but can be diagnosed by serological and virological tests.

For laboratory diagnosis, paired samples of serum and CSF samples are necessary for IgM antibody estimation by IgM capture ELISA (MAC-ELISA) for specific diagnosis. The test sensitivity reaches 100% when serum and CSF samples are collected after the first week of illness. JEV can be isolated from CSF and brain tissue during the early phase by intracerebral inoculation into suckling mice, but it is time consuming. Mosquito cell lines C6/36 from *Aedes albopictus* or *Aedes pseudoscutellaris* cell lines are sensitive and rapid methods for virus isolation from clinical specimens. Immunofluorescent localization of viral antigen in CSF mononuclear cells, and detection of soluble antigen in CSF by reverse passive hemagglutination are rapid methods for diagnosis during the first week of illness. Presently, polymerase chain reaction (PCR) has been developed as a molecular diagnostic method [8].

Neurophysiological investigations including electroencephalogram (EEG) and central motor conduction and neuroimaging such as computed tomography (CT), magnetic resonance imaging (MRI), and single photon emission computed tomography (SPECT) [14, 15] studies reveal a high frequency of thalamic involvement. CT and MRI show abnormal signal intensities in cerebral cortex, thalamus, basal ganglia (including putamen), and brainstem that are considered characteristic of JE. Hyperperfusion in the thalamus, cerebral cortex, and lentiform nucleus highlights the crucial role of the thalamus and the neuronal circuitry in the movement disorders seen in JE. EEG is abnormal, with bilateral slowing of background activity, asymmetry, and seizure activity.

On MRI, bilateral occasionally hemorrhagic thalamic lesions and hyperintensities in the cerebellum, midbrain, and basal ganglia are seen, similar to those in other arboviruses. The hemorrhagic lesions occur after 8–10 days and are likely to be a postinfectious complication. Coexisting parasitic infection

Infections of the Central Nervous System

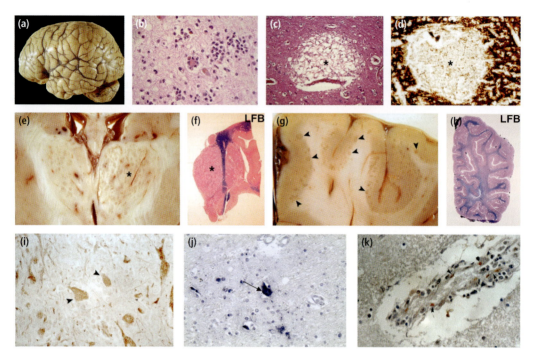

Figure 17.1 (a) Diffuse cerebral edema of the brain causing flattening of gyri (second day of illness). (b) Histology showing florid encephalitis with microglial reaction in the basal ganglia, and entrapped neurons with perivascular inflammation (hematoxylin & eosin [H&E] × Objective 10). (c) Rarefied necrolytic lesion (*) in the cerebral cortex with sparse inflammation (H&E × Objective 20). (d) Necrolytic lesion reveals axonal loss within the lesion (*) (Bodian Silver × 20). (e) Bilateral "punched-out" necrolytic lesions seen in the anterior thalamic nuclei (*). (f) Whole mount of the thalamus, subthalamic nucleus, and putamen revealing numerous necrolytic lesions (*) in nuclear areas extending into the internal capsule and white matter of frontal cortex. (Luxol fast blue [LFB] × 10). (g) The cortical ribbon of the frontal lobes on both sides show multiple tiny punched-out necrolytic lesions at the gray and white junctions (arrowheads). (h) Multiple necrolytic lesions seen along the cortical ribbon of the occipital lobe at the junction of gray and white matter (LFB × 10). (i) Japanese encephalitis (JE) viral antigen detectable within neuronal cytoplasm (arrowheads) and microglial cells by immunohistochemistry (Immunoperoxidase × 10). (j) JE viral genome detected by in situ hybridization within a neuron (arrow) × 40. [Source: 17] (k) JE viral antigen within vascular endothelium, detected by immunohistochemistry. (Immunoperoxidase × 20).

(such as neurocysticercosis) in tropical countries may modulate the encephalitis. Pathological changes of JE are more fulminant on the side harboring a solitary or multiple parasitic cyst(s), especially a degenerating one.

Pathology

The pathological lesions in JE are polymorphic, involving various anatomical areas of the brain. The brain is diffusely edematous with tonsillar herniation (Figure 17.1a). Small, circular necrolytic lesions in the superficial cortical ribbon and diencephalic nuclei are characteristic lesions seen on gross examination (Figure 17.1e, g).

Histologically, variable degrees of meningitis are seen, with a polymorph reaction and perivascular lymphocytic infiltration. During the initial stages, parenchymal inflammation is minimal. Subsequently, diffuse microglial reaction, neuronophagia, and formation of microglial nodules are found (Figure 17.1b). These features are characteristic of acute viral encephalitis. The gliomesenchymal nodules are found in the inferior olivary nucleus, pars compacta of the substantia nigra in midbrain, diencephalic nuclei, and cerebral cortex (frontal and temporal more than other areas). The viral antigen-positive-neurons are surrounded by microglial cells forming a satellite, without neuronophagia.

The second most characteristic microscopic feature of JE is discrete to confluent small, round "necrolytic regions" in the gray matter, including the deep nuclei (Figure 17.1c). Microscopically, these well-circumscribed areas are rarefied with infiltration by polymorphs, followed by lipid-containing macrophages. Subsequently, they transform into pale, relatively acellular zones with loss of axons and myelin (Figure 17.1c, d, f, h). Astroglial reaction is conspicuously absent. Though the pathology is confined to gray matter, occasionally necrolytic lesions are found in white matter fiber tracts. In rare cases, focal hemorrhagic lesions are found in the thalamus and brainstem, usually after 7–10 days. They probably represent allergic, hemorrhagic encephalitis and a "bystander" immune reaction.

In fulminant cases, when patients succumbed by day 3 or 4 of infection, their brains showed edema and vascular congestion. The microglial reaction was prominent between 4 and 10 days, associated with neuronophagia and necrolytic lesions. When associated with neurocysticercosis, the necrolytic lesions are florid in the vicinity of the cysts, and there is a high mortality.

In serologically confirmed cases, Ishii et al. [16] described persistent necrolytic lesions many years later within deep nuclear areas, representing the residual neuropathological stigmata of an earlier pathology [16]. The histopathological diagnosis can be confirmed by demonstration of viral antigens and RNA in neurons [16] and microglial cells by immunohistochemistry and in situ hybridization, respectively (Figure 17.1i, j) [17]. Oyanagi et al. [18] described the electron microscopic features of JE; viral particles were present in endoplasmic reticulum of neurons and more were seen in glial cells. Hematogenous spread of the virus is suggested by its presence in microvascular endothelial cells.

Pathogenesis and animal models

Despite its high incidence, the pathogenesis of human JEV infection and the mechanism of spread into the CNS are not well elucidated [19, 20]. Crossing the blood-brain barrier (BBB) is the most important factor in pathogenesis [21]. Following entry via a mosquito bite, the virus enters the CNS via T lymphocytes, where JEV virions bind to the endothelial surface of CNS vessels (Figure 17.1k) and are internalized by endocytosis [22]. Whether macrophages and B lymphocytes can also harbor JEV is unknown. Clathrin-coated endocytosis is the major route of entry for flaviviruses such as dengue and West Nile virus. An in vitro study however demonstrated that JEV infected fibroblasts in a clathrin-dependent manner, but used a clathrin-independent mechanism to infect neuronal cells using dynamin and plasma membrane cholesterol [23].

Recent studies suggest that JEV enters into the CNS, propagates in neurons, and induces the production of inflammatory cytokines and chemokines, which in turn disrupt the BBB. Involvement of dopaminergic-rich areas, such as thalamus and midbrain suggests that tissue tropism of JEV is associated with dopaminergic signaling pathways. JEV was found to increase dopamine levels during the early stage of infection. JE virus uses D2R-expressing cells via a phospholipase C (PLC)-mediated signaling pathway for entry and neuropathogenesis [24].

The role of the BBB during JEV infection and the role of endothelial and astrocytic cells for viral entry into the CNS are incompletely understood. A recent study by Li and colleagues, using a mouse model of intravenous JEV infection, revealed that viral entry into the CNS occurred 2–5 days post inoculation. This was followed by a dramatic increase in inflammatory cytokines, which preceded BBB permeability, demonstrating that viral entry and inflammation in the CNS preceded BBB damage [25]. Neutralization of interferon gamma (IFN-γ) ameliorated the BBB permeability in JEV-infected mice, suggesting that IFN-γ could be a potential therapeutic target.

The molecular pathogenesis of JEV infection is also unresolved. Neuronal apoptosis, one of the hallmarks of flaviviral infection, may occur in one of two ways, either by direct neuronal killing [26], wherein viral multiplication within neuronal cells leads to cell death, or by the indirect mode, wherein massive inflammatory response causes an upregulation of reactive oxygen species and cytokines such as TNF-α [27]. Activated microglia release proinflammatory cytokines interleukin 6 (IL-6), TNF-α, monocyte chemotactic protein 1 (MCP1), and RANTES, which induce CD4 and CD8+T lymphocyte migration into the brain, to form dense perivascular cuffs [28]. These predominant infiltrates of CD4+ and CD8+T cells may play a role in viral clearance.

Nitric oxide (NO) is an important mediator of neuronal damage, and CSF levels of NO are found to be elevated. In susceptible mice, the toll-like receptor (TLR7) was found to recognize ssRNA of the virus and mount a defensive mechanism by producing type-1 interferon (IFN) and proinflammatory mediators, initiating an innate immune response against the virus [29].

Proinflammatory cytokine and chemokine production is recognized by neurons and microglia, through a retinoic acid-inducible gene (RIG-1)-dependent pathway, TLRs, and pattern recognition receptors. Ablation of RIG-1 in neurons led to enhanced viral load and neuronal loss due to oxidative damage with subversion of antiviral innate immune response [30].

JEV-activated microglia produce inflammatory molecules, which are antiproliferative and antineuronal, contributing to neuropathogenesis [31]. Involvement of critical neuronal targets in the brainstem, thalamus, and reticular formation determine the mortality and clinical outcome. The destruction of reticular formation and thalamus account for deep coma, whereas brainstem, thalamus, and lentiform nuclei involvement account for dystonia and parkinsonian sequelae. Flaccid paralysis in children resembling poliomyelitis points to anterior horn cell involvement in the spinal cord [32]. The topographic distribution of neuronal pathology in the frontal cortex and hippocampus accounts for cognitive and intellectual deficits [33].

Association of movement disorders is well recognized in cases of JE [34]. Extrapyramidal signs like hypokinesia, hypophonia, rigidity, and parkinsonian facies are described, especially one to two months after the primary infection. Cranial CT scans in these patients reveal thalamic involvement, invariably bilateral. The movement disorders in JE are commonly the result of involvement of the thalamus, along with the basal ganglia and midbrain.

In a JE animal model, free radical levels in the brain were raised in the acute stage but declined in the subacute stage (more than three weeks) [35]. Regional and temporal variations in viral loads have been demonstrated in Wistar rats, with the cerebral cortex, corpus striatum, and thalamus showing prominent changes. The highest levels of JEV RNA copies were detected in thalamus and midbrain on days 3 and 10 postintracerebral inoculation in rodents [36].

Treatment, future perspective, and conclusions

No specific antiviral therapy is available. Open labeled clinical trial with recombinant IFNα has been tried in Thailand with good results. Maintenance of fluid and electrolyte balance, good nursing care, and management of cerebral edema are the mainstays of treatment. Recurrent convulsions and status epilepticus are treated by appropriate antiepileptic drugs. An effective way to counter the virus is to inhibit viral replication using antisense molecules directed against the viral genome. Administration of octaguanidium oligomer conjugated Morpholino (Vivo Morphalino) effectively facilitated enhanced survival of mice and neuroprotection in a murine model of JE [37].

Presently three types of vaccines are in large-scale use (a) mouse-brain–derived inactivated vaccine (b) cell-culture–derived inactivated vaccine (c) cell-culture–derived live attenuated vaccine. Among these, mouse-brain–derived inactivated vaccine is widely used in several Asian countries except China, which uses inactivated cell-culture vaccine. Two prototype strains are used for preparation, Nakayama strain and Beijing stain. The schedule is 0.5–1 ml subcutaneously, two doses one to two weeks apart, and a booster one year later, followed by a booster every three to four years in endemic areas. Seroconversion to neutralizing antibody titer of >10 is seen in 80–85% of subjects. Pox-virus–based recombinant virus, DNA viruses, chimeric vaccines, and subunit vaccines are being developed and tested.

References

1. Halstead, S.B. and Jacobson, J. (2003). Japanese encephalitis. *Adv. Virus Res.* 61: 103–138.
2. Hayashi, V.M. (1934). Ubertragung des virus von encephalitis epidemica auf affen. *Proc. Imp. Acad. Tokyo* 10: 41–44.

3. Das, S., Laxminarayana, S.V., Chandra, N. et al. (2009). Heat shock protein 70 on Neuro2a cells is a putative receptor for Japanese encephalitis virus. *Virology* 385: 47–57.
4. McMinn, P.C. (1997). The molecular basis of virulence of the encephalitogenic flaviviruses. *J. Gen. Virol.* 78: 2711–2722.
5. World Health Organization (WHO) (2015). *Summary of key points, position paper on vaccines against Japanese encephalitis (JE)*. http://www.who.int/immunization/documents/positionpapers (accessed 15 June 2018).
6. Wang, H. and Liang, G. (2015). Epidemiology of Japanese encephalitis: past, present, and future prospects. *Ther. Clin. Risk Manag.* 11: 435–448.
7. Basu, A. and Dutta, K. (2017). Recent advances in Japanese encephalitis [version1; referees: 4 approved] *F1000*Research 6 (F1000Faculty Rev):259.
8. Ravi, V., Desai, A., Shankar, S.K., and Gourie Devi, M. (2000). Japanese encephalitis. In: *Infectious Diseases of the Nervous System* (eds. L.E. Davis and P.G.E. Kennedy), 231–257. Oxford: Butterworth and Heinemann.
9. Singh, P., Kalra, N., Ratho, R.K. et al. (2001). Coexistent neurocysticercosis and Japanese B encephalitis: MR imaging correlation. *AJNR Am. J. Neuroradiol.* 22: 1131–1136.
10. Desai, A., Guru, S.C., Ravi, V. et al. (1994). Detection of autoantibodies to neural antigens in the CSF of Japanese encephalitis patients and correlation of findings with the outcome. *J. Neurol. Sci.* 122: 109–116.
11. Ravi, V., Parida, S., Desai, A. et al. (1997). Correlation of tumor necrosis factor levels in the serum and cerebrospinal fluid with clinical outcome in Japanese encephalitis patients. *J. Med. Virol.* 51: 132–136.
12. Babu, G.N., Kalita, J., and Misra, U.K. (2006). Inflammatory markers in the patients of Japanese encephalitis. *Neurol. Res.* 28: 190–192.
13. Ravi, V., Desai, A.S., Shenoy, P.K. et al. (1993). Persistence of Japanese encephalitis virus in the human nervous system. *J. Med. Virol.* 40: 326–329.
14. Misra, U.K., Kalita, J., Jain, S.K., and Mathur, A. (1994). Radiological and neurophysiological changes in Japanese encephalitis. *J. Neurol. Neurosurg. Psychiatry* 57: 1484–1487.
15. Kalita, J., Das, B.K., and Misra, U.K. (1999). SPECT studies of regional cerebral blood flow in 8 patients with Japanese encephalitis in subacute and chronic stage. *Acta Neurol. Scand.* 99: 213–218.
16. Ishii, T., Matsushita, M., and Hamada, S. (1977). Characteristic residual neuropathologic features of Japanese encephalitis. *Acta Neuropathol.* 38: 181–186.
17. Wong, K.T., Ng, K.Y., Ong, K.C. et al. (2012). Enterovirus 71 encephalomyelitis and Japanese encephalitis can be distinguished by topographic distribution of inflammation and specific intraneuronal detection of viral antigen and RNA. *Neuropathol. Appl. Neurobiol.* 38: 443–453.
18. Oyanagi, S., Ikuta, F., and Ross, E.R. (1969). Electron microscopic observations in mice infected with Japanese encephalitis. *Acta Neuropathol.* 13: 169–181.
19. Solomon, T. and Vaughn, D.W. (2002). Pathogenesis and clinical features of Japanese encephalitis and West Nile virus infections. In: *Japanese Encephalitis and West Nile Viruses* (eds. J.S. Mackenzie, A.D.T. Barrett and V. Deubel), 171–194. Berlin: Springer-Verlag Publishers.
20. Myint, K.S., Gibbons, R.V., Perng, G.C., and Solomon, T. (2007). Unravelling the neuropathogenesis of Japanese encephalitis. *Trans. R. Soc. Trop. Med. Hyg.* 101: 955–956.
21. King, N.J., Getts, D.R., Getts, M.T. et al. (2007). Immunopathology of flavivirus infections. *Immunol. Cell Biol.* 85: 33–42.
22. Mathur, A., Kulshreshtha, R., and Chaturvedi, U.C. (1989). Evidence for latency of Japanese encephalitis virus in T lymphocytes. *J. Gen. Virol* 70 (Pt 2): 461–465.
23. Kalia, M., Khasa, R., Sharma, M. et al. (2013). Japanese encephalitis virus infects neuronal cells through a clathrin-independent endocytic mechanism. *J. Virol.* 87: 148–162.
24. Simanjuntak, Y., Jian-Jong, L., Yi-Ling, L., and Yi-Ling, L. (2017). Japanese encephalitis virus exploits dopamine D2 receptor-phospholipase C to target dopaminergic human neuronal cells. *Front. Microbiol.* 8: 651.
25. Li, F., Wang, Y., Yu, L. et al. (2015). Viral infection of the central nervous system and neuroinflammation precede blood-brain barrier disruption during Japanese encephalitis virus infection. *J. Virol.* 89: 5602–5614.
26. Raung, S.L., Kuo, M.D., Wang, Y.M., and Chen, C.J. (2001). Role of reactive oxygen intermediates in Japanese encephalitis virus infection in muri neuroblastoma cells. *Neurosci. Lett.* 315: 9–12.
27. Ghoshal, A., Das, S., Ghosh, S. et al. (2007). Proinflammatory mediators released by activated microglia induces neuronal death in Japanese encephalitis. *Glia* 55: 483–449.
28. Chen, C.J., Chen, J.H., Chen, S.Y. et al. (2004). Upregulation of RANTES gene expression in neuroglia by Japanese encephalitis virus infection. *J. Virol.* 78: 12107–12119.

29. Nazmi, A., Mukherjee, S., Kundu, K. et al. (2014). TLR7 is a key regulator of innate immunity against Japanese encephalitis virus infection. *Neurobiol. Dis.* 69: 235–247.
30. Nazmi, A., Dutta, K., and Basu, A. (2011). RIG-I mediates innate immune response in mouse neurons following Japanese encephalitis virus infection. *PLoS One* 6: –C21761.
31. Nazmi, A., Dutta, K., and Basu, A. (2007). Antiviral and neuroprotective role of octaguaridiumdendrimer conjugated Morpholino oligomers in Japanese encephalitis. *PLoS Negl. Trop. Dis.* 51: 3367–3370.
32. Solomon, T., Kneen, R., Dung, N.M. et al. (1998). Poliomyelitis with illness due to Japanese encephalitis virus. *Lancet* 351: 1094–1097.
33. Chauhan, P.S., Khanna, V.K., Kalita, J., and Misra, U.K. (2017). Japanese encephalitis virus infection results in transient dysfunction of memory learning and cholinesterase inhibition. *Mol. Neurobiol.* 54: 4705–4715.
34. Misra, U.K. and Kalita, J. (1997). Movement disorders in Japanese encephalitis. *J. Neurol.* 244: 299–303.
35. Srivastava, R., Kalita, J., Khan, M.Y., and Misra, U.K. (2009). Free radical generation by neurons in rat model of Japanese encephalitis. *Neurochem. Res.* 34: 2141–2146.
36. Srivastava, R., Kalita, J., Khan, M.Y. et al. (2013). Temporal changes of Japanese encephalitits virus in different brain regions of rat. *Indian J. Med. Res.* 138: 219–223.
37. Das, S., Dutta, K., Kumawat, K.L. et al. (2011). Abrogated inflammatory response promotes neurogenesis in a murine model of Japanese encephalitis. *PLoS One* 6: –e17225.

18 CNS Disorders Caused by Hepatitis C and Hepatitis E Viruses

Melissa Umphlett, Clare Bryce, and Susan Morgello
Department of Pathology, Neurology, and Neuroscience, Icahn School of Medicine, Mount Sinai, New York, NY, USA

Abbreviations

CNS	central nervous system
CSF	cerebrospinal fluid
CSVD	cerebral small vessel disease
DAA	directly acting antivirals
ET	enterically transmitted
GBS	Guillain-Barré syndrome
HCV	hepatitis C virus
HEV	hepatitis E virus
LCM	laser capture microdissection
MRS	magnetic resonance spectroscopy
NA	neuralgic amyotrophy
NANB	non-A non-B
NCR	noncoding regions
ORF	open reading frame
PBMC	peripheral blood mononuclear cells
PET	positron emission tomography
PNS	peripheral nervous system
PT	parenterally transmitted
SVR	sustained virologic response

Definition of the disorder, major synonyms, and historical perspective

The "golden age" of research on hepatitis viruses was in the 1960s and 1970s, when hepatitis B and, later, hepatitis A were discovered, and serologic diagnostic assays developed [1]. Many individuals with hepatitis were seronegative, and non-A non-B (NANB) hepatitis became a significant and enigmatic entity. In 1981, hepatitis E virus (HEV) was discovered and subsequently identified as responsible for most enterically transmitted (ET)-NANB hepatitis. In 1989, hepatitis C virus (HCV) was cloned and identified as responsible for most parenterally transmitted (PT)-NANB hepatitis (1). With detection of these viruses in human biospecimens, appreciation grew of their extrahepatic manifestations, including nervous system disorders.

Both the CNS and peripheral nervous system (PNS) abnormalities are associated with HCV and HEV, but the literature must be interpreted with caution. First, liver disease, regardless of its origins, produces a variety of metabolic, immunologic, and cognitive-behavioral changes. Second, HCV and HEV have hematologic consequences, such as cryoglobulinemia and association with vascular wall pathologies; thus, nervous system disorders may be consequent to vasculopathy [2–7]. Finally, there is little published neuropathology for both viruses, and although human CNS infection has been demonstrated, much evidence for neurotropism relies on molecular analyses of cerebrospinal fluid (CSF) and blood.

Infections of the Central Nervous System: Pathology and Genetics, First Edition. Edited by Fabrice Chrétien, Kum Thong Wong, Leroy R. Sharer, Catherine (Katy) Keohane and Françoise Gray.
© 2020 John Wiley & Sons Ltd. Published 2020 by John Wiley & Sons Ltd.

The majority of HCV-associated neurologic disorders are cognitive and behavioral; however, mononeuritis multiplex, distal symmetrical polyneuropathy, encephalomyelitis, and CNS vasculitis with or without cryoglobulinemia are also reported [5–7]. HCV is associated with carotid atherosclerosis, cerebral small vessel disease (CSVD), and stroke with cardiolipin antibody syndrome, implicating virus in cerebrovascular disorders [3, 5–7].

The most common HEV-associated abnormalities are Guillain-Barré syndrome (GBS) and neuralgic amyotrophy (NA; also known as Parsonage-Turner syndrome or brachial plexus neuritis). Less commonly, encephalomyelitis, mononeuritis multiplex, myositis, vestibular neuritis, and Bell palsy are described [8, 9].

The main characteristics of both viruses are summarized in Table 18.1.

Microbiology

HCV is an enveloped, positive-sense, single-stranded RNA virus, 40–80 nm, in the family Flaviviridae, genus *Hepacivirus*. The genome is 9600 base pairs long, with 5′ and 3′ noncoding regions (NCR) and a single open reading frame (ORF) encoding a polyprotein precursor [10]. HCV has seven major genotypes and more than 60 subtypes, with extensive genetic heterogeneity, both worldwide and within an individual as quasispecies [10]. There are no studies relating genotype to neurologic dysfunction, with multiple genotypes represented in brain-derived sequences [11]. HCV cell entry is mediated by interactions with CD81, scavenger receptor-B1, claudin-1, and occludin, present on human cerebral endothelia but not glia [10, 12]. Once uncoated in cytoplasm, HCV acts directly as messenger RNA for transcription of viral proteins and in association with modified endoplasmic reticulum as a template for viral replication in a "membranous web." Replication produces a negative-strand RNA intermediate, serving as a template for production of new genomes; detecting this intermediate documents tissue-specific replication and has been seen in human peripheral blood mononuclear cells (PBMC) and brain [13].

HEV is a small (27–34 nm), positive-sense, single-stranded, nonenveloped RNA virus, of the family Hepeviridae, genus *Orthohepevirus*. Of four main genotypes, genotypes 1 and 2 are restricted to humans, and genotypes 3 and 4 are zoonotic, with a major reservoir in pigs. Less common zoonotic genotypes 5 through 8 are also recognized [14]. Most

Table 18.1 Main Characteristics of Hepatitis C and Hepatitis E Viruses.

	HCV	HEV
Family	Flaviviridae	Hepeviridae
Virion	enveloped	non-enveloped
Genome	Positive sense, single-strand RNA	Positive sense, single-strand RNA
Transmission	Blood borne (all genotypes)	Oral-fecal (genotypes 1 and 2); zoonotic (genotypes 3 and 4)
Course of liver disease	Chronic in up to 80%	Acute in greater than 90%
Neuropathogenesis	Possibly via infected monocytes	Unknown
CNS cell targets	Monocyte and macrophage Possibly astrocyte Possibly endothelia	Unknown
Neurologic syndromes	Nonspecific diffuse cognitive-behavioral deficits; mononeuritis multiplex; meningoencephalitis and encephalomyelitis	Guillain-Barré syndrome (GBS); neuralgic amyotrophy; mononeuritis multiplex; meningoencephalitis and encephalomyelitis

CNS, central nervous system; HCV, hepatitis C virus; HEV, hepatitis E virus.

neurologic disease is associated with genotype 3; genotypes 1 and 4 are also reported [8]. The HEV genome is 7200 base pairs long, with 3′ and 5′ NCRs, and three ORFs encoding nonstructural proteins (ORF1), capsid proteins (ORF2), and multifunctional proteins (ORF3). The HEV cell cycle is not characterized, and cell surface receptors are not identified. Although compartmentalized infection with CNS quasi-species is documented, it is unclear whether HEV is neurotropic or only neuroinvasive [8].

Epidemiology

Hepatitis C infection occurs worldwide and is chronic in up to 80% of individuals infected with the virus [10]. Approximately 71 million people have chronic HCV and 400 000 die annually from complications, commonly as a result of hepatocellular carcinoma and cirrhosis. In 2015, an estimated 23.7 new HCV infections per 100 000 people occurred globally [15, 16]. Prevalence in the World Health Organization (WHO) eastern Mediterranean and European regions is 2.3 and 1.5%, respectively. In other regions, prevalence ranges between 0.5 and 1%. It is a blood-borne pathogen; infection occurs via contaminated needles with intravenous drug use, contaminated blood products or inadequately sterilized medical equipment, sexual transmission, or vertical transmission from mother to infant [15, 16].

Worldwide, HEV is the most common cause of acute hepatitis with an estimated 20 million cases annually. Most infections are self-limited, resolving within six weeks [15, 16]. A minority of individuals and pregnant women in underdeveloped countries develop fulminant HEV. Chronic infection may occur in the setting of immunocompromise. In resource-poor areas with fecally contaminated water, genotypes 1 and 2 are prevalent. In areas with safe drinking water, infection is with genotypes 3 and 4 and is a porcine zoonosis [8, 15, 16]. Parenteral iatrogenic transmission via contaminated blood also occurs [8]. In contrast to HEV's widespread prevalence, neurologic complications are rare; by 2016, only 91 reports were identified in the literature [8]. However, in some series of GBS or NA, up to 10% of cases were related to HEV [8].

Clinical features

The majority of primary infections with HCV and HEV are asymptomatic. Liver disease may be mild or absent at the time of neurologic presentation [5, 8]. Direct infection is not strongly implicated in most HCV- and HEV-associated neurologic disorders.

In patients with chronic HCV, fatigue, depression, and cognitive impairment are extremely common (80% have fatigue), but it is unclear if these are HCV specific or reflect underlying hepatic or preexistent neuropsychiatric abnormalities [5, 17]. Putative evidence of viral neurobiology includes correlating neuropsychiatric symptoms with neuroinflammation on magnetic resonance spectroscopy (MRS) and HCV seropositivity with abnormal white matter. However, microglial activation quantified by positron emission tomography (PET) PK11195 binding has been related to preserved cognition, questioning the significance of HCV-associated brain inflammation to neuropsychiatric symptomatology [5, 12, 17, 18].

CNS and PNS manifestations of mixed cryoglobulinemia and cryoglobulin-negative vasculitis are more definitely HCV related [7]. Peripheral neuropathy is common and symptomatic in up to 10%, and possibly more than 70% in those with cryoglobulinemia [7, 17].

Most often, HCV-associated cryoglobulinemia results in mononeuritis multiplex and polyneuropathy; in brain, it is linked to ischemic damage and cognitive impairment [7, 19]. When clinical and neuroimaging features are compatible with vascular disease, implication of HCV rests with laboratory diagnosis by direct detection of HCV in serum and CSF by reverse transcriptase-polymerase chain reaction (RT-PCR), as well as serology.

In contrast to parainfectious HCV-associated manifestations, inflammatory disorders indicative of neuroinvasion (i.e. meningoencephalitis and myelitis) are limited to case reports and must be distinguished from the equally rare acute disseminated encephalomyelitis [5, 20, 21].

Similarly rare, there are 12 case reports of meningoencephalitis and myelitis associated with HEV, 5 in transplant recipients with immunosuppression [8, 9]. It is hard to discern a clinical pattern with so few published cases, but CSF pleocytosis is a feature, accompanying viral detection by RT-PCR.

The most common neurological manifestations of HEV are GBS and NA; both are clinically similar when occurring in other infectious etiologies. NA presents with neuropathic arm and shoulder pain and at onset individuals are often HEV RNA positive [8]. In GBS, HEV RNA is usually not detected, but serology remains positive, consistent with an immune pathogenesis.

Pathology

There is no specific viral neuropathology for any HCV- or HEV-related disorder. Reliable immunohistochemical reagents for tissue detection do not exist, and the few reports of tissue localization or CSF detection rely on molecular methods. A case of HCV encephalitis, confirmed by RT-PCR, showed predominantly T-cell perivascular and parenchymal infiltrates and prominent microglial activation with nodule formation; these are non-specific and typical of viral encephalitides [20]. In a series of individuals with brain-specific HCV evolution, the most frequent histopathology was Alzheimer type 2 gliosis, a manifestation of liver disease [22]. HCV has been detected in atheroma from carotid angioplasties and may be a risk factor for CSVD, but vascular phenomena may not reflect tissue tropism [3, 6].

Pathogenesis

A robust literature to explain neuroinvasion by HCV or HEV is not available, and pathogenesis of parainfectious complications is beyond the scope of this chapter. HCV infects and replicates in PBMC, and laser capture microdissection (LCM) has shown HCV RNA, including replication intermediates, from CD68+ cells in human brain samples [23]. Thus, it is plausible to postulate that neuroinvasion occurs through the blood-brain barrier (BBB) trafficking of infected monocytes; however, it is unclear how monocytes and microglia are infected because they lack specific receptors supporting HCV cell entry [12]. Astrocytes with low levels of HCV RNA (but not replication intermediates) have also been demonstrated; in culture systems, primary human astrocytes are inefficiently infected but do not support replication [23, 24].

The pathogenesis of HEV brain involvement is unknown. It is possible that direct viral infection of brain causes HEV-related encephalitis, largely based on observations in animal models [8].

Animal models

Chimpanzees are the only animal model of HCV replication and host immune responses. Immunodeficient mouse models with human chimeric livers or humanized mouse models have been used [10]. A variety of viruses related to HCV are found naturally in mammals, including dogs and horses. There are no animal models of neurologic disease.

Nonhuman primates are also ideal models for HEV infection, and zoonotic genotypes 3 and 4 can be studied in swine, chickens, rodents, and rabbits [14]. There are no models of neurologic disease, although mice and monkeys have demonstrated HEV infection of granule cell neurons [25].

Treatment

HCV therapy has been revolutionized by efficacious, direct-acting antivirals (DAA) such as sofosbuvir, daclatasvir, and ledipasvir, with sustained virologic response (SVR) occurring in more than 90% of treated individuals [15, 16]. Improved cognition and white matter integrity have been demonstrated in a subset of individuals with SVR, with reduced fatigue, depression, and better quality of life, but effects may be mediated through improved liver function [17, 26]. It is unclear why some fail to show reversal of cognitive and behavioral abnormalities with SVR. Parainfectious neurologic complications of HCV are treated following guidelines for specific disease processes (e.g. immunomodulation and plasma exchange for GBS) [8].

As HEV infection is usually self-limited, specific treatment is not warranted. Ribavirin monotherapy is used for acute on chronic liver failure and fulminant disease, but efficacy is documented in case reports and not systematic clinical trials [27].

PEGylated-interferon-α is also used [27]. As with HCV, treatment for parainfectious complications follows guidelines for the disease process.

Although therapeutic advances have enabled dramatic cures, there is no information regarding CNS penetrance and nervous system efficacy of DAAs. With time, it will become clear whether these neuroinvasive pathogens have significant neurotropism or transiently affect CNS because of manifestations of systemic disease.

References

1. Lemon, S.M. and Walker, C.M. (2018). Enterically transmitted non-A, non-B hepatitis and the discovery of hepatitis E virus. *Cold Spring Harb. Perspect. Med.* https://doi.org/10.1101/cshperspect.a033449.
2. Kamar, N., Dalton, H.R., Abravanel, F., and Izopet, J. (2014). Hepatitis E virus infection. *Clin. Microbiol. Rev.* 27: 116–138.
3. Morgello, S., Murray, J., Van Der Elst, S., and Byrd, D. (2014). HCV, but not HIV, is a risk factor for cerebral small vessel disease. *Neurol. Neuroimmunol. Neuroinflamm.* 1: e27.
4. Kamar, N., Marion, O., Abravanel, F. et al. (2016). Extrahepatic manifestations of hepatitis E virus. *Liver Int.* 36: 467–472.
5. Morgello, S. (2005). The nervous system and hepatitis C virus. *Semin. Liver Dis.* 25: 118–121.
6. Boddi, M., Abbate, R., Chellini, B. et al. (2010). Hepatitis C virus RNA localization in human carotid plaques. *J. Clin. Virol.* 47: 72–75.
7. Cacoub, P., Saadoun, D., Limal, N. et al. (2005). Hepatitis C virus infection and mixed cryoglobulinemia vasculitis: a review of neurological complications. *AIDS* 19: S128–S134.
8. Dalton, H.R., Kamar, N., van Eijk, J.J. et al. (2016). Hepatitis E virus and neurological injury. *Nat. Rev. Neurol.* 12: 77–85.
9. Mclean, B.N., Gulliver, J., and Dalton, H.R. (2017). Hepatitis E and neurological disorders. *Pract. Neurol.* 17: 282–288.
10. Bukh, J. (2016). The history of hepatitis C virus (HCV): basic research reveals unique features in phylogeny, evolution, and the viral life cycle with new perspectives for epidemic control. *J. Hepatol.* 65: S2–S21.
11. Fishman, S.L., Murray, J.M., Eng, F.J. et al. (2008). Molecular and bioinformatics evidence of hepatitis C virus evolution in brain. *J. Infect. Dis.* 197: 597–607.
12. Fletcher, N.F. and McKeating, J.A. (2012). Hepatitis C virus and the brain. *J. Viral Hepat.* 19: 301–306.
13. Laskus, T., Radkowski, M., Adair, D.M. et al. (2005). Emerging evidence of hepatitis C virus neuroinvasion. *AIDS* 19 (suppl 3): s140–s144.
14. Cao, D. and Meng, X.J. (2012). Molecular biology and replication of hepatitis E virus. *Emerg. Microbes Infect.* 1: e17.
15. World Health Organization (WHO) (2018). *Hepatitis C.* http://www.who.int/news-room/fact-sheets/detail/hepatitis-c (accessed 22 August 2018).
16. World Health Organization (WHO) (2018). *Hepatitis E.* http://www.who.int/news-room/fact-sheets/detail/hepatitis-e (accessed 22 August 2018).
17. Yeoh, S.W., Holmes, A.C.N., Saling, M.M. et al. (2018). Depression, fatigue and neurocognitive deficits in chronic hepatitis C. *Hepatol. Int.* 12: 294–304.
18. Pflugrad, H., Meyer, G.J., Dirks, M. et al. (2016). Cerebral microglia activation in hepatitis C virus infection correlates to cognitive dysfunction. *J. Viral Hepat.* 23: 348–357.
19. Petty, G.W., Duffy, J., and Huston, J. (1996). Cerebral ischemia in patients with hepatitis C virus infection and mixed cryoglobulinemia. *Mayo Clin. Proc.* 71: 671–678.
20. Seifert, F., Struffert, T., Hildebrandt, M. et al. (2008). *In vivo* detection of hepatitis C virus (HCV) RNA in the brain of a case of encephalitis: evidence for HCV virus neuroinvasion. *Eur. J. Neurol.* 15: 214–218.
21. Sim, J.E., Lee, J.B., Cho, Y.N. et al. (2012). A case of acute disseminated encephalomyelitis associated with hepatitis C virus infection. *Yonsei Med. J.* 53: 856–858.
22. Murray, J., Fishman, S.L., Ryan, E. et al. (2008). Clinicopathologic correlates of hepatitis C virus in brain: a pilot study. *J. Neurovirol.* 14: 17–27.
23. Wilkinson, J., Radkowski, M., and Laskus, T. (2009). Hepatitis C virus neuroinvasion: identification of infected cells. *J. Virol.* 83: 1312–1319.
24. Liu, Z., Zhao, F., and He, J.J. (2014). Hepatitis C virus (HCV) interaction with astrocytes: nonproductive infection and induction of IL-18. *J. Neurovirol.* 20: 278–293.
25. Zhou, X., Huang, F., Xu, L. et al. (2017). Hepatitis E virus infects neurons and brains. *J. Infect. Dis.* 215: 1197–1206.
26. Kuhn, T., Sayegh, P., Jones, J.D. et al. (2017). Improvements in brain and behavior following eradication of hepatitis C. *J. Neurovirol.* 23: 593–602.
27. European Association for the Study of the Liver (2018). EASL clinical practice guidelines on hepatitis E virus infection. *J. Hepatol.* 68: 1256–1271.

19 Alphaviral Equine Encephalomyelitis (Eastern, Western, and Venezuelan)

Kum Thong Wong
Department of Pathology, Faculty of Medicine, University of Malaya, Kuala Lumpur, Malaysia

Abbreviations

AEE	alphaviral equine encephalomyelitis
CNS	central nervous system
EEE	Eastern equine encephalomyelitis
EEG	electroencephalogram
NHP	nonhuman primate
MRI	magnetic resonance imaging
RNA	ribonucleic acid
VEE	Venezuelan equine encephalomyelitis
WEE	Western equine encephalomyelitis

Definition of the disorder, major synonyms, and historical perspective

Alphaviral equine encephalomyelitis (AEE) is a term used to describe mosquito-borne, zoonotic infections that include Eastern equine encephalomyelitis (EEE), Western equine encephalomyelitis (WEE), and Venezuelan equine encephalomyelitis (VEE) [1]. The causative alphaviruses mainly infect horses and other animals but occasionally spill over to involve humans as dead-end hosts. EEE and WEE viruses were first isolated in 1933 and 1930, respectively, from infected horses in the United States. VEE virus was also originally isolated from infected horses in 1938 in Venezuela. All three infections are confined to the Americas.

Microbiological characteristics

EEE, WEE, and VEE viruses belong to the genus *Alphavirus* in the Togaviridae family. They are called "new world" alphaviruses, being found only in the Americas, as opposed to "old world" alphaviruses (e.g. Sindbis virus, Ross Valley virus, and Chikungunya virus [2]). Like all alphaviruses, EEE, WEE, and VEE viruses are single-stranded, positive-sense RNA viruses with genome lengths of 11–12 kb that encode for three structural (capsid, E1, and E2) and four nonstructural proteins. The virions are icosahedral nucleocapsids with lipid envelopes that contain glycoprotein spikes comprising E viral proteins.

All three viruses have their own distinct genomes and antigenicities. Within the EEE virus antigenic complex, there are four lineages: lineage I (North American) and lineages II–IV (South American and newly renamed as Madariaga virus).

Infections of the Central Nervous System: Pathology and Genetics, First Edition. Edited by Fabrice Chrétien, Kum Thong Wong, Leroy R. Sharer, Catherine (Katy) Keohane and Françoise Gray.
© 2020 John Wiley & Sons Ltd. Published 2020 by John Wiley & Sons Ltd.

Lineage 1 is mainly responsible for human infections. In the WEE virus antigenic complex, which includes WEE, Highlands J, and Sindbis viruses, only the WEE virus is responsible for human CNS infections [2]. The VEE virus antigenic complex comprises at least eight species and seven antigenic subtypes [3, 4]. The species VEE virus is classified as antigenic subtype I and has four antigenic varieties (i.e. IAB, IC, ID, and IE). The IAB and IC antigenic varieties cause epidemics of human encephalomyelitis, whereas ID and IE are usually associated with endemic encephalomyelitis [3, 5].

Epidemiology

EEE was reported mainly in North America in the past, but in recent years, only a few cases have occurred annually; large epidemics have not been reported. In Central America, a few cases have been reported recently in Panama [6]. On the other hand, WEE has decreased dramatically in North America, but in South America, isolated cases have surfaced in Uruguay recently [7]. There is an apparent increasing incidence of VEE in South America where many cases may go unreported or undiagnosed. Nonetheless, in terms of human infection, current data already show it is the most prevalent and important of the three types of AEE [3]. Dual EEE and VEE infections have also been described [6].

In general, the AEE viruses have complex endemic and epidemic life cycles involving different mosquito species and mammalian hosts. In EEE and WEE, the endemic life cycles are mainly between birds (and also rodents in South America for EEE) and promiscuous feeding mosquitoes. During epidemic transmission cycles, both viruses are spread by the same mosquitoes (*Coquillettidia, Ochlerotatus, Aedes,* and *Culex*) to horses and humans which are dead-end hosts; viremia is very low [1]. In VEE, endemic life cycles are mainly maintained between rodents and *Culex* mosquitoes. The virus could spread by other mosquito species (*Psorophora* and *Ochlerotatus*) to horses and humans to trigger epidemics that can both involve and be maintained between these amplifying animal hosts. Person-to-person transmission has not been confirmed in VEE, although aerosol transmission has been reported in laboratories [8]. For more details of animal species involved in viral transmissions see [1].

Clinical features

The incubation period for AEE ranges from 2 to 10 days, but infections may be asymptomatic. Encephalitis occurs in probably less than 4% of symptomatic cases with a higher percentage in children [8]. Mild nonspecific symptoms include fever, headache, nausea, vomiting, anorexia, malaise, and myalgia. In more severe cases, there is alteration of mental status such as confusion, somnolence and coma, seizures, and respiratory symptoms. Neck stiffness is found in 36% of EEE [1, 9]. Clinical presentations may be confused with other equine encephalomyelitis and other arboviral infections [3, 6]. Other reported symptoms includes hematuria in EEE and watery diarrhea in VEE. In a recent fatal WEE case from Uruguay, the patient presented with headache, vomiting, neck stiffness, partial left seizures, raised intracranial pressure, and coma [7].

In EEE, leukocytosis was found in 69–93% of patients, with 57% neutrophilia. Hyponatremia was reported in 60% [9, 10]. The cerebrospinal fluid (CSF) findings included pleocytosis (97–100%) and elevated proteins (86–94%). The electroencephalogram (EEG) was characterized by generalized slowing and disorganization of background. Epileptiform discharges with or without periodic lateralizing discharges and status epilepticus may be seen in a few patients. T2-weighted brain magnetic resonance imaging (MRI) showed hyperintense lesions, most commonly in the basal ganglia, thalamus and cerebral cortex (63–88%), and in the brainstem. Lesions may be unilateral, asymmetric, and large, with mass effects. The subcortical white matter and meninges are also involved.

The highest mortality has been reported in EEE, ranging from 50 to 70% [10]. Mortality in VEE and WEE is much lower, ranging from 1 to 7%. In survivors of AEE, neurological sequelae were highest in EEE (50–90%) followed by WEE (15–30%) and VEE 4–14%) [11]. Neurological sequelae could include neuropsychiatric disorders (e.g. emotional instability, behavioral changes), intellectual disabilities, somnolence, epilepsy, paralysis, and visual disturbances.

Pathology

Apart from relatively few publications on pathology of EEE, there have been even fewer on VEE and WEE. The general pathological features of AEE in the CNS are those of an acute meningoencephalomyelitis and all three entities appear to share similar features. Macroscopically, there is diffuse brain edema, congestion, and focal hemorrhages [1, 12]. In a long-standing WEE case, bilateral lenticostriate region softening was recorded [13].

In EEE, inflammation is found mainly in neuronal areas of the cerebral cortex, basal ganglia, thalamus, brainstem, spinal cord, and cerebellum. In addition to perivascular and parenchymal inflammatory changes such as microglial nodules, intense focal necrosis can be found, resulting in rarefaction or islands of pallor (Figure 19.1a, b). Within these areas, degenerate neurons with eosinophilic cytoplasm can be seen (Figure 19.1c). There are no viral inclusions. Inflammatory cells are composed of lymphocytes, mononuclear cells, and neutrophils [10, 12]. Meningitis and focal hemorrhages have been described in the cerebral cortex and elsewhere. One distinctive feature that has been frequently described but seldom well illustrated in the literature is vasculitis. However, in monkey models and horses, vasculitis was convincingly demonstrated [8]. In 4 out of 20 VEE autopsy cases, vasculitis was reported [14]. Thus,

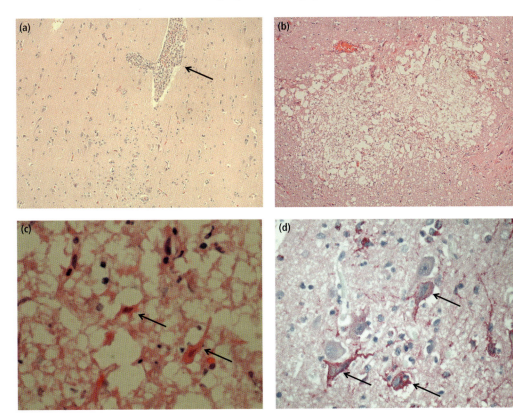

Figure 19.1 Eastern equine encephalomyelitis. (a) Mild perivascular (arrow) and parenchymal infiltration by inflammatory cells. (b) Areas of pallor or rarefaction in infected areas. (c) These areas are edematous and have degenerate eosinophilic neurons (arrows). (d) Infected neurons (arrows) stained for viral antigens (red). Magnification: a: ×4 objective; b: ×10 objective, c, d: ×40 objective. Hematoxylin and eosin (H&E) stains (a–c); Immunohistochemistry (d). (All figures photographed by the author using tissue glass slides courtesy of Dr. S. Zaki and Dr. W. J. Shieh, Centers for Disease Control and Prevention, Atlanta, USA).

vasculitis can be found in AEE; albeit it is likely to be a rare feature.

EEE viral antigens were localized mainly in neurons (Figure 19.1d). In the white matter, occasional glial cells may be positive for viral antigens [12, 14]. To date, there is no published information on immunohistochemical detection of viral antigens in VEE or WEE. Neither have viral antigens been demonstrated in blood vessel walls, including endothelium and smooth muscle. In VEE, inflammatory necrotizing lesions have been described in extra-CNS organs such as the lung, liver, lymphoid tissue, and spleen [14].

Genetics and pathogenesis

Generally, EEE has been largely confined to North America with only rare sporadic cases reported in South America. The reasons for this geographic variation in virulence and difference in human susceptibility are not clear, but different viral strains or mutations may be involved. However, recent increase of human EEE cases in South America has been detected and attributed to increased surveillance, viral circulation and virulence, and animal host range [6].

Enzootic and endemic strains of VEE subtypes ID and IE were thought to be able to undergo glycoprotein 2 (E2) gene mutations to give rise to IAB and IC subtypes that cause severe disease in horses with extensive spillover to human populations in South America [4].

Animal models and pathogenesis

Apart from equids, many other animal species can be infected by EEE, WEE, and VEE viruses, can develop fatal encephalitis, and indeed have been used as animal models. A comprehensive review of animal models in AEE is found in [8]. The pathological findings in horses infected by AEE are generally similar to those described in the human CNS, including meningoencephalitis and viral antigens in neurons [8, 15]. Vasculitis may also be found.

Among small animal models, mice, hamsters, guinea pigs and so on may, or may not, show much CNS pathology. The EEE mouse model demonstrated the presence of viral antigens mainly in neurons and provided evidence for direct CNS infection via the olfactory bulb following intranasal aerosol inoculation. However, vasculitis was not typical. [8]. Nonhuman primates (NHP) have also been used in studies to elucidate pathogenesis and for vaccine studies in EEE. The CNS pathology includes severe meningoencephalomyelitis with widespread neuronal necrosis and viral antigens, edema, hemorrhage, cerebral vasculitis, gliosis, and perivascular inflammatory cells.

WEE infection in the mouse and hamster model showed brain pathology consisting of neuronal necrosis, edema and parenchymal inflammation, gliosis, and meningitis. In the NHP, meningoencephalomyelitis was found and viral antigens localized to neurons and microglia [8]. Vasculitis was not reported.

VEE infection in the mouse model demonstrated neuronal viral antigens in the CNS and also extra-CNS lymphoid necrosis. NHP models of VEE showed pathological features in various parts of the brain and spinal cord comprising parenchymal inflammation, neuronal damage, and glial nodules but notably no vasculitis. These studies were also less informative than expected without application of more modern methods to localize virus such as immunohistochemistry [8].

Treatment, future perspective, and conclusions

There are increasing reports that the incidence of VEE is rising and, at the same time, grossly underdiagnosed in South America [4]. Together with the threat of its potential use in bioterrorism and the fact that AEE viruses could be spread by aerosols, there is a great concern that these viruses, especially VEE, could be developed for this purpose. Hence, there is an urgent need for effective vaccines because none exists at the moment [1, 8].

Following mosquito bites, the assumption is that viremia occurs, and virus crosses the blood-brain barrier to cause encephalitis. However, other pathways for neuroinvasion need further investigation. Findings in animal models and infections following accidental lab exposure suggest that transnasal neuroinvasion could occur [8]. Comparative studies of all three AEE viruses may be useful to further investigate neuropathogenesis, neuroinvasion, and extra-CNS organ involvement, particularly if NHP as animal models and modern histopathological techniques are applied. Whether viruses can directly infect endothelium or smooth muscle, and whether vasculitis plays a significant role in neuropathogenesis by causing thrombosis and microinfarction remains to be seen.

References

1. Arechiga-Ceballos, N. and Aguilar-Setien, A. (2015). Alphaviral equine encephalomyelitis (Eastern, Western and Venezuelan). *Rev. Sci. Tech. Int. Epiz.* 34: 491–501.
2. Iowa State University for Food Security and Public Health (2015). Eastern, Western and Venezuelan Equine Encephalomyelitis. Center for Food Security and Public Health Technical Factsheets 49. http://lib.dr.iastate.edu/cfsph_factsheets (accessed 17 July 2019).
3. Aguilar, P., Estrado-Franco, J.G., Navarro-Lopez, R. et al. (2011). Endemic Venezuelan equine encephalitis in the Americas: hidden under the dengue umbrella. *Futur. Virol.* 6: 721–740.
4. Forrester, N., Wertheim, J.O., Dugan, V.G. et al. (2017). Evolution and spread of Venezuelan equine encephalis complex alphavirus in the Americas. *PLoS Negl. Trop. Dis.* 11 (8): e0005693.
5. Vilcarromero, S., Aguilar, P.V., Halsey, E.S. et al. (2010). Venezuelan equine encephalitis and 2 human deaths, Peru. *Emerg. Infect. Dis.* 16: 553–556.
6. Carrera, J.P., Forrester, N., Wang, E. et al. (2013). Eastern equine encephalitis in Latin America. *N. Engl. J. Med.* 369: 732–744.
7. Delfraro, A., Burgueno, A., Morel, N. et al. (2011). Fatal human case of Western equine encephalitis, Uruguay. *Emerg. Infect. Dis.* 17: 952–954.
8. Steele, K.E. and Twenhafel, N.A. (2010). Pathology of animal models of alphaviral encephalitis. *Vet. Pathol.* 47: 790–805.
9. Deresiewicz, R.L., Thaler, S.J., Hsu, L., and Zamani, A.A. (1997). Clinical and radiologic manifestations of Eastern Equine Encephalitis. *N. Engl. J. Med.* 336: 1867–1874.
10. Silverman, M.A., Misasi, J., Smole, S. et al. (2013). Eastern equine encephalitis in children, Massachusetts and New Hampshire, USA, 1970–2010. *Emerg. Infect. Dis.* 19: 194–201.
11. Ronca, S.E., Dineley, K.T., and Paessler, S. (2016). Neurological sequelae resulting from encephalitic alphavirus infection. *Front. Microbiol.* 7: 959. https://doi.org/10.3389/fmicb.2016.00959.
12. Solomon, I.H., Ciarlini, P.D.S.C., Santagata, S. et al. (2017). Fatal Eastern equine encephalitis in a patient on maintenance Rituximab: a case report. *Open Forum Infect. Dis.* https://doi.org/10.1093/ofid/ofx021.
13. Quong, T.L. (1942). The pathology of Western equine encephalomyelitis: 18 human cases, Manitoba epidemic, 1941. *Can. Pub. Heal J* 33: 300–306.
14. De la Monte, S.M., Castro, F., Bonilla, N.J. et al. (1985). The systemic pathology of Venezuelan equine encephalitis virus infection in humans. *Am. J. Trop. Med. Hyg.* 34: 194–202.
15. Del Piero, F., Wilkins, P.A., Dubovi, E.J. et al. (2001). Clinical, pathologic and immunohistochemical, and virologic findings of Eastern Equine encephalitis in two horses. *Vet. Pathol.* 38: 451–456.

20 Chikungunya Virus

Cássia Shinotsuka[1], Michael Blatzer[2], Grégory Jouvion[1], and Fabrice Chrétien[1,3,4]

[1] Experimental Neuropathology Unit, Pasteur Institute, Paris, France
[2] Aspergillus and Experimental Neuropathology Units, Pasteur Institute, Paris, France
[3] Paris University, Paris, France
[4] Department of Neuropathology, Sainte Anne Hospital, Paris, France

Abbreviations

CHIKV	Chikungunya virus
CNS	central nervous system
CSF	cerebrospinal fluid
DENV	Dengue virus
GBS	Guillain-Barré syndrome
MRI	magnetic resonance imaging
NSAIDs	nonsteroidal anti-inflammatory drugs
RT-LAMP	reverse transcription loop-mediated isothermal amplification
RT-PCR	reverse transcription polymerase chain reaction
ZIKV	Zika virus

Introduction

Chikungunya virus (CHIKV) is an arthropod-borne virus (arbovirus) belonging to the family of Togaviridae and genus *Alphavirus*. Arboviruses are transmitted among vertebrate hosts by a variety of vectors, such as mosquitoes from the *Aedes* species (*Stegomyia*) for CHIKV or Zika virus (ZIKV). All arboviruses affecting human health are zoonotic pathogens that require animals as hosts or reservoirs, but some arboviruses can undergo direct human amplification and vertical transmission thereby bypassing enzootic hosts [1].

First isolated in Tanzania in 1952 [2], many outbreaks of CHIKV have since been reported in Asia in the 1950s and 1960s. However, CHIKV had not been considered a significant public health problem until 2004, when an outbreak in Kenya spread the virus initially to Indian Ocean Islands and India and, subsequently, to Europe, Asia, and the Americas, infecting millions of people [3]. This global epidemic is unprecedented and most likely driven by multiple factors. The spread of CHIKV began with the virus spillover from African zoonotic cycles [4], followed by spread via air travel and, finally, urban dissemination (probably like dengue virus [DENV]). The lack of herd immunity to CHIKV in humans in the Indian Ocean Basin region, coupled with the invasion of this area with *Aedes albopictus,* and increased adaptation of CHIKV to *A. albopictus,* which facilitated the virus replication, are additional factors that contributed to the global epidemic [5].

Virology and pathophysiology

Four CHIKV lineages with distinct genotypic and antigenic characteristics have been identified: isolates from the Indian Ocean outbreak, the Asian

Infections of the Central Nervous System: Pathology and Genetics, First Edition. Edited by Fabrice Chrétien, Kum Thong Wong, Leroy R. Sharer, Catherine (Katy) Keohane and Françoise Gray.
© 2020 John Wiley & Sons Ltd. Published 2020 by John Wiley & Sons Ltd.

lineage, the West African lineage, and the East, Central, and South African lineage [6, 7].

CHIKV consists of a single strand of positive-sense RNA genome of 11.4 kb, and a phospholipid envelope with hemagglutinin protein spikes. A mutation at residue 226 of the membrane fusion glycoprotein E1 (A226V) abrogated the virus cholesterol dependence, resulting in better viral uptake, replication, and transmission by *A. albopictus*, which has a wider geographical distribution than *Aedes aegypti*. This mutation led to a massive outbreak in the Indian subcontinent. Additional substitutions were found in the envelope proteins E2 and E3, indicating that the virus envelope changed over time and that these mutations enhanced the initial infection of *A. albopictus*, leading to increased vector competence [8, 9].

CHIKV is recognized as a cause of arthritis and neurological diseases throughout the world. After the bite of an infected mosquito, CHIKV infects epithelial cells and dermal fibroblasts, subsequently entering blood vessels [10]. Monocytes are then responsible for its dissemination and secondary infections. The principal secondary infection sites are muscles and joints, and in animal models, CHIKV infects the choroid plexus, the cerebrospinal fluid (CSF), and meningeal and ependymal cells [11].

Clinical features

Systemic presentation

After a mean incubation period of four to seven days, the disease usually starts with acute onset of fever (usually above 39 °C) associated with rashes, severe myalgia, and polyarthralgia. Viremia persists for five days from the onset of symptoms. The disease is usually self-limiting in patients, lasting one to two weeks. Chikungunya means "to walk bent over" in the Makonde language, which reflects the typical stooped walking position of infected people. The arthralgia is mostly symmetrical, affecting large joints, although smaller joints may also be affected. Up to 65% of patients develop a chronic, sometimes debilitating, relapsing polyarthralgia or arthritis predominantly in distal joints. A maculopapular rash occurs in 20–80% of patients, mainly on the trunk, but it may also affect the limbs (including soles and palms) and the head. Pruritus is present in 50% of cases. Other less common features include external ear redness (reflecting chondritis), lymphadenopathy, eye involvement (i.e. uveitis, iridocyclitis, retinitis, and conjunctivitis), myocarditis, pericarditis, pneumonia, and gastrointestinal disturbance.

Involvement of the CNS

In severe CHIKV disease there is multiorgan involvement, including the CNS. Neurological complications account for up to 25% of atypical cases and 60% of severe atypical cases, and are a significant cause of admission into the intensive care unit and death [12].

The most common CNS manifestations are encephalopathy and encephalitis. In the Indian Ocean Islands' outbreak, the CHIKV cumulative incidence of encephalitis was about 8.6 per 100 000 people, which is a twofold increase in the incidence of encephalitis in this area [13]. CHIKV encephalitis begins within two weeks of the onset of the infection, though postinfectious acute demyelinating encephalomyelitis and brainstem encephalitis have been reported. Clinical presentation varies widely and includes altered mental status, seizures, and focal neurological signs. Stimulus-sensitive myoclonus and cerebellar ataxia have also been reported [13].

Results of many investigations are often not abnormal in CHIKV encephalitis: CSF findings are nonspecific. Neuroimaging studies may be normal in up to 60% of cases, but abnormalities include edema and hemorrhage on computed tomography (CT) and diffusion restriction on magnetic resonance imaging (MRI). In one review, the mortality rate in patients with neurological involvement was 31.5%, 19.7% had neurological sequelae, and 48.8% had complete or near-complete recovery [14].

Other CHIKV-associated neurological disorders include acute myelopathy, myelitis, and Guillain-Barré syndrome (GBS).

In a review of CHIKV cases in India, 5% of patients had myelopathic involvement, which accounted for 27% of neurological cases [13]. Half the patients had a delayed-onset myelopathy, suggesting an immune-mediated postinfectious process. Several cases had concurrent encephalitis and encephalopathy. A recent case report details a patient traveling in the Dominican Republic who subsequently developed delayed onset of an intramedullary enhancing lesion and CSF lymphocytic pleocytosis. Serologic tests were positive for CHIKV, and the patients' symptoms improved with high-dose corticosteroids [15].

GBS is associated with arbovirus infections, including ZIKV. Increased incidence of GBS was reported during CHIKV outbreaks in French Polynesia and the Indian Ocean Islands. Some case series in Indian Ocean Islands also found elevated anti-CHIKV immunoglobulin M (IgM) in patients with GBS, further strengthening the link between CHIKV and GBS [16]. Of note, the majority of patients fully recovered, both in French Polynesia and in the Indian Ocean Islands.

Diagnosis

The diagnosis of CHIKV fever depends on laboratory tests because clinical manifestations of CHIKV are similar to, and overlap with, other viral fevers. The most important differential diagnosis is DENV, which can cause severe hemorrhagic disease. Cocirculation of DENV and CHIKV may complicate the diagnosis in a patient who is febrile. Patients infected with DENV have more thrombocytopenia and bleeding complications; patients infected with CHIKV have more arthralgia and arthritis. Unfortunately, it is difficult to distinguish DENV and CHIKV infection from each other and from other acute febrile illnesses. Both viruses must be included in the initial differential diagnosis for a patient with suspicious clinical symptoms who is living in, or returning from travel to, an endemic area. Early in the disease course, reverse transcription polymerase chain reaction (RT-PCR) can be used to differentiate DENV from CHIKV; later, serological assessment will help make a definite diagnosis.

Virus isolation is the gold standard diagnostic test; however, a result takes several days, and additionally, the virus can only be isolated in level-3 biosafety laboratories. The technique requires specific cell lines or infant mice exposed to whole-blood samples to identify CHIKV-specific responses. Test results are influenced by multiple factors, including adequate sample collection or cold chain maintenance during transport [17]. Early diagnosis can be obtained by detecting the virus's nucleic acid in blood using real-time PCR and reverse transcription loop-mediated isothermal amplification (RT-LAMP) methods [18, 19]. RT-LAMP has the advantage that it can be performed in a water bath and does not require any PCR instrument. Real-time PCR tests can be combined with the detection of other viruses, like DENV and ZIKV.

Serological diagnosis depends on demonstration of either serum IgM anti-CHIKV, or a fourfold increase of serum CHIKV immunoglobulin G (IgG) titer from the acute to the convalescent phase [20, 21]. To estimate CHIKV titers in blood, enzyme-linked immunosorbent assays (ELISAs) and immune chromatographic tests are usually more feasible tests for clinicians than PCR techniques. Cytokine or other biomarkers are heterogeneous and lack validation; however, cryoglobulinemia has been reported in some cases.

Pathology

Brain lesions have generally been described using MRI; very few macroscopic or histologic descriptions of human brains have been reported.

Macroscopic lesions include: edema, cerebellar hemorrhages, multifocal ischemia (cortex and internal capsule), and demyelination (subcortical white matter). Histological lesions are nonspecific. Perivascular lymphocytic infiltrates and gitter cells were detected in the basal ganglia, associated with rare microglial activation [22].

Experimental infections, carried out in *Cynomolgus* macaques, recently demonstrated that astrocytes could play a role in the disease pathogenesis [23].

Treatment and future perspectives

CHIKV fever is treated symptomatically, mainly with nonsteroidal anti-inflammatory drugs (NSAIDs) and corticosteroids. One study from South India demonstrated a beneficial outcome when NSAIDs and corticosteroids were combined to treat acute arthralgia and arthritis [24]; however, because of immunosuppressive effects, corticosteroids are relatively contraindicated in the acute viremic phase. Some patients who developed chronic rheumatic disease were successfully treated with methotrexate [25]. Chloroquine and arbidol were partly effective in vitro; however, in vivo studies were inconclusive [26].

Up to now, there is no licensed vaccine for CHIKV. A recent trial using a measles-virus–based CHIKV vaccine achieved 90% seroconversion, with an excellent safety profile [27]. Passive immunization tested in mouse models gave promising results, both for prophylaxis and treatment [28].

The recent CHIKV epidemic has demonstrated the virus's capacity to spread and infect large populations. Once herd immunity is achieved, CHIKV is seldom detected during the interepidemic period, which makes the development of a vaccine more difficult. Finally, avoiding mosquito bites and vector control are of paramount importance to limit the spread of CHIKV.

References

1. Paul, B.J. and Sadanand, S. (2018). Chikungunya infection: a re-emerging epidemic. *Rheumatol. Ther.* 5: 317–326.
2. Robinson, M.C. (1955). An epidemic of virus disease in Southern Province, Tanganyika Territory, in 1952–1953. I. Clinical features. *Trans. R. Soc. Trop. Med. Hyg.* 49: 28–32.
3. Chretien, J.P., Anyamba, A., Bedno, S.A. et al. (2007). Drought-associated chikungunya emergence along coastal East Africa. *Am. J. Trop. Med. Hyg.* 76: 405–407.
4. Weinbren, M.P. (1958). The occurrence of Chikungunya virus in Uganda. In man on the Entebbe peninsula. *Trans. R. Soc. Trop. Med. Hyg.* 52: 258–259.
5. Tsetsarkin, K.A., Chen, R., Yun, R. et al. (2014). Multi-peaked adaptive landscape for chikungunya virus evolution predicts continued fitness optimization in *Aedes albopictus* mosquitoes. *Nat. Commun.* 5: 4084.
6. Schuffenecker, I., Iteman, I., and Michault, A. (2006). Genome microevolution of chikungunya viruses causing the Indian Ocean outbreak. *PLoS Med.* 3: e263.
7. Mathew, A.J., Ganapati, A., Kabeerdoss, J. et al. (2017). Chikungunya infection: a global public health menace. *Curr Allergy Asthma Rep* 17: 13.
8. Tsetsarkin, K.A., Vanlandingham, D.L., McGee, C.E., and Higgs, S. (2007). A single mutation in chikungunya virus affects vector specificity and epidemic potential. *PLoS Pathog.* 3: e201.
9. Lounibos, L.P. and Kramer, L.D. (2016). Invasiveness of *Aedes aegypti* and *Aedes albopictus* and vectorial capacity for Chikungunya virus. *J. Infect. Dis.* 214 (Suppl 5): S453–S458.
10. Sourisseau, M., Schilte, C., Casartelli, N. et al. (2007). Characterization of reemerging chikungunya virus. *PLoS Pathog.* 3: e89.
11. Couderc, T., Chrétien, F., Schilte, C. et al. (2008). A mouse model for Chikungunya: young age and inefficient type-I interferon signaling are risk factors for severe disease. *PLoS Pathog.* 4: e29.
12. Economopoulou, A., Dominguez, M., Helynck, B. et al. (2009). Atypical Chikungunya virus infections: clinical manifestations, mortality and risk factors for severe disease during the 2005–2006 outbreak on Reunion. *Epidemiol. Infect.* 137: 534–541.
13. Chandak, N.H., Kashyap, R.S., Kabra, D. et al. (2009). Neurological complications of Chikungunya virus infection. *Neurol. India* 57: 177–180.
14. Mehta, R., Gerardin, P., de Brito, C.A.A. et al. (2018). The neurological complications of chikungunya virus: a systematic review. *Rev. Med. Virol.* 28: e1978.
15. Bank, A.M., Batra, A., Colorado, R.A., and Lyons, J.L. (2016). Myeloradiculopathy associated with chikungunya virus infection. *J. Neurovirol.* 22: 125–128.
16. Wielanek, A.C., Monredon, J.D., Amrani, M.E. et al. (2007). Guillain-Barré syndrome complicating a Chikungunya virus infection. *Neurology* 69: 2105–2107.
17. National Vector Borne Disease Control Programme. Chikungunya fever—national guidelines. http://nvbdcp.gov.in/Doc/National-Guidelines-Clinical-Management-Chikungunya-2016.pdf (accessed 27 November 2018).
18. Patel, P., Abd El Wahed, A., Faye, O. et al. (2016). A field-deployable reverse transcription recombinase polymerase amplification assay for rapid detection of the Chikungunya virus. *PLoS Negl. Trop. Dis.* 10: e0004953.
19. Parida, M.M., Santhosh, S.R., Dash, P.K. et al. (2007). Rapid and real-time detection of Chikungunya virus by reverse transcription loop-mediated isothermal amplification assay. *J. Clin. Microbiol.* 45: 351–357.
20. Staples, J.E., Breiman, R.F., and Powers, A.M. (2009). Chikungunya fever: an epidemiological review of a re-emerging infectious disease. *Clin. Infect. Dis.* 49: 942–948.
21. Prince, H.E., Seaton, B.L., Matud, J.L., and Batterman, H.J. (2015). Chikungunya virus RNA and antibody testing at a national reference laboratory since the

emergence of Chikungunya virus in the Americas. *Clin. Vaccine Immunol.* 22: 291–297.
22. Ganesan, K., Diwan, A., Shankar, S.K. et al. (2008). Chikungunya encephalomyeloradiculitis: report of 2 cases with neuroimaging and 1 case with autopsy findings. *AJNR Am. J. Neuroradiol.* 29: 1636–1637.
23. Inglis, F.M., Lee, K.M., Chiu, K.B. et al. (2016). Neuropathogenesis of Chikungunya infection: astrogliosis and innate immune activation. *J. Neurovirol.* 22: 140–148.
24. Padmakumar, B., Jayan, J.B., Menon, R.M.R. et al. (2009). Comparative evaluation of four therapeutic regimes in Chikungunya arthritis: a prospective randomized parallel-group study. *Indian J. Rheumatol.* 4: 94–101.
25. Hoarau, J.-J., Bandjee, M.-C.J., Trotot, P.K. et al. (2010). Persistent chronic inflammation and infection by Chikungunya arthritogenic alphavirus in spite of a robust host immune response. *J. Immunol.* 184: 5914–5927.
26. Gould, E.A., Coutard, B., Malet, H. et al. (2010). Understanding the alphaviruses: recent research on important emerging pathogens and progress towards their control. *Antivir. Res.* 87: 111–124.
27. Ramsauer, K., Schwameis, M., Firbas, C. et al. (2015). Immunogenicity, safety, and tolerability of a recombinant measles-virus-based chikungunya vaccine: a randomised, double-blind, placebo-controlled, active-comparator, first-in-man trial. *Lancet Infect. Dis.* 15: 519–527.
28. Couderc, T., Khandoudi, N., Grandadam, M. et al. (2009). Prophylaxis and therapy for Chikungunya virus infection. *J. Infect. Dis.* 200: 516–523.

21 Poliovirus Infection and Postpolio Syndrome

Catherine (Katy) Keohane[1], Leila Chimelli[2,3], and Aisling Ryan[4]

[1] Department of Pathology and School of Medicine, University College Cork, Brookfield Health Science Complex, Cork, Ireland
[2] Laboratory of Neuropathology and Molecular Genetics, State Brain Institute Paulo Niemeyer, Rio de Janeiro, Brazil
[3] Federal University of Rio de Janeiro (UFRJ), Rio de Janeiro, Brazil
[4] Department of Neurology, Cork University Hospital, Cork, Ireland

Abbreviations

CSF	cerebrospinal fluid
CDC	Centers for Disease Control and Prevention
EMG	electromyography
FcγR	receptors for the Fc part of IgG
GPEI	Global Polio Eradication Initiative
GIT	gastrointestinal tract
IFN	interferon
JNK	c-Jun NH2-terminal kinase
MRI	magnetic resonance Imaging
MUNE	Motor unit number estimation
PBA	poliovirus-binding associated
PPS	postpolio syndrome
PTPase	protein tyrosine phosphatase
PVR	poliovirus receptor
VDPV	vaccine-derived poliovirus
WPV	wild Poliovirus

Poliomyelitis and polioencephalitis virus infection

Definition of the disorder, major synonyms, and historical perspective

Poliomyelitis is defined as inflammation of the gray matter of the spinal cord, and polioencephalitis is its equivalent in the gray matter of the brain. They are commonly the result of infection by an enterovirus of the Picornaviridae family. Enteroviruses comprise poliovirus (PV) and nonpolio viruses (i.e. Group A and B Coxsackie virus, Echo virus, and enterovirus). The word "polio" comes from the Greek *polios* meaning "gray;" "myelitis" is derived from *muelos* meaning "marrow" and "itis" meaning "inflammation." Encephalitis refers to inflammation of the brain, from the Greek *encephalon*. Poliomyelitis was also known as "infantile paralysis" reflecting its prominence in young children.

Infections of the Central Nervous System: Pathology and Genetics, First Edition. Edited by Fabrice Chrétien, Kum Thong Wong, Leroy R. Sharer, Catherine (Katy) Keohane and Françoise Gray.
© 2020 John Wiley & Sons Ltd. Published 2020 by John Wiley & Sons Ltd.

PV has a predilection for motor neurons, hence the ensuing paralysis.

Images of humans from ancient times are believed to represent the effects of polio, but the first clinical description is ascribed to an English physician, Michael Underwood, in 1789. He wrote on "debility of the lower extremities" in children. A detailed description was given by Ivar Wickman in 1907 and 1911 [1], following an outbreak of 1031 cases in Scandinavia. Paralytic polio was recognized as nonbacterial and transmissible in 1908 by Karl Landsteiner and Erwin Popper. They suspected a viral cause when the infection was successfully transmitted to monkeys, by inoculation of spinal cord extract from a child who died of rapidly progressive paralysis [2]. Subsequent collaboration with Levanditi in the Pasteur Institute in Paris resulted in passage of the agent [3]. The importance of the gastrointestinal tract (GIT) in the natural history of human poliomyelitis was described by others, especially Albert Sabin and Robert Ward in 1941 [4]. For review of early milestones in PV research see [5].

The first US outbreak was in 1894 in Vermont but more than 9000 cases occurred in New York in 1916, causing 2343 deaths. Epidemics of polio have occurred worldwide, mostly in the summer months. In 1948 PV was grown in cells by Thomas Weller and Frederick Robbins. A successful injectable vaccine using killed virus was developed in 1952 by Jonas Salk, and in 1961 the oral live attenuated vaccine was developed by Albert Sabin. In the developed world, vaccination programs in children resulted in a huge reduction in cases. The Global Polio Eradication Initiative (GPEI) began in 1988. By the end of 2016 wild poliovirus (WPV) was eliminated from all but a few countries (i.e. Afghanistan, Nigeria, and Pakistan). It is estimated that the GPEI has saved more than 16 million people from paralysis.

Microbiology and genetics

The enteroviruses are nonenveloped icosahedral single-stranded positive sense RNA viruses in humans and mammals; disease is transmitted via fecal or oral contamination or respiratory secretions. Enteroviruses are approximately 30 nm in size, and their single-strand RNA is surrounded by a protein capsid with four virion proteins, VP1, VP2, VP3, VP4. The major capsid protein VP1 has approximately 900 nucleotides. Enteroviruses comprise PVs (of which there are three serotypes of WPV type 1, type 2, and type 3, each with a slightly different capsid protein) and non-polioviruses (i.e. Group A Coxsackieviruses, of which there are 31 serotypes; Group B Coxsackie viruses, 6 serotypes; Echo viruses, 28 serotypes; and 5 unclassified enteroviruses). Parechovirus is a more recently described related genus, to which some echoviruses have been reassigned (see Chapter 25). CD155 is the cell receptor for all three serotypes of PV; all can cause paralysis [6]. Immunity to one PV serotype does not give immunity to the other two.

WPV Type 2 has been eradicated, and the last case of type 3 was in 2012. Type 1 persists and causes infection in a small number of countries. WPV is defined as having no evidence of derivation from any vaccine strain, and a demonstrated capability of person-to-person transmission. Because live attenuated virus was used in vaccines, genetic alterations in the vaccine strain can rarely result in paralytic polio. Three types of vaccine-derived poliovirus (VDPV) are recognized, (i) circulating vaccine-derived poliovirus (cVDP) particularly when oral poliovaccine programs are incomplete; (ii) immunodeficiency-related vaccine-derived poliovirus (iVDPV); and (iii) ambiguous vaccine-derived poliovirus (aVDP), in which it is not possible to determine if the virus is either cVDPV or iVDPV. VDVPs have atypical genetic properties indicative of prolonged virus circulation or replication.

Epidemiology

Polio is usually acquired by fecal-oral contamination mainly from contaminated water, and outbreaks occur in conditions of overcrowding and poor sanitation. Cases decreased by more than 99% since 1988, from an estimated 350 000 cases to 37 reported cases in 2016 as a result of the success of the GPEI. This initiative was supported by national governments, the World Health Organization (WHO), Rotary International, the US Centers for Disease Control and Prevention (CDC), UNICEF, and key partners including the Bill & Melinda Gates Foundation. Noori et al.

correlated country-specific annual disease incidence with demographic, socioeconomic, and environmental factors and found that urban population density, access to improved sanitation facilities, and percentage of forest cover were the three most important variables [7]. WPV now occurs in very few countries, but can re-emerge with mass movement of people, such as in war-torn regions. Rare VDPV outbreaks occur when the live attenuated strain of virus in a vaccine genetically mutates and becomes neurovirulent. In undervaccinated communities VDVP can circulate, further mutate, and cause outbreaks. cVDPV cases occurred in 2017 in Syria and in the Democratic Republic of the Congo and in 2018 in Syria, Somalia, and Nigeria [8]. The WHO recommends that inactivated oral vaccine be used in countries where WPV has been eradicated. In some countries, such as Japan, cVDPV continued to occur up to the introduction of inactivated poliovirus vaccine in 2012 [9]. Poliomyelitis, encephalitis, and transverse myelitis can rarely be the result of non-polio enteroviruses, especially enteroviruses D68, D70, and A71 (see Chapter 22).

Clinical features, diagnosis, cerebrospinal fluid, and differentials
Clinical features

Clinical infections are categorized as abortive, nonparalytic, and paralytic. Most infections are in children; the majority are asymptomatic or have mild symptoms (i.e. abortive polio), but the virus is shed in the stool. Fever, pharyngitis, anorexia, nausea, vomiting, and malaise are the main symptoms related to viremia, with headache, neck stiffness, and Kernig's sign in those who develop aseptic meningitis (up to 5% of cases). The majority of patients recover (nonparalytic polio). The incubation period for paralytic polio is usually 7–21 days, but can be up to five weeks. In 1% of polio infections, flaccid paralysis develops within 18 days of the prodromal illness, often preceded by limb or back muscle pain. Weakness or paralysis involves the lower more than the upper limbs and is asymmetric. Deep tendon reflexes are lost, followed by atrophy of muscle within three weeks. Fasciculations can also be seen. With encephalitis, fever, headache, vomiting, and irritability are often present. Bulbar involvement occurs in 10–15% of such cases, with paralysis of the tongue and swallowing difficulty. If the brainstem reticular formation is affected, apnea and cardiac arrythmias occur. Respiratory muscle weakness necessitates ventilatory support, in the past using the "iron lung." External oculomotor weakness with sparing of the pupil is uncommon. Autonomic signs may occur, and some adults in particular may develop urinary retention that recovers. Sensation remains intact.

Laboratory investigations

Electromyography (EMG) shows features of acute motor axonal damage, with initial reduction in recruitment followed by reduced interference. Fibrillations and fasciculations develop later. Motor unit action potentials are reduced but following reinnervation, polyphasic motor units are present. Compound muscle action potential is reduced.

Magnetic resonance imaging (MRI) shows hyperintense T2 signal in anterior horns and, if involved, other areas including the brainstem [10], which may show enhancement post gadolinium [11, 12].

Diagnosis

In suspected cases, PV may be isolated from throat or pharyngeal swabs, fecal specimens, or blood. Fecal specimens are the most useful in the first two weeks of infection. The virus is shed at detectable levels for at least seven weeks post-oral polio vaccine [13]. Isolation from cerebrospinal fluid (CSF) or blood is less successful. WPV and VDPV are distinguished by real-time reverse transcription-polymerase chain reaction (RT-PCR). Paired sera taken three weeks apart can be tested for a fourfold rise in neutralizing antibodies in acute illness. The modified PV microneutralization assay, PV capture immunoglobulin M (IgM) and immunoglobulin A (IgA) enzyme-linked immunosorbent assays (ELISAs), and dried blood spot polio serology procedures for the detection of antibodies against PV serotypes 1, 2, and 3 can also be used in population surveillance to test immunity [14]. CSF examination shows a leukocytosis, initially mixed polymorphonuclear or lymphocytic but later mainly lymphocytes (10–100/mm^3), and increased protein

(40–50 mg/Dl). Higher protein levels are associated with more severe disease.

The main differential diagnoses are other virus infections (e.g. enterovirus and West Nile virus), botulism, tetanus, and Guillain-Barré syndrome.

Pathology histopathology, electron microscopy, and immunocytochemistry

Fatal cases in the acute phase show softening and brownish discoloration of the anterior horns of the spinal cord (Figure 21.1), microscopic vascular changes of congestion and edema (Figure 21.2a), lymphocytic inflammation, and degeneration of anterior horn cells (Figure 21.2 b and c), varying from chromatolysis to complete neurophagocytosis [15]. Perivascular lymphocytic inflammation, described as "a cellular collar following the vessels" (perivascular cuffing) sometimes extends to the meninges and is most marked in the spinal anterior horns (Figure 21.3a and b). In a vaccinated child with immunodeficiency who died five weeks post onset, asymmetric cystic areas of necrosis in the substantia nigra, reticular formation. and anterior horns were found, containing macrophages and surrounded by residual inflammatory cells [12]. Microglial clusters at sites of neuronal destruction are described in cases surviving weeks after inflammation has subsided. In the chronic phases, loss of anterior horn cells, thin atrophied anterior roots, and group atrophy of denervated affected muscles is evident (Figure 21.4). Immunocytochemistry and electron microscopy (EM) are not usually used in human studies. EM of in vitro studies of the cycle of viral replication in PV-infected Hela cells showed large ribosomal aggregates and accumulation of dense aggregates, designated viroplasm, in the cytoplasmic matrix, with numerous progeny particles seen as large virus crystals, and masses of small, membrane-enclosed bodies [16].

Genetics

Although PV infection requires exposure to the virus, not all those exposed become ill or develop paralysis. The increased incidence of PV infection in siblings and blood relatives of cases has long

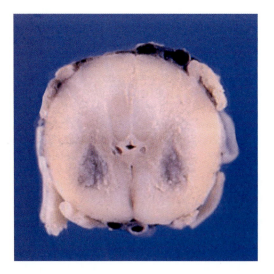

Figure 21.1 Transverse section of the spinal cord, which is swollen and shows brownish discoloration of the anterior horns. Source: (Courtesy of Prof. JEH Pittella, Brazil).

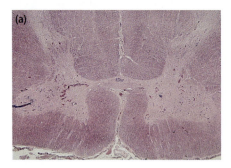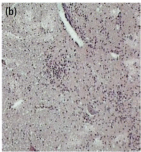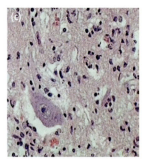

Figure 21.2 Lesions of the anterior horns of the spinal cord. (a) Transverse section of the spinal cord showing loose neuropil in the anterior horns as a result of edema and nerve cell loss. (b) Marked lymphocytic inflammation and neuronophagia in the anterior horn in fatal acute poliomyelitis. (c) High power showing a remaining viable anterior horn cell with adjacent neuronophagia.

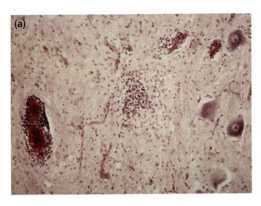
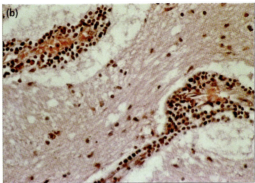

Figure 21.3 Perivascular lymphocytic inflammation. (a) Lymphocytes around vessels (lower left) in spinal anterior horn. Neuronophagia and chromatolysis of motor neurons is also visible. (b) Dense perivascular "cuffing" by lymphocytes and marked edema of spinal cord neuropil.

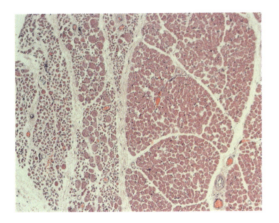

Figure 21.4 Groups of atrophic muscle fibers (denervation) as a result of motor nerve cell loss.

been known, but it is difficult to ascribe this to specific genetic or environmental exposure factors. A twin and triplet study of 46 families found statistically significant twin-pair concordance in more than 35.7% of monozygotic pairs, compared with 6.6% of dizygotic pairs [17]. A mutation in the polymorphism Ala67Thr, in the poliovirus receptor (PVR) CD155 was found in a higher percentage of patients with polio and regarded as a risk factor for both WPV and vaccine-associated polio [18]. This may also account for the differences in susceptibility among different races. Genetic investigations in simians (the only species susceptible to PV), suggested that amino-acid substitutions at the PV-binding associated (PBA) sites in the D1 domain of PVR CD155, occurring in evolution, influenced this susceptibility, possibly via another binding molecule [19]. Regarding mutations in PV strains, the genetic evolutionary relationships of PV isolate sequences are mainly determined by the VP1 protein, and PV strains located on the same branch of the phylogenetic tree contain the same mutation spots and mutation types [20]. For a review of genetic aspects see [21].

Pathogenesis

Following infection mainly via fecal-oral contamination, PV replicates in GIT lymphoid tissue, and enters the bloodstream, causing a minor viremia, followed by a second more severe viremia coinciding with increased viral replication. Virus can disseminate to the brain in both minor and more severe viremias and attaches to PVR present on neurons. Experimentally, PV enters the human brain vascular endothelial cells by a caveolin-dependent endocytosis, and specific PVR-mediated signals, including activation of a protein tyrosine phosphatase (PTPase), SHP-2, are essential for virus entry and infection [22]. Retrograde axonal transport, including from muscle motor end plates that express PVR [23], may be another entry mechanism. This has been suggested to explain "provocation poliomyelitis," which follows muscle trauma during PV infection. Viral uncoating and replication occurs in the cell body, preferentially within lower motor neurons. Strain-specific neurovirulence appears to depend on the ability to replicate in the CNS, rather than the entry route (hematogenous or axonal) [24]. A second infection with progeny virus appears necessary for neural cells to exhibit cytopathic changes, which can be blocked by anti-PV serum or monoclonal antibodies to PV and PVR [24]. Additionally, alpha and beta interferon (IFN) may be important in determining PV tropism for CNS neurons [25]. Relatively little is known of the exact mechanisms of the tissue response in humans to PV-induced neuronal cell degeneration and necrosis. In IMR5 neuroblastoma cells, c-Jun NH2-terminal kinase (JNK) is activated soon after PV infection and then triggers activation of Bax (i.e. the proapoptotic protein belonging to the Bcl family), which causes cytochrome c release from mitochondria and results in cell death [26]. PV infection can increase cytosolic calcium concentrations in IMR5 cells, which may also be related to PV-induced apoptosis [26].

Animal models

Oral infection by PV is restricted to humans and some primates and appears to relate largely but not entirely to PVR expression. Monkeys were originally used to study neurovirulence, but CD155-transgenic mouse models have more recently been used to study the role of productive PV infection in the GIT [27] and the brain [28] and to study the pathogenesis of, and immune responses to, various neurovirulence strains [29].

Treatment, future perspective, and conclusions

There is no effective specific antiviral treatment for PV infection, so prevention by vaccination and improved sanitation is the major focus of disease control, along with measures to control spread during outbreaks. Ventilatory supportive treatment and physiotherapy are used when required for the acute illness and for rehabilitation.

The goal of total global eradication should be achievable but depends on elimination of both WPV and VDPV and cooperation from all countries. This would mean that poliovirus should become a historic disease.

Postpolio syndrome

Definition and historical perspective

Decades following acute PV infection and stable disability, many patients develop progressive muscle weakens, with pain, fatigue, and bulbar and respiratory dysfunction known as the postpolio syndrome (PPS). First recognized in 1875 by Raymond and Charcot in France, PPS became accepted as a disease entity in the 1980s [30].

Epidemiology

The prevalence of PPS has been estimated at 15–80% of survivors of polio infection. The variance can be partly explained by including different study populations (i.e. patients with paralytic and nonparalytic polio) and applying differing diagnostic criteria. In a prospective, population-based study of 50 cases of paralytic polio in Minnesota, 60% reported new symptoms of pain, weakness, and fatigue decades later [31]. Studies from Denmark and Italy have reported prevalence figures of 63 and 42%, respectively [32, 33]. A population-based study in Pennsylvania (United States) found the prevalence of PPS was 28.5% of 40 paralytic cases, and the risk was higher in women and those with permanent impairment after the primary infection [34]. PPS incidence did not vary with age at acute onset, severity, or level of physical activity following recovery. With 15–20 million survivors of polio worldwide, PPS represents a significant global burden of illness impacting on healthcare provision and society.

Clinical diagnosis

PPS is a clinical diagnosis based on established criteria and exclusion of other diagnoses. The modern diagnostic criteria for PPS were established in 2000 by expert consensus at the March of Dimes international conference as follows:

1. Prior paralytic poliomyelitis with evidence of motor neuron loss, confirmed by history of the acute paralytic illness, signs of residual weakness, atrophy of muscles on neurological examination, and signs of denervation on EMG.
2. A period of partial or complete functional recovery after acute paralytic poliomyelitis,

followed by an interval (usually 15 years or more) of stable neurologic function.

3. Gradual or sudden onset of progressive and persistent muscle weakness or abnormal muscle fatigability (i.e. decreased endurance), with or without generalized fatigue, muscle atrophy, or muscle and joint pain. (Sudden onset may follow a period of inactivity, trauma, or surgery.) Less commonly, symptoms attributed to PPS include new problems with breathing or swallowing.

4. Symptoms persist for at least one year.

5. Exclusion of other neurologic, medical, and orthopedic problems as causes of symptoms.

New muscle weakness is a key feature, with or without additional pain, fatigue, or cold intolerance. This can involve previously affected or apparently clinically unaffected muscles. Focal atrophy or fasciculations may be observed. Even minor changes in muscle strength can cause significant disability because these patients have adapted to their existing deficit over many years.

Fatigue is an early disabling symptom for most patients with PPS. Generalized muscle weakness, decreased exercise tolerance, pain, sleep disturbance, and psychological factors may all be contributory.

New onset bulbar dysfunction has potential serious complications. It is most frequent and severe in those clinically affected during the acute illness but may occur independent of prior bulbar involvement. Clinical and subclinical bulbar dysfunction was detected in the majority of cases of PPS with dysphagia, mirroring the progressive deterioration of neurons innervating limb muscles [35].

Respiratory function compromise is largely the result of new respiratory muscle weakness. Worsening scoliosis, central hypoventilation due to medullary involvement, and sleep apnea may also contribute [36].

Paraclinical investigations can exclude other causes of fatigue. Serum CK may be normal or moderately elevated. Imaging with MRI may be required to exclude spinal stenosis.

EMG demonstrating ongoing denervation and reinnervation helps confirm evidence of prior poliomyelitis and exclude compressive neuropathies or radiculopathy. Importantly, EMG cannot accurately distinguish prior polio infection from PPS [37]. In the research setting, macro-EMG and motor unit number estimation (MUNE) may provide detailed evaluation of motor unit dysfunction over time [38].

Muscle biopsy is not required for diagnosis unless alternative pathology is suspected. The histopathological correlates of denervation and reinnervation including fiber type grouping, nuclear bag fibers, and small angulated fibers are seen in both PPS and stable patients after polio infection.

Pathogenesis

Why some survivors of polio develop PPS, but others do not is unknown. The most favored explanation is the Wiechers-Hubble hypothesis [39] of stress-induced degeneration of enlarged motor units. Neurons affected during the acute illness may be destroyed or recover incompletely. Terminal axons of the latter sprout in an attempt to reinnervate adjacent muscle fibers. A single motor unit can increase its number of innervated muscle fibers by approximately five times. This improves muscle strength but provides additional stress and metabolic demands on the cell. Ongoing active denervation and reinnervation in affected muscles leads to uncompensated denervation and gradual decline in muscle strength. Increased metabolic demands on an already stressed neuron, aging, or a combination of factors may all contribute to decompensation.

Another theory centers on reactivation of latent PV leading to further motor neuron loss. PV-specific genomic sequences were detected in 5 of 10 patients with PPS but not in controls [40, 41]. Another study examining serum, CSF, and muscle biopsies detected no evidence of PV RNA or a PV type-specific IgM response [42].

An inflammatory etiology was suggested by the observation of inflammatory cells in the spinal cords of survivors of poliomyelitis [43]. Oligoclonal IgM bands specific to PV were detected in CSF of 58% of patients with PPS but not in controls, supporting an intrathecal immune response [44]. A systemic inflammatory process is also postulated, with elevated levels of plasma tumor necrosis factor alpha (TNF-α), interleukin (IL)-6, IL-8, and leptin in patients with PPS [45] and increased CSF levels of proinflammatory cytokines (i.e. TNF-α,

IFN-γ, IL-4, and IL-10) [46]. The significance of these findings is uncertain.

Because of the already vulnerable enlarged motor units, there is a greater effect of normal biological aging in patients with PPS, leading to a decline in the number of motor units, muscle mass, and strength [47]. Interval following acute PV is a risk factor for the onset of PPS, with incidence peaking after 30–40 years [34].

Genetics

Antibody-mediated responses to infection are regulated through receptors for the Fc part of IgG (FcγR). Polymorphisms of the FcγR were investigated to determine susceptibility to, and course of, acute poliomyelitis, and development of PPS [48]. The FcγRIIIA V/V genotype occurred at a significantly lower frequency among patients with a history of acute poliomyelitis (5.4%) than among controls (15.1%), possibly related to microglial expression. No correlation was found for the FcγRIIIA V/F and F/F or the FcγRIIA and FcγRIIIB genotypes. There was insufficient evidence to support a pathogenetic role for IgG-FcγR polymorphisms in the development of PPS, but further studies may be of interest. A polymorphism Ala67Thr in the PVR gene was reported as a possible risk factor for development of PPS, although the mechanism is unknown [49].

Treatment

The mainstay of treatment is coordinated multidisciplinary rehabilitation with a tailored program of physiotherapy and nonfatiguing, strengthening exercises and avoidance of overuse [50].

Many pharmacological therapies failed to show significant benefit. Larger clinical trials are needed to test the role of IVIg in PPS in reducing CSF pro-inflammatory cytokines.

Respiratory dysfunction is managed by overnight oximetry; if ventilatory assistance is required, noninvasive bilevel positive airway pressure ventilation can help prevent respiratory tract infections and avoid the need for invasive mechanical ventilation.

Equipment to improve mobility, prevention of falls, management of osteoporosis to minimize fracture risk, and lifestyle modifications to conserve energy, manage weight, and cease smoking are all recommended.

Prognosis and future perspective

The natural history of PPS is that of slow gradual progression, possibly partly attributable to sarcopenia, normal aging, and increased loss of motor units. Functional impairment requires active management by the rehabilitation team. Long periods of stability are not uncommon. Identifying genetic or other risk factors together with therapeutic advances and tailored rehabilitation may improve quality of life for patients with PPS.

References

1. Wickman, I. (1911). *Die akute Poliomyelitis bzw. Heine-Medinsche Krankheit*. Berlin, Germany: Julius Springer.
2. Landsteiner, K. and Popper, E. (1909). Uebertragung der Poliomyelitis acuta auf Affen. *Z. Immunitätsforsch* 2: 377–390.
3. Landsteiner, K. and Levaditi, C. (1909). La paralysie infantile experimentale. *Compt. Rend. Soc. Biol.* 67: 787–789.
4. Sabin, A.B. and Ward, R. (1941). The natural history of human poliomyelitis. I. Distribution of virus in nervous and non-nervous tissues. *J. Exp. Med.* 73: 771–793.
5. Eggers, H.J. (1999). Milestones in early poliomyelitis research (1840 to 1949). *J. Virol.* 73: 4533–4535.
6. Racaniello, V.R. (2006). One hundred years of poliovirus pathogenesis. *Virology* 344: 9–16.
7. Noori, N., Drake, J.M., and Rohani, P. (2017). Comparative epidemiology of poliovirus transmission. *Sci. Rep.* 7: 17362. https://doi.org/10.1038/s41598-017-17749-5.
8. Polio Global Eradication Initiative (PGEI) (2018). Polio today. http://polioeradication.org (accessed 21 June 2018).
9. Shimizu, H. (2016). Development and introduction of inactivated poliovirus vaccines derived from Sabin strains in Japan. *Vaccine* 34: 1975–1985.
10. Choudhary, A., Sharma, S., Sankhyan, N. et al. (2010). Midbrain and spinal cord magnetic resonance imaging (MRI) changes in poliomyelitis. *J. Child Neurol.* 25: 497–449.
11. Kornreich, L., Dagan, O., and Grunebaum, M. (1996). MRI in acute poliomyelitis. *Neuroradiology* 38: 371–372.

12. Wasserstrom, R., Mamourian, A.C., McGary, C.T. et al. (1992). Bulbar poliomyelitis: MR findings with pathologic correlation. *Am. J. Neuroradiol.* 13: 371–373.
13. Mas Lago, P., Gary, H.E. Jr., Pérez, L.S. et al. (2003). Poliovirus detection in wastewater and stools following an immunization campaign in Havana, Cuba. *Int. J. Epidemiol.* 32: 772–777.
14. Weldon, W.C., Oberste, M.S., and Pallansch, M.A. (2016). Standardized methods for detection of poliovirus antibodies. *Methods Mol. Biol.* 1387: 145–176.
15. Erb, I.H. (1931). Pathology of poliomyelitis. *Can. Med. Assoc. J.* 25: 547–555.
16. Dales, S., Eggers, H., Tamm, I. et al. (1965). Electron microscopic study of the formation of poliovirus. *Virology* 26: 379–389.
17. Herndon, C.N. and Jennings, R.G. (1951). A twin-family study of susceptibility to poliomyelitis. *Am. J. Hum. Genet.* 3: 17–46.
18. Kindberg, E., Ac, C., Fiore, L. et al. (2009). Ala67Thr mutation in the poliovirus receptor CD155 is a potential risk factor for vaccine and wild-type paralytic poliomyelitis. *J. Med. Virol.* 81: 933–936.
19. Suzuki, Y. (2006). Ancient positive selection on CD155 as a possible cause for susceptibility to poliovirus infection in simians. *Gene* 373: 16–22.
20. Liu, Y., Ma, T., Liu, J. et al. (2014). Bioinformatics analysis and genetic diversity of the poliovirus. *J. Med. Microbiol.* 63: 1724–1731.
21. Wyatt, H.V. (2014). Genetic susceptibility: a forgotten aspect of poliomyelitis. *J. Mol. Genet. Med.* 8: 131.
22. Coyne, C.B., Kim, K.S., Jeffrey, M., and Bergelson, J.M. (2007). Poliovirus entry into human brain microvascular cells requires receptor-induced activation of SHP-2. *EMBO J.* 26: 4016–4028.
23. Leon-Monzon, M.E., Illa, I., and Dalakas, M.C. (1995). Expression of poliovirus receptor in human spinal cord and muscle. *Ann. N. Y. Acad. Sci.* 753: 48–57.
24. Nomoto, A. (2007). Molecular aspects of poliovirus pathogenesis. *Proc. Jpn. Acad Ser. B Phys. Biol. Sci.* 83: 266–275.
25. Ida-Hosonuma, M., Iwasaki, T., Yoshikawa, T. et al. (2005). The alpha/beta interferon response controls tissue tropism and pathogenicity of poliovirus. *J. Virol.* 79: 4460–4469.
26. Huang, H.-I. and Shih, S.-R. (2015). Review: neurotropic enterovirus infections in the central nervous system. *Viruses* 7: 6051–6066.
27. Iwasaki, A., Welker, R., Mueller, S. et al. (2002). Immunofluorescence analysis of poliovirus receptor expression in Peyer's patches of humans, primates, and CD155 transgenic mice: implications for poliovirus infection. *J. Infect. Dis.* 186: 585–592.
28. Ren, R. and Racaniello, V.R. (1992). Human poliovirus receptor gene expression and poliovirus tissue tropism in transgenic mice. *J. Virol.* 66: 296–304.
29. Koike, S. and Nagata, N. (2016). A transgenic mouse model of poliomyelitis. *Methods Mol. Biol.* 1387: 129–144.
30. Halstead, L.S. and Rossi, C.D. (1985). New problems in old polio patients: results of a survey of 539 polio survivors. *Orthopedics* 8: 845–850.
31. Windebank, A.J., Litchy, W.J., and Daube, J.R. (1995). Prospective cohort study of polio survivors in Olmsted County, Minnesota. *Ann. N. Y. Acad. Sci.* 753: 81–86.
32. Lønnberg, F. (1993). Late onset polio sequelae in Denmark. Results of a nationwide survey of 3,607 polio survivors. *Scand. J. Rehabil. Med. Suppl.* 28: 1–32.
33. Bertolasi, L., Danese, A., Monaco, S. et al. (2016). Polio patients in northern Italy, a 50 year follow-up. *Open Neurol. J.* 10: 77–82.
34. Ramlow, J., Alexander, M., LaPorte, R. et al. (1992). Epidemiology of the post-polio syndrome. *Am. J. Epidemiol.* 136: 769–786.
35. Sonies, B.C. and Dalakas, M.C. (1991). Dysphagia in patients with the post-polio syndrome. *N. Engl. J. Med.* 324: 1162–1167.
36. Bach, J.R. and Tilton, M. (1997). Pulmonary dysfunction and its management in post-polio patients. *NeuroRehabilitation* 8: 139–153.
37. Cashman, N.R., Maselli, R., Wollmann, R.L. et al. (1987). Late denervation in patients with antecedent paralytic poliomyelitis. *N. Engl. J. Med.* 317: 7–12.
38. Sorenson, E.J., Daube, J.R., and Windebank, A.J. (2006). Motor unit number estimates correlate with strength in polio survivors. *Muscle Nerve* 34: 608–613.
39. Wiechers, D.O. and Hubbell, S.L. (1981). Late changes in the motor unit after acute poliomyelitis. *Muscle Nerve* 4: 524–528.
40. Leparc-Goffart, I., Julien, J., Fuchs, F. et al. (1996). Evidence of presence of poliovirus genomic sequences in cerebrospinal fluid from patients with postpolio syndrome. *J. Clin. Microbiol.* 34: 2023–2026.
41. Julien, J., Leparc-Goffart, I., Lina, B. et al. (1999). Postpolio syndrome: poliovirus persistence is involved in the pathogenesis. *J. Neurol.* 246: 472–476.
42. Melchers, W., de Visser, M., Jongen, P. et al. (1992). The postpolio syndrome: no evidence for poliovirus persistence. *Ann. Neurol.* 32: 728–732.

43. Pexeshkpour, G.H. and Dalakas, M.C. (1988). Long-term changes in the spinal cord of patients with old poliomyelitis: signs of continuous disease activity. *Arch. Neurol.* 45: 505–508.
44. Sharief, M.K., Hentges, R., and Ciardi, M. (1991). Intrathecal immune response in patients with the post-polio syndrome. *N. Engl. J. Med.* 325: 749–755.
45. Bickerstaffe, A., Beelen, A., Lutter, R., and Nollet, F. (2015). Elevated plasma inflammatory mediators in post-polio syndrome: no association with long-term functional decline. *J. Neuroimmunol.* 289: 162–167.
46. Gonzalez, H., Khademi, M., Andersson, M. et al. (2002). Prior poliomyelitis-evidence of cytokine production in the central nervous system. *J. Neurol. Sci.* 205 (1): 9–13.
47. Fielding, R.A., Vellas, B., Evans, W.J. et al. (2011). Sarcopenia: an undiagnosed condition in older adults. Current consensus definition: prevalence, etiology, and consequences. International working group on sarcopenia. *J. Am. Med. Dir. Assoc.* 12: 249–256.
48. Rekand, T., Langeland, N., Aarli, J.A., and Vedeler, C.A. (2002). Fcgamma receptor IIIA polymorphism as a risk factor for acute poliomyelitis. *J. Infect. Dis.* 186: 1840–1843.
49. Bhattacharya, S., Sarkar, A., and Sengupta, S. (2014). Ala67Thr mutation in the human polio virus receptor (PVR) gene in post-polio syndrome patients. *J. Microb. Biochem. Technol.* 6: 4.
50. Farbu, E., Gilhus, N.E., Barnes, M.P. et al. (2006). EFNS guideline on diagnosis and management of post-polio syndrome. Report of an EFNS task force. *Eur. J. Neurol.* 13: 795–801.

22 Enterovirus A71 Infection

Kum Thong Wong[1,*], Kien Chai Ong[2,*], Thérèse Couderc[3,4], and Marc Lecuit[3,4,5,6]

[1] Department of Pathology, Faculty of Medicine, University of Malaya, Kuala Lumpur, Malaysia
[2] Department of Biomedical Science, Faculty of Medicine, University of Malaya, Kuala Lumpur, Malaysia
[3] Biology of Infection Unit, Pasteur Institute, Paris, France
[4] Inserm U1117, Paris, France
[5] Department of Infectious Diseases and Tropical Medicine, Necker-Sick Children University Hospital and Imagine Institute, APHP, Paris, France
[6] Paris University, Paris, France

Abbreviations

AFP	acute flaccid paralysis
CNS	central nervous system
CSF	cerebrospinal fluid
EV-A71	enterovirus A71
HFMD	hand-foot-mouth disease
IVIG	intravenous immune globulin
MRI	magnetic resonance imaging
RNA	ribonucleic acid
SCARB2	scavenger receptor class B member 2

Definition of disorder, major synonyms, and historical perspective

Enterovirus A71 (EV-A71) is a major cause of hand-foot-and-mouth disease (HFMD) in young children, which is characterized by self-limiting fever, skin rashes and vesicles, mainly in the extremities and oral cavity. Rarely, less than 0.01% of EV-A71 infections (the true incidence remains unknown) may be complicated by aseptic meningitis, acute flaccid paralysis (AFP), and encephalomyelitis [1]. AFP is similar to poliomyelitis, and the more serious and often fatal EV-A71 encephalomyelitis has similar features to the bulbar or encephalitic forms of poliovirus (PV) infection (See Chapter 21).

First isolated from the feces of an infant with fatal encephalitis in the United States in 1969 [2], HFMD outbreaks with serious neurological complications have since been reported in Europe, Australia, and United States, but the largest outbreaks have so far occurred in Asia [3].

Microbiological characteristics

EV-A71 belongs to a large group of enteroviruses that includes PV, coxsackievirus A and B, echovirus, and numerous other enteroviruses. Although serotypes had traditionally been classified by antibody neutralizing tests, the classification of the

*These authors contributed equally.

Infections of the Central Nervous System: Pathology and Genetics, First Edition. Edited by Fabrice Chrétien, Kum Thong Wong, Leroy R. Sharer, Catherine (Katy) Keohane and Françoise Gray.
© 2020 John Wiley & Sons Ltd. Published 2020 by John Wiley & Sons Ltd.

genus *Enterovirus* (family Picornaviridae) has recently been further refined using genomic sequences. Within the genus there are nine species groups (A to H and J), each group comprising a varying number of serotypes [4]. EV-A71 as a serotype is in the species group A (formerly called human enterovirus A), together with some coxsackievirus A viruses, including coxsackievirus A16 (CV-A16). Species group C consists of the three PV and other enteroviral serotypes. The nomenclature "Enterovirus A71," rather than "Enterovirus 71" as previously written, indicates its current species group.

Like other enteroviruses, EV-A71 is a naked, icosahedral virion of about 30 nm in diameter. The virus capsid comprises 60 repeating protomer units, each composed of four viral structural proteins, VP1 to VP4. The genome is a single-stranded, positive (+) sense RNA molecule of approximately 7.5 kb. In general, enteroviruses are relatively stable, insensitive to organic solvents, resistant to acidic pH and, thus, can survive in the gastrointestinal tract [5]. Several putative host cell membrane virus receptors enable EV-A71 attachment and entry, but the most important receptor is probably human scavenger receptor class B member 2 (SCARB2), a ubiquitously expressed transmembrane lysosomal protein.

Epidemiology

Humans are the only natural hosts for EV-A71. Person-to-person transmission is usually through fecal-oral or oral-oral routes and sometimes via droplets [5]. Viral antigens and RNA are detected in tonsillar crypt squamous epithelium (but not in other parts of the gastrointestinal tract), and the higher isolation rate from throat swabs compared to rectal swabs or stools suggest that the palatine tonsil or oral mucosa are major sources of viral shedding into both the oral cavity and into feces [6, 7]. Viable viruses from skin vesicles suggest that cutaneous-oral transmission is possible, but its significance is unknown. Figure 22.1 summarizes the possible routes for viral entry, replication sites and shedding.

After its first isolation in 1969 in the United States [2], HFMD resulting from EV-A71 was first reported in Japan [8]. Since then, EV-A71 infections have been reported worldwide, although recent outbreaks have predominantly emerged in the Asia-Pacific region [9]. In the past two decades, the series of EV-A71 epidemics in this region (i.e. Australia, Japan, Malaysia, Taiwan, Vietnam, and China) have raised concerns about the potential worldwide dissemination of EV-A71. Moreover, these epidemics were associated with higher rates of morbidity and mortality among young children than any previous EV-A71 outbreaks [1]. China reported between 9.8 million and 11.3 million HFMD cases to the World Health Organization (WHO) from 2010 to 2014, with an estimated incidence of 1.2 per 1000 person-years and a case-fatality rate of 0.03% [10]. A pattern of cyclic epidemics every two to three years has been identified in the Asia-Pacific region. Outside this region, EV-A71 circulates at low levels in North America, Europe, and Africa, causing sporadic cases or small outbreaks [3].

Phylogenetic analysis of EV-A71, based on VP1, has been used to study the molecular epidemiology of outbreaks. Based on these variations, EV-A71 has been divided into four distinct genogroups (A, B, C, and D) [9, 11]. Genogroup A comprises the prototype EV-A71 strain isolated in 1969. Genotype B (subgenotypes B0–B5) has been circulating globally. Subgenotypes B1 and B2 were predominant in Japan, Europe, Australia, and the United States from the 1970 to the 1990s, whereas B3-B5 had circulated in Southeast Asia since 1997. Genogroup C has five lineages: C1, which replaced B as the dominant genotype in Europe and America from 1987; C2, which emerged in 1995; and C3–C5, which had been involved in epidemics in Southeast Asia since 1997. Genogroup D is represented by virus strains isolated in India in the 2000s [12]. Two additional genogroups have been proposed: genogroup E for isolates from African countries and genogroup F for isolates from Madagascar [12, 13].

No particular genotype has been conclusively associated with an increased risk of EV-A71 neurological disease, but generally, large epidemics are associated with genotype replacement [9, 11]. The largest outbreak that occurred in China between 2008 and 2011 was caused by extensive spread of EV-A71 subgenogroup C4. Subsequently, C4

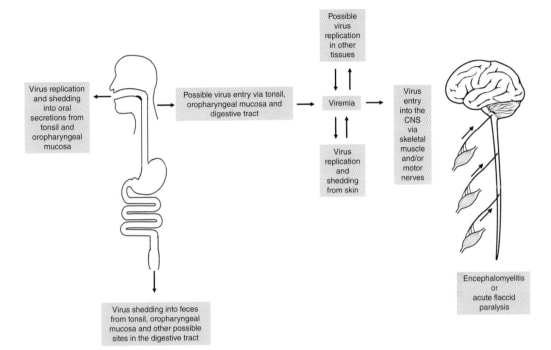

Figure 22.1 Possible routes of viral entry into the body and CNS, viral replication sites and viral shedding in Enterovirus A71 encephalomyelitis, based on available data from human and animal studies. Person-to-person transmission is mainly via fecal-oral and oral-oral routes. The portal(s) for viral entry are unknown but are likely to be via the palatine tonsil and oropharyngeal mucosa, following viral replication in the squamous epithelia of these tissues. Viral entry through the gastrointestinal tract could possibly also occur. Viremia spreads infection to the skin and perhaps other organs, where there is further viral replication. Retrograde axonal transport in cranial and spinal motor nerves enables neuroinvasion of brainstem motor nuclei and spinal cord anterior horn cells, respectively. Within the CNS, motor and other neural pathways spread virus further. Gastrointestinal tract replication sites have not been identified, so the source of fecal viral shedding may be mainly from infected squamous epithelia in the tonsil crypt, oropharynx, and esophagus. Source: Reproduced with permission from [29].

emerged and spread in Vietnam in 2011 and in Cambodia in 2012, causing large epidemics with fatal cases in these and subsequent years [14, 15].

Subgenotype emergence and global expansion are associated with recombinations of EV-A71 genome encoding the nonstructural proteins [16], particularly of the more recent EV-A71 subgenotypes. Recombination events occur between strains belonging to the same genogroup or to different genogroups. They have also been observed between EV-A71 and CV-A16 or other human enterovirus A viruses ([17]. Recombination likely plays a crucial role in EV-A71 evolution.

In China from 2008 to 2012, young children younger than five years old had the highest risk of disease. The highest incidence and mortality rates were among children ages 12–23 months (38.2 cases per 1000 and 1.5 deaths per 100 000 in 2012), followed by 6–11 months of age (28.9 cases per 1000 and 1.3 deaths per 100 000 in 2012) and 24–59 months of age (23.1 cases per 1000 and 0.4 deaths per 100 000 in 2012) [10]. The incidence is low among infants younger than six months, older children (ages 5–14 years), and adults (ages ≥ 15 years). It has been suggested that the lower incidence in the youngest infants is to the result of the presence of maternal antibodies [18]. A 10-year study in Taiwan reported similar data and revealed that males have a higher incidence of HFMD than females (4.24 vs. 2.99) [3]. Besides host factors, climatic factors may influence EV-A71 infection because the highest number of cases are from May to October, and quantitative evidence showed that warmer temperature and higher humidity increased the rate of infection [3, 10]. Several other risk factors have been identified as predictors for mortality, including polymorphisms in chemokine genes, sanitary conditions, and demographic factors.

Clinical features

The incubation period is three to six days [19]. Typically, HFMD is an acute febrile illness presenting with oral ulcers on the tongue and buccal mucosa and vesicular or erythematous maculopapular rashes on the hands, feet, knees, or buttocks. Herpangina is another variant of HFMD, in which oral ulcers are confined to the posterior oral cavity and soft palate.

The rare neurological complications occur during the febrile period in the setting of HFMD or herpangina, although oro-cutaneous manifestations may be absent or missed on examination. Patients with aseptic meningitis typically have meningism. AFP presents with limb weakness and hyporeflexia without sensory loss. It is the result of a limited infection of spinal cord anterior horn cells. Encephalomyelitis is the most serious CNS involvement. It typically presents with a few days of fever, lethargy and an acute catastrophic onset of neurological symptoms and signs, cardiopulmonary collapse, and fatal outcome within hours of hospital admission. Neurological signs include hyporeflexia, flaccid muscle weakness, myoclonic jerks, ataxia, nystagmus, oculomotor and bulbar palsies, and coma [20]. Terminally, autonomic dysregulation (i.e. cold sweating, tachycardia, hypertension, hyperglycemia, tachypnea), fulminant pulmonary edema and myocardial dysfunction occurs. Four clinical stages have been described: stage 1, HFMD/herpangina; stage 2, CNS involvement; stage 3, cardiopulmonary collapse; stage 4, convalescence or sequelae. Patients with stage 4 infection may recover or develop neurological sequelae such as severe cerebellar, cognitive, respiratory and motor impairment, and delayed neurodevelopment [20].

In encephalomyelitis, the T2-weighted magnetic resonance imaging (MRI) shows hyperintense lesions of the entire spinal cord involving bilateral anterior horns, medulla, posterior pons, and midbrain [20] and apparently also the thalamus, frontal and parietal lobes, and other areas [21]. In AFP, lesions are confined to the anterior horns of the spinal cord and ventral nerve roots [20].

Serological diagnosis of EV-A71 infection using serum or cerebrospinal fluid (CSF) and immunoglobulin G (IgG) or immunoglobulin M (IgM) enzyme-linked immunoassays have been attempted but generally not recommended because specific antibodies may not be found during the acute disease, and a high prevalence of antibodies in the general population from previous exposure negates clinical specificity [22]. Virus isolation and identification in clinical specimens; throat swabs, stools, and CSF is still the gold standard for diagnosis. Isolated viruses can be identified by immunofluorescence staining using EV-A71 specific monoclonal antibodies or reverse transcription-polymerase chain reaction (RT-PCR) using specific primers.

Pathology

EV-A71 encephalomyelitis is characterized by a stereotyped distribution of inflammation, invariably found in the spinal cord, brainstem, hypothalamus, and cerebellar dentate nucleus (Figure 22.2) [23, 24]. The most severe inflammation is in the spinal cord (anterior horns), medulla oblongata (including reticular formation and nucleus ambiguus), pontine-tegmentum/floor of fourth ventricle (Figure 22.3(a)), midbrain posterior to the corticospinal tracts, hypothalamus, subthalamic nucleus, and cerebellar dentate nucleus. The cerebral cortex, especially the motor area, may show mild inflammation. The inflammatory cells form perivascular cuffs and parenchymal infiltrates composed mainly of macrophages, lymphocytes, and plasma cells with occasional neutrophils. The parenchyma also shows microglial nodules, neuronophagia, edema, and necrosis often appearing as spotty necrolytic lesions (Figure 22.3b, c, and d). There are no viral inclusions. Inflammation is absent in the corpus striatum, thalamus,

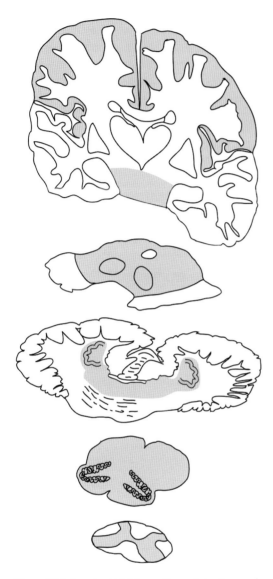

Figure 22.2 Areas in which inflammation or viral antigens and RNA can be consistently found include the brainstem, spinal cord, hypothalamus, cerebellar dentate nucleus, and occasionally, the cerebral cortex. Source: Reproduced with permission from [24].

hippocampus, anterior pons (Figure 22.3a), and cerebellar cortex. Mild meningitis is found throughout the CNS.

Viral antigens and RNA are localized to neuronal bodies and processes in the inflamed areas but may be very focal (Figure 22.3e and f). Some inflammatory cells around infected neurons contain phagocytosed viral antigens and RNA, but meninges, glial cells, blood vessels, and choroid plexus are all negative. In AFP, the inflammation is probably restricted to localized spinal cord anterior horn cells and is likely to be similar to that seen in encephalomyelitis. In nonfatal aseptic meningitis, the meningeal inflammatory infiltrate is also assumed to be similar.

In fatal encephalomyelitis, the lungs show severe pulmonary edema, multifocal hemorrhage, congestion, and occasionally mild inflammation. Myocarditis is either absent or very mild [6, 25]. The mesenteric lymph nodes, Peyer patches, spleen, and thymus show congestion or reactive hyperplasia. Significant inflammation is not observed in other systemic organs. Viral antigens and RNA are localized to squamous epithelium in the palatine tonsil crypt but are not found in other lymphoid organs or tissues, gastrointestinal tract, liver, pancreas, lungs, myocardium, kidney, and skeletal muscle [6].

Pathogenesis

Localization of viral antigens or RNA in neurons undergoing neuronophagia or degeneration in inflamed areas suggests that neuronotropism and viral cytolysis are important mechanisms for tissue injury. These findings have been confirmed in animal models [26, 27]. The stereotypic distribution and varying intensity of inflammation in human encephalomyelitis and the supportive findings in animal models make it likely that viral entry into the CNS may be via cranial and peripheral motor nerves [27, 28] (Figure 22.3g and h). According to this hypothesis, anterior horn cells and brainstem motor nuclei are the first CNS neurons to be infected, and from these neurons, the virus spreads to the motor cortex and other parts of the CNS, probably via existing neural pathways (Figure 22.1) [29]. Like poliomyelitis, it is assumed that AFP is the result of a localized, focal infection of spinal anterior horn neurons. Hematogenous spread of virus through the blood-brain-barrier has not been well studied and still cannot be excluded.

Terminal pulmonary edema and cardiopulmonary collapse in encephalomyelitis may be related to neurogenic pulmonary edema, a phenomenon

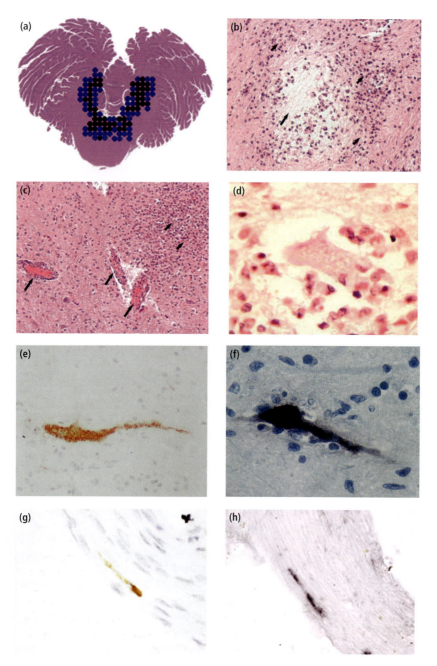

Figure 22.3 Neuropathology of enterovirus A71 (EV-A71) infection. (a) Horizontal section of the whole cerebellum at the mid-pons level from an autopsy of EV-A71 encephalomyelitis showing the distribution of moderate (blue dots) and severe inflammation (black dots). (b–f). Microscopy inflammation is confined to the dentate nucleus (b), tegmentum or floor of fourth ventricle (c, arrows), sparing the anterior pons, and cerebellar cortex. Intense parenchymal inflammation, necrosis, and perivascular cuffing is seen in the medulla (d). In inflamed areas, viral antigens (e) and RNA (f) are localized to infected neuronal bodies and processes with or without evidence of neuronophagia. In an encephalomyelitis mouse model infected by intramuscular injection into jaw or facial muscles, viral antigens (g) and RNA (h) were demonstrated in cranial nerves. Source: Figures a–f reproduced with permission from [23]; Figures g, h reproduced with permission from [28].

previously described in bulbar poliomyelitis and other CNS diseases. There may be a complex interplay of various pathogenetic mechanisms involving excessive sympathetic hyperactivity or catecholamine release consequent on brainstem encephalitis and a cytokine storm of inflammatory mediators [1]. Proinflammatory mediators, such as TNF-α, IL-1β, and many others, are increased in the CSF or plasma in patients with encephalitis with or without pulmonary edema [30].

So far, viral genomic sequence analyses from fatal and nonfatal cases have not clearly identified any mutations that confer neurovirulence. Nevertheless, several animal studies have demonstrated that mutations in structural and nonstructural genes may be associated with neurovirulence [31]. As mentioned previously, other factors like the infective viral dose, host immune status, diminishing protective maternal antibodies [18], gender, and host genetic predisposition may be important.

Treatment, future perspectives, and conclusions

Although many antiviral agents have been tested for effectiveness against EV-A71, including type 1 interferons, ribavirin, suramin, and pleconaril, as far as we are aware, none has been approved for use.

Intravenous immune globulin (IVIG), given for established EV-A71 infection with CNS complications, may be useful [32]. A few approved inactivated whole-EV71 vaccines are now in commercial production [33]. Unfortunately, these vaccines do not protect against CV-A16 infection, the other major cause of HFMD.

Neurotropic enteroviruses such as PV, EV-A71, and enterovirus D68, and to a lesser extent, CV-A16, are diverse in terms of virological characteristics (e.g. different virus receptors) and the initial illnesses they cause (e.g. HFMD in EV-A71 and CV-A16; respiratory illness in EV-D68). Yet observations in human autopsies and brain MRIs, and animal models suggest that these viruses share a common pathway via peripheral motor nerves to invade the CNS and cause encephalomyelitis [29]. The mechanisms responsible for pulmonary edema that is associated with a fatal outcome in children infected with EV-A71 remain unclear. With the impending global eradication of poliovirus, EV-A71 may emerge as the most important neurotropic enterovirus.

Acknowledgments

This study was supported in part, by the University of Malaya/Ministry of Education High Impact Research Grant (H-20001-00-E000004), Fundamental Research Grant Scheme (FP19/2016, FP038/2015A), Pasteur Institute, Inserm and LabEx IBEID.

Disclosure/conflict of interest

The authors declare no conflict of interest.

References

1. Solomon, T., Lewthwaite, P., Perera, D. et al. (2010). Virology, epidemiology, pathogenesis, and control of enterovirus 71. *Lancet Infect. Dis.* 10: 778–790.
2. Schmidt, N.J., Lennette, E.H., and Ho, H.H. (1974). An apparently new enterovirus isolated from patients with disease of the central nervous system. *J. Infect. Dis.* 129: 304–309.
3. Chang, P.C., Chen, S.C., and Chen, K.T. (2016). The current status of the disease caused by Enterovirus 71 infections: epidemiology, pathogenesis, molecular epidemiology and vaccine development. *Int. J. Environ. Res. Public Heath* 13: 890.
4. King, A.M.Q., Adams, M.J., Carstens, E.B., and Lefkowitz, E.J. (2012). *Virus taxonomy: classification and nomenclature of viruses: Ninth Report of the International Committee on Taxonomy of Viruses*. San Diego: Academic Press.
5. Pallansch, M.A. and Roos, R.P. (2001). Enteroviruses: poliovirus, coxsackieviruses, echoviruses, and newer enteroviruses. In: *Field Virology* (eds. D.M. Knipe, P.M. Howley, D.E. Griffin, et al.), 723–775. Philadelphia: Lippincott Williams & Wilkins.
6. He, Y., Ong, K.C., Gao, Z. et al. (2014). Tonsillar crypt epithelium is an important extra-nervous system site for viral replication in EV71 encephalomyelitis. *Am. J. Pathol.* 184: 714–720.

7. Ooi, M.H., Solomon, T., Podin, Y. et al. (2007). Evaluation of different clinical sample types in diagnosis of human enterovirus 71-associated hand-foot-and-mouth disease. *J. Clin. Microbiol.* 45: 1858–1866.
8. Ishimaru, Y., Nakano, S., Yamaoka, K., and Takami, S. (1980). Outbreaks of hand, foot, and mouth disease by enterovirus 71. High incidence of complication disorders of central nervous system. *Arch. Dis. Child.* 55: 583–588.
9. McMinn, P.C. (2012). Recent advances in the molecular epidemiology and control of human enterovirus 71 infection. *Curr. Opin. Virol.* 2: 199–205.
10. Xing, W., Liao, Q., Viboud, C. et al. (2014). Hand, foot, and mouth disease in China, 2008-12: an epidemiological study. *Lancet Infect. Dis.* 14: 308–318.
11. Yip, C.C., Lau, S.K., Woo, P.C., and Yuen, K.Y. (2013). Human enterovirus 71 epidemics: what's next? *Emerg. Health Threats J.* 6: 19780.
12. Bessaud, M., Razafindratsimandresy, R., Nougairede, A. et al. (2014). Molecular comparison and evolutionary analyses of VP1 nucleotide sequences of new African human enterovirus 71 isolates reveal a wide genetic diversity. *PLoS One* 9: e90624.
13. Bessaud, M., Pillet, S., Ibrahim, W. et al. (2012). Molecular characterization of human enteroviruses in the Central African Republic: uncovering wide diversity and identification of a new human enterovirus A71 genogroup. *J. Clin. Microbiol.* 50: 1650–1658.
14. Horwood, P.F., Andronico, A., Tarantola, A. et al. (2016). Seroepidemiology of human Enterovirus 71 infection among children, Cambodia. *Emerg. Infect. Dis.* 22: 92–95.
15. Khanh, T.H., Sabanathan, S., Thanh, T.T. et al. (2012). Enterovirus 71-associated hand, foot, and mouth disease, Southern Vietnam, 2011. *Emerg. Infect. Dis.* 18: 2002–2005.
16. McWilliam Leitch, E.C., Cabrerizo, M., Cardosa, J. et al. (2012). The association of recombination events in the founding and emergence of subgenogroup evolutionary lineages of human enterovirus 71. *J. Virol.* 86: 2676–2685.
17. Zhang, Y., Zhu, Z., Yang, W. et al. (2010). An emerging recombinant human enterovirus 71 responsible for the 2008 outbreak of hand foot and mouth disease in Fuyang city of China. *Virol. J.* 7: 94.
18. Zhu, F.C., Liang, Z.L., Meng, F.Y. et al. (2012). Retrospective study of the incidence of HFMD and seroepidemiology of antibodies against EV71 and CoxA16 in prenatal women and their infants. *PLoS One* 7: e37206.
19. Ma, E., Fung, C., Yip, S.H. et al. (2011). Estimation of the basic reproduction number of enterovirus 71 and coxsackievirus A16 in hand, foot, and mouth disease outbreaks. *Pediatr. Infect. Dis. J.* 30: 675–679.
20. Chang, L.Y. (2008). Enterovirus 71 in Taiwan. *Pediatr. Neonatol.* 49: 103–112.
21. Shen, W.C., Chiu, H.H., Chow, K.C., and Tsai, C.H. (1999). MR imaging findings of enteroviral encephalomyelitis: an outbreak in Taiwan. *Am. j. neuroradiol.* 20: 1889–1895.
22. Harvala, H., Broberg, E., Benschop, K. et al. (2018). Recommendations for enterovirus diagnostics and characterization in Europe and beyond. *J. Clin. Virol.* 101: 11–17.
23. Wong, K.T., Badmanathan, M., Ong, K.C. et al. (2008). The distribution of inflammation and virus in human enterovirus 71 encephalomyelitis suggests possible viral spread by neural pathways. *J. Neuropathol. Exp. Neurol.* 67: 162–169.
24. Wong, K.T., Ng, K.Y., Ong, K.C. et al. (2012). Enterovirus 71 encephalomyelitis and Japanese encephalitis can be distinguished by topographic distribution of inflammation and specific intraneuronal detection of viral antigen and RNA. *Neuropathol. Appl. Neurol.* 38: 443–453.
25. World Health Organization (WHO) (2011). *A guide to clinical management and public heath response for hand, foot and mouth disease (HFMD)*. Geneva, Switzerland: World Health Organization.
26. Nakata, N., Iwasaki, T., Ami, Y. et al. (2004). Different localization of neurons susceptible to enterovirus 71 and poliovirus type 1 in the central nervous system of cynomolgus monkeys after intravenous inoculation. *J. Gen. Virol.* 85: 2981–2989.
27. Ong, K.C., Munisamy, B., Leong, K.L. et al. (2008). Pathologic characterization of a murine model of human enterovirus 71 encephalomyelitis. *J. Neuropathol. Exp. Neurol.* 67: 532–542.
28. Tan, S.H., Ong, K.C., and Wong, K.T. (2014). Enterovirus 71 can directly infect the brainstem via cranial nerves and infection can be ameliorated by passive immunization. *J. Neuropathol. Exp. Neurol.* 73: 999–1009.
29. Ong, K.C. and Wong, K.T. (2015). Understanding Enterovirus 71 neuropathogenesis and its impact on other neutrotropic enteroviruses. *Brain Pathol.* 25: 614–624.
30. Wang, S.M., Lei, H.Y., and Liu, C.C. (2012). Cytokine immunopathogenesis of enterovirus 71 brain stem encephalitis. *Clin. Dev. Immunol.*: 876241.

31. Huang, H.I., Weng, K.F., and Shih, S.R. (2012). Viral and host factors that contribute to pathogenicity of enterovirus 71. *Future Microbiol.* 7: 469–479.
32. Chea, S., Cheng, Y., Chokephaibulkit, K. et al. (2015). Workshop on use of intravenous immunoglobulin in hand, foot and mouth disease in Southeast Asia [online report]. *Emerg. Infect. Dis.* http://dx.doi.org/10.3201/eid2101.140992.
33. Yi, E.J., Shin, Y.J., Kim, J.H. et al. (2017). Enterovirus 71 infection and vaccines. *Clin. Exp. Vaccine Res.* 6: 4–14.

23 Human Immunodeficiency Virus Infection of the CNS

Françoise Gray[1,2] and Leroy R. Sharer[3]

[1] Retired from Department of Pathology, Lariboisière Hospital, APHP, Paris, France
[2] University Paris Diderot (Paris 7), Paris, France
[3] Division of Neuropathology, Department of Pathology, Immunology, and Laboratory Medicine, Rutgers New Jersey Medical School and University Hospital, Newark, NJ, USA

Abbreviations

AIDS	acquired immunodeficiency syndrome
ANI	asymptomatic neurocognitive impairment
ART	antiretroviral therapy
BBB	blood-brain barrier
CART	combined antiretroviral therapy
CMV	cytomegalovirus
CNS	central nervous system
CSF	cerebrospinal fluid
DNA	deoxyribonucleic acid
DPD	diffuse poliodystrophy
FIV	feline immunodeficiency virus
HAART	highly active antiretroviral therapy
HAD	HIV-associated dementia
HAND	HIV-associated neurocognitive disorder
HIV	human immunodeficiency virus
HIVE	HIV encephalitis
HIVL	HIV leukoencephalopathy
HTLV-III	human T-cell leukemia/lymphoma virus type III
IRIS	immune reconstitution inflammatory syndrome
MGC	multinucleated giant cells
MND	minor neurocognitive disorder
MRI	magnetic resonance imaging
OI	opportunistic infections
PML	progressive multifocal leukoencephalopathy
RNA	ribonucleic acid
SIV	Simian immunodeficiency virus
VM	vacuolar myelopathy

Definition of the disorder, major synonyms, and historical perspective

Compared with other neurological diseases, the description of involvement of the CNS in acquired immunodeficiency syndrome (AIDS) is relatively recent. In the early 1980s, the medical community became alarmed by a new "epidemic" of Kaposi sarcoma and unusual opportunistic infections (OIs) in men who were homosexual and in Haitians. A new disorder with T-cell depletion was identified, called "acquired immunodeficiency syndrome"; a viral origin was rapidly suspected and confirmed by identification of the responsible

Infections of the Central Nervous System: Pathology and Genetics, First Edition. Edited by Fabrice Chrétien, Kum Thong Wong, Leroy R. Sharer, Catherine (Katy) Keohane and Françoise Gray.
© 2020 John Wiley & Sons Ltd. Published 2020 by John Wiley & Sons Ltd.

virus. Originally known as "lymphadenopathy-associated virus" [1] or "human T cell leukemia/lymphoma virus type III" (HTLV-III) [2], by consensus it was finally named "human immunodeficiency virus" (HIV) [3].

Involvement of the nervous system was quickly recognized as a major cause of disability and death in patients with AIDS [4]. Because the disease was invariably fatal, the spectrum of HIV neuropathology was described in many concordant autopsy series [5].

Since the early 1990s, introduction of antiretroviral therapy (ART), particularly highly active antiretroviral therapy (HAART), or combined antiretroviral therapy (cART) including protease inhibitors, has dramatically improved the course and prognosis of HIV disease. In countries where treatment is widely available, morbidity and mortality in patients with HIV has greatly reduced, and their quality of life has improved. However, the CNS is still a major target of the infection and new types of complication have emerged [6], including those related to drug toxicity. People with undiagnosed or unsuspected HIV infection may present with CNS involvement, as can individuals with HIV who are not compliant with therapy or those who develop HIV mutations that are resistant to antiretroviral agents. CNS involvement in AIDS is still a major problem in developing countries, where effective treatment and prevention are often not available.

Microbiological and genetic characteristics specific to the agent

HIV-1 is a retrovirus of the Lentivirus subfamily, properly classified as an immunodeficiency virus, a subgroup of lentiviruses that also includes HIV-2 and the closely related simian immunodeficiency virus (SIV) [7]. Recent molecular archeology studies showed that HIV-1 first crossed into man accidentally in Central Africa about 1920, from a chimpanzee infected with SIV. The West African HIV-2 crossed from sooty mangabey monkeys into man in the early twentieth century [8].

HIV is a nontransforming virus, which replicates by generating proviral DNA, mediated by the action of a retroviral enzyme, RNA-directed DNA polymerase (reverse transcriptase). In vivo, persistent infection is established following integration of proviral DNA into the host genome. HIV-1 consists of two single-stranded copies of RNA, noncovalently linked to the core proteins, closely associated with the RNA-directed DNA-reverse transcriptase. The viral envelope contains a viral-encoded transmembrane glycoprotein (gp41), which noncovalently anchors the extravirion spike glycoprotein gp-120. The HIV genome includes three principal structural genes, *gag, pol,* and *env,* and the nonstructural genes *tat, nef,* and *rev.*

HIV-1 infects cells that express CD4 antigen on their surface. CD4 antigen is present both on CD4+ helper T lymphocytes and monocytes and macrophages, and the chemokine receptor CCR5 is an important coreceptor for HIV-1 on monocyte and macrophage cells. Infection of CD4+ lymphocytes leads to their destruction and cell-mediated immunodeficiency. HIV-1 can invade the CNS via infected macrophages. These are the major cell type capable of supporting viral replication. Thus, they potentially act both as a reservoir for the virus and as a vehicle for its spread. Viral particles can also freely cross the blood-brain barrier (BBB), gaining entry into the CNS parenchyma.

The presence of HIV within a cell does not necessarily result in viral replication and new virus formation; there are three possible outcomes: (i) productive infection; (ii) latent infection, a situation in which the DNA provirus is blocked at the stage of transcription; (iii) nonproductive (or restricted) infection, in which unintegrated or integrated viral DNA does not proceed to viral reproduction.

HIV evolves continuously in vivo; this property has important implications for replication of the virus and its cytopathic effects.

Epidemiology

Transmission of HIV is mainly sexual, but transmission by blood and breast milk is also possible.

HIV infection was first described in men who were homosexual, but it soon spread to other groups, including intravenous drug users, recipients of blood transfusion and organ transplant, women undergoing artificial insemination, and children born to parents who were HIV-positive or breast-fed by women who were seropositive. Although recognized from the outset, heterosexual transmission has more recently become the predominant route of infection, particularly in sub-Saharan regions.

From the outset, the AIDS epidemic spread dramatically worldwide, but in each region there are different risk factors, coinfections, and medical responses. The following epidemiologic data are, therefore, necessarily a generalization.

More than 70 million people have been infected by HIV and about 35 million have died from HIV disease. Globally, 36.7 million people including 1.8 million children worldwide were living with HIV at the end of 2016. Most of the children live in sub-Saharan Africa and were infected through transmission from their mothers who were HIV-positive during pregnancy, childbirth, or breast-feeding. As a result of better access to antiretroviral (ART), individuals who are HIV-positive now live longer healthier lives. In addition, ART prevents onward transmission of HIV. In 2016, 19.5 million people living with HIV were receiving ART globally. Progress has also been made in preventing and eliminating mother-to-child transmission and keeping mothers alive. In 2015, almost 8 out of 10 pregnant women living with HIV, or 1.1 million women, received ART. The estimated annual number of new HIV infections in 2016 was 1.8 million (including 150 000 children), versus 3.0 million in 2000 (39% lower). One million people died of HIV-related illnesses worldwide in 2016, representing half the number of deaths in 2005.

The burden of the epidemic varies considerably between countries and regions; sub-Saharan Africa is the most severely affected, where nearly 1 in every 25 adults (4.2%) are living with HIV, accounting for nearly two-thirds of people living with HIV worldwide. However, the epidemic has decreased in Africa, while in Eastern Europe and Central Asia, new infections have increased by 60% [9].

Clinicopathological presentation of CNS involvement in HIV infection

CNS changes in early HIV infection

CNS changes at the time of seroconversion

Early invasion of the CNS by HIV-1 has been demonstrated by many cerebrospinal fluid (CSF) studies. In a case of iatrogenic infection by accidental HIV-1 inoculation, the virus was isolated from the brain 15 days after inoculation and 1 day after the virus was recovered from blood [10]. Primary infection by HIV is usually clinically silent, but there are occasional reports of transient symptomatic meningitis, encephalopathy, or myelopathy coinciding with seroconversion for the virus. Very rarely, acute encephalopathy can occur, revealing or coinciding with HIV seroconversion, with neuropathological features of acute inflammatory demyelinating leukoencephalopathy [11] (Figure 23.1) or autoimmune limbic encephalitis [12]. In such patients, it seems likely that acute HIV infection in a genetically susceptible host produces florid inflammatory disease.

CNS changes in asymptomatic HIV carriers

Despite persistent CSF abnormalities [13], most carriers of HIV appear neurologically unimpaired in the so-called "asymptomatic" period lasting from seroconversion to symptomatic AIDS. However, a number of psychometric, radiological, and electrophysiological studies suggest that neurological abnormalities are present in these patients [14].

Brain examination in asymptomatic individuals who are HIV-positive and who died accidentally—mainly heroin addicts who died from heroin overdose—compared with individuals who were seronegative with similar causes of death, revealed an inflammatory T-cell reaction with vasculitis and leptomeningitis (Figure 23.2a and b) and immune activation of brain parenchyma, with increased numbers of microglial cells, upregulation of major histocompatibility complex class II antigens, and local production of cytokines. Myelin pallor and gliosis of the white matter were usually found, most likely secondary to BBB disruption resulting from vasculitis (Figure 23.2c and d). In contrast, cortical damage seems to be a late

Infections of the Central Nervous System

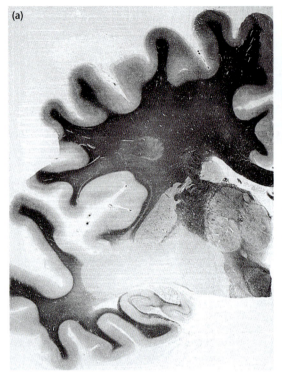
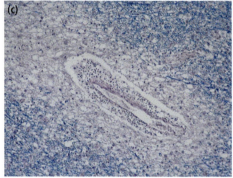

Figure 23.1 Acute inflammatory demyelinating leukoencephalopathy coinciding with human immunodeficiency virus (HIV) seroconversion [11]. (a) Macroscopic appearance (Loyez stain). Large well-defined area of recent demyelination involving the left temporal lobe around the temporal horn of the lateral ventricle and extending to the internal capsule. Note less-circumscribed multifocal lesions in the centrum semiovale. (b) Multifocal perivenous demyelinated lesions, acute disseminated encephalomyelitis (ADEM) type in the centrum semiovale (Klüver- Barrera/cresyl violet). (c) Microscopic perivenous demyelinated area surrounding an inflammatory vessel in the parietal white matter (Bodian-Luxol).

event in the course of HIV infection. Cortical astrocytosis or significant neuronal loss is not seen at the early stage of HIV infection, and neuronal apoptosis is exceptional. HIV proviral DNA was identified in a number of brains, but viral replication was very low in the asymptomatic stage of HIV infection (for review see [15]).

Neurological complications in patients with AIDS

Neurological complications of HIV infection are common at the stage of full-blown AIDS and result from various mechanisms. They include lesions related to direct infection of the CNS by HIV and OIs and lymphomas that occur as a result of immunodeficiency. HIV-associated systemic disorders may also cause secondary CNS involvement.

HIV-induced CNS lesions

HIV-induced CNS lesions are defined as original and specific changes that had never been observed before the AIDS epidemic and are found only in individuals with HIV without evidence of another cause. Clinically, HIV-associated neurocognitive disorder (HAND) is a common primary neurological disorder associated with HIV infection of the CNS [16]. HAND is a specific subcortical cognitive disorder; psychomotor slowing is its most salient feature. The clinical severity of HAND ranges from asymptomatic neurocognitive impairment (ANI) and minor neurocognitive disorder (MND), through to the most severe form of HIV-associated dementia (HAD). Neuropathological changes include HIV encephalitis (HIVE), resulting from direct infection of the CNS by the virus; HIV

Human Immunodeficiency Virus Infection of the CNS Chapter 23

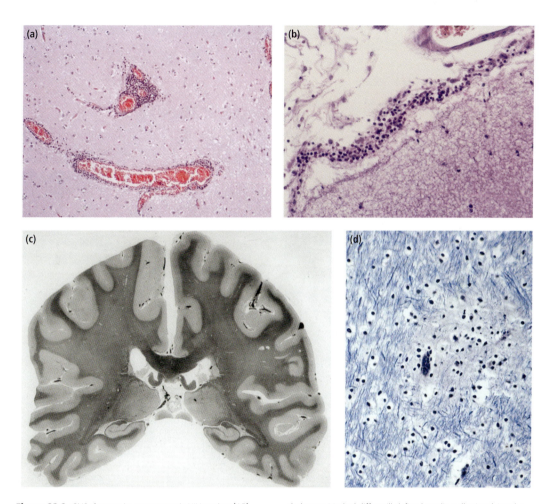

Figure 23.2 CNS changes in asymptomatic HIV carriers [15]. (a) Several parenchymal perivascular inflammatory infiltrates (hematoxylin and eosin [H&E]). (b) Lymphocytic meningitis (H&E). (c) Coronal section of the cerebral hemispheres at the level of the thalamus: Marked diffuse ill-defined myelin pallor involving the deep white matter tending to spare the U fibers, corpus callosum, and optic radiations (Loyez stain). (d) Perivascular demyelination in the deep white matter (Bodian-Luxol).

leukoencephalopathy (HIVL); and diffuse poliodystrophy (DPD), all of which may occur together.

HIV encephalitis

HIVE, due to a productive HIV infection of the CNS, is the most characteristic neuropathological HIV-induced lesion. It includes marked astrocytic and microglial activation with many multinucleated giant cells (MGC) (Figure 23.3a) [17] and abundant viral load demonstrated by immunocytochemistry or in situ hybridization. MGCs (Figure 23.3b and c) have been proposed as the hallmark of HIVE. They are of macrophage lineage, contain HIV in their cytoplasm and result from the virus's fusing capacity. Their presence provides evidence of productive HIV infection and of its cytopathic effect [18]. The lesions consist of multiple disseminated foci (Figure 23.3d) that may affect any part of the CNS but are mostly found in the deep white matter and basal ganglia.

Involvement of the white matter, HIV leukoencephalopathy, and diffuse axonal damage

HIVL is characterized by diffuse myelin pallor, particularly severe in the centrum semiovale and usually sparing the U fibers (Figure 23.4a) [19].

Infections of the Central Nervous System

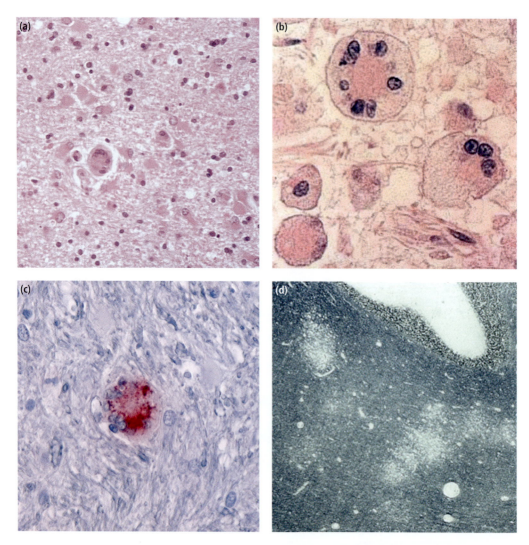

Figure 23.3 Human immunodeficiency virus encephalitis (HIVE). (a) An area in the white matter shows marked astrocytic and microglial activation with multinucleated giant cells (hematoxylin and eosin [H&E]). (b) Multinucleated giant cells (H&E). (c) Immunohistochemistry showing HIV antigens in the cytoplasm of a multinucleated giant cell. (d) Multiple disseminated foci of HIVE in the cerebellar white matter (Loyez stain).

It is frequently associated with HIVE. Both types of lesion (HIVE and HIVL) were regarded by some authors as extremes of a spectrum of HIV-induced pathology, which overlap in one-third of cases. However, brain microvasculature is abnormal in HIVL [20], and the diffuse myelin pallor was shown to be secondary to alterations of the BBB and not to demyelination [21]. This was confirmed by immunohistochemical demonstration of loss of the tight junction protein, zonula occludens-1, in patients with HAD [22]. Widespread axonal damage was identified by beta-amyloid protein precursor immunocytochemistry (Figure 23.4b) and was also extremely frequent in AIDS [23].

Involvement of the gray matter and diffuse poliodystrophy

DPD is characterized by diffuse reactive astrocytosis and microglial activation in the cerebral gray

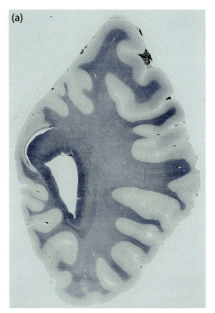 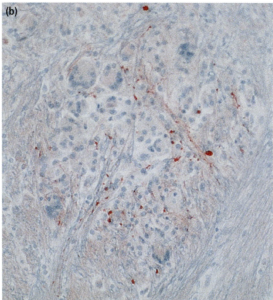

Figure 23.4 White matter changes. (a) Human immunodeficiency virus leukoencephalopathy (HIVL; Loyez stain). (b) Axonal dilatation demonstrated by bAPP immunostaining and human immunodeficiency virus encephalitis focus with numerous multinucleated giant cells.

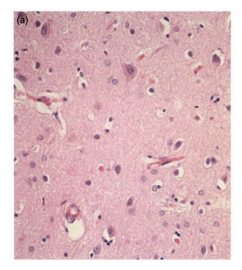 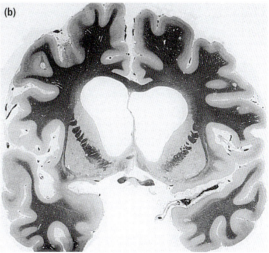

Figure 23.5 Diffuse poliodystrophy (DPD). (a) Microscopic aspect: Diffuse reactive astrocytosis and microglial activation in the cerebral gray matter (hematoxylin and eosin [H&E]). (b) Macroscopy: Atrophy of the cerebral cortex and striatum with widening of the sulci and marked ventricular dilatation. Note the absence of white matter pallor (Loyez stain).

matter (Figure 23.5a) [24]. It is associated with neuronal loss [25], resulting, at least partly, from apoptosis [26]. When severe, it may cause macroscopic cortical atrophy (Figure 23.5b).

HIV-Induced CNS lesions in children

CNS lesions in children differ significantly from adults. The most common clinical manifestation is a progressive encephalopathy with developmental delay, apathy, spastic quadriparesis, and convulsions. Radiological examination reveals brain atrophy and prominent calcifications especially in the basal ganglia.

Neuropathology confirms microcephaly and basal ganglia mineralization. HIVE and HIVL are not uncommon. Corticospinal tract degeneration, in the absence of inflammation or evidence of the local presence of HIV, is the most common pathological finding [5].

Opportunistic infections

OIs were the first identified CNS complication of AIDS. Their incidence has decreased following the introduction of HAART, but they remain a major cause of morbidity and mortality in patients with AIDS and are the presenting sign in many cases. Multiple OIs may involve the brain. The four most frequent are toxoplasmosis, progressive multifocal leukoencephalopathy (PML), cryptococcosis, and cytomegalovirus (CMV). Primary brain lymphomas strongly related to Epstein–-Barr virus infection can also be included in this group. These infections are described in specific chapters (Chapters 3, 6, 7, 9, and 44). It is worth highlighting that OIs in AIDS often have a misleading, atypical clinical presentation for the following reasons: (i) A wide range of organisms is involved; (ii) a particular patient may have successive or simultaneous infections by different agents (Figure 23.6) [5]; (iii) there can be involvement of several organs at the same time; and (iv) there is generally a reduced inflammatory reaction. Also, the type of infection depends on the severity of immunodeficiency; toxoplasmosis (a frequent presenting disease) occurs in patients with milder immunodeficiency (CD4<200) than PML, and CMV infection and primary brain lymphomas that are all found in severely immunodeficient patients (CD4<5).

In patients with AIDS, OIs of the CNS vary between different geographic regions and between different age groups.

Cerebral toxoplasmosis is more frequent in France and Germany than in the United States or United Kingdom. Toxoplasmosis has also been reported in patients from sub-Saharan Africa, South America, and India. CNS histoplasmosis, blastomycosis, and coccidioidomycosis are much more frequent in America than in Europe. Acute or

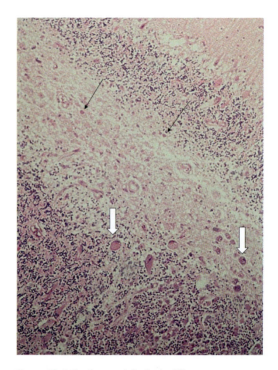

Figure 23.6 Simultaneous infection by different agents (cytomegalovirus [CMV] and progressive multifocal leukoencephalopathy [PML]) within the same site. Cytomegalic cells (white large arrows) characteristic of CMV are present close to a demyelinated focus containing inclusion-bearing oligodendrocytes (thin black arrows) characteristic of PML in the cerebellar cortex (hematoxylin and eosin [H&E]).

reactivated cerebral trypanosomiasis causing devastating lesions occurs only in South America. CNS *Mycobacterium tuberculosis* infection is especially common in patients with AIDS living in developing countries that have a high incidence of tuberculosis, particularly in Africa.

In general, children up to 13 years of age have a lower incidence of CNS OIs than adults, probably because children have had less time to be exposed to opportunistic pathogens. This is especially true for toxoplasmosis, which is a less common cause of CNS mass lesion than primary brain lymphoma in children with AIDS. For this reason, it is recommended that children with AIDS who have a CNS mass lesion be biopsied at presentation, rather than after a trial of anti-*Toxoplasma* therapy [27]. Cryptococcal meningitis and PML are also rare in children with AIDS. CMV continues to be the most common opportunistic pathogen in this age group, even in young children.

Secondary CNS lesions in AIDS

Apart from HIV-induced lesions and OIs, a variety of changes may be found in the CNS of patients with AIDS. Their pathogenesis is not well understood, but most are secondary to general or systemic complications of AIDS [5].

Vascular changes include hypercoagulable states (noninfectious "marantic" thrombotic endocarditis, disseminated intravascular coagulation, and venous thrombosis), probably related to the patients' general debility and hemorrhages, often related to spontaneous or drug-induced thrombocytopenia.

Metabolic and nutritional abnormalities are frequently observed, particularly at the preterminal stage of the disease. These include hypoxia, electrolyte disturbances, and vitamin deficiencies.

Electrolyte disturbances may be responsible for central pontine myelinolysis. Mineral deposits may be particularly severe in patients with disturbances in phosphate or calcium metabolism resulting from HIV nephropathy.

Wernicke encephalopathy resulting from thiamin deficiency may occur preterminally and has been associated with onset of zidovudine treatment [28].

Vacuolar myelopathy is characterized by intramyelinic and periaxonal vacuoles, some containing macrophages, within the lateral, posterior and, less prominently, anterior columns of the spinal cord, though not limited to any specific tract [29]. The pathology usually starts in the mid-low thoracic cord and spreads in both rostral and caudal directions with increasing severity. The incidence varies considerably among studies and its etiology is unclear. MGCs, HIV antigens, and HIV particles have sporadically been found in the lesions [30], but attempts to correlate the presence of HIV in the spinal cord with the development of myelopathy have not yielded significant results [31]. The strong similarity with subacute combined degeneration suggested a possible role for vitamin B_{12} deficiency. Normal vitamin B_{12} and folic acid levels were found in patients with AIDS with vacuolar myelopathy (VM), but the vitamin B_{12}-dependent transmethylation pathway was abnormal in all cases [32]. This abnormality, possibly induced by HIV or cytokine activation, is considered the most likely cause of VM associated with AIDS.

Hepatic encephalopathy is relatively common in patients with terminal liver failure.

Multifocal pontine leukoencephalopathy characterized by multiple microscopic asymmetric foci of necrosis within the basis pontis has been described in patients with AIDS [33] and is likely to be the result of increased levels of circulating proinflammatory cytokines.

CNS changes in patients receiving HAART

Introduction of HAART has dramatically changed the course and prognosis of HIV disease. In the developed world, HAART is readily available and the management of OIs in general has improved, so the incidence of CNS OIs has declined significantly. Epidemiological studies show that AIDS-defining events are no longer the major causes of death in patients infected with HIV [34]. The benefit is mainly due to a decrease in HIV viral load and a restored functioning immune system. However, new types of complications now occur (for review see [6, 35]).

"Scar lesions" and "burnt out lesions" in treated infections

Scar lesions with no evidence of inflammation or the original infectious agent have become more frequent (Figure 23.7) in patients who were clinically and biologically cured and died from other causes. In other instances although "burnt out" inactive lesions were present, secondary Wallerian degeneration developed when irreversible cerebral destruction had occured. In those patients, despite appropriate treatment, disease continued to progress clinically and often radiologically. This pattern was particularly prevalent in patients with severe, multifocal toxoplasmosis, PML or HIVE when treatment had been administered late in the course of the disease.

New inflammatory lesions related to restoration of the immune system

An "immune reconstitution inflammatory syndrome" (IRIS), was identified with four diagnostic

Infections of the Central Nervous System

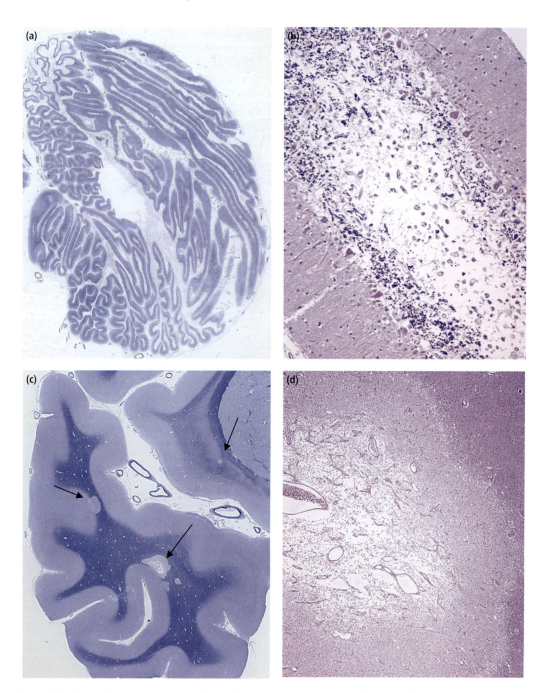

Figure 23.7 "Burnt out" lesions in patients receiving highly active antiretroviral therapy (HAART). (a and b) "Burnt out" progressive multifocal leukoencephalopathy (PML). The white matter of the cerebellar folia has disappeared (a, Klüver-Barrera/cresyl violet). At higher magnification the white matter of a folium is cavitated. Inflammation or infectious agents are no longer evident (b, hematoxylin and eosin [H&E]). (c and d) "Burnt out" varicella-zoster encephalitis. Coronal section of the left temporal pole showing several necrotic foci at the corticosubcortical junction (arrows) (c, Klüver-Barrera/cresyl violet). At higher magnification one lesion shows the typical "target" pattern. Note the absence of inflammation (d, H&E).

criteria: (i) Patients with AIDS; (ii) efficiently treated by HAART; (iii) presenting symptoms consistent with an infectious or inflammatory condition that appeared while the patient was on ART; (iv) symptoms that could not be explained by a newly acquired infection, the expected course of a previously recognized infection or side effects of therapy [36]. In the CNS, IRIS caused paradoxical exacerbation of tuberculosis, cryptococcal infection, and CMV retinitis. In some patients with PML or HIVE, starting HAART led to onset or worsening of neurological signs, associated with contrast enhancement on magnetic resonance imaging (MRI), suggesting an unusually intense inflammation with impairment of the BBB (for review see [37]). Neuropathological studies confirmed intense inflammation with an influx of CD8+ lymphocytes (Figure 23.8) variably associated with an acute aggravation of the underlying infection (HIV or John Cunningham [JC] virus) and a nonspecific immunopathologic reaction similar to acute disseminated encephalomyelitis or multiple sclerosis. In most cases, IRIS correlates with prolonged survival, interpreted as a marker of both improved immune status and outcome; rarely, IRIS coincided with clinical and radiological deterioration and death [37].

HAART and HAND
Clinically, the impact of HAART on HAND is not straightforward. Although HAART has reduced the incidence of HAD, there is a continued and increasing prevalence of ANI and MND in patients who are efficiently treated. Most patients who continue to be virally suppressed remain stable, but some improve and a small number deteriorate (for review see [38]).

Animal models and pathogenesis

Animal models
Transgenic mice, rats, and rabbits expressing the proteins that are necessary for HIV-1 replication or HIV-1 proviruses have been generated, but their utility is limited. The best small-animal models for HIV and AIDS are based on "humanized mice," which are genetically immunocompromised mice engrafted with human tissues to reconstitute the human immune system. A mouse model using a chimeric virus with the HIV-1 genome with the substitution with the envelope of murine leukemia virus, to allow mice to be infected, has proved to be useful to study CNS disease, with regard to functional impairment [39].

Cats are not susceptible to HIV-1, but feline immunodeficiency virus (FIV) infection in domestic cats can serve as a surrogate model for human HIV-1 infection and has the advantage of being noninfectious to man. Infected cats develop behavioral abnormalities and the neuropathology resembles HAD. However, the cat FIV model has limitations and is not widely used.

Nonhuman primate models of AIDS and neuroAIDS are important to study CNS neuropathogenesis and HIV and the effects of ART. Asian macaques, particularly the rhesus macaque *(Macaca mulatta)*, the pig-tailed macaque *(Macaca nemestrina)*, and the cynomolgus macaque *(Macaca fascicularis)*, infected with SIV have become the most commonly used and widely accepted models for HIV/AIDS (for review see [40]).

Pathogenesis
The dramatic spread of the AIDS epidemic, which was invariably fatal before the introduction of effective treatment, generated enormous clinical and pathological research. This provided essential insights into the pathogenesis of CNS lesions and natural history of the disease [35]. However, there are still a number of unsolved issues.

The most puzzling is the precise mechanism of neuronal damage and the neuropathological changes underlying HAND.

Are neurons directly infected by HIV? This is controversial. Despite evidence that a number of cell types within the CNS appear to become infected, and that glial cells, particularly astrocytes, may provide a reservoir for HIV, in all these cell types, HIV establishes a persistent, rather than productive, infection. Within the CNS, HIV establishes a productive infection only in microglial cells and monocytes, which are the undisputed reservoir and source of transmission (for review see [35]).

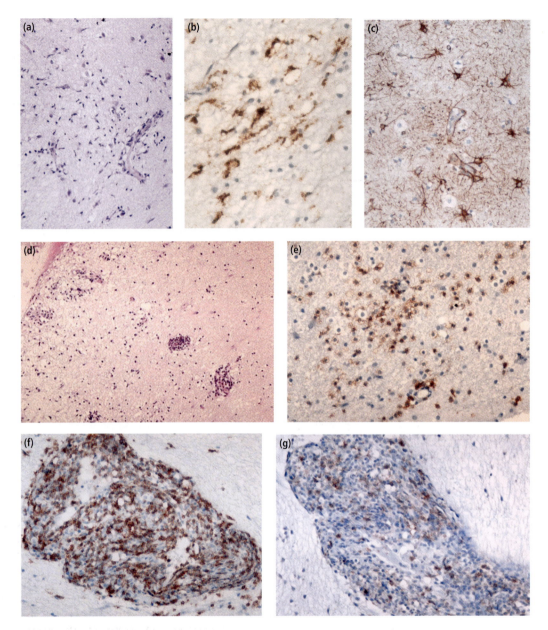

Figure 23.8 Encephalitic changes and CD8+ lymphocytic infiltration in brain biopsies of patients with immune reconstitution inflammatory syndrome (IRIS) [36]. (a) Rod cell microglial proliferation (hematoxylin and eosin [H&E]). (b) Microglial activation (HLA-DR immunostain). (c) Reactive astrocytic gliosis (glial fibrillary acidic protein [GFAP]). (d) Diffuse and perivascular lymphocytic infiltration (H&E). (e) Diffuse parenchymal infiltration by CD8+ lymphocytes (CD8 immunostain). (f and g) Massive perivascular and intramural "pseudo-lymphocytic" infiltration. The lymphocytes are predominantly CD8+ lymphocytes (f, CD8 immunostain), but there are also a few CD4+ lymphocytes (g, CD4 immunostain).

None of the HIV-induced CNS lesions can be regarded as the absolute pathological counterpart of HAND, although they are frequently found in patients with characteristic cognitive disorders (for review see [41]). Some cognitive disorders in treated patients are reversible; this, together with lack of improvement or even paradoxical deterioration of the neurological status in others, suggests that HAND is not the direct consequence of HIV infection of the CNS. More likely it reflects a specific neuronal dysfunction resulting from the combined effects of several neurotoxic factors. These include factors produced by HIV itself and substances produced by activated glial and microglial cells, perhaps mediated by oxidative stress and glutamate-mediated excitotoxicity [42, 43], some of which may be reversible.

It is clear that HAND relates to the different forms of HIV-induced neuropathology [41]. Indeed, the neuropathological changes may all result from the same mechanisms: HIVE reflects productive HIV infection, and HIVL is secondary to an alteration of the BBB resulting either from the effect of circulating factors or factors locally produced by activated macrophages. The same applies for axonal damage. Neuronal apoptosis and consequent DPD may result from the neurotoxicity of all of these combined factors or from axonal damage through retrograde degeneration. It is also possible that deafferentation of neurons may induce apoptosis in nerve cells. This hypothesis is supported by the description of synaptic and dendritic simplification in the brains of patients with AIDS with severe HAD [44] and in those with mild to moderate neurocognitive disorders [45].

The importance of the different factors can vary from one individual to another, resulting in variable histological features. This could explain why no single type of HIV-induced neuropathologies (i.e. HIVE, HIVL, or DPD), on its own, correlates with the cognitive impairment, although all these lesions are more frequent in patients with HAD.

Treatment, future perspective, and conclusions

In the absence of effective vaccination, preventive measures including education, HIV screening in the population and in blood donors, safe sex, use of needle-exchange programs, and prevention of mother-to-child transmission have been promoted and significantly reduced the incidence of HIV infection in specific risk groups.

HAART is the current standard treatment for HIV infection. It is a customized combination of different classes of antiretroviral agents, including nucleoside reverse transcriptase inhibitors (i.e. non-nucleoside reverse transcriptase inhibitors, protease inhibitors, integrase inhibitors, and entry inhibitors). The development of therapeutic vaccines as a strategy to safely eliminate or control viral reservoirs is under investigation.

Although HAART has changed the course of neurological complications of HIV infection, new problems have emerged such as the lack of improvement or even paradoxical deterioration of neurological status in treated patients. In some patients, HAND is becoming a chronic disease and remains a burden. Recent data must be interpreted as speculative because there are very few neuropathological studies related to the beneficial consequences of HAART. There is still a need for new and more effective therapies. Future studies should focus on effective delivery of drugs to the CNS compartment, suppression of viral replication in the CNS, reduction of drug toxicity, and new approaches to reduce HIV-associated neuroinflammation [38].

References

1. Barré-Sinoussi, F., Cherman, J.C., Rey, F. et al. (1983). Isolation of T-lymphotropic retrovirus from a patient at risk for acquired immune deficiency syndrome. *Science* 220: 868–871.
2. Popovic, M., Sarngadharan, M.G., Read, E., and Gallo, R.C. (1984). Detection, isolation and continuous production of cytopathic retrovirus (HTLV-III) from patients with AIDS and pre-AIDS. *Science* 224: 497–500.
3. Coffin, J., Haase, A., Levy, J.A. et al. (1986). What to call the AIDS virus? *Nature* 321: 10.
4. Snider, W.D., Simpson, D.M., Nielsen, S. et al. (1983). Neurological complications of acquired immune deficiency syndrome: analysis of 50 patients. *Ann. Neurol.* 14: 403–418.

5. Gray, F. (ed.) (1993). *Atlas of the Neuropathology of HIV Infection*, 290. Oxford, New York, Tokyo: Oxford University Press.
6. Gray, F., Chretien, F., Vallat-Decouvelaere, A.V., and Scaravilli, F. (2003). The changing pattern of HIV neuropathology in the HAART era. *J. Neuropathol. Exp. Neurol.* 62: 429–440.
7. Weiss, R. (1985). Human T-cell retroviruses. In: *RNA Tumor Viruses*, Supplements and Appendices, 2e, vol. 2 (eds. R. Weiss, N. Teich, H. Varmus and J. Coffin), 405–485. New York: Cold Spring Harbor Laboratory.
8. Pépin, J. (2013). The origins of AIDS: from patient zero to ground zero. *J. Epidemiol. Community Health* 67: 473–475.
9. ONUSIDA (2016). le rapport pour l'année 2016. http://www.francetvinfo.fr/sante/sida/onusida-le-rapport-pour-l-annee-2016_2292151.html (accessed 17 July 2019).
10. Davis, L.E., Hjelle, B.L., Miller, V.E. et al. (1992). Early viral brain invasion in iatrogenic human immunodeficiency infection. *Neurology* 42: 1736–1719.
11. Gray, F., Chimelli, L., Mohr, M. et al. (1991). Fulminating multiple sclerosis-like leukoencephalopathy revealing human immunodeficiency virus infection. *Neurology* 41: 105–109.
12. Ferrada, M.A., Xie, Y., and Nuermberger, E. (2015). Primary HIV infection presenting as limbic encephalitis and rhabdomyolysis. *Int. J. STD AIDS* 26: 835–836.
13. Chiodi, F., Keys, B., Albert, J. et al. (1992). Human immunodeficiency virus type 1 is present in the cerebrospinal fluid of a majority of infected individuals. *J. Clin. Mocrobiol.* 30: 1768–1771.
14. Post, M.J.D., Berger, J.R., Duncan, R. et al. (1993). Asymptomatic and neurologically symptomatic HIV seropositive subjects: results of a long term MR imaging and clinical follow-up. *Radiology* 188: 727–733.
15. Gray, F., Scaravilli, F., Everall, I. et al. (1996). Neuropathology of early HIV infection. *Brain Pathol.* 6 (1): 1–15.
16. Janssen, R.S., Cornblath, D.R., Epstein, L.G. et al. (1991). Nomenclature and research case definition for neurological manifestations of human immunodeficiency virus type −1 (HIV-1) infection. Report of a working group of the American Academy of Neurology AIDS Task Force. *Neurology* 41: 778–785.
17. Sharer, L.R., Cho, E.-S., and Epstein, L.G. (1985). Multinucleated giant cells and HTLV-III in AIDS encephalopathy. *Hum. Pathol.* 16: 760.
18. Budka, H. (1986). Multinucleated giant cells in brain: a hallmark of the acquired immune deficiency syndrome (AIDS). *Acta Neuropathol.* 69: 253–258.
19. Kleihues, P., Lang, W., Burger, P.C. et al. (1985). Progressive diffuse leukoencephalopathy in patients with acquired immune deficiency syndrome (AIDS). *Acta Neuropathol.* 68: 333–339.
20. Smith, T.W., De Girolami, U., Hénin, D. et al. (1990). Human immunodeficiency virus (HIV) leukoencephalopathy and the microcirculation. *J. Neuropathol. Exp. Neurol.* 49: 357–370.
21. Power, C., Kong, P.A., Crawford TO et al. (1993). Cerebral white matter changes in acquired immunodeficiency syndrome dementia: alterations of the blood-brain-barrier. *Ann. Neurol.* 34: 339–350.
22. Boven, L.A., Middle, J., Verhoef, J. et al. (2000). Monocyte infiltration is highly associated with loss of the tight junction protein zonula occludens in HIV-a-associated dementia. *Neuropathol. Appl. Neurobiol.* 26: 356–360.
23. Giometto, B., An, S.F., Groves, M. et al. (1997). Accumulation of beta-amyloid precursor protein in HIV encephalitis: relationship with neurophysiological abnormalities. *Ann. Neurol.* 42: 34–40.
24. Budka, H., Costanzi, G., Cristina, S. et al. (1987). Brain pathology induced by the infection with the human immunodeficiency virus (AIDS). *Acta Neuropathol.* 75: 186–198.
25. Everall, I.P., Luthert, P., and Lantos, P.L. (1993). A review of neuronal damage in human immunodeficiency virus infection: its assessment, possible mechanism and relationship to dementia. *J. Neuropathol. Exp. Neurol.* 52: 561–556.
26. Adle-Biassette, H., Levy, Y., Colombel, M. et al. (1995). Neuronal apoptosis in HIV infection in adults. *Neuropathol. Appl. Neurobiol.* 21: 218–227.
27. Epstein, L.G., DiCarlo, F.J., Joshi, V.V. et al. (1988). Primary lymphoma of the central nervous system in children with acquired immunodeficiency syndrome. *Pediatrics* 82: 355–363.
28. Davtyan, D.G. and Vinters, H.V. (1987). Wernicke's encephalopathy in AIDS patient treated with zidovudine. *Lancet* 1 (8538): 919–920.
29. Petito, C.K., Navia, B.A., Cho, E.-S. et al. (1985). Vacuolar myelopathy pathologically resembling subacute combined degeneration in patients with acquired immunodeficiency syndrome. *N. Engl. J. Med.* 312: 874–879.
30. Maier, H., Budka, H., Lassmann, H., and Pohl, P. (1989). Vacuolar myelopathy with multinucleated giant cells in the acquired immunodeficiency syndrome (AIDS). Light and electron microscopic dis-

tribution of the human immunodeficiency virus (HIV) antigens. *Acta Neuropathol.* 78: 497–503.
31. Petito, C.K., Vecchio, D., and Chen, Y.T. (1994). HIV antigen and DNA in AIDS spinal cords correlate with macrophage infiltration but not with vacuolar myelopathy. *J. Neuropathol. Exp. Neurol.* 53: 86–94.
32. Di Rocco, A., Bottiglieri, T., Werner, P. et al. (2002). Abnormal cobalamin-dependent transmethylation in AIDS-associated myelopathy. *Neurology* 58: 730–735.
33. Vinters, H.V., Anders, K.H., and Barach, P. (1987). Focal pontine leukoencephalopathy in immunosuppressed patients. *Arch. Pathol. Lab. Med.* 111: 192–196.
34. D'Arminio Monforte, A., Duca, P.G., Vago, L. et al. (2000). Decreasing incidence of CNS AIDS defining events associated with antiretroviral therapy. *Neurology* 54: 1856–1859.
35. Scaravilli, F., Bazille, C., and Gray, F. (2007). Neuropathologic contributions to understanding AIDS and the central nervous system. *Brain Pathol.* 17: 197–208.
36. Shelburne, S.A. 3rd, Hamill, R.J., Rodriguez-Barradas, M.C. et al. (2002). Immune reconstitution inflammatory syndrome: emergence of a unique syndrome during highly active antiretroviral therapy. *Medicine* 81: 213–227.
37. Gray, F., Lescure, F.X., Adle-Biassette, H. et al. (2013). Encephalitis with infiltration by CD8+ lymphocytes in HIV patients receiving combination antiretroviral treatment. *Brain Pathol.* 23: 525–533.
38. Carroll, A. and Brew, B. (2017). HIV-associated neurocognitive disorders: recent advances in pathogenesis, biomarkers, and treatment. *F1000Res.* 6: 312.
39. Potash, M.J., Chao, W., Bentsman, G. et al. (2005). A mouse model for study of systemic HIV-1 infection, antiviral immune responses, and neuroinvasiveness. *Proc. Natl. Acad. Sci. U.S.A.* 102: 3760–3765.
40. Williams, K., Lackner, A., and Mallard, J. (2016). Non-human primate models of SIV infection and CNS neuropathology. *Curr. Opin. Virol.* 19: 92–98.
41. Gray, F., Adle-Biassette, H., Chretien, F. et al. (2001). Neuropathology and neurodegeneration in human immunodeficiency virus infection. Pathogenesis of HIV-induced lesions of the brain, correlations with HIV associated disorders and modifications according to treatment. *Clin. Neuropathol.* 20: 146–145.
42. Kaul, M., Garden, G.A., and Lipton, S.A. (2001). Pathways to neuronal injury and apoptosis in HIV associated dementia. *Nature* 410: 988–994.
43. Vallat-Decouvelaere, A.V., Chrétien, F., Gras, G. et al. (2003). Expression of excitatory amino acid-transporter-1 in brain macrophages and microglia of HIV patients. A neuroprotective role for microglia? *J. Neuropathol. Exp. Neurol.* 62: 475–485.
44. Masliah, E., Eaton, R.K., Marcotte, T.D. et al. (1997). Dendritic injury is a pathological substrate for human immunodeficiency virus-related cognitive disorders. HNRC group. The HIV neurobehavioral research center. *Ann. Neurol.* 42: 963–972.
45. Everall, I.P., Heaton, R.K., Marcotte, T.D. et al. (1999). Cortical synaptic density is reduced in mild to moderate human immunodeficiency virus neurocognitive disorder. HNRC group. HIV neurobehavioral research center. *Brain Pathol.* 9: 209–217.

24 HTLV-1 and Neurological-Associated Disease

Antoine Gessain[1,2], Olivier Cassar[1,2], and Philippe V. Afonso[1]

[1] Oncogenic Virus Epidemiology and Pathophysiology, Department of Virology, Pasteur Institute, Paris, France
[2] CNRS, UMR3569, Paris, France

Abbreviations

ATLL	adult T-cell leukemia/lymphoma
ATLV	adult T-cell leukemia/lymphoma virus (ATLV)
BBB	blood-brain barrier
BLV	bovine leukemia virus
CNS	central nervous system
CSF	cerebrospinal fluid
CT scan	computed tomography scan
DNA	deoxyribose nucleic acid
GLUT-1	glucose transporter 1
HAM	HTLV-1 associated myelopathy (HAM)
HAM/TSP	HTLV-1 associated myelopathy/tropical spastic paraparesis
HBZ	HTLV-1 basic zipper factor
HSPG	heparan sulfate proteoglycan
HTLV-1	human T-cell leukemia/lymphoma virus type 1
LTR	long terminal repeat
MRI	magnetic resonance imaging
NRP1	neuropilin 1
ORF	open reading frame
PCR	polymerase chain reaction
PET	positron emission tomography
PTLVs	T-lymphotropic viruses that infect primates
PVL	proviral load
RNA	ribonucleic acid
SNP	single nucleotide polymorphism
STLV	Simian T-lymphotropic virus
TSP	tropical spastic paraparesis
TSP/HAM	tropical spastic paraparesis/HTLV-1 associated myelopathy

Infections of the Central Nervous System: Pathology and Genetics, First Edition. Edited by Fabrice Chrétien, Kum Thong Wong, Leroy R. Sharer, Catherine (Katy) Keohane and Françoise Gray.
© 2020 John Wiley & Sons Ltd. Published 2020 by John Wiley & Sons Ltd.

Definition of the disorder, major synonyms, and historical perspective

In 1980, a team at the National Institutes of Health headed by Dr. RC Gallo, reported the isolation of the first human oncoretrovirus [1]. It was present in peripheral blood cells of an African American patient suffering from a T lymphoproliferative disease, originally considered to be a cutaneous T-cell lymphoma with a leukemic phase. The virus was named human T-cell leukemia/lymphoma virus (HTLV). In 1981, a virus, called adult T-cell leukemia/lymphoma virus (ATLV) was isolated in Japan from an adult T-cell leukemia/lymphoma (ATLL), a severe T-cell lymphoproliferative disorder originally described in Japan in 1977 [2]. Later, it was recognized that the so-called cutaneous lymphoma was actually an ATLL, and Japanese and American scientists rapidly demonstrated that both isolates were the same virus and agreed to name it HTLV-1 [3].

In 1983, a French team of virologists, epidemiologists, and neurologists demonstrated the association of HTLV-1 with a chronic neuromyelopathy, endemic in the Caribbean and originally called tropical spastic paraparesis (TSP) [4, 5]. This association was quickly confirmed in Colombia and Jamaica [6]. A year later, the association of HTLV-1 with a chronic spastic myelopathy of unknown etiology was also documented in southern Japan; the clinical entity was named HTLV-1–associated myelopathy (HAM) [7]. Soon after, it was recognized that TSP and HAM were the same disease [8], and the hybrid terms TSP/HAM or HAM/TSP were adopted. The etiological link between TSP/HAM and HTLV-1 was further demonstrated when the disease rapidly developed following viral transmission through contaminated blood in France, Japan, and the United States [9, 10].

Later, HTLV-1 infection was also linked with other inflammatory conditions, including infective dermatitis and certain forms of uveitis, myositis, and pulmonary disorders (Table 24.1).

Microbiological characteristics of HTLV-1

HTLV-1 belongs to the *Retroviridae* family, the *Orthoretrovirinae* subfamily, and the *Deltaretrovirus* genus, which includes bovine leukemia virus (BLV) and T-lymphotropic viruses that infect primates (PTLVs). PTLVs comprise simian T-lymphotropic viruses (STLVs) types 1–4,

Table 24.1 HTLV-1-associated diseases.

Diseases	Association
Adulthood	
Adult T-cell leukemia/lymphoma (ATLL)	++++
Tropical spastic paraparesis/HTLV-1–associated myelopathy (TSP/HAM)	++++
Intermediate uveitis (Japan/Caribbean)	+++
Myositis (polymyositis and SIBM)	+++
Infective dermatitis (very rare)	+++
HTLV-1–associated arthritis (Japan)	++
Bronchiectasis (Central Australia)	++
Childhood	
Infective dermatitis (Jamaica/Brazil/Africa)	++++
TSP/HAM (very rare)	++++
ATLL (very rare)	++++

The strength of association is based on epidemiological studies as well as molecular data, animal models, and intervention trials.
++++, proven association; +++, probable association; ++: likely association.
HTLV-1, human T-cell leukemia/lymphoma virus-1; SIBM, sporadic inclusion body myositis.

which infect nonhuman primates (NHPs), and human T-lymphotropic viruses type 1–4.

Retroviruses are enveloped viruses with an average diameter of 110 nm (Figure 24.1). The envelope consists of a lipid bilayer incorporating the viral envelope glycoproteins. The envelope surrounds matrix proteins and a capsid of icosahedral symmetry. The capsid contains a diploid, single-stranded, positive-polarity RNA. The genomic organization of HTLV-1 is typical of retroviruses. The genome is approximately 9 kb in size and is flanked by two long terminal repeat (LTR) regions. LTRs contain the viral promoters. The region between the two LTRs includes 10 overlapping open reading frames (ORFs). Some correspond to the canonical retroviral genes: *gag* encodes the nucleocapsid, capsid, and matrix; *pro* and *pol* encode the enzymes necessary for nucleic acid manipulation (i.e. reverse transcriptase, which synthesizes double-stranded deoxyribose nucleic acid [DNA] from viral RNA) and integrase; and *env* gene encodes the two subunits of the virus envelope protein. The pX region, located between the *env* gene and the 3′ LTR, contains additional ORFs, which encode the regulatory genes *tax* and *rex*. Thus, HTLV-1 is considered to be a "complex" retrovirus. The pX region also encodes auxiliary proteins (p8/p12, p13, and p30), which are not fully required for *in vitro* replication but are necessary for persistence in vivo. Finally, the anti-sense strand of the genome encodes a regulatory protein called HTLV-1 basic zipper factor (HBZ), which is a negative regulator of viral transcription. Tax and HBZ both have oncogenic properties [11–14].

The replication cycle of the virus can be divided into two major phases. During the early phase, the viral envelope protein interacts with the receptor complex located on the surface of target cells, composed of a ternary complex consisting of glucose transporter 1 (GLUT-1), neuropilin 1 (NRP1), and heparan sulfate proteoglycan (HSPG) [15]. This step allows fusion of the viral and cellular membranes and internalization of the viral capsid. The viral RNA genome is retrotranscribed, accesses the nucleus, and is integrated as a provirus, into the host-cell DNA through the action of viral integrase. During the late phase, the provirus is transcribed. Initially, basal transcription takes place and fully spliced mRNA, encoding Tax and Rex, is synthesized. Tax is the viral transactivator and increases transcription. Rex interacts with viral mRNA and allows nonfully spliced RNA, encoding the structural proteins, to reach the cytoplasm. The structural proteins assemble and the virus buds at the plasma membrane. Cell-free virus particles are generally undetectable in vivo and transfusion of leuko-reduced blood products is not responsible for HTLV-1 transmission.

HTLV-1 is mainly transmitted during close contact between an infected cell and a target cell, through viral synapse, viral conduits, or biofilms [15]. Except during the primo-infection phase, the virus appears to propagate mostly by clonal expansion of infected lymphocytes rather than the production of new virions. Some clones can be followed for up to a decade in an individual. Despite a vigorous cellular and humoral immune response, HTLV-1 is never eliminated from the infected host.

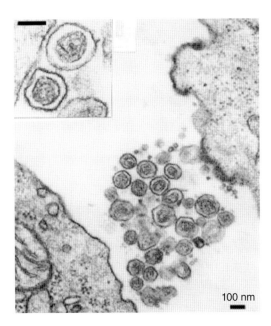

Figure 24.1 Electron microscopy of human T-cell leukemia/lymphoma virus-1 (HTLV-1) virus particles. Retroviral particles in the extracellular compartment of a HTLV-1 producing line established from long-term culture of lymphocytes from the peripheral blood of a patient with tropical spastic paraparesis/HTLV-1–associated myelopathy (TSP/HAM).

Epidemiology

Epidemiology of HTLV-1

HTLV-1 is not ubiquitous. Although it is present throughout the world, highly endemic clusters are located near areas where the virus is almost absent [16]. In endemic clusters, HTLV-1 seroprevalence in adults is higher than 1–2%; it can reach 20–40% in people older than 50 years of age in some regions. The areas of highest prevalence are southwestern Japan, parts of the Caribbean and surroundings regions, foci in South America, particularly in Colombia and French Guyana, parts of intertropical Africa (such as southern Gabon) and the Middle East (such as the Mashhad region in Iran), and some isolated groups in Australo-Melanesia (aboriginal people living in Central Australia). In Europe, only Romania appears to have an endemic region for HTLV-1 (Figure 24.2) [16]. The explanation for this puzzling geographical and ethnic distribution is not known but is probably linked to a founder effect associated with local traditional or environmental factors favoring high viral transmission in these populations.

HTLV-1 seroprevalence gradually increases with age, especially among women, in all highly endemic areas. The current estimate of individuals infected with HTLV-1 worldwide is at least 5–10 million [16]. This is probably an underestimate because it is based on only 1.5 billion people living in known endemic areas. The situation in densely populated regions such as China, India, and North and East Africa is still largely unknown.

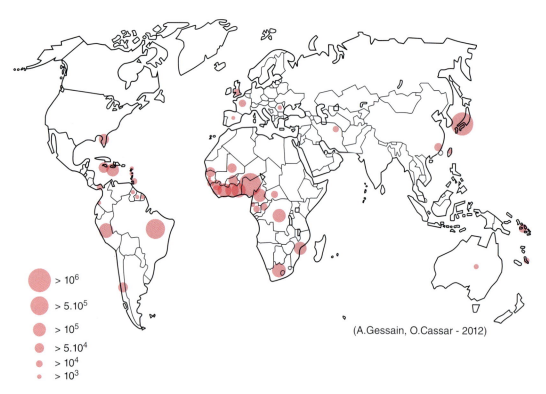

Figure 24.2 Estimates of the number of carriers infected with human T-cell leukemia/lymphoma virus-1 (HTLV-1) (Source: reproduced from [16]). Geographical distribution of the main sites of HTLV-1 infection. Estimates of the number of carriers with HTLV-1, based on approximately 1.5 billion individuals from known endemic areas and reliable epidemiological data from studies among pregnant women, blood donors, or different adult populations. In a few countries, HTLV-1 endemic areas are limited to certain regions such as Mashhad in Iran, the Fujian Province in China, Tumaco in Colombia, and Alice Springs in Central Australia.

Three modes of transmission between humans have been demonstrated for HTLV-1.

1. Mother-to-child transmission occurs mainly during breastfeeding. Indeed, 10–25% of children who are breastfed by mothers infected with HTLV-1 will become infected. A high HTLV-1 proviral load in milk or blood, high HTLV-1 antibody titers in serum, and long breastfeeding period (>6 months) are major risk factors for mother-to-child transmission.

2. Sexual transmission occurs mainly (but not exclusively) from men to women and may explain the higher seroprevalence among women and its increase with age [17].

3. Transmission by contaminated blood products (containing HTLV-1–infected lymphocytes) is responsible for acquired HTLV-1 infection in a high proportion (15–60%) of blood recipients. Organ transplantation (i.e. kidney, liver, heart) has also resulted in transmission [18]. HTLV-1 infection is also present among intravenous drug users, although to a lesser extent than HTLV-2 infection. Zoonotic acquisition of STLV-1, the simian counterpart of HTLV-1, also occurs in central and West Africa. This has been reported mainly in male hunters who were severely bitten by NHPs [19].

From a molecular viewpoint, HTLV-1 exhibits remarkable genetic stability, an unusual feature among retroviruses. Viral spread by clonal expansion of infected cells (rather than neo-infection) may explain this striking genetic stability. The low sequence variation of HTLV-1 and its limited transmission within a given population can be used as molecular tools to monitor migrations of infected populations in the recent or distant past [20]. Therefore, the few nucleotide substitutions observed among viral strains are often specific to the patients' geographical origin, rather than to the pathology.

Four major geographical subtypes (genotypes) have been reported: the cosmopolitan a-subtype, the Central African b-subtype, the Central African/Pygmies d-subtype, and the Australo-Melanesian c-subtype (Figure 24.3). A limited number of strains present in central Africa belong to other rare subtypes (e, f, g). The cosmopolitan a-subtype is the most widespread and is found in Japan, the Caribbean, Central and South America, north and west Africa, and part of the Middle East. In this subtype, sequences are often grouped into geographical subgroups. The sequence variability within a-subtype is very low and probably reflects relatively recent dissemination (a few centuries to a few millennia) of this genotype by a common ancestor. The Australo-Melanesian c-subtype is the most divergent. This reflects a long period of evolution (at least several millennia) in isolated populations living in different Pacific-zone islands [16, 21, 22]. To date, there is no evidence that specific mutations or genotypes are associated with the development of TSP/HAM or ATLL.

Epidemiology of TSP/HAM

As expected, many cases of TSP/HAM have been reported in areas endemic with HTLV-1, including Japan, the Caribbean islands (especially Jamaica, Trinidad and Tobago, and Martinique), South and Central American countries (Brazil, Peru, and Colombia), and central and South Africa, as well as Iran. In addition, several TSP/HAM cases have also been described in Australo-Melanesia, north and west African countries, Romania, and among immigrants from HTLV-1- endemic areas living in Europe (mainly in France and the United Kingdom) and in the United States. It is difficult to estimate the true prevalence of TSP/HAM. Studies in Brazil, some African countries, and French Guiana concluded that the prevalence of TSP/HAM will remain underestimated until a study specifically designed to determine its prevalence is conducted. Diagnosis (especially in mild and early cases) is difficult and can be confused with similar neuromyelopathy of other cause. Laboratory tests, such as HTLV-1 Western blot, and molecular tests, such as polymerase chain reaction (PCR), are not always available in endemic countries and remote areas. In Japan, with approximately one million people infected with HTLV-1, a TSP/HAM registry has been set up, and more than 450 cases have been reported. The authors speculate that approximately 2000–2500 people in Japan suffer from TSP/HAM [23]. The lifetime risk of developing TSP/HAM in HTLV-1 carriers is estimated at 0.25–4%, depending on the endemic area.

The incidence of TSP/HAM appears to be higher in the Caribbean and South America than in

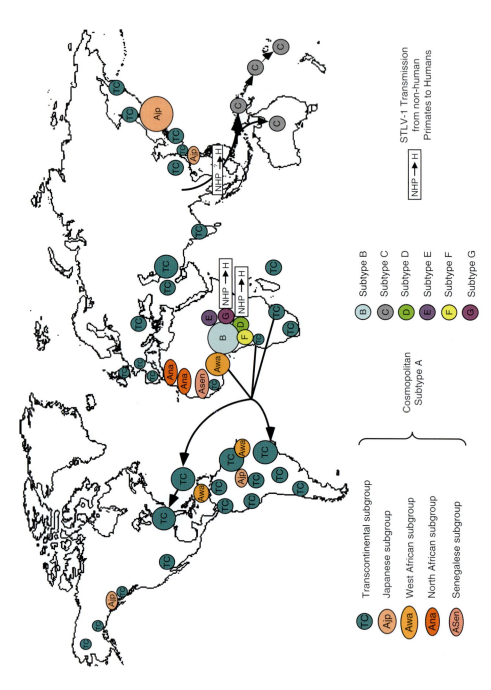

Figure 24.3 Geographical distribution of the seven main molecular subtypes of human T-cell leukemia/lymphoma virus-1 (HTLV-1, A–G) and major pathways for its spread through the movements of infected populations. Arrows indicate the likely interspecies transmission of Simian T-lymphotropic virus-1 (STLV-1) from nonhuman primates (NHPs) to humans (H) as the source for some current HTLV-1 subtypes. The main subtypes include the Cosmopolitan subtype A with its different subgroups, TC (transcontinental, the most frequent and widespread), Ajp (Japanese), Awa (West Africa), Ana (North Africa), Sen (Senegal); the Central African subtype B (the most frequent in this large endemic area), the Australo-Melanesian subtype C; the subtype D also from Central Africa and present mainly in certain Pygmy groups; and subtypes E, F, and G with very few strains yet reported, all in Central Africa.

southern Japan. The situation is less clear in Africa. Although the risk of developing TSP/HAM appears lower than that of ATLL, the disease burden of TSP/HAM in some areas can be higher because of its long progressive evolution. TSP/HAM occurs mainly in adults, with an average age of onset of 40–50 years. Some cases have occurred in children, particularly in Peru and Brazil [24, 25]. In contrast to ATLL (male-to-female ratio = 1.4), TSP/HAM occurs more frequently in women (male-to-female ratio = 0.4).

Sexually acquired infection seems more strongly associated with TSP/HAM than other modes of viral acquisition. Acquisition of the virus by blood transfusion can also promote development of TSP/HAM. In a case-control study in Japan, more patients with TSP/HAM reported a history of blood transfusion (20%) than controls (3–5%) [26]. In the first two years following HTLV-1 screening in blood donors in Japan, the number of TSP/HAM cases reported decreased by 16%. In Peru, Martinique, and Brazil, 20–30% of patients with TSP/HAM reported a blood transfusion [27], and several posttransfusion TSP/HAM cases have been documented in France and the United States, with molecular evidence linking donor and recipient [9, 10]. Infection by organ transplantation also appears to favor development of TSP/HAM. The incubation period between the primary infection (which occurs mainly in adults) and the onset of myelopathy signs ranges from a few years to several decades, but TSP/HAM developed in 3.3 years in 50% of post-transfusion–associated cases [26].

The proviral load (PVL) is the most important predictor of the development of TSP/HAM. PVL load is measured by the number of copies of HTLV-1 DNA per mononuclear cell in peripheral blood [28]. Patients with TSP/HAM have a high PVL (>1%) and the incidence increases exponentially with PVL. However, few HTLV-1 carriers with high PVL will develop TSP/HAM. Furthermore, monitoring PVL levels in asymptomatic carriers infected with HTLV-1 did not appear to help predict the development of TSP/HAM in a prospective study, and changes in clinical status did not coincide with significant changes in peripheral blood PVL [29].

Sporadic TSP/HAM is the most common form. Family groups of patients with TSP/HAM have been described, suggesting host genetic susceptibility factors such as HLA genotype (which modifies the immune response) [30]. A protective effect of the class 1 allele HLA-A*02 has been reported, but HLA-DRB1*0101 and HLA-B*07 are associated with a higher risk of TSP/HAM. Similarly, a series of single nucleotide polymorphisms (SNPs) within the promoter of cytokine-encoding genes (e.g. interleukin (IL)-6, IL-10, tumor necrosis factor [TNF]) are also associated with TSP/HAM.

Clinical features of TSP/HAM

The initial diagnostic criteria for TSP/HAM established in Martinique in 1984 included: (i) chronic spastic paraparesis, usually slowly progressive with bilateral pyramidal tract signs manifested by increased patellar reflexes, ankle clonus, and extensor plantar responses; (ii) minor sensory signs of posterior column and spinothalamic tract damage; (iii) a history of insidious onset with gait disturbance without an episode of complete remission; (iv) absence of compression or swelling of the spinal cord on magnetic resonance imaging (MRI), myelography, or computed tomography (CT) scan; or (v) the presence of anti-HTLV-1 antibodies in serum or plasma and cerebrospinal fluid (CSF) [4, 5].

World Health Organization (WHO) criteria were defined in 1989, but the WHO criteria are rarely met during the early stages of the disease. In 2006, a large group of neurologists proposed modifying the diagnostic criteria of TSP/HAM [31]. They suggested that a specific case of TSP/HAM should correspond to non-remitting progressive spastic paraparesis with a gait sufficiently altered to be perceived by the patient. Symptoms or sensory signs may be present. When present, they remain subtle and without a precise sensory level. Urinary and anal sphincter signs or symptoms may or may not be present [31, 32]. The disease onset is often insidious, and the main symptoms reported are lower limb weakness, lumbar pain, and sensory and urinary disorders (i.e. nocturia and urinary loss). Generally, the disease progresses, with an increase in disability without remission. Rapidly and slowly progressive groups have been characterized: cases progressing to severe paraplegia in less than two years have been reported post transplantation and transfusion. The mean age at disease onset is older in patients with rapid progression than those with slow progression. After years of evolution, the neurological characteristics of TSP/HAM are lower limb spasticity or hyperreflexia, urinary bladder disturbances such as nocturia, urgency, frequency, and infections, often associated with lower limb muscle weakness, sensory disturbances, and low back pain. Constipation and impotence are also frequent. Central functions and cranial nerves are generally spared. Approximately 50% of patients require a wheelchair after 15–20 years of evolution. For a review of the clinical aspects, see [32–34]. Although the disease is not directly life threatening, a report in Martinique showed that life expectancy is considerably reduced [35].

Cerebral MRI of patients with TSP/HAM most often reveals multiple high intensities in the periventricular and subcortical white matter, and these are also common in asymptomatic carriers with HTLV-1. One study reported that the number, size, and location of lesions were no different between carriers and patients with TSP/HAM [36]. In some cases white matter lesions may be indistinguishable from other demyelinating disorders. MRI may show slight atrophy of the thoracic spinal cord in patients who have had TSP/HAM for many years.

Combined clinical and biological features facilitate the diagnosis of TSP/HAM. High levels of anti-HTLV antibodies are present in both blood (i.e. plasma and serum) and CSF. Intrathecal production of HTLV-1 antibody provides additional support for the diagnosis. Patients often have mild lymphocytic pleocytosis (usually no more than 50 cells/mm^3), and ATLL-like cells (flower cells) can sometimes be detected in the blood smear. PVL may be considered as a marker of disease progression: PVL is higher in patients with rapid progression than in those with slow progression. Lastly, other differential diagnoses must be excluded [37].

Pathology and pathogenesis

The pathology of TSP/HAM is characterized by chronic inflammation with perivascular lymphocyte cuffs and mild parenchymal lymphocytic infiltrates, foamy macrophages, astrocyte proliferation, and fibrillary gliosis [38] (Figure 24.4). Pyramidal tract lesions with myelin and axonal loss are also observed, mainly in the lower thoracic spinal cord.

Neurodegeneration is linked to inflammatory foci in the CNS, which can be detected early in the disease (and even in some asymptomatic cases) by positron emission tomography (PET) scan. Inflammatory infiltrates are essentially composed of T lymphocytes. CD4$^+$ T-cells are predominant in early active lesions. The proportion of CD8$^+$ T-cells (and macrophages) then gradually increases in areas where astrocyte gliosis and vascular fibrosis are observed.

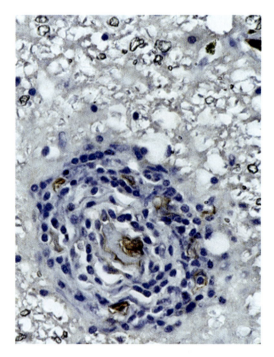

Figure 24.4 Section of thoracic spinal cord of a patient with tropical spastic paraparesis/HTLV-1–associated myelopathy (TSP/HAM). Perivascular infiltration by CD4 lymphocytes infected with human T-cell leukemia/lymphoma virus-1 (HTLV-1) in a paraffin section of the thoracic spinal cord from a patient with TSP/HAM. Immunostain (DAB substrate, brown). Nuclei were counterstained with Harris hematoxylin (blue). Magnification: 75 ×.

The first cells to enter the CNS are CD4+ T lymphocytes infected with HTLV-1; these become capable of overcoming the blood-brain barrier (BBB). Infected lymphocytes (i) have increased adhesion capacity, (ii) secrete inflammatory factors that can disrupt the tight junctions that seal the BBB endothelium, and (iii) overexpress molecules (e.g. ALCAM, JAM-A) that promote transmigration. Within the CNS, infected lymphocytes can then activate astrocytes by secreting interferon gamma (IFN-γ) and tumor necrosis factor alpha (TNF-α) and induce astrocytic CXCL10 secretion, which acts as a chemotactic signal for the recruitment of CXCR3+ leukocytes into the CNS [33, 39, 40].

Although mononuclear infiltrates may be found in many CNS regions, perivascular infiltrates are mostly present in the upper thoracic spinal cord, where demyelination and axonal lesions are the most severe. The reasons for such localized infiltration are not clear. Endothelial cells may locally express various surface molecules or develop weaker tight junctions. Local astrocytes may be more inclined to secrete CXCL10. Some have suggested that local blood flow is slower, promoting interactions between infected cells and the endothelium.

Although the mechanisms linking infiltration to neurodegeneration are still uncertain, three have been proposed [33] (Figure 24.5).

The first is the cytotoxic model. Patients with TSP/HAM have an abundance of activated anti-HTLV cytotoxic lymphocytes (CTLs) (mostly directed against the Tax protein), but neurons and glial cells can still be infected with HTLV-1 *in vitro* but there is no strong direct evidence of such infection *in vivo*. It has been proposed that neural tissue is infected by infiltrating infected cells and that CTLs then lyse the neural cells. However, this would require massive infection of nervous tissue, which seems unlikely.

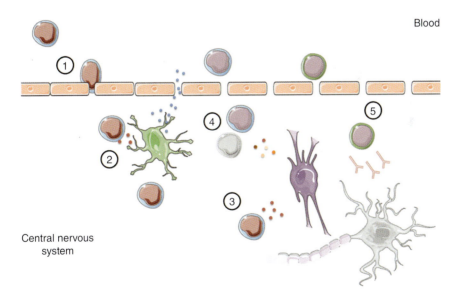

Figure 24.5 Proposed tropical spastic paraparesis/HTLV-1–associated myelopathy (TSP/HAM) pathogenesis. Human T-cell leukemia/lymphoma virus-1 (HTLV-1)-infected lymphocytes (red nuclei) disrupt and cross the endothelial blood-brain barrier (BBB) (1). Infected lymphocytes secrete IFNγ. In response, astrocytes (in green) secrete CXCL10 (2). CXCL10 is a chemoattractant facilitating recruitment of T-cells (blue) and B cells (green) into the CNS. Infected lymphocytes secrete a range of inflammatory cytokines, and soluble viral Tax protein. These induce cellular stress in glial cells, especially oligodendrocytes (3). In the CNS, infected cells may be lysed directly by anti-HTLV cytotoxic lymphocytes (CTLs), with resulting release of cellular factors that also induce stress on glial cells (4). Inflammation leads to oligodendrocyte cell death, demyelination, and neuronal death. In addition, B-lymphocytes secrete anti-Tax antibodies, which cross-react with neural proteins (such as hnRNP-A1) (5). This may also contribute directly to neuronal death. *This figure was generated using drawings from Servier Medical Art.*

The second model involves autoimmunity. Anti-HTLV-1 antibody titer is high in patients with TSP/HAM and antibodies against Tax have been detected in CSF. Anti-Tax antibodies have also been shown to interact with neural proteins, such as hnRNP-A1, a specific glial antigen. It has been proposed that the anti-HTLV response could generate antibody-mediated autoimmune damage in TSP/HAM because of molecular mimicry. Antibodies specific to hnRNPA1 in CSF do not appear specific to TSP/HAM and may be a more generic marker of neurodegenerative diseases.

The third model involves bystander toxicity. HTLV-1-infected lymphocytes secrete a wide range of factors such as inflammatory cytokines (TNF-α, IL-6), IFN-γ, and Tax protein (either soluble or within exosomes) that can be detrimental to nervous system cells. In addition, the intrathecal immune response against infiltrated HTLV-1-infected lymphocytes can lead to the release of factors toxic to neural cells. Together, these elements would stress glial cells and induce demyelination and neuronal loss [33, 40].

The absence of a good animal model hinders efforts to understand the pathogenesis.

Treatment

Curative treatment

The treatment of TSP/HAM is largely symptomatic, and there is currently no disease-modifying therapy with a known long-term clinical benefit. In general, two therapeutic strategies have been tested.

First, immunosuppressive therapy should hypothetically limit disease progression, especially in the early stages. Corticosteroids have been extensively used, and although general improvement has been reported in some cases, it has never been sustained. Interferon alpha has also been commonly prescribed, particularly in Japan but without evidence of efficacy.

Second, therapies to reduce PVL have also been explored. Conventional antiviral drugs (i.e. zidovudine, lamivudine, tenofovir,) had little effect on PVL in vivo. A strategy called "kick and kill" has also been tested. It consists of promoting HTLV expression (using histone deacetylase inhibitors, such as valproic acid) to make infected cells more sensitive to the immune response. A decrease in PVL has been reported in patients with TSP/HAM during the first months of treatment. However, the decrease was not sustained, and the clinical status did not improve.

The inefficacy of treatment may relate to the fact that neuronal loss had already occurred. Good predictive factors or early markers of TSP/HAM are needed to test patients as early as possible. For a recent review of therapies, see [33].

Recently, an anti-CCR4 monoclonal antibody (mogamulizumab) was used in a small, short, uncontrolled phase 1-2a study in Japanese patients with corticoid steroid–refractory TSP/HAM [41]. The number of HTLV-1-infected cells and the levels of inflammatory markers decreased. Clinically, spasticity was reduced and motor disability decreased. These results offer some hope but need to be validated in larger controlled studies.

Prevention

To date, there is no evidence that TSP/HAM can be prevented in people already infected with HTLV-1, so avoidance of infection is crucial [42]. This can be achieved by screening blood donors, as already occurs in Japan, several European countries, the United States, Canada, Brazil, and most Caribbean islands. Africa should be included next, but screening is rarely carried out, although African countries represent the largest endemic area for HTLV-1. Prevention of HTLV-1 transmission through organ donor screening is also crucial, at least for people from highly endemic areas [18]. Prevention of sexual transmission should also be considered. Avoiding long-term breastfeeding is also important but raises major issues in most resource-limited areas.

Information is absolutely crucial for all health workers to raise awareness of this truly neglected disease, which represents a significant burden on public health in most regions where the virus is endemic.

References

1. Poiesz, B.J., Ruscetti, F.W., Gazdar, A.F. et al. (1980). Detection and isolation of type C retrovirus particles from fresh and cultured lymphocytes of a patient with cutaneous T-cell lymphoma. *Proc. Natl. Acad. Sci. U. S. A.* 77: 7415–7419.
2. Takatsuki, K., Uchiyama, T., Sagawa, K., and Yodoi, J. (1977). Adult T cell leukemia in Japan. In: *Topics in Hematology* (eds. S. Seno, F. Takaku and S. Irino), 73–77. Amsterdam: Excerpta Medica.
3. Gallo, R.C. (2005). The discovery of the first human retrovirus: HTLV-1 and HTLV-2. *Retrovirology* 2: 17.
4. Gessain, A., Barin, F., Vernant, J.C. et al. (1985). Antibodies to human T-lymphotropic virus type-I in patients with tropical spastic paraparesis. *Lancet* 2: 407–410.
5. Gessain, A. and Gout, O. (1992). Chronic myelopathy associated with human T-lymphotropic virus type I (HTLV-I). *Ann. Intern. Med.* 117: 933–946.
6. Rodgers-Johnson, P., Gajdusek, D.C., Morgan, O.S. et al. (1985). HTLV-I and HTLV-III antibodies and tropical spastic paraparesis. *Lancet* 2: 1247–1248.
7. Osame, M., Usuku, K., Izumo, S. et al. (1986). HTLV-I associated myelopathy, a new clinical entity. *Lancet* 1: 1031–1032.
8. Roman, G.C. and Osame, M. (1988). Identity of HTLV-I-associated tropical spastic paraparesis and HTLV-I-associated myelopathy. *Lancet* 1: 651.
9. Gout, O., Baulac, M., Gessain, A. et al. (1990). Rapid development of myelopathy after HTLV-I infection acquired by transfusion during cardiac transplantation. *N. Engl. J. Med.* 322: 383–388.
10. Kaplan, J.E., Litchfield, B., Rouault, C. et al. (1991). HTLV-I-associated myelopathy associated with blood transfusion in the United States: epidemiologic and molecular evidence linking donor and recipient. *Neurology* 41 (Pt 1): 192–197.
11. Bangham, C.R.M. and Matsuoka, M. (2017). Human T-cell leukaemia virus type 1: parasitism and pathogenesis. *Philos. Trans. R. Soc. Lond. Ser. B Biol. Sci.* 372.
12. Enose-Akahata, Y., Vellucci, A., and Jacobson, S. (2017). Role of HTLV-1 tax and HBZ in the pathogenesis of HAM/TSP. *Front. Microbiol.* 8 (2563).
13. Ma, G., Yasunaga, J., and Matsuoka, M. (2016). Multifaceted functions and roles of HBZ in HTLV-1 pathogenesis. *Retrovirology* 13 (16).
14. Tanaka, A. and Matsuoka, M. (2018). HTLV-1 alters T cells for viral persistence and transmission. *Front. Microbiol.* 9: 461.
15. Pique, C. and Jones, K.S. (2012). Pathways of cell-cell transmission of HTLV-1. *Front. Microbiol.* 3: 378.
16. Gessain, A. and Cassar, O. (2012). Epidemiological aspects and world distribution of HTLV-1 infection. *Front. Microbiol.* 3: 388.
17. Roucoux, D.F., Wang, B., Smith, D. et al. (2005). A prospective study of sexual transmission of human T lymphotropic virus (HTLV)-I and HTLV-II. *J. Infect. Dis.* 191: 1490–1497.
18. Taylor, G.P. (2013). Editorial commentary: lessons on transplant-acquired human T-cell lymphotropic virus infection. *Clin. Infect. Dis.* 57: 1425–1426.
19. Filippone, C., Betsem, E., Tortevoye, P. et al. (2015). A severe bite from a non-human primate is a major risk factor for HTLV-1 infection in hunters from Central Africa. *Clin. Infect. Dis.* 60: 1667–1676.
20. Gessain, A., Gallo, R.C., and Franchini, G. (1992). Low degree of human T-cell leukemia/lymphoma virus type I genetic drift in vivo as a means of monitoring viral transmission and movement of ancient human populations. *J. Virol.* 66: 2288–2295.
21. Proietti, F.A., Carneiro-Proietti, A.B., Catalan-Soares, B.C., and Murphy, E.L. (2005). Global epidemiology of HTLV-I infection and associated diseases. *Oncogene* 24: 6058–6068.
22. Verdonck, K., Gonzalez, E., Van Dooren, S. et al. (2007). Human T-lymphotropic virus 1: recent knowledge about an ancient infection. *Lancet Infect. Dis.* 7: 266–281.
23. Coler-Reilly, A.L., Yagishita, N., Suzuki, H. et al. (2016). Nation-wide epidemiological study of Japanese patients with rare viral myelopathy using novel registration system (HAM-net). *Orphanet J. Rare Dis.* 11: 69.
24. Kendall, E.A., Gonzalez, E., Espinoza, I. et al. (2009). Early neurologic abnormalities associated with human T-cell lymphotropic virus type 1 infection in a cohort of Peruvian children. *J. Pediatr.* 155: 700–706.
25. Varandas, C.M.N., da Silva, J.L.S., Primo, J.R.L. et al. (2018). Early juvenile human T-cell lymphotropic virus type-1-associated myelopathy/tropical spastic paraparesis: study of 25 patients. *Clin. Infect. Dis.* 67: 1427–1433.
26. Osame, M., Janssen, R., Kubota, H. et al. (1990). Nationwide survey of HTLV-I-associated myelopathy in Japan: association with blood transfusion. *Ann. Neurol.* 28: 50–56.
27. Gotuzzo, E., Cabrera, J., Deza, L. et al. (2004). Clinical characteristics of patients in Peru with human T cell lymphotropic virus type 1-associated tropical spastic paraparesis. *Clin. Infect. Dis.* 39: 939–944.
28. Matsuzaki, T., Nakagawa, M., Nagai, M. et al. (2001). HTLV-I proviral load correlates with progression of

motor disability in HAM/TSP: analysis of 239 HAM/TSP patients including 64 patients followed up for 10 years. *J. Neurovirol.* 7: 228–234.
29. Iwanaga, M., Watanabe, T., Utsunomiya, A. et al. (2010). Human T-cell leukemia virus type I (HTLV-1) proviral load and disease progression in asymptomatic HTLV-1 carriers: a nationwide prospective study in Japan. *Blood* 116: 1211–1219.
30. Jeffery, K.J., Usuku, K., Hall, S.E. et al. (1999). HLA alleles determine human T-lymphotropic virus-I (HTLV-I) proviral load and the risk of HTLV-I-associated myelopathy. *Proc. Natl. Acad. Sci. U. S. A.* 96: 3848–3853.
31. De Castro-Costa, C.M., Araujo, A.Q., Barreto, M.M. et al. (2006). Proposal for diagnostic criteria of tropical spastic paraparesis/HTLV-I-associated myelopathy (TSP/HAM). *AIDS Res. Hum. Retrovir.* 22: 931–935.
32. Sato, T., Yagishita, N., Tamaki, K. et al. (2018). Proposal of classification criteria for HTLV-1-associated myelopathy/tropical spastic paraparesis disease activity. *Front. Microbiol.* 9: 1651.
33. Bangham, C.R., Araujo, A., Yamano, Y., and Taylor, G.P. (2015). HTLV-1-associated myelopathy/tropical spastic paraparesis. *Nat. Rev. Dis. Primers.* 1: 15012.
34. Cooper, S., van der Loeff, M.S., McConkey, S. et al. (2009). Neurological morbidity among human T-lymphotropic-virus-type-1-infected individuals in a rural West African population. *J. Neurol. Neurosurg. Psychiatry* 80: 66–68.
35. Olindo, S., Cabre, P., Lezin, A. et al. (2006). Natural history of human T-lymphotropic virus 1-associated myelopathy: a 14-year follow-up study. *Arch. Neurol.* 63 (11): 1560–1566.
36. Morgan, D.J., Caskey, M.F., Abbehusen, C. et al. (2007). Brain magnetic resonance imaging white matter lesions are frequent in HTLV-I carriers and do not discriminate from HAM/TSP. *AIDS Res. Hum. Retrovir.* 23: 1499–1504.
37. Cooper, S.A., van der Loeff, M., and Taylor, G.P. (2009). The neurology of HTLV-1 infection. *Pract. Neurol.* 9: 16–26.
38. Izumo, S. (2010). Neuropathology of HTLV-1-associated myelopathy (HAM/TSP): the 50th anniversary of Japanese society of neuropathology. *Neuropathology* 30: 480–485.
39. Bangham, C.R. (2003). The immune control and cell-to-cell spread of human T-lymphotropic virus type 1. *J. Gen. Virol.* 84: 3177–3189.
40. Sato, T., Coler-Reilly, A., Utsunomiya, A. et al. (2013). CSF CXCL10, CXCL9, and neopterin as candidate prognostic biomarkers for HTLV-1-associated myelopathy/tropical spastic paraparesis. *PLoS Negl. Trop. Dis.* 7: e2479.
41. Coler-Reilly, A.L.G., Sato, T., Matsuzaki, T. et al. (2017). Effectiveness of daily prednisolone to slow progression of human T-lymphotropic virus type 1-associated myelopathy/tropical spastic paraparesis: a multicenter retrospective cohort study. *Neurotherapeutics* 14: 1084–1094.
42. Olindo, S., Jeannin, S., Saint-Vil, M. et al. (2018). Temporal trends in Human T-Lymphotropic virus 1 (HTLV-1) associated myelopathy/tropical spastic paraparesis (HAM/TSP) incidence in Martinique over 25 years (1986–2010). *PLoS Negl. Trop. Dis.* 12: e0006304.

25 Parechovirus A

Clayton A. Wiley
Division of Neuropathology, UPMC Presbyterian Hospital, Pittsburgh, PA, USA

Abbreviations

CSF   cerebrospinal fluid
CNS   central nervous system
IVIG intravenous immunoglobulin
MRI   magnetic resonance imaging
PCR   polymerase chain reaction
PeVA Parechovirus A
RNA   ribonucleic acid

Definition of parechovirus A and historical perspective

Picornaviruses are a large family of positive single-stranded nonenveloped RNA viruses. Of the 31 genera, 7 contain important human pathogens [1]. Of these, the enteroviruses are perhaps the most common human pathogens mediating up to 10 million infections per year in the United States alone. Although the vast majority of these infections are clinically asymptomatic, several agents have the capacity to inflict severe neurological disease (see Chapters 21 and 22). As with other RNA viruses, enteroviruses have a proven capacity to undergo intra- and intergenotypic recombination, setting the stage for emergence of new potentially deadly pathogens.

Like many other viruses, enteroviruses were originally classified on the basis of serology. As one of the most common infections of mankind, there are more than 100 different enteroviral serotypes. The advent of high-speed sequencing has permitted a more consistent molecular-based classification of enteroviruses. Sequence analysis required reclassification of echoviruses 22 and 23 into a new genus: *Parechovirus,* the human strains of which were most recently classified in the species *Parechovirus* A (PeVA) [2].

Since their original isolation more than 50 years ago, the number of genetically distinct PeVA strains (as defined by at least 73% nucleic acid or 81% amino-acid identity in VP1 gene) has grown to 19 [2–4]. Human *Parechovirus* (HPeV) 1, 2, and 3 are the most common types identified in infected patients. Type 1 has been associated with a broad spectrum of diseases. Although most commonly linked to mild gastrointestinal and upper respiratory disease, more severe infections with encephalomyocarditis have been seen in some populations [5]. However, the vast majority of reported neurological disease cases have been linked to HPeV3.

Virology

The molecular biology of PeVA is analogous to the other picornaviruses, with some distinguishing features. Like the other Picornaviruses, protein translation occurs off a single genomic transcript,

---

Infections of the Central Nervous System: Pathology and Genetics, First Edition. Edited by Fabrice Chrétien, Kum Thong Wong, Leroy R. Sharer, Catherine (Katy) Keohane and Françoise Gray.
© 2020 John Wiley & Sons Ltd. Published 2020 by John Wiley & Sons Ltd.

with later cleavage to make individual structural and enzymatic proteins. Unlike the enteroviruses, rather than producing four virion capsid proteins, only three proteins are cleaved (P0, P1, and P3), with the P0 protein being retained as a solitary molecule rather than being cleaved into P2 and P4 proteins.

Picornaviruses use a wide variety of cell surface receptors to mediate infection. Individual viruses have a more limited but still varied set of host proteins that bind virion capsids. Structure of the virion capsid P1 protein has been associated with significant differences in cell surface binding, particularly the presence or absence of arginine-glycine-aspartic acid (RGD) motif critical to integrin binding.

Molecular estimates suggest that parechoviruses diverged from other picornaviruses as recently as 400 years ago [6]. The important human pathogen HPeV3 may have diverged a mere 150 years ago and emerged as a worldwide infection as recently as 20–30 years ago [7]. Since that time there have been several outbreaks and "epidemics" associated with clinical disease [8–10]. Some of these outbreaks have been traced back to specific recombinant events.

Seroepidemiology

Estimates of seroprevalence vary depending upon the strain of HPeV and the age and nationality of subjects. In general, seroconversion occurs early, within months of birth for HPeV1, and within weeks of birth for HPeV3. Seropositivity for HPeV1 is as high as 99% in Finnish and 92% in Dutch adult populations [11]. HPeV2, 5, and 6 show similar but lower percentage seropositivities, whereas seropositivity to HPeV3 is low (10–13%) in adult populations, presumably reflecting its more recent emergence.

Exposure to HPeV occurs soon after birth. By 6 months, 40% of infants are seropositive, by 1 year 70%, and by 5 years up to 100% are seropositive. But seropositivity also varies by strain of HPeV. The mean ages of HPeV1 and 2 positivity are 14.6 and 6.3 months, respectively, and the mean age of HPeV3 positivity is 0.7 months. Exposure to HPeV also shows a curious biennial pattern, with infection in Europe occurring in even years and infection in North America occurring in odd years. In all continents, infection peaks during summer months.

A recent study in Japan has attempted to better understand the seroprevalence of HPeV3 infection and the role of maternal antibody in blocking disease in newborns [12]. These investigators measured neutralizing antibody in 175 cord blood samples. They found an overall seroprevalence of approximately 60%; however, titer was dependent on maternal age, with those younger than the age of 35 having a seroprevalence of approximately 70%, and those 35–44 years of age had a seroprevalence of approximately 30%. Infants born with low cord blood neutralizing antibody had a higher incidence of serious HPeV infection than those born with higher titer of pre-existing maternal antibodies.

HPeV detection

It is important to recognize that PeVA is not detected by general clinical enteroviral polymerase chain reaction (PCR). Additionally, PeVA is difficult to culture and only limited cell lines support replication. Specific reverse transcriptase-PCR is 100- to 1000-fold more sensitive than culture. (Sequencing of VP1 is used for viral typing.) Also, choice of bodily fluids for assaying is critical as PeVA is excreted from the gastrointestinal system for prolonged times, whereas its presence in blood and cerebrospinal fluid (CSF) is limited to intervals of disease.

A recent study of CSF from 239 infants in Colorado [13] detected enterovirus in approximately 12% and HPeV in approximately 3%. HPeV infections occurred between July and October, and the infants averaged 24 days of age. A similar study in Kansas and Missouri [8] identified 35 cases of HPeV infection in infants 5–56 days old. Seven infants required intensive care and six of these had neurological complications.

First isolated in 1999 and reported in 2004 [14], HPeV3 has emerged as an important human nervous system pathogen. Given its recent emergence, the exact seroprevalence has been difficult to pin down and probably varies geographically. Nevertheless, it has become clear that absence of maternal antibody is a significant risk factor in newborns for severe neurological disease [12].

PeVA clinical disease

Most PeVA infections are subclinical, but those that are apparent show: fever and irritability (95%), rash (17–60%), gastrointestinal symptoms (29%), and respiratory symptoms (26%). Transmission can be fecal-oral or respiratory and potentially from ambient environmental water sources [15]. High viral titers are detected in stool with shedding lasting for five months. Less common respiratory disease is associated with viral shedding for one to three weeks. Different PeVA subtypes are associated with clinical disease: lymphadenitis (HPEV4), myositis (HPeV3), myocarditis and enterocolitis (HPeV1), hepatitis, steatosis, and hemorrhage (HPeV5 and 6).

A retrospective review of 133 cases of suspected encephalitis in newborns showed that 13 were related to HPeV infection [16]. Although short-term outcome analysis indicated no or minor sequelae in two-thirds of the children, assessment at one year post infection showed significant developmental concerns in two-thirds of the children, with 2 of the 13 having a diagnosis of cerebral palsy.

HPeV3 neurological disease
Clinical features

Neurological disease associated with HPeV3 infection is peculiar from a variety of perspectives. The infant exhibits signs of neonatal sepsis with a clinical impression of "meningitis." Nevertheless, there is no increased intracranial pressure and CSF analysis is mostly normal with only rare and mild pleocytosis. More severe disease manifests as an encephalitis (i.e. seizures in 84%, rash in 66%, and apnea in 55%) and is exclusively seen in neonates and young infants. Full-term infants show an onset in the first two weeks, whereas premature infants show an onset at two to three months. This suggests a possible delayed exposure to an environmental pathogen in premature infants who are retained in hospital. Yet even in these severe cases, CSF is mostly normal, directing the differential away from an infectious etiology. Imaging shows periventricular echogenicity with ultrasonography, and on magnetic resonance imaging (MRI), 90% demonstrate deep white matter lesions. There are reports of acute flaccid paralysis with HPeV3, similar to those observed in classic poliomyelitis; however, reports of death are exceptional. At discharge there may be no clinical residual; however, on later follow up, developmental abnormalities (including seizures, cerebral palsy, visual impairment, and learning disability) are more prevalent.

One of the first intensive studies of newborns with HPeV3 assessed 10 infants who developed neonatal sepsis and seizures [17]. Three of the infants were preterm and presented with sepsis several weeks after birth, whereas the 7 term infants all presented within two weeks of birth. Despite a clinical impression of meningitis, CSF was mostly acellular with a normal protein and glucose. (CSF cytokine analysis in infants with HPeV demonstrates a less-robust cytokine response than that observed with enterovirus infection [18]). HPeV3 RNA was detected in the CSF of eight, blood of one, and feces of one. Soon after clinical onset, MRI showed abnormal water content and diffusion pattern predominantly in periventricular white matter. None of these subjects died, but one developed cerebral palsy, and another, seizures. Half were described as neurologically normal at discharge.

Pathology

Given the difficulties of diagnosing CNS HPeV3 infection during life and the rarity of lethal infection, it is not surprising that autopsy studies are almost unique. Two infants who died of HPeV3 infection showed histopathology fully compatible with the clinical findings [19]. Both infant brains showed gross pathology consistent with periventricular leukomalacia (Figure 25.1). Despite white matter necrosis there was minimal evidence of a cell-mediated immune response except for a modest mononuclear meningitis. Tissue inflammation was limited to a perivascular distribution along with infiltration into necrotic regions and phagocytosis of cellular debris. In situ hybridization showed HPeV3 nucleic acids limited to blood vessel smooth muscle cells in brain parenchyma, meninges, and

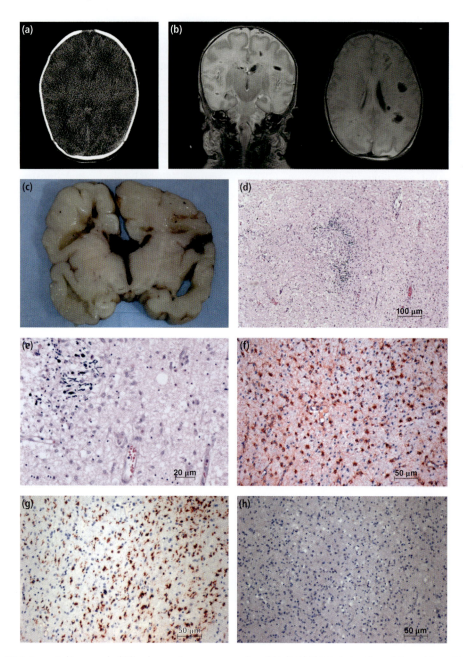

Figure 25.1 Computed tomography (CT) and magnetic resonance imaging (MRI) scans and neuropathology of human parechovirus-3 (HPeV3) infection [19]. (a) Horizontal CT scan from a patient admitted with acute HPeV3 infection. At one day of illness, there is no evidence of structural abnormality. (b) T2 Fast Spin Echo MRI without contrast two days after admission when seizures were observed. Coronal and horizontal sections demonstrate multifocal cavitation in deep white matter bilaterally, left side of patient greater than right. (c) Gross photograph of brain from autopsy. Coronal section at the level of the thalamus demonstrates dilated ventricles containing some blood and surrounded by cavitated white matter, left side of brain greater than right. (d–h) Histological sections of deep white matter. (d) Low-power hematoxylin and eosin (H&E) demonstrates mineralized white matter with mild increase in cellularity. (e) Higher-power H&E adjacent to mineralization demonstrates spongiform hypercellular white matter without evidence of viral inclusions. (f) Immunohistochemical stain for glial fibrillary acidic protein (GFAP) demonstrates reactive astrocytosis with delicate starlike fibrillary processes along with foci of beadlike dissolution consistent with clasmatodendrosis. (g) Immunohistochemical stain for CD68 highlights macrophages with reactive ameboid morphology. (h) Immunohistochemical stain for CD3 demonstrates absence of T cells.

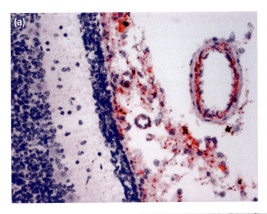
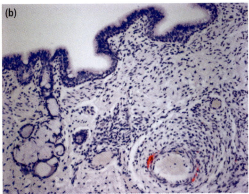
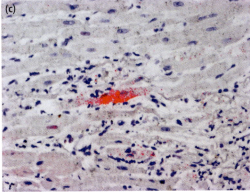

Figure 25.2 In situ hybridization (ISH) for human parechovirus-3 (HPeV3) in the meninges, smooth muscle of lung blood vessels, and cardiomyocytes. (a–c) Paraffin sections were hybridized with the chromogenic HPeV3 RNA probe (red) and counterstained with hematoxylin (blue). (a) Hypercellular meninges overlying the cerebellum hybridized extensively to HPeV3 RNA probe. (b) Sections of lung show hybridization of HPeV3 RNA probe to smooth muscle of large blood vessels. Endothelium and adjacent bronchial and cartilaginous tissues do not hybridize. (c) ISH for HPeV demonstrates the presence of viral RNA within cardiomyocytes (red).

lung arterioles (Figure 25.2). This distribution suggests that HPeV3 mediates neurological damage indirectly by compromising blood flow and causing ischemic damage to susceptible regions.

Chronic HPeVA infection of immunosuppressed

Although most commonly seen in neonates, HPeV3 disease has occurred rarely in adults. Mardekian et al. [20] reported a young woman with systemic lupus erythematosus treated with Rituximab and cyclophosphamide, who developed a chronic HPeV3 infection. This patient exhibited cardiomyopathy, aseptic meningitis, and diffuse symmetrical deep white matter and brainstem diffusion abnormalities on MRI. HPeV3 was detected by PCR in CSF and serum and by in situ hybridization in cardiomyocytes (Figure 25.2). Despite intensive antiviral and intravenous immunoglobulin (IVIG) therapy, the patient remained incapacitated and chronically infected.

Acute HPeVA infection of adults

Given the recent emergence and dissemination of HPeV3, there was an interesting report of an "epidemic of myalgia" in an adult population in Japan [21]. From June to August of 2008, 22 previously healthy adults developed acute muscle pain and weakness. Laboratory findings confirmed elevated creatinine phosphokinase and acute HPeV3 infection in 14 of these. A recent follow-up study in children suggests this disease is not limited to adults [22]. It is presumed these patients were newly exposed and infected, but the pathogenesis of the disease is unknown. In 2017, another epidemic of HPeV3 infection was reported in 18 Australian neonates [10]. All of the subjects were infected between 2012 and 2015. Phylogenetic and network analysis suggested this outbreak was the result of a recombination event.

Animal models

Given the limited capacity to replicate in human cells in vitro, it is not surprising that no animal models exist at the current time.

Health threat, vaccines, and therapy

From the preceding discussion, it would be expected that individuals with immunocompromise, especially those with hypogammaglobulinemia are at particular risk. Logically, IVIG has been tried and shown to have some efficacy in treatment of PeVA infections. Unfortunately, limited blood-brain barrier permeability of IVIGs makes treatment of CNS infections problematic. There are a variety of experimental drugs that disrupt picornavirus pathogenesis; however, none of them have proven efficacious for treating PeVA infections.

As infection with individual picornaviruses leads to lifelong immunity, it is only logical to attempt to design vaccines for these important human pathogens. Because humoral immunity appears to be critical in preventing viremia and spread to the CNS, most vaccines have focused on this arm of immunity. The development of the polio vaccine is considered nothing less than one of man's greatest accomplishments. But that vaccine was directed against a limited repertoire of three strains of the poliovirus. There is substantial need to develop new vaccines to other important human pathogens from this family of viruses like EV71, EV-68, coxsackievirus A16, and HPeV3. Most of these vaccine strategies target the development of high neutralizing antibody under the theory that prolonged viremia is the sine qua non for the development of neurological disease. Fortunately, good humoral immunity can be achieved with safe inactivated vaccines, viruslike proteins, and even recombinant proteins. Because of limited cross-neutralization of different viral species, vaccines need to target genotype-specific neutralization epitopes.

Pooled serum immunoglobulin had been used in IVIG therapy for a variety of viral infections. The success of IVIG treatment is presumably dependent on the titer of neutralizing antibody for the infecting virus. This complicates the use of IVIG in the treatment of the relatively recent emergent HPeV3. Aizawa recently assayed IVIG from Japan, the United States, and Germany [12]. Depending on the source population, not all IVIG will have high titer to HPeVs and HPeV3 in particular.

The armamentarium of drugs to suppress viral infection is gradually expanding. Some of the most successful drugs (e.g. acyclovir) would not be expected to have any efficacy in treatment of RNA viruses. Of those drugs more specifically designed to treat RNA viral infections, Pleconaril's capacity to bind virion capsid and prevent infection shows some promise.

References

1. Adams, M.J., Lefkowitz, E.J., King, A.M. et al. (2015). Ratification vote on taxonomic proposals to the international committee on taxonomy of viruses (2015). *Arch. Virol.* 160: 1837–1850.
2. Pirbright Institute. *Parechovirus A in the Picornaviridae.* http://www.picornaviridae.com/parechovirus/parechovirus_a/parechovirus_a.htm (accessed 18 August 2017).
3. Romero, J.R. and Selvarangan, R. (2011). The human parechoviruses: an overview. *Adv. Pediatr. Infect. Dis.* 58: 65–85.
4. Chuchaona, W., Khamrin, P., Yodmeeklin, A. et al. (2015). Detection and characterization of a novel human parechovirus genotype in Thailand. *Infect. Genet. Evol.* 31: 300–304.
5. Wildenbeest, J.G., Benschop, K.S., Bouma-de Jongh, S. et al. (2016). Prolonged shedding of human parechovirus in feces of young children after symptomatic infection. *Pediatr. Infect. Dis. J.* 35: 580–583.

6. Faria, N.R., de Vries, M., van Hemert, F.J. et al. (2009). Rooting human parechovirus evolution in time. *BMC Evol. Biol.* 9: 164.
7. Calvert, J., Chieochansin, T., Benschop, K.S. et al. (2010). Recombination dynamics of human parechoviruses: investigation of type-specific differences in frequency and epidemiological correlates. *J. Gen. Virol.* 91 (Pt 5): 1229–1238.
8. Midgley, C.M., Jackson, M.A., Selvarangan, R. et al. (2017). Severe parechovirus 3 infections in young infants-Kansas and Missouri, 2014. *J. Pediatr. Infect. Dis. Soc.* https://doi.org/10.1093/jpids/pix010.
9. Khatami, A., McMullan, B.J., Webber, M. et al. (2015). Sepsis-like disease in infants due to human parechovirus type 3 during an outbreak in Australia. *Clin. Infect. Dis.* 60: 228–236.
10. Alexandersen, S., Nelson, T.M., Hodge, J., and Druce, J. (2017). Evolutionary and network analysis of virus sequences from infants infected with an Australian recombinant strain of human parechovirus type 3. *Sci. Rep.* 7: 3861.
11. Westerhuis, B., Kolehmainen, P., Benschop, K. et al. (2013). Human parechovirus seroprevalence in Finland and the Netherlands. *J. Clin. Virol.* 58: 211–215.
12. Aizawa, Y., Watanabe, K., Oishi, T. et al. (2015). Role of maternal antibodies in infants with severe diseases related to human parechovirus type 3. *Emerg. Infect. Dis.* 21: 1966–1972.
13. Messacar, K., Breazeale, G., Wei, Q. et al. (2015). Epidemiology and clinical characteristics of infants with human parechovirus or human herpes virus-6 detected in cerebrospinal fluid tested for enterovirus or herpes simplex virus. *J. Med. Virol.* 87: 829–835.
14. Ito, M., Yamashita, T., Tsuzuki, H. et al. (2004). Isolation and identification of a novel human parechovirus. *J Gen Virol* 85 (Pt 2): 391–398.
15. Reynolds, K.A., Mena, K.D., and Gerba, C.P. (2008). Risk of waterborne illness via drinking water in the United States. *Rev. Environ. Contam. Toxicol.* 192: 117–158.
16. Britton, P.N., Dale, R.C., Nissen, M.D. et al. (2016). Parechovirus encephalitis and neurodevelopmental outcomes. *Pediatrics* 137: e20152848.
17. Verboon-Maciolek, M.A., Groenendaal, F., Hahn, C.D. et al. (2008). Human parechovirus causes encephalitis with white matter injury in neonates. *Ann. Neurol.* 64: 266–273.
18. Fortuna, D., Cardenas, A.M., Graf, E.H. et al. (2017). Human parechovirus and enterovirus initiate distinct CNS innate immune responses: pathogenic and diagnostic implications. *J. Clin. Virol.* 86: 39–45.
19. Bissel, S.J., Auer, R.N., Chiang, C.H. et al. (2015). Human parechovirus 3 meningitis and fatal leukoencephalopathy. *J. Neuropathol. Exp. Neurol.* 74: 767–777.
20. Mardekian, S.K., Fortuna, D., Nix, A. et al. (2015). Severe human parechovirus type 3 myocarditis and encephalitis in an adolescent with hypogammaglobulinemia. *Int. J. Infect. Dis.* 36: 6–8.
21. Mizuta, K., Kuroda, M., Kurimura, M. et al. (2012). Epidemic myalgia in adults associated with human parechovirus type 3 infection, Yamagata, Japan, 2008. *Emerg. Infect. Dis.* 18: 1787–1793.
22. Mizuta, K., Yamakawa, T., Kurokawa, K. et al. (2016). Epidemic myalgia and myositis associated with human parechovirus type 3 infections occur not only in adults but also in children: findings in Yamagata, Japan, 2014. *Epidemiol. Infect.* 144: 1286–1290.

26 Acute Disseminated Encephalomyelitis and Acute Hemorrhagic Leukoencephalomyelitis

Romana Höftberger[1] and Hans Lassmann[2]

[1] Institute of Neurology, Medical University of Vienna, Vienna, Austria
[2] Center for Brain Research, Medical University of Vienna, Vienna, Austria

Abbreviations

ADEM	acute disseminated encephalomyelitis
AHLE	acute hemorrhagic leukoencephalitis
ANE	acute necrotizing encephalopathy
CNS	central nervous system
CSF	cerebrospinal fluid
MHC	major histocompatibility complex
MOG	myelin oligodendrocyte glycoprotein
MRI	magnetic resonance imaging
MS	multiple sclerosis
NMOSD	neuromyelitis optica spectrum disorders
RANBP2	RAN binding protein 2

Introduction

Acute disseminated encephalomyelitis (ADEM) and acute hemorrhagic leukoencephalomyelitis (AHLE) were originally classified as human inflammatory demyelinating diseases because of the association of brain and spinal cord inflammation with the presence of perivenous primary demyelination [1]. These diseases are rare; they may occur spontaneously, following infections or vaccinations [2]. Because similar changes are seen in humans or experimental animals after active sensitization with brain antigens, they are believed to be autoimmune diseases and can be induced by molecular mimicry between proteins of infectious agents and the tissue of the CNS. In the majority of patients, they are severe monophasic diseases with rapid evolution of clinical deficits and a high mortality rate when untreated [3–5]. Depending on disease severity, patients who survive the acute attack may have permanent neurological deficits. Recent data suggest that ADEM and AHLE may represent clinical syndromes, which may be elicited by different pathogenetic triggers and may involve different immunological mechanisms.

Infections of the Central Nervous System: Pathology and Genetics, First Edition. Edited by Fabrice Chrétien, Kum Thong Wong, Leroy R. Sharer, Catherine (Katy) Keohane and Françoise Gray.
© 2020 John Wiley & Sons Ltd. Published 2020 by John Wiley & Sons Ltd.

Acute disseminated encephalomyelitis (ADEM)

Epidemiology

ADEM is a severe acute neurological disease, with an incidence of 0.1–0.7 per 100 000 population. This incidence is similar in Europe, the United States, and Asia [3, 6, 7]. It is more frequent in children than in adults and affects males and females in similar proportion. In children the average age at presentation is between five and eight years, but cases can occur in any age group. Precipitating events are active immunizations against brain antigens, as has been seen for instance following rabies vaccination with immunogen containing brain tissue. They may also develop after exposure to brain tissue-free vaccines (postvaccinial ADEM) [8] and following infectious diseases (postinfectious ADEM) [9]. A very large spectrum of different infections has been shown to give rise to ADEM, but certain infections, such as measles, mumps, and rubella (MMR), are particularly frequent [4]. The incidence of ADEM following infection is higher than that seen after vaccination with the respective virus. In general, postinfectious ADEM occurs at the peak of the immune response against the infectious agent, when the agent is already cleared from the sites of original infection. Thus, attempts to isolate virus or other infectious agents from patients with ADEM are mostly unsuccessful.

Clinical and paraclinical findings

In the majority of patients, ADEM is a rapidly evolving acute monophasic disease. The peak of clinical disease is reached between two and five days after disease onset [3]. The clinical presentation is highly variable and diverse between patients, giving rise to symptoms related to nearly any functional system of the brain or spinal cord. Nevertheless, there are some highly characteristic features, enabling defined diagnostic criteria, at least in children [10]. Criteria include multifocal clinical CNS events of presumed inflammatory demyelinating cause, together with encephalopathy and multiple focal but ill-demarcated magnetic resonance imaging (MRI) abnormalities in the forebrain white matter and the corticosubcortical junctions [11]. In addition, there may be associated lesions in the deep gray nuclei, cerebellum, brainstem, and spinal cord. Additional criteria are the monophasic nature of the disease and the absence of new MRI findings three months or more after the clinical onset [11]. However, there are rare variants of multiphasic or even relapsing–remitting ADEM [10]. These variants appear to include diseases such as myelin oligodendrocyte glycoprotein (MOG) autoantibody-associated disease [12] or neuromyelitis optica [13], which are now regarded as separate from classical ADEM. Such cases can be distinguished by identification of serum antibodies against MOG or aquaporin 4.

There is no serological test for the diagnosis of ADEM. In the cerebrospinal fluid (CSF), there is a mild pleocytosis, mainly consisting of lymphocytes and monocytes, together with increased protein levels. Intrathecal immunoglobulin synthesis and oligoclonal bands may be present in a small subset of patients [3].

Pathology

The hallmark of ADEM pathology (Figure 26.1) is a widespread inflammatory process in the brain and spinal cord, predominantly affecting the white matter, but it may spread into the deep gray nuclei and the corticosubcortical layers [1]. The inflammatory cells are mainly composed of T lymphocytes, whereas B cells are rare or absent. In addition, activated macrophages and microglia are seen in high numbers, particularly in perivascular areas, which show demyelination and axonal injury. The inflammatory process is associated with profound leakage of serum proteins, suggesting massive blood-brain barrier (BBB) damage. The most characteristic feature of ADEM pathology is the presence of small perivascular sleeves of demyelination with acute axonal injury [14]. In contrast to multiple sclerosis (MS) lesions, these do not result in confluent plaques of primary demyelination. When patients recover from the acute disease episode, inflammation resolves and pathology regresses to some perivascular glial scaring. There is no systematic study regarding immunophenotyping of inflammatory cells in ADEM cases. Because of their similarities to the

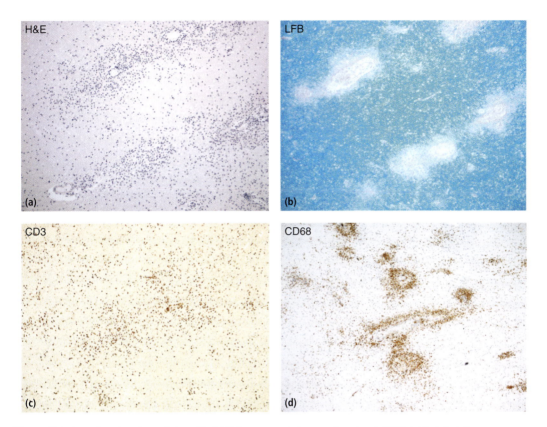

Figure 26.1 Acute disseminated encephalomyelitis (ADEM), which developed in a boy at the time of clearance of the skin rash of measles: massive perivenous inflammatory reaction, the infiltrates mainly being composed of lymphocytes and macrophages (a, hematoxylin and eosin [H&E] staining); the inflammatory process is associated with perivenous demyelination (b, Luxol fast blue [LFB] myelin stain); the inflammatory infiltrates are mainly composed of T cells (c, CD3) and macrophages (d, CD68).

lesions seen in experimental models of autoimmune encephalomyelitis, it is generally assumed that major histocompatibility complex (MHC) Class II restricted CD4+ T lymphocytes drive the inflammatory reaction in ADEM [1]. Unexpectedly, we recently found that the T cells were nearly exclusively composed of MHC Class I restricted CD8+ cells in a case of postinfectious ADEM. This may indicate that in some patients the pathogenesis of postinfectious ADEM could be different from that seen in ADEM-like disease driven by autoimmunity.

A fundamentally different pathology is seen in ADEM cases associated with anti-MOG antibodies (Figure 26.2). ADEM with anti-MOG antibodies occurs mainly in children and is rare in adults, in whom the clinical spectrum of MOG-antibody associated disease more likely reflects neuromyelitis optica spectrum disorders (NMOSD) [15]. Although the core clinical features in patients with MOG-positive ADEM overlap with classical ADEM, some differences are seen on MRI [16]. Patients with MOG-positive ADEM have large, more focal, and better-demarcated lesions compared to classical ADEM cases. In addition, MOG-positive cases have a higher risk of developing a relapsing or recurrent disease course [12, 16, 17]. The pathology in such cases is characterized by profound inflammation, associated with confluent demyelination, resulting in large plaques of primary demyelination, similar to those seen in MS [18]. However, distinct from MS, even within these lesions, there is marked perivenous accentuation of demyelination, resulting in

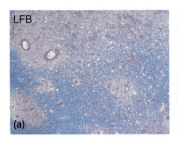 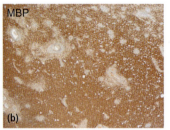 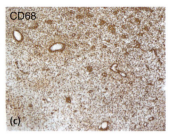

Figure 26.2 Spontaneous anti-myelin oligodendrocyte glycoprotein (anti-MOG) antibody-associated inflammatory demyelinating disease in a 53-year-old female patient with a large diffuse confluent lesion in the forebrain; although the demyelination is accentuated in perivascular spaces, similar to classical ADEM, the lesions show confluent demyelination, as typically seen in multiple sclerosis. (a, Luxol fast blue (LFB) myelin stain; b, immunocytochemistry for myelin basic protein [MPB]); active demyelination is associated with dense macrophage infiltration (c, CD68).

a phenotype intermediate between ADEM and MS lesions. It is important to note that MOG antibody-associated inflammatory demyelination differs in clinical presentation, pathology, and response to therapy, from classical MS [17].

Pathogenesis of ADEM and experimental models

At least three different pathogenetic scenarios may merge into the same clinical phenotype seen in patients with ADEM. The first is T-cell mediated autoimmunity. This view is supported by the close similarity of ADEM to both clinical disease and pathological changes induced by active sensitization of experimental animals with brain tissue [19]. The disease can be induced in all vertebrates tested so far, including humans. In humans, the incidence was 1 in 1000 following rabies vaccination with a vaccine containing brain tissue [8] or in slaughterhouse workers, who were chronically exposed to aerosols containing brain tissue [20]. Pathogenetic studies in experimental models show that this disease is induced by CD4+ MHC Class II restricted T-lymphocytes directed against brain auto-antigens. To date, most brain proteins tested were able to induce a T-cell response, which gives rise to brain inflammation after systemic T-cell transfer [21]. Thus, the number of potentially encephalitogenic brain antigens is very high. It is likely that postvaccinial ADEM is also driven by a T-cell mediated autoimmune response. Up to now, a specific brain antigen or antigenic peptide has not been successfully identified. This is not surprising, considering that large numbers of different brain protein peptides are potentially encephalitogenic and that T cells recognize three dimensional structures bound to the MHC molecules, which may be shared between peptides with completely different amino-acid sequences [22]. It would be extremely lucky to succeed in identifying such a cross-reactive epitope, recognized by disease-driving T lymphocytes.

The pathogenesis may be different in cases with postinfectious ADEM. Although a mechanism similar to that described above may play a role, the dominance of MHC Class I restricted CD8+ T cells in the lesions differs from that seen in classical models of autoimmune encephalomyelitis. Whether postinfectious ADEM is driven by autoreactive CD8+ T cells, a possibility shown in some experimental models, or whether it is the result of a massively overreacting antiviral immune response in a brain with a very low degree of local infection remains unresolved [4, 23].

Finally, ADEM associated with anti-MOG autoantibodies has a different pathogenesis as described previously. It is very well reflected in experimental models in rats, guinea pigs, and primates, where it is induced by active sensitization with naturally folded full-length MOG protein [24]. The disease is induced by a combination of an encephalitogenic T cells response against MOG, which starts disease and inflammation, and a demyelinating antibody response against a conformational epitope of MOG [25]. Although

MOG-antibody associated inflammatory demyelinating disease is clearly an autoimmune disease, it remains to be determined how it is triggered.

AHLE or acute necrotizing encephalopathy

Epidemiology

The incidence of AHLE or acute necrotizing encephalopathy (ANE) is much lower than that of ADEM, and thus, no reliable demographic data are available [5, 11]. Children are more likely to be affected than adults. As with ADEM, a high proportion of cases develop the disease following a systemic infection, mostly an upper respiratory tract infection. Infection with influenza virus is among the most prevalent inciting factors.

Clinical and paraclinical findings

Clinical disease is very severe and aggressive; the patients progressing from initial focal neurological symptoms to seizures and coma within a few days [5, 26]. In most cases acute neurological disease is associated with fever. In untreated patients, mortality is very high. In surviving patients, clinical assessment one month after disease onset helps to define a prognosis for long-term outcome [26]. MRI changes are similar to those seen in ADEM but show more severe brain edema, and in contrast to ADEM, there are petechial hemorrhages [11]. CSF analysis reveals evidence of inflammation with increased leukocyte counts and increased protein levels, but absence of intrathecal immunoglobulin synthesis or oligoclonal bands. A characteristic feature in the CSF is the presence of red blood cells (up to 1000/µl).

Pathology

Similar to ADEM, the characteristic feature of AHLE is the presence of inflammation with perivenous demyelination or tissue damage (Figure 26.3). Overall, however, the degree of lymphocytic infiltration is less pronounced. In contrast to ADEM, numerous granulocytes are present and the walls of some veins show fibrinoid necrosis and small perivascular hemorrhages [11].

Pathogenesis and experimental models

Originally, AHLE was thought to be a variant of ADEM with a particularly severe disease course and aggressive lesions. This view is supported by the observation in experimental animals that autoimmune encephalomyelitis may develop into a very severe aggressive variant, called hyperacute autoimmune encephalitis [27]. Its pathology is similar to that seen in AHLE. Methods to induce hyperacute experimental autoimmune encephalomyelitis (EAE) in animals involve the use of specific animal strains (genetic background), changes in the immunization protocol (e.g. choice of the immune-stimulating adjuvant), or manipulation of the immune system prior to immunization. However, AHLE and ADEM in humans may have different pathogenetic backgrounds. The dominant association of AHLE with influenza virus infections [28] differs from the spectrum of infectious diseases associated with ADEM. Recent genetic studies provided evidence that in AHLE the infection-triggered inflammatory response may be modified by genetically determined alterations in the immune system or the target tissue. Genetic polymorphisms in a gene coding for the complement factor 1 were identified in a family with two children affected by AHLE [29]. Complement plays a major role in inflammation and immune-mediated tissue injury, and its activation has been described in hyperacute EAE lesions [30], so this association could explain the particularly severe inflammatory CNS disease seen in these patients. A series of other studies describe an association between ANE following common viral infections (mainly influenza and parainfluenza), and mutations in the gene for the RAN binding protein 2 (RANBP2) [31]. RANBP2 is a nuclear pore protein and its malfunction leads to energy deficiency in tissues challenged by an acute infection. Although the exact mechanism of how these mutations affect the inflammatory mechanisms is not clear, these data suggest that AHLE could be the result of an infection-triggered (potential autoimmune) inflammatory reaction, which is massively augmented by the malfunction of genes involved in the regulation of immune-mediated tissue damage.

Infections of the Central Nervous System

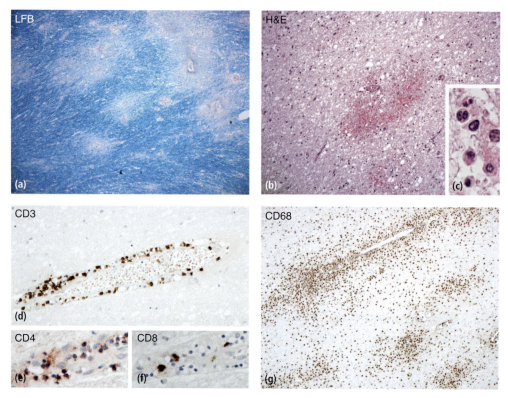

Figure 26.3 Acute hemorrhagic leukoencephalitis (AHLE) in an adult patient following a respiratory infection (possibly influenza); the perivenous demyelination is similar to classical acute disseminated encephalomyelitis (ADEM) (a, Luxol fast blue [LFB] myelin stain); within the lesions there is fibrinoid change in the vessel wall, perivascular hemorrhage and infiltration with lymphocytes and granulocytes (b, c, hematoxylin and eosin [H&E] staining); the inflammatory infiltrates are composed of T cells (d, CD3), with a dominance of CD4+ T cells (e, CD4) over CD8+ cells (f, CD8); demyelination and tissue damage is associated with profound macrophage infiltration (g, CD68).

References

1. Alvord, E.C. (1970). Acute disseminated encephalomyelitis and "allergic" neuroencephalopathies. In: *Handbook of Clinical Neurology*; Vol. 9 (eds. P.Y. Vinken and G.W. Bruyn), 500–571. New York: Elsevier.
2. Tenembaum, S., Chamoles, N., and Fejerman, N. (2002). Acute disseminated encephalomyelitis: a long term follow-up study of 84 pediatric patients. *Neurology* 59: 1224–1231.
3. Pohl, D., Alper, G., Van Haren, K. et al. (2016). Acute disseminated encephalomyelitis. Updates on inflammatory CNS syndromes. *Neurology* 87 (Suppl 2): S38–S45.
4. Steiner, I. and Kennedy, P.G.E. (2015). Acute disseminated encephalomyelitis: current knowledge and open questions. *J. Neurovirol.* 21: 473–479.
5. Sonneville, R., Klein, I.F., and Wolff, M. (2010). Update on investigation and management of postinfectious encephalitis. *Curr. Opin. Neurol.* 23: 300–304.
6. Leake, J.A.D., Albani, S., Kao, A.S. et al. (2004). Acute disseminated encephalomyelitis in childhood: epidemiologic, clinical and laboratory features. *Pediatr. Infect. Dis. J.* 23: 756–764.
7. Torisu, H., Kira, R., Ishizaki, Y. et al. (2010). Clinical study of childhood acute disseminated encephalomyelitis, multiple sclerosis, and acute transverse myelitis in Fukuoka Prefecture, Japan. *Brain and Development* 32: 454–462.

8. Stuart, G. and Krikorian, K.S. (1928). The neuro-paralytic accidents of anti-rabies treatment. *Ann. Trop. Med. Parasitol.* 22: 327–377.
9. Bale, J.F. (2015). Virus and Immune-mediated encephalitides: Epidemiology, Diagnosis, Treatment, and Prevention. *Pediatr. Neurol.* 53: 3–12.
10. Krupp, L.B., Tardieu, M., Amato, M.P. et al. (2013). International Pediatric Multiple Sclerosis Study Group criteria for pediatric multiple sclerosis and immune-mediated central nervous system disorders: revisions to the 2007 definitions. *Mult. Scler.* 19: 1261–1267.
11. Hardy, T.A., Reddel, S.W., Barnett, M.H. et al. (2016). Atypical inflammatory demyelinating syndromes of the CNS. *Lancet Neurol.* 15: 967–981.
12. Hennes, E.M., Baumann, M., Schanda, K. et al. (2017). Prognostic relevance of MOG antibodies in children with an acquired demyelinating syndrome. *Neurology* 89: 900–908.
13. Banwell, B., Tennembaum, S., Lennon, V.A. et al. (2008). Neuromyelitis optica-IgG in childhood inflammatory demyelinating CNS disorders. *Neurology* 70: 344–352.
14. Young, N.P., Weinshenker, B.G., Parisi, J.E. et al. (2010). Perivenous demyelination: association with clinically defined acute disseminated encephalomyelitis and comparison with pathologically confirmed multiple sclerosis. *Brain* 133: 333–348.
15. Sepulveda, M., Amangue, T., Martinez-Hernandez, E. et al. (2016). Clinical spectrum assicated with MOG autoimmunity in adults: significance of sharing rodent MOG epitopes. *J. Neurol.* 263: 1349–1360.
16. Baumann, M., Sahin, K., Lechner, C. et al. (2015). Clinical and neuroradiological differences of pediatric acute disseminating encephalomyelitis with and without antibodies to the myelin oligodendrocyte glycoprotein. *J. Neurol. Neurosurg. Psychiatry* 86: 265–272.
17. Jarius, S., Ruprecht, K., Kleiter, I. et al. (2016). MOG-IgG in NMO and related disorders: a multicenter study of 50 patients. Part 2: Epidemiology, clinical presentation, radiological and laboratory features, treatment responses, and long-term outcome. *J. Neuroinflammation* 13: 280.
18. Spadaro, M., Gerdes, L.A., Mayer, M.C. et al. (2015). Histopathology and clinical course of MOG-antibody associated encephalomyelitis. *Ann. Clin. Transl. Neurol.* 2: 295–301.
19. Lassmann, H. (1983). Comparative neuropathology of chronic experimental allergic encephalomyelitis and multiple sclerosis. *Schriftenr. Neurol.* 25: 1–135.
20. Lachance, D.H., Lennon, V.A., Pittock, S.J. et al. (2010). An outbreak of neurological autoimmunity with polyradiculoneuropathy in workers exposed to aerosolised porcine neural tissue: a descriptive study. *Lancet Neurol.* 9: 55–66.
21. Wekerle, H., Kojima, K., Lannes-Vieira, J. et al. (1994). Animal models. *Ann. Neurol.* 36 (Suppl): S47–S53.
22. Wucherpfennig, K.W. and Strominger, J.L. (1995). Molecular mimicry in T-cell mediated autoimmunity: viral peptides activate human T-cell clones specific for myelin basic protein. *Cell* 80: 695–705.
23. Johnson, R.T., Griffin, D.E., Hirsch, R.L. et al. (1984). Measles encephalomyelitis – clinical and immunological studies. *N. Engl. J. Med.* 19: 137–141.
24. Lassmann, H. and Bradl, M. (2017). Multiple sclerosis: experimental models and reality. *Acta Neuropathol.* 133: 223–244.
25. Reindl, M., DiPauli, F., Rostasy, K., and Berger, T. (2013). The spectrum of MOG antoantibody-associated demyelinating diseases. *Nat. Rev. Neurol.* 9: 455–461.
26. Lim, H.Y., Ho, V.P., Thomas, T., and Chan, D.W. (2016). Serial outcomes in acute necrotizing encephalopathy of childhood: A medium and long term study. *Brain and Development* 38: 928–936.
27. Levine, S. (1965). Hyperacute allergic encephalomyelitis. Electron microscopic observations. *Am. J. Pathol.* 47: 209–221.
28. Wang, G.F., Li, W., and Li, K. (2010). Acute encephalopathy and encephalitis caused by influenza virus infection. *Curr. Opin. Neurol.* 23: 305–311.
29. Broderick, L., Gandhi, C., Mueller, J.L. et al. (2013). Mutations of complement factor I and potential mechanisms of neuroinflammation in acute hemorrhagic leukoencephalitis. *J. Clin. Immunol.* 33: 162–171.
30. Grundke-Iqbal, I., Lassmann, H., and Wisniewski, H.M. (1980). Chronic relapsing experimental allergic encephalomyelitis: Immunohistochemical studies. *Arch. Neurol.* 37: 651–656.
31. Singh, R.R., Sedani, S., Lim, M. et al. (2015). RANB2 mutation and acute necrotizing encephalopathy: 2 cases and a literature review of the expanding clinic-radiological phenotype. *Eur. J. Pediatr. Neurol.* 19: 106–113.

27 Miscellaneous Inflammatory Disorders of the CNS of Possible Infectious Origin

Mari Perez-Rosendahl[1], Jamie Nakagiri[1], Xinhai R. Zhang[2], and Harry V. Vinters[3]

[1] Department of Pathology and Laboratory Medicine, UC Irvine Medical Center, Orange, CA, USA
[2] Department of Pathology RUSH University Medical Center, Chicago, IL, USA
[3] Department of Pathology and Laboratory Medicine (Neuropathology) and Neurology, David Geffen School of Medicine UCLA and Ronald Reagan UCLA Medical Center, Los Angeles, CA, USA

Abbreviations

BS	Behçet's syndrome
CD	cortical dysplasia
CNS	central nervous system
CSF	cerebrospinal fluid
EEG	electroencephalogram
EL	encephalitis lethargica
EPC	epilepsia partialis continua
MRI	magnetic resonance imaging
NBS	neuro-Behçet's syndrome
RE	Rasmussen encephalitis
RS	Rasmussen syndrome
TSC	tuberous sclerosis complex

Introduction

This chapter will deal with several fairly rare entities that may be encountered in surgical pathology specimens or at autopsy. Any neuropathologist is likely to see only a small number of these entities unless he or she works at a center specializing in the diagnosis and treatment of unusual inflammatory CNS conditions, or pediatric epilepsy. Some of these diseases are of interest more from an historical perspective (e.g. encephalitis lethargica [EL]). Meaningful research on these uncommon conditions requires the pooling of resources and talent. There is a concerted effort to set up multicenter international registries that include a detailed database and cerebrospinal fluid (CSF) and brain tissue bank or repository, supplying data or specimens for research that would not be possible at a single institution; this has been done, for example, with cases of Rasmussen syndrome (RS)/Rasmussen encephalitis (RE) [1].

Rasmussen syndrome/Rasmussen encephalitis

RS/RE is a rare, medically intractable seizure disorder characterized clinically by epilepsia partialis

Infections of the Central Nervous System: Pathology and Genetics, First Edition. Edited by Fabrice Chrétien, Kum Thong Wong, Leroy R. Sharer, Catherine (Katy) Keohane and Françoise Gray.
© 2020 John Wiley & Sons Ltd. Published 2020 by John Wiley & Sons Ltd.

continua (EPC) and progressive unilateral neurologic deficit (usually hemiparesis). Neuropathologic features in the affected brain include chronic inflammatory and destructive changes, almost always confined to one cerebral hemisphere. Corticectomy or hemispherectomy is often the treatment of choice for affected patients, yielding abundant material for detailed neuropathologic and molecular study. Despite this, a definitive etiology for RS/RE has yet to be established. This entity was described in detail in a recent International Society of Neuropathology (ISN) volume focusing on *Developmental Neuropathology* [2]. RS/RE is also known as smoldering encephalitis and chronic (pathogen-free) encephalitis. Rasmussen et al. [3, 4] described the first cases more than 60 years ago at the Montreal Neurologic Institute. He and colleagues observed the enigmatic chronic localized encephalitis, after documenting the inflammatory features in cortical tissue from some young patients with intractable epilepsy, treated by surgical resection.

Epidemiology, demographics, and genetics

The age range at presentation with first seizure is usually 5–10 years, although first occurrence of initial clinical symptoms outside this range is not inconsistent with the diagnosis. A small percentage of affected patients have their onset in adulthood. There is no apparent sex predominance. The true underlying etiology of RS/RE remains unknown and is frequently debated. Some reports suggest a possible link to an initial viral infection, including reports of associated iritis at presentation. No particular risk factors are reported. There is one report of brothers with alternating bilateral EPC, in whom a brain biopsy showed chronic inflammation [5]. However, the limited morphologic information and uncharacteristic semiology in these cases renders the diagnosis uncertain.

Clinical features

Children usually present with focal seizures, typically focal (unilateral) motor seizures, which prove resistant to anticonvulsant medication. The seizures are associated with evidence of a progressive hemiparesis and, in many cases, with associated cognitive decline. EPC ultimately occurs in 60%. The rate of progression is variable, ranging from months to many years [6]. On neuroimaging, it appears that early involvement of the head of the caudate nucleus may be pathognomonic. Thereafter, signal change and progressive atrophy of one cerebral hemisphere is consistent with the clinical diagnosis. Uniformly progressive change is not seen in all cases, and it is not unusual for there not to be direct correlative progressive change linked to the clinical presentation.

Neuropathologic features

Macroscopy

The majority of neuropathologic observations have been gained from surgical material, both diagnostic biopsy and hemispherectomy, either anatomical or functional [7, 8]. Gyral damage is patchy and varies from indiscernible, through slight granularity or discoloration and thinning in the early stages, to extensive hemi-atrophy, striatal atrophy, and ventricular dilatation in longstanding cases. Multifocal neuronal loss resulting in laminar necrosis and microcystic change may be macroscopically visible.

Microscopy

Microscopic changes (Figures 27.1 and 27.2) are much more extensive than is evident macroscopically, though patchy and often sharply demarcated from normal areas. Early changes may be subtle and include microgliosis within the brain; microglial aggregates may form into inflammatory nodules (Figures 27.1a, b). Destructive and inflammatory change may be abundant and extensive in large cortical resections. Active lesions show perivascular lymphomonocytic cuffs (Figure 27.1c) in the leptomeninges, randomly scattered through the cortical layers and less often in subjacent white matter. In the cortex there are activated microglia [9], microglial nodules, and prominent neuronophagia with a variable degree of neuronal loss and gliosis. The neuropathologic substrate of cerebral atrophy is multifocal neuronal loss with astrocytic gliosis, sometimes with laminar necrosis or pancortical neuronal loss, microcystic change, and astrocytic gliosis. Long-standing "burnt-out" lesions have little inflammation but show spongy destruction

Miscellaneous Inflammatory Disorders of the CNS of Possible Infectious Origin Chapter 27

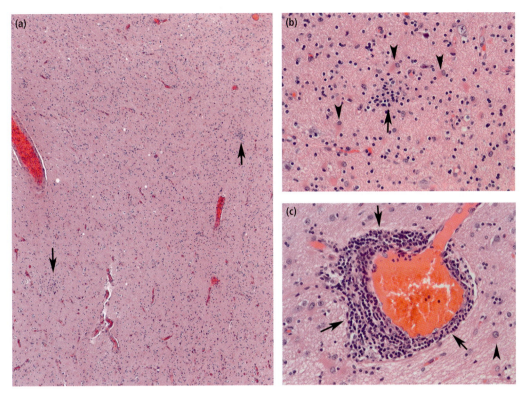

Figure 27.1 Rasmussen syndrome/Rasmussen encephalomyelitis (RS/RE), microscopic features; all panels are from hematoxylin and eosin (H&E)-stained sections. (a) Subtle (and probably early) abnormalities, including a modestly increased cellularity throughout brain parenchyma (a mixture of microglia and astrocytes) and poorly defined microglial (inflammatory) cell aggregates, indicated by arrows. (b) Magnified view of an inflammatory (microglial) nodule (arrow). The surrounding brain parenchyma shows gemistocytic astrocytes (indicated by arrowheads). (c) Perivascular cuffing by mononuclear cells (arrows). Despite the prominent inflammatory infiltrate centered on blood vessels, there is no evidence of injury to the vessel wall. Arrowhead indicates astrocyte in the adjacent neuropil.

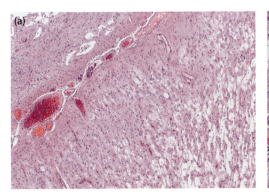
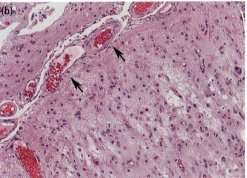

Figure 27.2 Advanced Rasmussen syndrome/Rasmussen encephalomyelitis (RS/RE), microscopic features; both panels are from hematoxylin and eosin (H&E)-stained sections. (a) Marked microcystic cavitation of the cortex and dense reactive gliosis; chronic inflammation is relatively minimal. (b) Magnified view of the subpial region of affected cortex (arrows indicate the overlying subarachnoid space, including an artery and a venule). Pronounced astrogliosis and microcavitation is present throughout the cortex.

of the cortical ribbon, marked capillary proliferation and gliosis (Figures 27.2a, b). Active and burnt-out areas can occur in close proximity in the same biopsy. Rare postmortem studies have confirmed that the inflammatory process is, with rare exceptions [10], strictly unilateral, involving the cerebral hemisphere very widely from frontal pole to occipital pole. These unilateral neuropathologic features distinguish RS/RE from other immune-mediated CNS disorders [11]. The basal ganglia and, occasionally, the brainstem may be involved. There is also cerebellar atrophy (but no inflammation), some of which may be secondary to the neocortical destruction (i.e. a trans-synaptic phenomenon), to hypoxia resulting from seizures, or a combination of the two.

It has been proposed that the neuropathologic features of RS/RE comprise four merging stages [12–14]. The earliest stage is characterized by inflammation, especially the presence of perivascular lymphocytes and accumulation of microglial nodules within the brain but with little evidence of neuronal loss or injury. In the second stage, lymphocytic inflammation becomes more prominent and both astrogliosis and microgliosis become widespread, involving all cortical layers; patchy neuronal loss may be present. In the third stage, severe neocortical degeneration becomes apparent with a patchy panlaminar pattern and astrocytic gliosis. In the fourth stage, there is profound cortical atrophy with gliosis and vacuolation of the neuropil and, (in many cases), cystic cavitation, especially within the neocortex. It bears emphasis that areas of almost normal cortex can separate areas with severe abnormalities; the occipital cortex may be relatively spared.

Immunohistochemical and ultrastructural findings

CD68 and Iba1 positive microglia and CD3 positive T cells are readily apparent in RS/RE brain, though variable in different segments of the neocortex. B cells are present in smaller numbers [8, 14, 15]. A quantitative analysis of microglial activation in RS/RE brain, as compared to that in cortical dysplasia (CD) and tuberous sclerosis complex (TSC) tubers, has shown clear evidence of accentuated Iba1+ immunoreactivity in RS/RE [9].

On ultrastructural examination, generally there is no evidence of definite viral particles, deposition of immune complexes or damage to the blood-brain barrier (BBB), though some curious electron microscopic findings have been described, including rare endothelial tubuloreticular inclusions [15, 16].

Differential diagnosis and pathogenesis

The major clinical and morphologic differential diagnoses are any neocortical lesion that may be epileptogenic (e.g. CD), though neuroimaging features of RS/RE are quite distinct from those of CD. A European consensus conference on RS/RE has formulated helpful diagnostic criteria that incorporate clinical, electroencephalogram (EEG), magnetic resonance imaging (MRI), and histopathologic findings [12, 13].

Overall, the pathological features of RS/RE brain suggest a chronic viral infection or autoimmunity. Reviews and references of RS/RE pathogenesis (especially immunopathogenesis) and relevant experimental models are found in [2, 17, 18].

Very low levels of *Herpesviridae* genomic sequences that may be of pathological significance have been detected in some patients. A search for RNASeq data from six RS/RE brain specimens failed to find any evidence for actively transcribed viral genes. However, after clearance of a virus from the brain, some persisting memory T cells may cross-react with a brain-specific self-antigen because of molecular mimicry. Autoreactive bystander T cells that have escaped tolerance could also traffic to the brain during the response to an infection. Many of the T cells in resected brain tissue are resident memory T cells, consistent with an acute immune response occurring at a very early stage of the disease.

Circulating autoantibodies against the glutamate ionotropic receptor α-amino-3-hydroxy-5-methyl-4-isoxazolepropionic acid (AMPA) type subunit 3(GRIA3) detected in subjects with RS/RE supported an autoimmune pathogenesis. These antibodies also occur in other seizure disorders, leading to the conclusion that they form when receptors are "shed" into the circulation during seizures. Autoantibodies to the glutamate ionotropic receptor N-methyl-D-aspartate (NMDA) type subunit 2 (GRIN2B) and the synaptic protein Munc18 have also been described in some patients with RS/RE, sometimes accompanied by a

B lymphocyte and plasma cell infiltrate. Aggressive plasmapheresis treatment and anti-CD20 monoclonal antibody therapy have been tried in some affected individuals.

Cellular immunity also plays a role. The lymphocytic infiltrates in RS/RE brain consist predominantly of CD8+αβ T cells and CD4-/CD8-γδ T cells. Polarized T cells containing granzyme B have been described in close apposition to neurons and astrocytes. With rare exceptions, B lymphocytes, immunoglobulins, and complement are usually not found in RS/RE brain tissue. The T cell infiltrate is of comparatively restricted clonality. CD8+ clones observed within brain infiltrates in RS/RE tissue, and their persistence in the periphery, suggested that RS/RE may be caused by an antigen-driven major histocompatibility (MHC) class-I restricted CD8+T-cell–mediated attack on CNS astrocytes and neurons. γδ T immune cells also appear involved. They are early responders to an inflammatory reaction and produce proinflammatory cytokines such as interferon gamma (IFN-γ). Resected RS/RE brain tissue has shown increased levels of IFN-γ mRNA compared with focal cortical dysplasia (FCD), and elevated levels of IFN-γ and tumor necrosis factor alpha (TNF-α) have been measured in CSF from patients with RS/RE. Transcripts for CCL5, CXCL9, and CXCL10, chemokines that attract cytotoxic CD8+ T cells, are also increased in RS/RE brain tissue compared with focal CD. It likely that activated microglia also produce proinflammatory cytokines and chemokines, resulting in an inflammatory milieu that may promote seizures. Activated microglia may also influence neuron excitability by forming hemichannels with pyramidal neurons. The arterial intimal thickening seen in patients with RS/RE who have undergone serial corticectomies over months or years may be related to an autoimmune mechanism directed against blood vessel wall components.

Future directions and therapy

Many RE subjects have shown a response to steroid therapy. In view of the possible autoimmune etiology, various immunosuppressive therapies have been proposed, including high-dose steroids and intravenous immunoglobulin [19, 20]. Surgery (i.e. hemispherectomy or more focal corticectomy) still appears to be the only long-term cure for such seizures. Further evaluation of possible autoimmune mechanisms and alternative immunosuppressive therapy is required and ongoing.

Neuro-Behçet's disease and syndrome

Behçet's syndrome (BS), originally described in 1937 by Hulusi Behçet, is a rare idiopathic chronic, relapsing, multisystem, vascular inflammatory disorder that most commonly presents as recurrent ulceration of the mouth and genitalia accompanied by uveitis or iridocyclitis. An encephalitic syndrome may occur occasionally, as well as symptoms related to involvement of various other organs [21–23].

Epidemiology

The prevalence of neuro-Behçet's syndrome (NBS) is 3–9% among patients with BS, although rates up to 59% have been reported in areas where BS is rare. One study of a cohort of 728 BS cases showed neurological involvement in only 3.6% of patients. The mean age of onset is between 25 and 33 years, with neurologic involvement usually occurring three to five years later. BS is very rare in the pediatric population. Although no gender differences are noted, the male-to-female ratio for neurological symptoms is about 4:1. In general, men tend to have more serious complications from BS. However, once neurologic involvement develops, its severity does not differ between genders. Because of the variable nature of BS, the prognosis is highly dependent on disease severity and the associated complications.

Clinical features

In general, BS does not present with neurological symptoms. The two most common neurological manifestations in NBS are parenchymal involvement of the CNS and cerebral venous sinus thrombosis. Intra-axial NBS is due to small vessel disease leading to focal or multifocal CNS involvement. It can have a relapsing and remitting course initially, with secondary progression. Extra-axial NBS as a result of large vessel disease has a better prognosis than intra-axial vascular involvement and may have a different pathogenesis, which is largely unknown [21–23].

CSF examined during the acute stage of intra-axial NBS shows inflammatory changes with an increased number of cells (neutrophilic predominance) and modestly elevated protein levels. CSF in patients with extra-axial NBS generally show normal cellular and chemical composition but with an increased opening pressure on lumbar puncture.

MRI generally reveals lesions in the brainstem, diencephalon, and basal ganglia. The most commonly affected areas are the mesencephalic-diencephalic junction and the pontobulbar region. Lesion distribution can help to differentiate NBS from multiple sclerosis and systemic lupus erythematosus but can overlap with many other entities including chronic brainstem meningoencephalitis. Evaluation for the presence of mucocutaneous-ocular symptoms in NBS must be used to distinguish it from other disorders.

Neuropathology
There is a paucity of histopathologic data on NBS. The most frequent findings include multifocal necrotizing lesions, predominantly involving the thalamus, hypothalamus, and midbrain. The inflammatory changes are often necrotic and sometimes hemorrhagic. Neutrophilic perivascular infiltrates as well as chronic nodular inflammation leading to tissue destruction and subsequent gliosis have been reported. Necrotic lesions, without specific features, can also occur [22, 23]. Vasculitis is considered to be the underlying lesion, but cerebral blood vessel changes are non-specific.

Etiology
The etiology of BS is not completely understood. Attempts to demonstrate a virus as the cause of BS have failed. It is thought that genetic predisposition, HLA type, infectious agents, autoantigens, cellular and humoral immunological hyperactivity, endothelial cell dysfunction, and oxidative stress may all play a role.

Treatment
Steroids are the treatment of choice for the acute treatment of both types of neurologic symptoms. Other immunosuppressants may be used for long-term treatment of BS.

Encephalitis lethargica

Definition of the disorder, major synonyms, and historical perspective
EL also called von Economo disease, epidemic encephalitis, or postencephalitic parkinsonism describes a perplexing neuropsychiatric disorder that occurred in epidemic proportions between 1917 and 1930. The disorder is also called "von Economo disease," named after the psychiatrist and neurologist Constantin von Economo (1876–1931), who authored the first paper on EL in 1917. The exact etiology is still unknown and is a source of longstanding debate; the most prevalent theory implicated influenza, which was pandemic during a similar time period (1918–1919), as a causal agent. However, just as von Economo first proposed, several features of EL substantiate its distinction from influenza, including epidemiology, transmission, symptomatology, neuropathology, and outcome. Furthermore, contemporary study has not revealed influenza RNA within archived EL brain tissue [24–27].

Epidemiology and clinical features
During the 1917–1930 epidemic, EL was reported around the world, most evident in Europe, North America, and the Soviet Union and most commonly affecting persons 12–35 years of age. Reports of transmission of EL were very rare. Although some reports described the number of affected males being twice that of females, others showed an even distribution between genders. Flulike symptoms were often seen at the onset (including fever, somnolence, diplopia, and pharyngitis). However, subsequent symptomatology was distinct from influenza and included sleep disorders, basal ganglia signs (including parkinsonism), and neuropsychiatric sequelae (often behavioral problems in younger patients and parkinsonism or oculogyria in the older population). Sleep derangements comprised days to weeks of increasing somnolence, with some cases progressing to a comatose state, at which point recovery was unlikely [24, 25]. Death occurred acutely in about one-third of patients with EL, one-third recovered completely, and one-third

developed neuropsychiatric sequelae, most commonly postencephalitic parkinsonism.

Neuropathologic features

The most common macroscopic findings reported during the epidemic included cerebral swelling and multiple petechial or patchy cortical or meningeal hemorrhages. Microscopically, inflammation, hemorrhage, gliosis, thrombosis, and necrosis were often found in many cortical areas, and a subset also showed similar pathology in the thalamus, basal ganglia, brainstem, and cerebellum. Of the cases with midbrain pathologic alterations, about half were oculomotor nerve abnormalities and 12% had substantia nigra lesions [25, 26].

In chronic cases, most of whom had postencephalitic parkinsonian syndromes, severe brainstem lesions with complete discoloration of the substantia nigra and tegmental atrophy were observed. Extensive or total nerve cell loss was accompanied by severe astrocytosis. Neurofibrillary tangles were widespread but particularly affected the substantia nigra, locus coeruleus, nuclei of the reticular formation, hypothalamus, and the nucleus basalis of Meynert [27]. Perivascular inflammatory mononuclear infiltrates were rare.

Current perspectives

Since the EL epidemic of the 1900s, sporadic cases with EL-like phenotypes continue to be reported; some of these have shown intrathecal oligoclonal bands and improvement with steroid treatment. Recent data in EL-like cases has shown autoantibodies against human basal ganglia antigens. Although further investigation is required to determine whether these antibodies are pathogenic, these findings suggest EL may represent a postinfectious autoimmune disorder, with antibodies directed against deep gray matter neurons [28].

Hashimoto's encephalopathy

This is a rare and poorly characterized inflammatory disorder of the brain. The clinical manifestations include decreased consciousness, confusion and disorientation, cognitive deficit, seizures, ataxia, myoclonus, and a variety of focal neurologic deficits [29–31]. There are three diagnostic criteria: (i) the presence of clinical neurological abnormalities after exclusion of other causes of encephalopathy; (ii) the presence of antithyroid antibodies; and (iii) clinical improvement following the administration of "immunomodulatory therapy."

Neuropathologic studies are few. Because this is not a fatal condition, autopsy studies are lacking, and brain biopsy has been performed usually when another lesion (e.g. brain tumor) is suspected [30]. In such cases, there is reactive gliosis and a T-cell predominant perivascular lymphocytic infiltrate within the brain parenchyma.

References

1. Kruse, C.A., Pardo, C.A., Hartman, A.L. et al. (2016). Rasmussen encephalitis tissue transfer program. *Epilepsia* 57: 1004–1006.
2. Vinters, H.V., Magaki, S.D., and Owens, G.C. (2018). Rasmussen encephalitis. In: *Developmental Neuropathology*, seconde (eds. H. Adle-Biassette, B.N. Harding and J.A. Golden), 531–536. Oxford, England: Wiley Blackwell.
3. Rasmussen, T. (1978). Further observations on the syndrome of chronic encephalitis and epilepsy. *Appl. Neurophysiol.* 41: 1–12.
4. Rasmussen, T., Olszewski, J., and Lloyd-Smith, D. (1958). Focal seizures due to chronic localized encephalitis. *Neurology* 8: 435–445.
5. Silver, K., Andermann, F., and Meagher, V.K. (1998). Familial alternating epilepsia partialis continua with chronic encephalitis: another variant of Rasmussen syndrome? *Arch. Neurol.* 55: 733–736.
6. Oguni, H., Andermann, F., and Rasmussen, T.B. (1992). The syndrome of chronic encephalitis and epilepsy. A study based on the MNI series of 48 cases. *Adv. Neurol.* 57: 419–433.
7. Honavar, M., Janota, I., and Polkey, C.E. (1992). Rasmussen's encephalitis in surgery for epilepsy. *Dev. Med. Child Neurol.* 34: 3–14.
8. Robitaille, Y. (1991). Neuropathologic aspects of chronic encephalitis. In: *Chronic Encephalitis and Epilepsy: Rasmussen's Syndrome* (ed. F. Andermann), 79–110. London: Butterworth-Heinemann.
9. Wirenfeldt, M., Clare, R., Tung, S. et al. (2009). Increased activation of Iba1+ microglia in pediatric

epilepsy patients with Rasmussen's encephalitis compared with cortical dysplasia and tuberous sclerosis complex. *Neurobiol. Dis.* 34: 432–440.
10. Tobias, S.M., Robitaille, Y., Hickey, W.F. et al. (2003). Bilateral Rasmussen encephalitis: postmortem documentation in a five-year-old. *Epilepsia* 44: 127–130.
11. Junker, A. and Bruck, W. (2012). Autoinflammatory grey matter lesions in humans: cortical encephalitis, clinical disorders, experimental models. *Curr. Opin. Neurol.* 25: 349–357.
12. Bien, C.G., Granata, T., Antozzi, C. et al. (2005). Pathogenesis, diagnosis and treatment of Rasmussen encephalitis: a European consensus statement. *Brain* 128: 454–471.
13. Bien, C.G., Urbach, H., Deckert, M. et al. (2002). Diagnosis and staging of Rasmussen's encephalitis by serial MRI and histopathology. *Neurology* 58: 250–257.
14. Pardo, C.A., Vining, E.P.G., Guo, L. et al. (2004). The pathology of Rasmussen syndrome: stages of cortical involvement and neuropathological studies in 45 hemispherectomies. *Epilepsia* 45: 516–526.
15. Farrell, M.A., Droogan, O., Secor, D.L. et al. (1995). Chronic encephalitis associated with epilepsy: immunohistochemical and ultrastructural studies. *Acta Neuropathol.* 89: 313–321.
16. Park, S.-H. and Vinters, H.V. (2002). Ultrastructural study of Rasmussen encephalitis. *Ultrastruct. Pathol.* 26: 287–292.
17. Owens, G.C., Erickson, K.L., Malone, C.C. et al. (2015). Evidence for the involvement of gamma delta T cells in the immune response in Rasmussen encephalitis. *J. Neuroinflammation* 12: a134.
18. Owens, G.C., Huynh, M.N., Chang, J.W. et al. (2013). Differential expression of interferon-gamma and chemokine genes distinguishes Rasmussen encephalitis from cortical dysplasia and provides evidence for an early Th1 immune response. *J. Neuroinflammation* 10: a56.
19. Andrews, P.I., Dichter, M.A., Berkovic, S.F. et al. (1996). Plasmapheresis in Rasmussen's encephalitis. *Neurology* 46: 242–246.
20. Andrews, P.I. and McNamara, J.O. (1996). Rasmussen's encephalitis: an autoimmune disorder? *Curr. Opin. Neurol.* 6: 673–678.
21. Saip, S., Akman-Demir, G., and Siva, A. (2014). Neuro-Behcet syndrome. *Handb. Clin. Neurol.* 121: 1703–1723.
22. Arai, Y., Kohno, S., Takahashi, Y. et al. (2006). Autopsy case of neuro-Behcet's disease with multifocal neutrophilic perivascular inflammation. *Neuropathology* 26: 579–585.
23. Yamada, H., Saito, K., Hokari, M., and Toru, S. (2017). Brain biopsy to aid diagnosis of neuro-Behcet's disease: case report and literature review. *eNeurologicalSci.* 8: 2–4.
24. Foley, P.B. (2009). Encephalitis lethargica and the influenza virus. II. The influenza pandemic of 1918/19 and encephalitis lethargica: epidemiology and symptoms. *J. Neural Transm. (Vienna)* 116: 1295–1308.
25. Foley, P.B. (2009). Encephalitis lethargica and the influenza virus. III. The influenza pandemic of 1918/19 and encephalitis lethargica: neuropathology and discussion. *J. Neural Transm. (Vienna)* 116: 1309–1321.
26. Anderson, L.L., Vilensky, J.A., and Duvoisin, R.C. (2009). Review: neuropathology of acute phase encephalitis lethargica: a review of cases from the epidemic period. *Neuropathol. Appl. Neurobiol.* 35: 462–472.
27. Escourolle, R., de Recondo, J., and Gray, F. (1971). Etude anatomo-pathologique des syndromes parkinsoniens. In: *Monoamines, noyaux gris centraux et syndrome de Parkinson* (eds. J. de Ajuriaguerra and G. Gauthier), 173–229. Genève: Georges et Cie SA.
28. Dale, R.C., Church, A.J., Surtees, R.A. et al. (2004). Encephalitis lethargica syndrome: 20 new cases and evidence of basal ganglia autoimmunity. *Brain* 127: 21–33.
29. Pinedo-Torres, I. and Paz-Ibarra, J.L. (2018). Current knowledge on Hashimoto's encephalopathy: a literature review. *Medwave* 18: e7298.
30. Uwatoko, H., Yabe, I., Sato, S. et al. (2018). Hashimoto's encephalopathy mimicking a brain tumor and its pathological findings: a case report. *J. Neurol. Sci.* 394: 141–143.
31. Amanat, M., Thijs, R.D., Salehi, M., and Sander, J.W. (2019). Seizures as a clinical manifestation in somatic autoimmune disorders. *Seizure* 64: 59–64.

28 Mycoplasmal and Rickettsial Infections of the CNS

Roy H. Rhodes
School of Medicine, Department of Pathology, Louisiana State University, New Orleans, LA, USA

Abbreviations

CNS	Central nervous system
CSF	Cerebrospinal fluid
EM	Electron microscopy
EPM(s)	Extrapulmonary manifestation(s)
G6PD	Glucose-6-phosphate dehydrogenase
GFAP	Glial fibrillary acidic protein
IHC	Immunohistochemistry
MRI	Magnetic resonance imaging
MSF	Mediterranean spotted fever
PCR	Polymerase chain reaction
RMSF	Rocky Mountain spotted fever
SFG	Spotted fever group
TG	Typhus group

Mycoplasmal infections of the CNS

Mycoplasma pneumoniae
Definition of the disorder, microbiological characteristics, and epidemiology

M. pneumoniae (class Mollicutes), the best-studied mycoplasmal species and known since the 1940s, is a major cause of atypical (community-acquired, "walking") pneumonia. Infrequently, it causes extrapulmonary manifestations (EPMs) affecting the CNS of children and adults worldwide. Spherical mycoplasmal cells (as small as 0.1 μm) are the smallest bacteria living a cell-free existence, but they can become 2 μm or longer. They lack a cell wall, allowing them to be pleomorphic (i.e. fusiform, flask-shaped) and unaffected by beta-lactam antibiotics. They usually attach to respiratory epithelial or urothelial cell surfaces. When living as facultative intracellular parasites, they may be protected from extracellular host immunity and antibiotics. *Mycoplasma* species rely on host cells for nutritional requirements because they have a minimal genome due to reductive evolution [1–5].

Encephalitis is the most common and severe EPM of *M. pneumoniae*. Standard serologic diagnosis is problematic in establishing causality because of the high population frequency of serum anti-*M. pneumoniae* immunoglobulin G (IgG). CNS mycoplasmal lesions evolve hematogenously, by immunomodulation, or rarely through inoculation or contamination [1, 2, 5].

There are three proposed mechanisms of lesion formation: (i) Direct infection, with a *Mycoplasma*-induced inflammatory cytokine response, (ii) indirect infection through immunomodulation, and (iii) vascular occlusion with direct or indirect effects on blood flow obstruction. These mechanisms are not mutually exclusive and they may operate concomitantly during vascular endothelial cell invasion (i.e. the relevant host cell invaded by *M. pneumoniae*), through

---

Infections of the Central Nervous System: Pathology and Genetics, First Edition. Edited by Fabrice Chrétien, Kum Thong Wong, Leroy R. Sharer, Catherine (Katy) Keohane and Françoise Gray.
© 2020 John Wiley & Sons Ltd. Published 2020 by John Wiley & Sons Ltd.

immunopathogenesis (i.e. molecular mimicry, immune complex formation), and blood-flow compromise. Pneumonia is frequently absent in patients with clinical evidence of mycoplasmal CNS disease, providing an additional challenge in diagnosis [1–3, 5, 6].

Although neurologic disease is a rare complication of *M. pneumoniae* infection, it is suspected in up to 10% of acute childhood encephalitis cases [7] and can affect people who are immunocompetent and immunocompromised[3].

Clinical features

Direct CNS infection usually presents as aseptic meningitis or early-onset encephalitis or myelitis. Indirect involvement includes late-onset encephalitis or myelitis, Guillain-Barré syndrome, cranial or peripheral neuropathies, cerebellitis, acute cerebellar ataxia, and the opsoclonus-myoclonus syndrome. Evidence of vascular occlusion includes altered mental status, cerebral infarct, striatal necrosis, and thalamic necrosis. Optic neuritis and transient parkinsonism are reported.

Computed tomography (CT) without contrast enhancement may show progressive brain calcific deposits in mycoplasmal encephalitis (Figure 28.1a–c) [3]. Magnetic resonance imaging (MRI) of *M. pneumoniae* encephalomyelitis in children reveals focal abnormalities in white matter, neocortex, and basal ganglia relatively often, with fewer lesions in thalamus, limbic regions, cerebellum, and brainstem [8].

M. pneumoniae serology, often using enzyme immunoassay to detect immunoglobulin M (IgM) and IgG, requires a fourfold antibody titer increase in comparing acute and convalescent sera over two to three weeks. A throat swab for culture or polymerase chain reaction (PCR) is also suggested for diagnosis. The diagnosis of *M. pneumoniae* encephalitis usually requires both seroconversion and positive cerebrospinal fluid (CSF) PCR. Evidence of intrathecal antibody production may be a specific infection indicator. CSF antiganglioside antibody detection may be a clue to indirect CNS lesions.

Pathology

Bilateral lesions occur in the splenium of the corpus callosum and in the brainstem. Bickerstaff brainstem encephalitis, which is severe, is associated with anti-GQ1b antibodies. Acute necrotizing encephalopathy may be reversible, an indication of poor understanding of its pathologic basis. Acute demyelinating encephalomyelitis and acute hemorrhagic leukoencephalitis have suggested both direct and indirect *M. pneumoniae* involvement [1, 3, 6, 7].

Microscopically, mycoplasmal meningoencephalomyelitis can produce mild leptomeningitis and perivasculitis with lymphocytes and macrophages. Focal microvascular endothelial cell clustering with nuclear and cytoplasmic enlargement (atypia) can be striking and is reminiscent of viral changes (Figure 28.1d–f). Chronic microvascular damage with vascular looping and adventitial thickening resembles animal models of hypoxic damage (Figure 28.2a, b) [3]. Cerebral gliosis even with longstanding mycoplasmal encephalitis can be mild, and chronic perivasculitis can remain active (Figure 28.2c, d). Immunohistochemistry (IHC) demonstrates mycoplasmal antigen in endothelial cells (Figure 28.2e–f). Microcalcifications may be found in CNS parenchyma. Electron microscopy (EM) demonstrates microvascular changes including nuclear atypia of endothelial cells and to a lesser extent of smooth muscle cells and swollen endothelial cytoplasm that frequently narrows capillary lumina (Figure 28.3a–c). The mycoplasmal cells are in the cytoplasm of some endothelial cells, within occasional microvascular lumina, and in some perivascular macrophages. Not all capillaries have demonstrable parasitic invasion, yet many possibly uninfected capillaries show nuclear atypia and swollen endothelial cytoplasm, suggesting both direct (possibly including a *M. pneumoniae* exotoxin) and indirect (i.e. induced cytokine production, hypoxic consequences) mechanisms of infection. Rarely, instead of only spherical, fusiform, and dumbbell shapes indistinguishable from some other Mollicutes, flask-shaped and other pleomorphic mycoplasmal cells are seen. Unique terminal and attachment organelles, present in mycoplasmal species, used for gliding movement and for host cell attachment, have been documented in human CNS specimens (Figure 28.3d–i) [1–4].

Treatment

Antibiotic treatment for *Mycoplasma* species includes macrolides, tetracycline, and quinolones. Encephalitis often also requires corticosteroids and intravenous immunoglobulin. Macrolide-resistant *M. pneumoniae* cases have been reported [1, 6, 7].

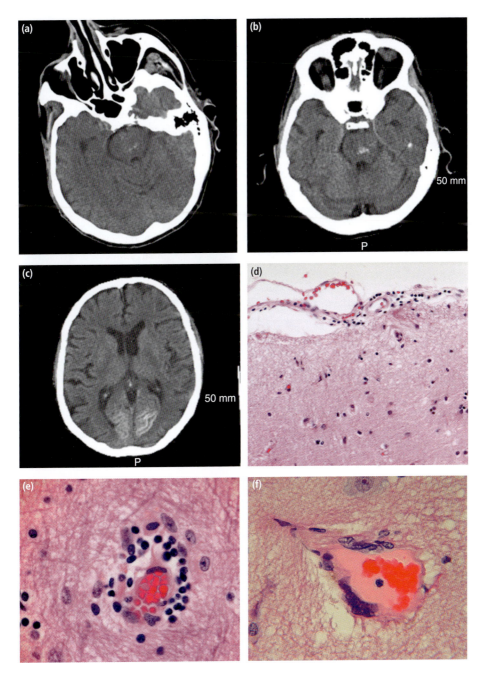

Figure 28.1 Mycoplasmal encephalitis. (a) An unenhanced computed tomography (CT) scan of a 73-year-old man with episodic altered mental status and ataxia shows focal pontine calcifications 15 months after the initial episode [3]. (b) An unenhanced CT scan of the same patient 10 years later shows progression of the pontine calcifications. The midbrain also had calcifications. Source: courtesy of Dr. Bruce T. Monastersky. (c) Bilateral stippled occipital lobe calcifications in this patient are present in the latter study. The patient had good cognition and had been employed during most of the 10 years after the first study. He died with hepatic cirrhosis of uncertain etiology soon after the latter CT study. Source: Courtesy of Dr. Bruce T. Monastersky. (d) There is mild leptomeningitis over the inferior temporal lobe of a 31-year-old man who died after four years with mycoplasmal encephalitis (×200, hematoxylin and eosin [H&E] stain) [4]. (e) Chronic perivasculitis in cerebellar white matter involves a dilated microvessel from the 31-year-old man with mycoplasmal encephalitis (×400, H&E stain). (f) Right frontal lobe cerebral biopsy from a 73-year-old patient, 15 months after symptom onset, shows three clusters of enlarged venular endothelial cell nuclei (×600, H&E stain) [3].

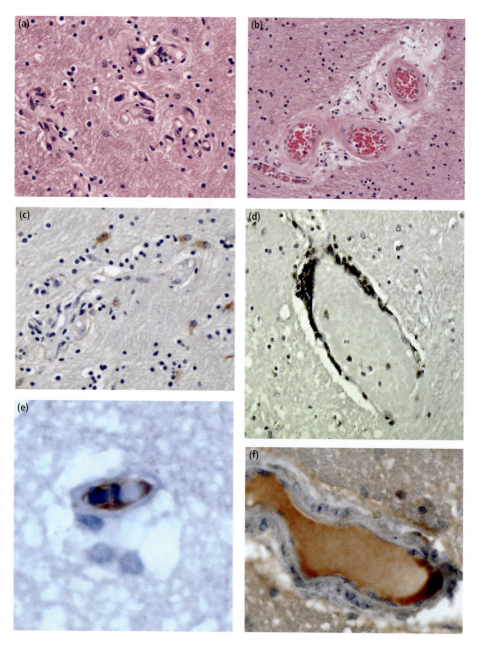

Figure 28.2 (a) Cerebral white matter of a 31-year-old man with mycoplasmal encephalitis shows microvascular proliferation (vascular looping, vascular wickerworks) with nuclear atypia (×200, hematoxylin and eosin [H&E] stain). (b) The right parietal white matter of a 31-year-old man with mycoplasmal encephalitis has significant vascular wall sclerosis, luminal dilation, and widening of the perivascular space. There were adjacent foci of white matter demyelination and axonal loss (×200, H&E stain). (c) Subcortical white matter of a 31-year-old man who died of mycoplasmal encephalitis has very mild gliosis demonstrated by immunostaining for glial fibrillary acidic protein (GFAP) (×200, GFAP immunohistochemistry [IHC]). (d) A dilated midbrain venule from a 31-year-old man with mycoplasmal encephalitis has chronic perivasculitis with lymphocytes and perhaps macrophages immunostained for leukocyte common antigen (×200, CD45 IHC). (e) Frontal lobe biopsy from a 73-year-old man with mycoplasmal encephalitis shows a dilated capillary with mycoplasmal antigen immunostained in endothelial cells. Note the large endothelial cell nuclei (×600, anti-*Mycoplasma pneumoniae* antibody, unabsorbed, IHC; may react with related microorganisms per manufacturer's note). (f) Cerebellar white matter of a 31-year-old man who died of mycoplasmal encephalitis shows residual endothelial cells positive for mycoplasmal antigen in a dilated arteriole. Light luminal staining above negative controls indicates possible luminal mycoplasmal antigen (×600, anti-*M. pneumoniae* antibody, unabsorbed, IHC; may react with related microorganisms).

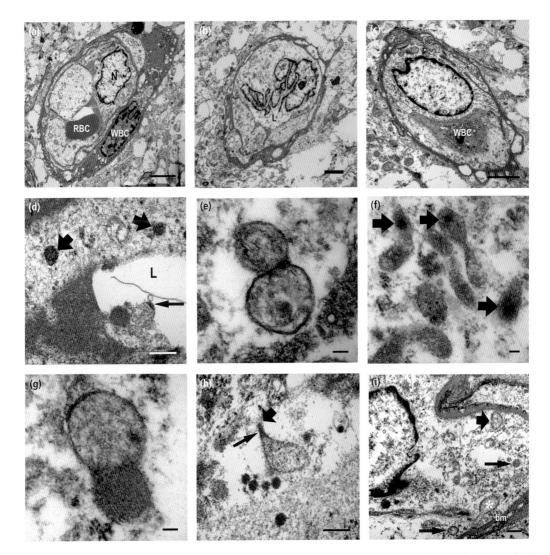

Figure 28.3 (a) Electron microscopy (EM) of a capillary in the frontal lobe biopsy shows endothelial cell cytoplasmic swelling. A small red blood cell (RBC) profile fills most of the reduced lumen. The nuclear profile (N) is enlarged and the nuclear envelope is irregular (atypia). A white blood cell (WBC) that appears to be a macrophage lies in the perivascular space (EM, scale bar 2 μm). (b) A frontal lobe biopsy capillary has an atypical endothelial cell nucleus with deep invaginations or complex lobulations of its nuclear envelope. The lumen (L) is a thin slit filled with fine, electron-dense granular material (EM, scale bar 2 μm) [3]. (c) This capillary in the frontal lobe biopsy has an atypical nucleus and a WBC profile fills its small lumen (EM, scale bar 2 μm). (d) Bacterial cells from the frontal lobe biopsy vary in density. Two small, dense spherical intraendothelial mycoplasmal cells (arrowheads) are seen. A more electron-lucent mycoplasmal cell in the capillary lumen (L) has a dense attachment organelle (arrow) (EM, scale bar 500 nm) [3]. (e) Two intraendothelial bacterial cells in the frontal biopsy have trilaminar plasma membranes and the appearance of having undergone binary fission (EM, scale bar 100 nm) [3]. (f) Bacterial cells within a large phagocyte in a microvascular perivascular space of the biopsied frontal lobe are fusiform and dumbbell shaped. Three have nucleoids (arrowheads). This is a common appearance of Mollicutes, including *Mycoplasma* species, but only mycoplasmal cells get significantly larger and have further pleomorphism (EM, scale bar 100 nm) [3]. (g) This bacterial cell within the same phagocyte as those seen in (f) has a prominent constriction that separates regions of different densities, a distinctive appearance of some mycoplasmal cells (EM, scale bar 100 nm) [3]. (h) In the cytoplasm of a frontal lobe biopsy capillary endothelial cell, the smallest of the dense, spherical bacterial cells, about 100 nm in diameter, contrasts with the large, flask-shaped cell with a terminal organelle (arrow) ending in an attachment organelle (arrowhead), emphasizing the size range and pleomorphism of mycoplasmal cells (EM, scale bar 500 nm) [3]. (i) Spherical (arrows) and oblong bacterial cells (arrowhead) are in an endothelial cell in the frontal biopsy. An oblong bacterial cell (*) is attached at the plasma membrane, and possibly to the underlying basement membrane (bm), by its dense attachment organelle at the end of a long terminal organelle. The upper oblong bacterial cell may have a similar attachment without a terminal organelle (EM, scale bar 500 nm) [3].

Mycoplasma hominis

M. hominis, a urogenital tract colonizer, rarely causes CNS lesion- or wound-site infections (i.e. brain abscess, meningitis), most likely from a genitourinary source. These *M. hominis* lesions are reported after craniotomies with head trauma or immunodeficiency and in newborns after delivery manipulation. *M. hominis* is usually not recovered from blood cultures. Real-time PCR has identified this species in brain abscesses [5]. A unique finding supported by IHC and EM has suggested direct *M. hominis* infection of neurons, glial cells, and macrophages in addition to endothelial cells, reported in a child with mycoplasmal encephalitis [9].

Rickettsial infections of the CNS

Definition and general microbiological, epidemiological, and clinical characteristics of rickettsiosis

The α-proteobacteria in the order Rickettsiales consists of four pathogenic groups of zoonotic infections with significant CNS complications. Three groups come from the genus *Rickettsia* in the family Rickettsiaceae, including the spotted fever group (SFG) and the typhus group (TG). Most potentially severe rickettsioses are in the SFG, including tick-borne Rocky Mountain spotted fever (RMSF; due to *Rickettsia rickettsii*) and Mediterranean spotted fever (MSF; *Rickettsia conorii*). The TG consists of louse-borne epidemic typhus *(Rickettsia prowazekii)* and flea-borne murine endemic typhus *(Rickettsia typhi)*. Mite-borne scrub typhus (tsutsugamuchi disease), principally caused by *Orientia tsutsugamuchi*, forms the third group [10–13]. The fourth disease group, from the family Anaplasmataceae (order Rickettsiales), includes tick-borne *Ehrlichia chaffeensis*, the agent of human monocytic ehrlichiosis, and *Anaplasma phagocytophilum*, the cause of human granulocytic anaplasmosis (previously known as human granulocytic ehrlichiosis). Both rickettsial families consist of small, Gram-negative, obligate intracellular bacteria that manipulate potential host cells for entry and then for metabolic support in order to grow and replicate [12, 14].

Rickettsial infections are found worldwide with geographic restrictions that define regions of endemic disease. However, the boundaries are not static and domestic animal reservoirs and human travelers can bring rickettsioses into locales not endemic for the disease, making clinical suspicion a key element in diagnosis. The emerging and re-emerging aspects of rickettsioses are important in rickettsial epidemiology. For example, for some SFG rickettsioses the previously documented restriction of limited tick vectors for the diseases in certain geographic regions is incorrect; epidemic (classic louse-borne) typhus has been identified in ticks; and scrub typhus, previously known only in the "tsutsugamuchi triangle" of the Asia-Pacific region, has been identified in the Middle East and Chile [15, 16].

Rickettsioses result from skin bite-site inoculations or from conjunctival or mucous membrane contamination with a rickettsial species carried by arthropods. The infections are often seasonal because of the needs of the arthropods (i.e. climate, habitat, vertebrate reservoir). Arthropod vector and rickettsial contacts with human hosts have been increasing as jungle and woodlands are cleared for plantations, farming, housing, and outdoor activities and as travel for ecotourism expands [10, 11, 14, 15].

Most rickettsioses have an incubation period of 6–20 days. They are difficult to diagnose close to symptom onset, when antibiotic treatment should be started. Disease is marked by an abrupt high fever, severe headache, malaise, myalgia, weakness, sometimes chills and gastrointestinal symptoms, and often a rash that initially is macular or maculopapular. The rash is caused by vasculitis from the infection of microvascular endothelial cells. Tick or mite bites may cause focal dermal and epidermal necrosis under a scab (i.e. eschar or tache noire). Infected endothelial cells become activated, and along with leukocytes, they produce cytokines that provide a proinflammatory, procoagulant environment. For most rickettsioses, thrombus formation is not a major problem, but microvascular permeability is a significant cause of morbidity. As the infection advances in vascular walls, the rash spreads, and it may become petechial or purpuric. Platelets are consumed locally. The vasculitis may involve the lungs, CNS, liver, and other organs, causing noncardiogenic pulmonary edema, hypotension, focal hepatic necrosis, and sometimes renal failure. Neurologic complications follow systemic hypotension or direct endothelial infection of CNS vessels [10, 11, 17, 18].

A rash may never appear, an arthropod bite may not be reported, and early symptoms may be mild even in a case that soon takes a severe or fatal course. The early course may resemble a viral disease, meningococcal infection, or other vasculitides [17].

SFG tick-borne rickettsioses
RMSF

The most severe rickettsiosis is tick-borne RMSF (*R. rickettsii*), first described more than a century ago. RMSF is found in most of North America and in parts of Central and South America. It varies cyclically, presumably from activities placing human hosts at greater risk [15]. Some tick vectors are more aggressive in hot weather when most infections occur [13]. Bacteria in salivary secretions are injected by feeding ticks at the bite site [11, 19].

Following phagocytosis by an endothelial cell and replication, *R. rickettsii* uses host-cell actin to move to the plasma membrane for exit. Exit may be into an adjacent endothelial cell, allowing the bacterium to avoid the extracellular host immune system while spreading through the vascular tree [11, 12, 14]. Fever, headache, gastrointestinal symptoms, and malaise develop. A rash is found in most cases, usually by days 3–5 of symptoms and appears on the wrists and ankles, spreads to the trunk, and then to palms and soles (Figure 28.4a) [14, 20, 21]. A bite-site eschar is rarely seen in RMSF [22]. CSF usually has lymphocytic and sometimes polymorphonuclear pleocytosis, while elevated protein is not often found, and low glucose is usually not seen [11, 21]. Cerebral MRI T2-weighted images might show meningeal enhancement, scattered, punctate areas of increased signal from perivascular inflammation, and infarcts [22].

CNS-related findings in RMSF can include ankle clonus, extensor plantar responses, hyperreflexia, spasticity, dysarthria, aphasia, nystagmus, cranial nerve palsies, hearing loss, severe vertigo, unilateral corticospinal tract signs, hemiplegia, paraplegia, complete paralysis, athetotic movements, fasciculations, and neurogenic bladder. Encephalitis with stupor, confusion or delirium occurs in roughly a quarter of cases. Seizures, ataxia, and coma are less common, although coma usually precedes a fatal outcome [14, 23]. Fatalities are seen most often in children younger than 10 years of age, the most common age for RMSF to occur, and in adults older than 70 years of age [22]. Mortality is also high for men and for black men with glucose-6-phosphate dehydrogenase (G6PD) deficiency. Untreated RMSF has a fatality rate of 25% or higher [11, 13, 19].

In endemic regions, empirical treatment with doxycycline is often provided for suspected RMSF before confirming the diagnosis with serology or PCR [11, 24]. This is usually true for every rickettsiosis, as is the non-specificity of routine laboratory findings. Thrombocytopenia from platelet consumption, elevated serum transaminases from focal hepatic necrosis, and leukopenia commonly occur [10, 19, 23, 25, 26].

Biopsies in RMSF reveal vasculitis and perivascular inflammation. In the CNS a characteristic angiocentric pattern of chronic inflammation (lymphocytes and macrophages) and microglial nodules are seen. *R. rickettsii* antigen can be immunostained in vascular walls (Figure 28.4b–d). Chronic leptomeningitis and infarcts are often present. EM can show *R. rickettsii* invasion of cerebrovascular endothelial and smooth muscle cells (Figure 28.4e, f) and phagocytosis by perivascular macrophages. Bacterial culture provides results slowly. Diagnostic confirmation of seroconversion for all rickettsioses requires both acute and convalescent serum for IgM and IgG findings (fourfold increase in antibody titer). Because both antibodies may take up to three weeks to appear in the serum in rickettsioses, real-time PCR assay is preferred for any patient sample, including skin and eschar biopsies and CSF. PCR is not universally available in endemic areas, where direct and indirect immunofluorescence assays, microimmunofluorescence assay, or enzyme-linked immunosorbent assay (ELISA) is performed for immunoglobulin comparisons. Species confirmation requires adsorption steps or Western blot analysis. For the rest of the SFG, ehrlichiosis, anaplasmosis, the typhus group (TG), and scrub typhus, the clinical laboratory studies, IHC where available, and antibiotic therapy parallel those in the management of RMSF [11, 14, 15].

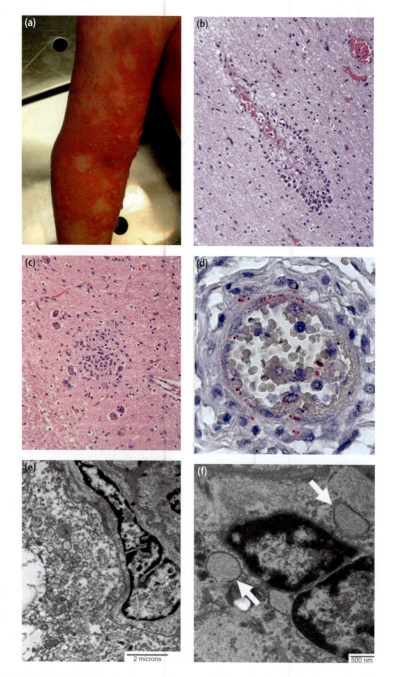

Figure 28.4 Rickettsial encephalitis. (a) An extensive purpuric and bullous rash is seen in an upper extremity of a 3-year-old boy who died with multiorgan failure, including encephalitis, 12 days after a tick bite. The differential diagnosis was meningococcemia versus Rocky Mountain spotted fever (RMSF). Autopsy specimens were polymerase chain reaction (PCR)-positive for *Rickettsia rickettsii* DNA. (b) A small, dilated blood vessel in the cerebrum of the 3-year-old boy has angiocentric inflammation consisting of lymphocytes and macrophages (×100, hematoxylin and eosin [H&E]). (c) A microglial nodule is present in the inferior olivary nucleus of the medulla in the boy with RMSF (×100, H&E). (d) A pulmonary blood vessel in a 3-year-old girl dying of RMSF shows *R. ricketsii* antigen using a red chromogen. Note the positive immunostaining associated with endothelial cells and with the medial layer smooth muscle cells (original magnification ×158, immunohistochemistry [IHC]) [20]. (e) A cerebral arteriole inner wall from the 3-year-old boy reveals numerous *R. rickettsii* cells within the endothelial cell on the left, while none are seen in the smooth muscle cells on the right (electron microscope [EM], scale bar 2 μm). (f) An arteriolar smooth muscle cell from the 3-year-old boy shows nuclear atypia and two invasive *R. rickettsii* cells (arrows) in the cytoplasm (EM, scale bar 500 nm).

MSF

MSF, also known as boutonneuse fever, is found mostly during warm weather in Europe and the Mediterranean islands, with fewer cases in both North and South Africa, and some identified in Asia and the United States. Onset and symptoms resemble RMSF, except that an eschar is commonly seen at the tick-bite site and the rash is usually in the extremities, sometimes involving palms and soles. The course of MSF is usually mild or moderate [11, 15]. In severe MSF, with rapid multiorgan failure and encephalopathy, there may be underlying alcoholism, old age, G6PD deficiency, or immunodeficiency. A recent regional report found a 13% fatality rate. CNS complications in MSF include cerebral infarction, meningoencephalitis, sensorineural hearing loss, acute quadriplegia secondary to an axonal polyneuropathy, and motor and sensory polyneuritis. Uveitis, retinopathy, and retinal vasculitis may also occur [15].

African tick bite fever

After malaria, the second-most reported travel-related infection is African tick bite fever *(R. africae)*. This is usually a benign disease. Nevertheless, a more severe course is described in older persons, with complications such as chronic fatigue, subacute cranial or peripheral neuropathy, and internuclear ophthalmoplegia [15].

Ehrlichial and anaplasmal tick-borne rickettsioses

In ehrlichiosis *(E. chaffeensis)*, circulating blood monocytes are infected, whereas in anaplasmosis *(A. phagocytophilum)* granulocytes are infected. Early presentation can resemble that of SFG rickettsioses or a viral infection. A mild febrile illness is often seen and rash is uncommon. Multiorgan failure and death can occur, particularly in patients who are immunosuppressed and have a higher rate of severe and fatal infection. Occasional neurologic findings in both infections include headache, altered mental status, hyperactive reflexes, and seizures. Other findings in ehrlichiosis include lymphocytic or neutrophilic CSF pleocytosis, meningismus, photophobia, optic neuritis, lymphocytic meningitis, ankle clonus, ataxia, cranial neuropathies, unilateral arm weakness, Bell palsy, and demyelinating polyneuropathy. In CSF, elevated protein or low glucose are not commonly found. CSF granulocytic pleocytosis has been reported in anaplasmosis. Laboratory investigations in ehrlichiosis and anaplasmosis include a blood smear and CSF cytology to find membrane-bound rickettsial colonies (morulae) in monocytes or granulocytes, respectively (Figure 28.5a) [31, 32].

Louse-borne rickettsiosis

Epidemic louse-borne classic typhus *(R. prowazekii)* is historically a severe disease associated with war, famine, and migrations when the human body louse parasitizes crowded human hosts to take a blood meal. Transmission is facilitated during cold weather (from infested clothing) and with reduced hygiene and poverty. *R. prowazekii* infects louse intestinal epithelial cells. Human infection occurs at louse-bite sites, conjunctivae, and mucous membranes contaminated with feces or crushed bodies of infected lice. Dried louse feces enter pruritic inoculation sites by scratching or they are inhaled as an aerosol. Epidemic typhus is now seen in rural highlands of Africa and Central and South America, especially in cold months [10, 25, 26]. Recently, it has been spread by a tick vector in Ethiopia, the southwestern United States, and Northern Mexico as an emerging disease that, because of vector and locale, can cause clinical confusion [19].

Unlike the bacteria of the SFG, *R. prowazekii* is immobile within endothelial cells and it exits following excessive proliferation causing lytic necrosis of the host cell (Figure 28.5b) [11, 12, 17]. There is a severe headache and vomiting. The rash often begins in the axilla and spreads mostly on the trunk and then the extremities. Eschars are not seen in epidemic typhus. *R. prowazekii* can re-emerge from a subclinical infection in patients under stress or with immune compromise, as a recrudescent infection after years or decades (Brill-Zinsser disease). This has been a source of local epidemics. At least one CNS complication is often seen, causing drowsiness, confusion, or seizures. In severe cases, hearing loss, meningismus, meningoencephalitis, or coma can occur. Survivors may have peripheral neuropathy, hemiparesis, or transverse myelitis. The fatality is about 4% with, and >50% without antibiotic treatment. Some organs, including the CNS, contain scattered typhus nodules consisting

Infections of the Central Nervous System

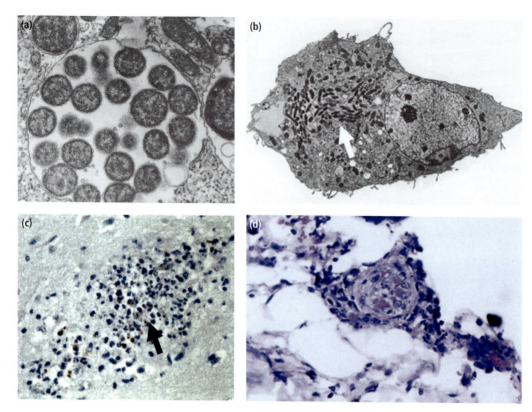

Figure 28.5 Rickettsial encephalitis. (a) Electron microscopy (EM) shows a colony of *Ehrlichia chaffeensis* cells within a cytoplasmic vacuole of a monocyte. From [27]. Source: courtesy of Dr. Vsevolod L Popov. (b) EM of a cell infected with *Rickettsia prowazekii* reveals early cytoplasmic accumulation of the intracellular parasites of epidemic typhus (arrow). The ultrastructural appearance of cells infected with typhus group rickettsiae remains normal until the abundance of replicating bacteria causes the host cells to burst. (Modified [replaced the arrowhead with a larger arrow] from Figure 40.2 in [27]). (c) *R. prowazekii* antigen is found in endothelium of a damaged capillary (arrow) and in surrounding chronic inflammatory cells in a developing typhus nodule in the brain (original magnification ×200, anti-*R. prowazekii* lipopolysaccharide monoclonal antibody Immunohistochemistry (IHC). [Modified by adding an arrow, from [28]]. (d) In a patient with murine endemic typhus, the endothelial cells of this small dermal blood vessel are swollen and injured by infection with *Rickettsia typhi*. Note the perivascular lymphocytic infiltrate. Source: from [29] Photomicrograph 5D was reproduced by and taken from: Figure 40.2 in [30].

of thrombosed microvessels surrounded by lymphocytes and macrophages. The lytic necrosis of infected endothelial cells activates humoral and cellular immunity and coagulation to form typhus nodules (Figure 28.5c) [10, 25, 26].

Flea-borne rickettsiosis

Murine endemic flea-borne typhus (*R. typhi*) is found in tropical and temperate climates, in parts of Europe, the Southeast Asia-Pacific region, China, North and South Americas, and Africa. It occurs most often in summer and early autumn, and many patients live in rural areas [18, 25, 33]. It has emerged in suburban areas of the United States where opossums and their cat fleas are found [24]. *R. typhi* in flea feces is inoculated at the bite site by scratching, or often it is inhaled, and it can infect directly from a flea bite. Clinical presentation resembles that of tick-borne diseases, and the course is usually mild. The rash, when present, begins on the trunk and is macular or maculopapular, mostly sparing palms and soles [18, 24, 33]. Disseminated intravascular coagulation, septic shock with multiorgan failure, and the hemophagocytic syndrome can occur [33]. The mortality in patients who are hospitalized is 4% [10, 24]. CNS involvement is infrequent but typically occurs in the second week of illness, with altered mental status, stupor, meningismus, seizures, ataxia, meningitis, encephalitis, meningoencephalitis, and ocular findings [18, 33, 34]. *R. typhi* shows erratic intraendothelial mobility [12]. It elicits perivasculitis but not typhus nodules (Figure 28.5d) [34].

Mite-borne rickettsiosis

Orientia tsutsugamuchi is the most important cause of mite-borne scrub typhus. As noted, with rare exception, scrub typhus is found in a restricted region of warm weather, the tsutsugamuchi triangle. It is transmitted from the bite of larval mites (chiggers) living on high grass, often growing in previously cleared jungle, around villages and plantations in rural Southeast Asia, India, Japan, and northern Australia. An estimated one million cases of scrub typhus occur annually, with significant mortality among the one billion-plus population of the affected Asia-Pacific triangle [10, 16, 25].

Clinical findings of scrub typhus are nonspecific in resembling other rickettsioses, except for the frequent eschar (up to 80% of cases), typically in the axilla or groin, that is characteristic to local practitioners. Macrophages rather than endothelial cells may be the main hosts [10, 25]. Most cases are mild and recovery is complete, but severe cases with multiorgan failure have a mortality rate as high as 24%. Some strains of *O. tsutsugamuchi* are resistant to standard treatment [35].

The most common neurologic complications in scrub typhus include headaches, meningitis, meningoencephalitis, and encephalitis. Also seen are cerebral venous thrombosis, Guillain-Barré syndrome, transient parkinsonism, myoclonus, opsoclonus, cerebellitis, transverse myelitis, polyneuropathy, facial palsy, abducens nerve palsy, and optic neuritis [35].

References

1. Atkinson, T.P., Balish, M.F., and Waites, K.B. (2013). Epidemiology, clinical manifestations, pathogenesis and laboratory detection of *Mycoplasma pneumoniae* infections. *FEMS Microbiol. Rev.* 32: 956–973.
2. Razin, S. and Hayflick, L. (2010). Highlights of mycoplasma research – an historical perspective. *Biologicals* 38: 183–190.
3. Rhodes, R.H., Monastersky, B., Tyagi, R., and Coyne, T. (2011). Mycoplasmal cerebral vasculopathy in a lymphoma patient: presumptive evidence of *Mycoplasma pneumoniae* microvascular endothelial cell invasion in a brain biopsy. *J. Neurol. Sci.* 309: 18–25.
4. Rhodes, R.H. and Anderson, B.A. (2012). Correspondence regarding: a novel cerebral microangiopathy with endothelial cell atypia and multifocal white matter lesions: a direct mycoplasmal infection? *J. Neuropathol. Exp. Neurol.* 2007;66:1100–1117. *J. Neuropathol. Exp. Neurol.* 71: 931–932.
5. Bergin, S.M., Mendis, S.M., Young, B., and Binti Izharuddin, E. (2017). Postoperative *Mycoplasma hominis* brain abscess: keep it in mind! *BMJ Case Rep* 2017: pii: bcr2016218022. https://doi.org/10.1136/bcr-2016-21802.
6. Narita, M. (2016). Classification of extrapulmonary manifestations due to *Mycoplasma pneumoniae* infection on the basis of possible pathogenesis. *Front. Microbiol.* 7: 23.
7. Meyer Sauteur, P.M., Jacobs, B.C., Spuesens, E.B.M. et al. (2014). Antibody responses to *Mycoplasma pneumoniae*: role in pathogenesis and diagnosis of encephalitis? *PLoS Pathog.* 10: e1003983.
8. Francis, D.A., Brown, A., Miller, D.H. et al. (1988). MRI appearances of the CNS manifestations of *Mycoplasma pneumoniae*: a report of two cases. *J. Neurol.* 235: 441–443.
9. Powers, J.M. and Johnson, M.D. (2012). Mycoplasmal panencephalitis: a neuropathologic documentation. *Acta Neuropathol.* 124: 143–148.
10. Cowan, G. (2000). Rickettsial diseases: the typhus group of fevers – a review. *Postgrad. Med. J.* 76: 269–272.
11. Mahajan, S.K. (2012). Rickettsial diseases. *J. Assoc. Physicians India* 60: 37–44.
12. Mansueto, P., Vitale, G., Cascio, A. et al. (2012). New insight into immunity and immunopathology of rickettsial diseases. *Clin. Dev. Immunol.* 2012: 967852.
13. Merhej, V., Angelakis, E., Socolovschi, C., and Raoult, D. (2014). Genotyping, evolution and epidemiological findings of *Rickettsia* species. *Infect. Genet. Evol.* 25: 122–137.
14. Fang, R., Blanton, L.S., and Walker, D.H. (2017). Rickettsiae as emerging infectious agents. *Clin. Lab. Med.* 37: 383–400.
15. Parola, P., Paddock, C.D., Socolovschi, C. et al. (2013). Update on tick-borne rickettsioses around

the world: a geographic approach. *Clin. Microbiol. Rev.* 26: 657–702.
16. Weitzel, T., Dittrich, S., López, J. et al. (2016). Endemic scrub typhus in South America. *N. Engl. J. Med.* 375: 954–961.
17. Rathi, N. and Rathi, A. (2010). Rickettsial infections: Indian perspective. *Indian Pediatr.* 47: 157–164.
18. Aung, A.K., Spelman, D.W., Murray, R.J., and Graves, S. (2014). Rickettsial infections in Southeast Asia: implications for local populace and febrile returned travelers. *Am. J. Trop. Med. Hyg.* 91: 451–460.
19. Walker, D.H., Paddock, C.D., and Dumler, J.S. (2008). Emerging and re-emerging tick-transmitted rickettsial and ehrlichial infections. *Med. Clin. N. Am.* 92: 1345–1361.
20. Álvarez-Hernández, G., Roldán, J.F.G., Milan, N.S.H. et al. (2017). Rocky Mountain spotted fever in Mexico: past, present, and future. *Lancet Infect. Dis.* 17: e189–e196.
21. Walker, D.H. (1989). Rocky Mountain spotted fever: a disease in need of microbiological concern. *Clin. Microbiol. Rev.* 2: 227–240.
22. Woods, C.R. (2013). Rocky Mountain spotted fever in children. *Pediatr. Clin. N. Am.* 60: 455–470.
23. Walker, D.H. (1995). Rocky Mountain spotted fever: a seasonal alert. *Clin. Infect. Dis.* 20: 1111–1117.
24. Blanton, L.S. and Walker, D.H. (2017). Flea-borne rickettsioses and rickettsiae. *Am. J. Trop. Med. Hyg.* 96: 53–56.
25. Watt, G. and Parola, P. (2003). Scrub typhus and tropical rickettsioses. *Curr. Opin. Infect. Dis.* 16: 429–436.
26. Bechah, Y., Capo, C., Mege, J.L., and Raoult, D. (2008). Epidemic typhus. *Lancet Infect. Dis.* 8: 417–426.
27. Walker, D.H. and Yu, X.J. (2012). *Rickettsia*, *Orientia*, *Ehrlichia*, *Anaplasma* and *Coxiella*: typhus; spotted fevers; scrub typhus; ehrlichioses; Q fever. In: *Medical Microbiology*, 18e (eds. D. Greenwood, M. Barer, R. Slack and W. Irving), 390–399. Edinburgh; New York: Churchill Livingstone/Elsevier.
28. Walker, D.H., Feng, H.M., Ladner, S. et al. (1997). Immunohistochemical diagnosis of typhus rickettsioses using an anti-lipopolysaccharide monoclonal antibody. *Mod. Pathol.* 10: 1038–1042.
29. Connor, D.H., Chandler, F.W., Schwartz, D.Q. et al. (1997). *Pathology of Infectious Diseases*. Stamford CT: Appleton & Lange.
30. Ryan, K.J., Ray, C.G., and Sherris, J.C. (2014). *Rickettsia*, *Ehrlichia*, *Anaplasma*, and *Bartonella*. In: *Sherris Medical Microbiology*, 6e (eds. K.J. Ryan and C.G. Ray). New York: McGraw Hill; chapter 40.
31. Frohman, L. and Lama, P. (2000). Annual update of systemic disease-1999: emerging and re-emerging infections (Part II). *J. Neuroophthalmol.* 20: 48–58.
32. Hongo, I. and Bloch, K.C. (2006). *Ehrlichia* infection of the central nervous system. *Curr. Treat. Options Neurol.* 8: 179–184.
33. Tsioutis, C., Zafeiri, M., Avramopoulos, A. et al. (2017). Clinical and laboratory characteristics, epidemiology, and outcomes of murine typhus: a systematic review. *Acta Trop.* 166: 16–24.
34. Masalha, R., Merkin-Zaborsky, H., Matar, M. et al. (1998). Murine typhus presenting as subacute meningoencephalitis. *J. Neurol.* 245: 665–668.
35. Peter, J.V., Sudarsan, T.I., Prakash, J.A., and Varghese, G.M. (2015). Severe scrub typhus infection: clinical features, diagnostic challenges and management. *World J. Crit. Care Med.* 4: 244–250.

29 Pathogenesis and Pathophysiology of Bacterial Infections of the CNS

Loic Le Guennec[1,2] and Sandrine Bourdoulous[1]

[1] Inserm, U1016, Institut Cochin, CNRS, UMR8104, Paris University, Paris, France
[2] La Pitie-Salpetriere Hospital, APHP, Paris, France

Abbreviations

ACP	alpha C protein
β2AR	beta-2-adrenergic receptor
BBB	blood-brain barrier
CNS	central nervous system
CSF	cerebrospinal fluid
E. coli	Escherichia coli
EMPRINN	extracellular matrix metalloproteinase inducer for N. meningitidis
EoD	early-onset disease
fHBP	factor H-binding protein
GBS	group B Streptococcus
H. influenzae	Haemophilus influenzae
HvgA	hypervirulent GBS adhesin
IL	interleukin
ICP	intracranial pressure
L. monocytogenes	Listeria monocytogenes
LoD	late-onset disease
LTA	lipoteichoic acid
N. meningitidis	Neisseria meningitidis
MMP	matrix metalloproteinase
MRI	magnetic resonance image
M. tuberculosis	Mycobacterium tuberculosis
PAF	platelet-activating factor
PCR	polymerase chain reaction
Pcho	Phosphorylcholine
pIgR	polymeric immunoglobulin receptor
PMNL	polymorphonuclear leukocyte
SCID	severe combined immunodeficient
SOL	space-occupying lesion
Sfb	streptococcal fibronectin-binding
S. pneumoniae	Streptococcus pneumoniae
Srr	serine-rich repeat
T4P	type IV pili
TNF-α	tumor necrosis factor alpha
TRL	toll-like receptor
ZO1	zona occludens 1

Introduction

Bacterial infections of the CNS pose a unique challenge to physicians because of their potential morbidity and mortality and inherent difficulties involved in their treatment. Rapid diagnosis and prompt treatment are mandatory, but despite advances in antibacterial therapy and vaccines, complications frequently occur, resulting in an

---

Infections of the Central Nervous System: Pathology and Genetics, First Edition. Edited by Fabrice Chrétien, Kum Thong Wong, Leroy R. Sharer, Catherine (Katy) Keohane and Françoise Gray.
© 2020 John Wiley & Sons Ltd. Published 2020 by John Wiley & Sons Ltd.

unfavorable outcome in a high proportion of patients and neurological sequelae in survivors [1].

The most important infections are meningitis, encephalitis, and brain abscesses. They differ considerably from systemic infections, due to the particular structure and function of the CNS. Structurally, the CNS is covered by three protective membranes: the skull, the spine, and the meninges. Additionally the blood-brain barrier (BBB) constitutes a selective filter that controls the entry of toxic compounds or pathogens [2]. The presence of a lymphatic vasculature within the brain is still controversial [3]. Consequently, leukocytes (i.e. granulocytes and T and B cells) stay within blood vessels and usually do not enter healthy brain tissue. Within the CNS, host defenses rely on innate immune cells including parenchymal (microglia) and nonparenchymal macrophages and perivascular blood-derived monocytes [4]; these defenses are not sufficient to control bacterial proliferation and pathogenicity. During CNS infection or disease, peripheral blood immune cells cross the BBB and reach the nervous system parenchyma. The host inflammatory response then plays a central role in contributing to local complications. Depending on the pathogen involved, systemic complications such as septic shock, pneumonia, and disseminated intravascular coagulation also contribute to a poor outcome.

In this chapter, we will briefly review the most common clinical and pathological features of bacterial CNS infections.

Clinical presentation of bacterial infections of the CNS

The clinical features of CNS infections depend on the bacterial agent, the site of infection, and host characteristics, such as underlying risk factors and immune status. In a patient who is febrile, the common neurologic manifestations suggesting CNS infection are disturbance of consciousness, behavioral changes, headache, symptoms of raised intracranial pressure (ICP), seizures, and focal neurologic deficits. Overall, fever associated with neurological impairment should suggest one of the following medical emergencies.

Acute meningitis

Acute meningitis is the most frequent and life-threatening bacterial infection of the CNS, characterized by an acute purulent infection of the meninges [5]. It is usually caused by *Streptococcus pneumoniae, Neisseria meningitidis,* or *Haemophilus influenzae* in children and adults and by *Escherichia coli* and group B *Streptococcus* (GBS) during the neonatal period. *Listeria monocytogenes* can affect neonates and patients who are immunocompromised. The main route of infection is hematogenous, but the responsible bacteria can also spread contiguously from adjacent tissues or gain entry as a complication of trauma, surgery, or developmental malformations. Usually, patients present with fever associated with acute or subacute meningeal syndromes (i.e. headache, stiff neck, Kernig and Brudzinski signs, nausea, vomiting, and phono- or photophobia) [5].

Assuming clinical guidelines for safe lumbar puncture are followed, in a patient with suspected meningitis, rapid examination of the cerebrospinal fluid (CSF) is the cornerstone of diagnosis. Typical CSF examination for bacterial meningitis shows a cloudy and turbid fluid with pleocytosis (white blood cell count >10 cells/mm^3) with marked predominance of polymorphonuclear leukocytes (PMNL) (>50%), low or absent glucose (<40% of serum glucose), and an elevated protein levels (>50 mg/dl). Direct microscopy with appropriate stains for organisms, followed by culture and antibiotic sensitivity tests, allow identification of the responsible bacteria. Blood culture is also useful, especially when CSF sampling is precluded by significant raised ICP.

Chronic meningitis

Chronic meningitis is defined as an inflammatory CSF profile and meningitis symptoms that persist for at least one month. Worldwide, the main causative pathogen is *Mycobacterium tuberculosis*, the agent responsible for tuberculosis, which continues to cause high morbidity and mortality. It is frequently associated with spinal tuberculosis and CSF analysis reveals elevation of PMNL early in the infection, later followed by lymphocytic meningitis with high CSF protein. Early detection of *M. tuberculosis* in the CSF of patients with tuberculous meningitis still remains a challenge for clinicians, mainly because of the lack of rapid, efficient and practical detection methods. Isolation of *M. tuberculosis* from the CSF is complicated as culture is unacceptably slow and requires specialized laboratory safety procedures (see Chapter 35). Polymerase chain reaction (PCR) assays were found to be insensitive at detecting *M. tuberculosis* in CSF samples, and interferon gamma (IFN-γ) release assays are not recommended for diagnosis of active tuberculous disease [6].

Less commonly, other intracellular or extracellular bacteria can cause chronic meningitis. These include *Brucella* spp., which causes brucellosis (see Chapter 38); *Treponema pallidum*, the causative agent of syphilis (see Chapter 37); and *Borrelia burgdorferi*, which causes Lyme disease (see Chapter 38). For these pathogens, CSF analysis usually shows a lymphocytic meningitis, and direct microscopy and culture are negative because they cannot be cultivated in culture media. Diagnosis is mostly based on the patient's history, positive serology, and extraneurological symptoms.

In all cases, repeat CSF examination is required over time to survey bacterial infection and inflammation within the meninges.

Brain abscess

Abscess is the second-most frequent infection of the CNS and the most frequent infective cause of intracranial space-occupying lesion (SOL). When formed, it is a focal brain parenchymal suppurative infection, generally enclosed by a capsule of granulation tissue. At the early stage, following local vascular injury after inoculation of bacteria, brain abscess is characterized by cerebritis with PMNL infiltration, edema, and a perivascular fibrinous exudate causing raised ICP. The sequential changes in the following days are described in detail in Chapter 31.

In 75% of cases, the abscess is single. Microorganisms reach the brain (i) from an adjacent cranial or extracranial focus of infection, (ii) from distant foci via the bloodstream, or (iii) when introduced by trauma (Figure 29.1) or via a congenital defect (see Chapter 31 for more details). Infections of paranasal sinuses, ears, lungs, and odontogenic foci were regarded as the sources of infection in approximately 70% in a series of 45 cases [7].

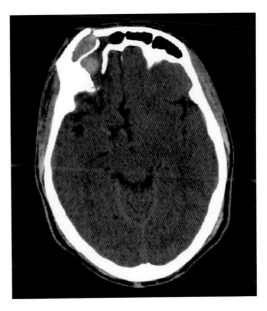

Figure 29.1 Axial computed tomography (CT) brain scan showing right frontal sinusitis in an adult with past medical history of open right frontal bone fracture in childhood, complicated by right frontal lobe brain abscess. Bacterial culture of the abscess was positive for *Streptococcus pneumoniae*.

The abscess location depends on the site of the initial infective focus: frontotemporal regions for the sinuses, cerebellar and temporal regions for the middle ear, and frontoparietal regions for hematogenous spread. Post-traumatic abscesses occur at the sites of craniocerebral injury. Multiple abscesses tend to be found at the gray and white matter junctions and should suggest an embolic cause, such as an infective endocarditis (Figure 29.2).

Neurological examination shows clinical signs of raised ICP associated with focal neurologic signs (i.e. seizures, alteration of behavior or consciousness, sensorimotor deficit). Forty percent of patients have fever and only 25% have a meningeal syndrome. Magnetic resonance imaging (MRI) shows a ring-enhancing SOL associated with edema and mass effect. Imaging can also demonstrate complications such as subdural empyema or epidural abscess. In the presence of significant raised ICP, lumbar puncture is contraindicated. Neurosurgical drainage and antibiotic therapy following microbiological analysis are usually necessary for treatment.

Infections of the Central Nervous System

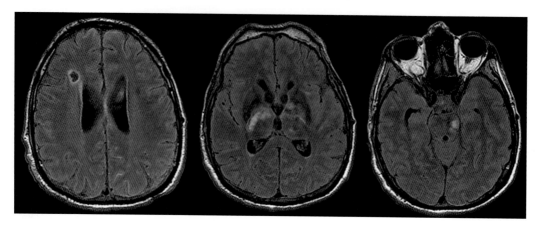

Figure 29.2 Brain magnetic resonance image (MRI) (axial plane, T2 fluid attenuated inversion recovery [FLAIR] sequence) showing multiple embolic abscesses within the right frontal lobe, the basal ganglia, and the brainstem in a patient with *Streptococcus pneumoniae* endocarditis.

The causative agent depends on the primary site of infection and on host factors, particularly the immune status. Immunosuppression is a well-established risk factor and is reported in 80% of patients. The most common pathogens are anaerobic streptococci (e.g. *Streptococcus milleri*) and anaerobic Gram-negative bacilli (e.g. *Bacteroides fragilis*). In patients who are immunocompetent, when the primary source is a dental infection, a mixed growth of bacteria is commonly found in the brain abscess. In patients who are immunocompromised, other species such as *Actinomyces israelii* and *Nocardia* spp. can be responsible for brain abscesses. *L. monocyogenes* can also cause abscesses within the brainstem with or without meningitis. Finally, intracranial tuberculous abscesses (tuberculomas) are an uncommon manifestation of CNS tuberculosis. The initial empirical antibiotic treatment depends on the immunological status of the host, adjusted following bacterial identification and results of sensitivity.

Epidural abscess

Infection of the epidural space is rare. It is located in the virtual space between the skull (or the spine) and the outer layer of the dura mater. These infections mainly affect immunocompromised adults older than 50 years of age. The abscess is caused by an adjacent infection (i.e. osteomyelitis, or following cranial or spinal trauma, epidural anesthesia, or surgery) or by bacteremia (Figure 29.3) because of distant-site infections (endocarditis, furuncle, or soft-tissue abscess) [8].

The clinical picture is similar to spinal cord compression with intense spinal pain, radicular signs, and paraparesis associated with sensory, bladder, and bowel sphincter disturbance. MRI shows a biconvex extra-axial lesion outlined by the bony skull or vertebra. On T1-weighted sequences the

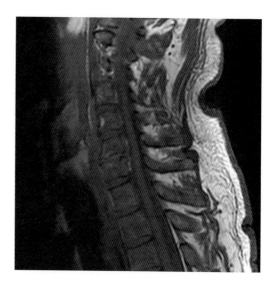

Figure 29.3 Cervicomedullary magnetic resonance image (MRI) (sagittal plane, T1 sequence) showing anterior epidural abscess contiguous with cervical spondylodiscitis resulting from embolism in a patient with *Staphylococcus aureus* endocarditis.

lesion is iso- or hypodense and hyperdense on T2-weighted sequences with peripheral or diffuse contrast enhancement. Bacterial identification can be from blood cultures, from the primary site of infection, from CSF, or by ultrasound-guided or neurosurgically acquired biopsy from the epidural abscess.

Treatment consists of urgent surgical drainage together with broad spectrum antibiotics against *Staphylococcus aureus*, *Streptococcus* spp., and Gram-negative rod-shaped bacteria and anaerobes. *M. tuberculosis* can also be responsible for epidural abscess, as a complication of tuberculosis of the spine (Pott's disease).

Subdural empyema

The mode of development and bacteriology of subdural empyema is similar to that of epidural abscess. Subdural empyema is a collection of pus between the dura and the subarachnoid membrane. The subdural space is traversed by veins and divided into several large compartments. Subdural empyema is usually caused by aerobic and anaerobic bacteria, which reach the subdural space from veins draining the skull. The primary sites of infection are mainly in the sinuses, followed by mastoid and middle ear infections. Usually, the empyema is located above the tentorium or adjacent to the falx cerebri and rarely in the spinal canal. Treatment includes antibiotics and surgical intervention.

Ventriculitis

Ventriculitis generally occurs as a complication of a previous CNS bacterial infection such as meningitis or a brain abscess that ruptures into the cerebral ventricles. The main complication is hydrocephalus. Clinical symptoms are due to raised ICP because of hydrocephalus.

Bacterial invasion of the CNS

In the past few decades, our knowledge of the mechanisms of bacterial invasion of the CNS has greatly improved because of basic research and experimental animal models.

The routes of entry by which bacteria access the CNS are: (i) hematogenous dissemination, by crossing the BBB transcellularly, paracellularly or in infected phagocytes (the so-called Trojan horse mechanism); (ii) by retrograde axonal transport to the brain via cranial or peripheral nerves; and (iii) by direct invasion.

The most common route of entry to the CNS for extracellular bacteria is via the bloodstream. Most pathogens responsible for CNS infections can asymptomatically colonize skin and mucosa of healthy individuals. These pathogens can reach the bloodstream, survive within the blood, and ultimately cross the BBB. Extracellular pathogens that can cause meningitis are well-adapted to survive in the extracellular environment: they can all resist killing by PMNLs or complement and can obtain the ferric iron required for their growth and survival. Sustained bacteremia seems to be required to cause meningeal invasion [9]. The duration of bacteremia is also important, for example in *H. influenzae* meningitis, both the density and duration of bacteremia correlate with meningeal invasion [10]. Furthermore, autopsies have shown that most extracellular bacteria can interact directly with brain endothelial cells [11]. A dense bacteremia probably increases the likelihood of bacterial interaction with the components of CNS barriers, which is a prerequisite for meningeal invasion.

Numerous in vitro studies using brain-derived endothelial cell lines expressing tight junctions have investigated how circulating bacteria responsible for meningitis interact with the BBB. These studies have identified bacterial adhesins and their specific endothelial cell receptors such as platelet activating factor receptor for *S. pneumoniae* [12] or CD147 (also known as Basigin or extracellular matrix metalloproteinase inducer [EMPRINN]) for *N. meningitidis* [13]. Relevant in vivo experimental models have been set up to study how pathogens such as *E. coli*, GBS, *S. pneumoniae*, or *N. meningitidis* can reach the CNS, but the precise site or method of entry by which they cross into the CSF is still unknown. The choroid plexus is suggested as one site where bacteria could cross. If this were the case, bacterial meningitis might be expected to be associated with ventriculitis, which is not always present. Another theory suggests bacteria cross the BBB through postcapillary perforating venules because of their proximity to the subarachnoid space. Bacteria crossing the endothelial monolayer at this site would be close to the Virchow Robin space. Also, the low blood flow in these venules could facilitate bacterial adhesion to endothelial cells [11].

There are several hypotheses as to how bacteria cross the endothelial cell barrier. One possibility is a facilitated transport occurring during diapedesis of infected leukocytes, but extracellular bacteria responsible for meningitis probably do not use this route to cross the BBB because several studies have shown a specific interaction between bacteria and endothelial cells [13]. Many studies hypothesized that bacterial adhesion to endothelial cells induces intracellular signaling that could cause disruption of intercellular tight junctions, allowing bacteria to cross between or across cells (transcytosis) of the endothelial monolayer. Transcytosis across this monolayer has been demonstrated for *S. pneumoniae* [14], *E. coli* [15], GBS [16], and through human umbilical vein endothelial cells for *H. influenzae* [17]. In vitro, although *N. meningitidis* internalized in human brain microvascular endothelial cells [18], the pathway used by meningococci to cross endothelial cells is still debated. Another hypothesis is that bacteria exert a direct cytotoxic effect resulting in disruption of the endothelial barrier, but BBB leakage because of bacterial cytotoxicity might be expected to cause subarachnoid hemorrhage, which is a rare event in bacterial meningitis. These pathogens seem to respect the architecture of the BBB [19]. Inflammation may also play a role in bacterial entry into the CNS. The innate immune response induced by bacteremia, with or without septic shock, may increase BBB permeability, thereby promoting bacterial entry into the CNS.

The following section describes the most frequent bacteria responsible for acute meningitis and their respective pathophysiological mechanisms leading to mucosal colonization, dissemination, and crossing of the BBB (Table 29.1).

S. pneumoniae

S. pneumoniae (pneumococcus) is an alpha-hemolytic Gram-positive extracellular coccus. It frequently resides in the upper respiratory tract of humans and other related mammalian species. It is the most frequent organism responsible for community-acquired bacterial meningitis worldwide, affecting young children and the elderly. It can colonize the nasopharyngeal mucosa in asymptomatic individuals but is responsible for otitis media, sinusitis, and for severe invasive infections, such as pneumonia, bacteremia, and acute meningitis (Figure 29.4). Findings regarding the pathophysiology of pneumococcal meningitis are either derived from brain autopsies or from animal models.

To reach the meninges, pneumococci have to escape ear-nose-throat or respiratory mucosal defenses and either cause sinusitis or mastoiditis, with local spread through the skull, or survive within the bloodstream and be carried into the CNS (Figure 29.5). The pneumococcal capsule provides protection against phagocytosis, complement-mediated immunity, and opsonophagocytic killing. The capsule also reduces pneumococcal capture by neutrophil extracellular traps and interferes with innate immune responses by masking several toll-like receptor (TLR) ligands associated with the pneumococcal cell wall. These include lipoteichoic acid and lipopeptides. Furthermore, its ability to form biofilms is important in nasopharyngeal colonization, pneumonia, and otitis

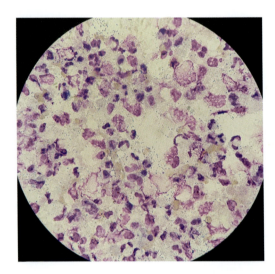

Figure 29.4 Bronchioalveolar lavage (BAL), stained with May-Grünwald Giemsa, showing diplococci within altered polymorphonuclear neutrophils in a patient with acute community-acquired pneumonia and clinical meningitis. Blood cultures were positive for Gram-positive cocci. The patient also had purpura fulminans with coagulopathy, so lumbar puncture was contraindicated. BAL and blood cultures were positive for *Streptococcus pneumoniae*.

Table 29.1 Main bacterial pathogens responsible for acute meningitis.

	Streptococcus pneumoniae	Neisseria meningitidis	Haemophilus Influenzae type b	Group B Streptococcus	Escherichia coli K1	Listeria monocytogenes
Type of bacteria	Gram-positive diplococcus	Gram-negative diplococcus	Gram-negative rod shaped	Gram-positive diplococcus	Gram-negative rod shaped	Gram-positive rod shaped
Population affected	Between 2 months and 5 years, and >50 years	Between 2 months and 5 years, and young adults	Children <5 years	<3 months	<3 months	<3 months, and adults
Risk factors	Splenectomy or functional hyposplenia	Alternative and terminal complement pathway deficiencies	Insufficient access to vaccines	Maternal carriage and prematurity	Maternal carriage and prematurity	Ingestion of contaminated food in pregnant women or patients with immunocompromise
Carriage site/ Site of entry	Nasopharynx, lung	Nasopharynx	Nasopharynx	Rectal or vaginal	Rectal	Digestive tract
Virulence factors	Capsule, CbpA, PCho (PAF), pneumolysin	Capsule, LOS, Type IV pili	Capsule, gA1 protease LOS, Hib Type I pili, Omp	Capsule, lipotechoic acid, ScpB, FbsA, b-hemolysin	Capsule, O-LPS, OmpA, type 1 fimbriae, CNF1	Capsule, InlA, InlB, Listeriolysin O
Host cell receptors	pIgR, laminin receptor, PAF receptor	CD147, β2-adrenergic receptor	Mucin, Lactoferrin	Fibronectin, fibrinogen and laminin	Laminin receptor	E-cadherin, Met

CbpA, Choline-binding protein A; CNF1, cytotoxic necrotizing factor 1; LOS, lipooligosaccharide; LPS, lipopolysaccharide; Omp, outer member protein; PAF, platelet-activating factor; PCho, phosphorylcholine (mimics the chemokine PAF); pIgR, polymeric immunoglobulin receptor.

Infections of the Central Nervous System

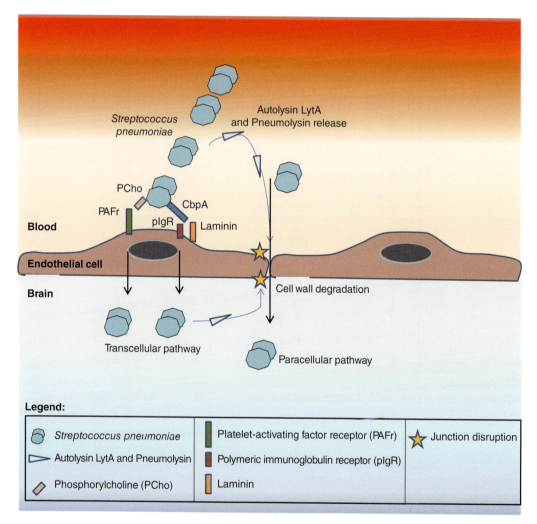

Figure 29.5 Mechanism of CNS invasion by *Streptococcus pneumoniae*. *S. pneumoniae* adheres to endothelial cells by the bacterial choline-binding protein CbpA (also called PspC, SpsA or Hic), which binds to human cell laminin and polymeric immunoglobulin receptor (pIgR), and bacterial phosphorylcholine (PCho), which mimics the chemokine platelet-activating factor (PAF) and binds to the cell receptor PAF receptor (PAFr), enabling transcytosis across the endothelium. Additional release of pneumococcus autolysin LytA and pneumolysin promote cell wall degradation and endothelial monolayer disruption, allowing paracellular bacterial invasion.

media. Pneumolysin, a key virulence factor secreted by *S. pneumoniae*, binds to cholesterol in cell membranes. This pore-forming toxin, produced by virtually all clinical isolates of *S. pneumoniae*, contributes significantly to its virulence by inducing tissue damage and plays a role in biofilm formation [20].

The first step in pneumococcal invasion is the interaction between the bacterial choline-binding protein CbpA (also called PspC, SpsA or Hic) and a polymeric immunoglobulin receptor (pIgR) at the cell surface of nasopharyngeal or respiratory epithelial cells. This interaction promotes bacterial transcytosis across the epithelial barrier [20]. Once in the bloodstream, bacterial CbpA binds brain endothelial cells through laminin receptor. Pneumoccoci can also anchor to human epithelial and endothelial cells through an interaction between bacterial phosphorylcholine (PCho), which mimics the chemokine platelet-activating factor (PAF) and binds its cell receptor (PAF receptor [PAFr]), the first known host cell receptor for *S. pneumoniae*. This interaction promotes bacterial transcytosis, through a clathrin-mediated endocytosis in brain endothelial cells [20]. Pneumococcus has an additional important property of undergoing autolysis, characterized by cell wall degradation by a peptidoglycan hydrolase (autolysin Lyt A), leading to pneumolysin release (and its associated virulence). In a microvascular endothelial cell culture model, pneumococci expressing pneumolysin could breach endothelial cells, whereas mutant pneumococci deficient in pneumolysin could not [21]. This effect on brain endothelial cells could potentially induce apoptosis and disruption of BBB, favoring bacterial entry into the CNS. Pneumolysin impairs PMN leukocyte activity and also activates different proinflammatory signaling pathways, which may accentuate brain inflammation and neuronal damage. Both CbpA and pneumolysin seem essential for pneumococcal pathogenesis. In mice, immunization against CbpA and pneumolysin can protect against pneumococcal infection and prevent nasopharyngeal carriage [22]. Finally, nasal cavity infection in a mouse model suggests that pneumococci may enter the brain directly by axonal transport through olfactory nerves [23]. Teichoic acid in the pneumococcal cell wall can interact with gangliosides, so it has been suggested that pneumococcal carriage can induce olfactory tissue infection and bacterial entry into the brain in the absence of bacteremia. However, these colonizing bacteria fail to cause extensive brain infection. Whether these events occur in humans remains to be proven, so further studies are required to determine the precise pathophysiology of pneumococcal meningitis.

N. meningitidis

N. meningitidis (meningococcus) is an extracellular Gram-negative diplococcus. It is one of the most virulent bacteria, responsible for 10% of meningitis deaths. Systemic complications, such as septic shock, purpura fulminans, and disseminated intravascular coagulation, contribute to the unfavorable outcome. *N. meningitidis* is restricted to humans; it is a frequent nasopharynx commensal with asymptomatic carriage in healthy individuals in 8- 20% of the population and up to 25% in children [24]. Meningococci are transmitted by respiratory secretions, saliva, or by inhalation of contaminated aerosol droplets. Nasopharyngeal acquisition may be transient, lead to colonization, or result in invasive disease. Blood-borne infections can rapidly progress to septic shock. As meningococci adhere to, and proliferate in, systemic microvessels, vascular colonization leads to abnormal inflammation and coagulation, endothelial dysfunction and, in severe cases, to vascular leakage associated with the typical extensive necrotic purpuric rash. Interaction with brain microvessels allows bacteria to cross the BBB, reach the meninges, and cause meningitis (Figure 29.6), while brain endothelial cell junctions are relatively intact with no signs of hemorrhage or thrombosis [13].

The prerequisite for meningococcal pathogenicity is its interaction with the nasopharyngeal epithelial surface and transfer across this mucosal barrier to reach the circulation [25]. Mucosal colonization and crossing mechanisms are poorly described. Once in the bloodstream, many virulence factors enable bacterial growth and immune escape from host effectors and the complement system. They include the iron chelation systems, the polysaccharide capsule, the sialylated lipooligosaccharide, and factor H-binding protein (fHBP). Pathogenesis is also linked to some bacterial genetic factors (e.g. expression of a gene encoding a hemoglobin receptor and the expression of a filamentous prophage were detected at a higher frequency in pathogenic isolates than in carriage isolates) [26].

However, meningococcal pathogenicity principally relies on the capacity to interact with human microvessels. This was elegantly demonstrated in vivo in a severe combined immunodeficient (SCID) mouse model, grafted with human skin. The grafted human vessels connected with the mouse vasculature and remained functional. Following infection with *N. meningitidis*, circulating meningococci specifically colonized human endothelial cells within the grafts and promoted vascular lesions similar to purpuric lesions in humans [27]. Mouse vessels were not colonized and remained intact. The model also demonstrated that pathogenic capsulated meningococci required

Infections of the Central Nervous System

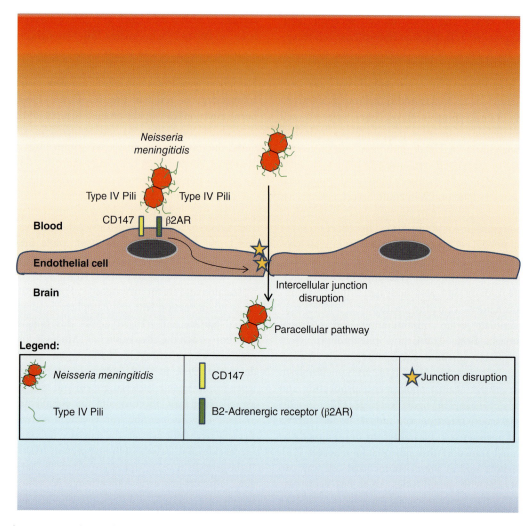

Figure 29.6 Mechanism of CNS invasion by *Neisseria meningitidis*. Type IV pili (T4P) of *N. meningitidis* interact with endothelial cell receptor CD147, leading to the activation of both β2-adrenergic receptor (β2AR) and downstream signaling cascades. In vitro, infection promotes the disruption of intercellular junctions, which could favor paracellular bacterial entry into the CNS across the blood-brain barrier.

type IV pili (T4P) to colonize and induce vascular damage. T4P are long dynamic filamentous structures extending from the bacterial surface through the capsule. Nonpiliated mutants failed to target human graft vessels or induce vascular damage [27]. This model also showed that the vascular cell wall provided an environment for meningococcal multiplication promoting a sustained bacteremia and mouse lethality. These studies highlighted the importance of pilus-mediated vascular colonization in the development and outcome of meningococcal sepsis.

At the molecular level, to colonize human endothelium, meningococcal T4P interact with two key endothelial cell receptors: CD147 (also called EMMPRIN or Basigin), a member of the immunoglobulin superfamily, and endothelial beta-2-adrenergic receptor (β2AR) leading to its bias activation [25]. β2AR activation promotes local recruitment and activation of cytoskeleton-associated and signaling proteins. This results in (i) forming protrusions of the apical plasma membrane, which stabilize bacterial colonies at the endothelial cell surface (Figure 29.7), and

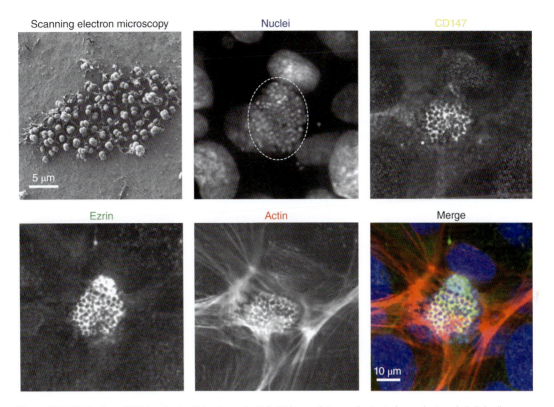

Figure 29.7 Mechanism of CNS invasion by *Neisseria meningitidis*. Right panel: Upon adhesion to human brain endothelial cells (hCMEC/D3 cells) meningococci proliferate at the endothelial cell surface forming compact microcolonies observed by scanning electron microscopy (left panel). Subsequently, local membrane protrusions form which stabilize bacterial colonies at the endothelial cell surface upon shear stress. The protrusions result from local changes in endothelial cytoskeletal architecture. Immunofluorescence microscopy (right panels) shows surface microcolonies, with local accumulation of the endothelial cell receptor CD147, of the membrane-cytoskeleton linker Ezrin and of cortical actin polymerization, all involved in protrusion formation.

(ii) opening of intercellular junctions that contribute to vascular changes [25]. Colonization also favors endothelial cell survival, the expression of adhesion molecules, and the secretion of cytokines [28].

Although the affinity of T4P for CD147 and β2AR is weak, these receptors are assembled into multimers [29], and CD147 expression on brain endothelial cells is strong, thus enhancing avidity [13]. The low levels of shear stress in the cerebral microcirculation also favor bacterial adhesion [11]. Other meningococcal factors can reinforce or modulate adhesion (detailed in [30]).

Colonization of brain capillaries in the subarachnoid space, the parenchyma and the choroid plexus suggested that *N. meningitidis* actively crosses the BBB by disrupting cell-cell junctions. In vitro studies indicate that meningococcal adhesion to human brain endothelium induces signaling events leading to altered endothelial permeability. *N. meningitidis* actively disrupts cell-cell junctions and promotes sequestration of cell-cell junction molecules, such as VE-cadherin, zona occludens 1 (ZO1), or claudin 5, to the sites of bacterial adhesion [25]. Meningococcus also activates matrix metalloproteinase 8 (MMP8) production, which promotes proteolytic cleavage of the tight junction protein occludin, favoring cell detachment. Because *N. meningitidis* infection is specific to humans, there is no relevant in vivo animal model of CNS invasion to test whether the same process occurs in vivo at the human BBB.

Infections of the Central Nervous System

GBS

GBS is a Gram-positive extracellular coccus and is the main cause of bacterial meningitis in babies younger than two months of age. Contamination usually occurs by maternal-fetal transmission from the birth canal at the time of delivery. Mothers are frequently asymptomatic. About 30–70% of neonates born to mothers with GBS-colonization become transiently colonized by their mother's organisms. Neonates, particularly if premature, have an increased risk for bacterial meningitis because of small numbers of alveolar macrophages and PMNL and low levels of immunoglobulin A/immunoglobulin G (IgA/IgG). The most common route of entry is inhalation or ingestion of amniotic fluid contaminated by the maternal genital tract, which itself can be contaminated by pelvic examination during the peripartum period. Bacteria then cross the fetal respiratory or gastrointestinal mucosa, proliferate in the blood, and enter the CNS (Figure 29.8). GBS is responsible for early-onset disease (EoD), typically occurring within the first

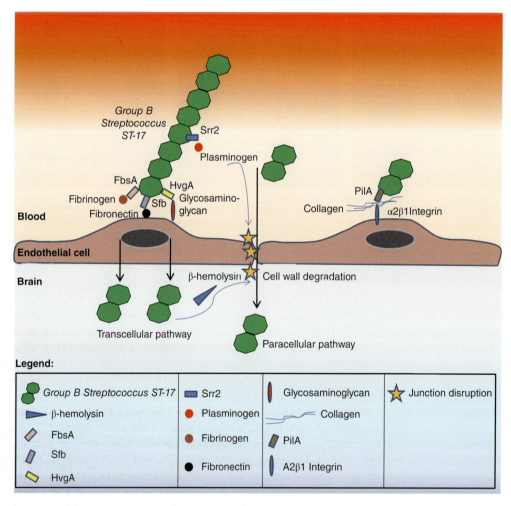

Figure 29.8 Mechanism of CNS invasion in Group B *Streptococcus* (GBS) meningitis. GBS adheres to brain endothelial cells through interaction of the adhesins Srr2, HvgA, and FbsA with components of the extracellular matrix (ECM). GBS adhesin pilA binds to collagen and indirectly interacts with α2β1 integrins at the endothelial cell surface. Following interaction, GBS can invade brain endothelial cells, allowing transcellular crossing of the blood-brain barrier (BBB) by an unknown mechanism. Additional release of β-hemolysin promotes cell wall degradation and endothelial monolayer disruption, allowing bacterial invasion through a paracellular pathway.

week of life, with pneumonia, bacteremia, and sometimes meningitis. Late-onset disease (LoD) occurs in infants up to two months of age, with fewer symptoms related to bacteremia and a higher incidence of meningitis. A single clone, GBS ST-17, is strongly associated with LoD [31].

GBS possesses multiples adhesins [31], including lipoteichoic acid (LTA), pili, serine-rich repeat (Srr) proteins, streptococcal fibronectin-binding protein (Sfb), the surface protein hypervirulent GBS adhesin (HvgA), found in hypervirulent ST-17 strains, and alpha C protein (ACP; encoded by *bca*), which binds to glycosaminoglycan. These components enable GBS to interact with various human cell types, including vaginal epithelium, placental membranes, airways, and brain endothelial cells. Adhesion to epithelial cells is mediated by lipoteichoic acid associated with the bacterial wall, and by GBS surface proteins. The pilus protein PilA, Srr1, Sfb, and ACP also mediate GBS interaction with basement membrane components. GBS binds to extracellular matrix components, including fibronectin, fibrinogen, and laminin, which facilitate mucosal colonization [31]. This interaction is mediated by ScpB, a homolog of the Lra1 adhesin family, and by FbsA, a surface-anchored protein. ST-17 strains specifically express Srr2, a cell wall-anchored protein, which binds plasminogen and plasmin, increases bacterial survival from phagocytic killing and bacterial persistence in a murine model of meningitis. This suggests that Srr2 hijacks ligands of the host coagulation system, contributing to GBS dissemination, invasiveness, and ultimately to meningitis [32].

GBS has also developed strategies to penetrate and cross host cell barriers and to avoid immunological clearance and inflammatory response because its sialylated capsular polysaccharide limits host complement activation and phagocytosis. Animal models and in vitro culture systems have shown that GBS can invade brain endothelial cells, supporting the transcellular theory of BBB crossing. Recent data support a Snail1-dependent mechanism of BBB disruption and penetration [33]. GBS can promote the induction of host transcriptional repressor Snail1, which impedes expression of tight junction genes, facilitating tight junction disruption and promoting BBB permeability to allow bacterial passage. In addition, GBS β-hemolysin/cytolysin is directly cytolytic for human brain endothelial cells and may contribute to BBB disruption.

E. coli

E. coli is an extracellular Gram-negative bacillus. It is the second cause of meningitis in neonates and the leading cause in premature infants [34]. Rectal carriage of *E. coli* in women of childbearing age is up to 50%. Maternal-fetal colonization affects about 70% of their newborns, without necessarily causing pathogenicity. About 80% of *E. coli* strains isolated from pregnant women and newborns possess the K1 capsular polysaccharide antigen that protects the bacterial cell from immune attack. *E. coli* K1 meningitis starts with gastrointestinal mucosa colonization, followed by invasion, survival, and proliferation within the blood [35]. *E. coli* K1 can induce high-level bacteremia [35]. At the brain level, *E. coli* K1 binds to cerebral capillaries via bacterial surface structures such as OmpA and type 1 fimbriae. The interaction induces host cell actin cytoskeleton rearrangement and microvilli-like protrusions that facilitate bacterial internalization. *E. coli* K1 is then stored in cell vacuoles and reaches the subarachnoid space after its release at the basal membrane of microvascular endothelial cells.

L. monocytogenes

L. monocytogenes is a facultative intracellular Gram-positive bacillus, which can survive at freezing temperatures and proliferates at very low (refrigeration) temperatures. For this reason, it is associated with foodborne illness. *L. monocytogenes* crosses the intestinal and fetoplacental barriers via the interaction of bacterial proteins InlA and InlB with cell surface proteins E-cadherin and Met respectively [36]. *L. monocytogenes* spreads through the CNS by the diapedesis of infected monocytes (Trojan horse mechanism) across the BBB, and by direct invasion of endothelial cells [36]. After entering endothelial cells, the bacteria escape from phagosomes via a hemolysin called listeriolysin O or LLO, a pore-forming molecule. Once in the cytoplasm, *L. monocytogenes* highjacks actin cytoskeleton of the infected cell for its own propulsion (comet tails), and spreads in adjacent cells. Direct intra-axonal spread along lower cranial nerves and within the brain has been demonstrated in animal models and may also be important in human listeria brainstem and rhomboencephalitis [37].

Inflammation

Inflammation plays a central role during bacterial CNS infection. Although mandatory for host protection against pathogens, inflammation is also responsible for several crucial steps of bacterial invasion and inflammation-induced adverse events, such as BBB rupture, CSF cytokine production, leukocyte invasion in the CSF, and neuronal injury.

A wide range of innate sensors are expressed by all neuronal and nonneuronal cells within the CNS. Locally, in response to bacterial invasion, endothelial, glial, and resident immune cells produce pro-inflammatory factors, including the cytokines tumor necrosis factor alpha (TNF-α), interleukin (IL)-1β, IL-8/CXCL-8, and IL-6. These initiate an inflammatory cascade and attract immune cells. Matrix metalloproteinases (MMPs) are also produced, which degrade the extracellular matrix, allow cell migration, and increase BBB permeability [38]. In the inflammatory state, adhesion molecules such as VCAM-1 and ICAM-1 are expressed at the endothelial cell surface, facilitating leukocyte adhesion [39]. PMNL are locally recruited in the acute phase, and a mix of T and B cells, monocytes, and dendritic cells in the chronic stage; all are required for microbial control. Several portals of entry into the brain exist for inflammatory cells, including the fenestrated vasculature within the subarachnoid space and the choroid plexus, across epithelial and ependymal cells of the choroid plexus or astrocyte endfeet of BBB.

Inflammation affects cerebral blood flow during bacterial infection of the CNS. In acute meningitis, endothelin, a strong vasoconstrictor, is secreted by brain endothelial cells, and contributes to cerebral blood flow reduction and ischemia [40]. Reactive oxygen species (ROS) and reactive nitrogen species produced by granulocytes, endothelial cells, and microglial cells are responsible for vascular damage within the brain [41].

Conclusions

Many clinical syndromes are encountered in CNS infections. Accurate diagnosis and prompt treatment are mandatory. The pathophysiology is complex, contributed to by both direct bacterial damage and the host inflammatory response. A full understanding of these infections may help the design of new therapies to block bacterial invasion and reduce inflammation response-induced injuries.

References

1. Leber, A.L., Everhart, K., Balada-Llasat, J.M. et al. (2016). *Multicenter evaluation of biofire filmarray meningitis/encephalitis panel for detection of bacteria, viruses, and yeast in cerebrospinal fluid specimens. J. Clin. Microbiol.* 54: 2251–2261.
2. Weiss, N., Miller, F., Cazaubon, S., and Couraud, P.O. (2009). *Biology of the blood-brain barrier: Part I. Rev. Neurol. (Paris)* 165: 863–874.
3. Aspelund, A., Antila, S., Proulx, S.T. et al. (2015). *A dural lymphatic vascular system that drains brain interstitial fluid and macromolecules. J. Exp. Med.* 212: 991–999.
4. Prinz, M. and Priller, J. (2017). *The role of peripheral immune cells in the CNS in steady state and disease. Nat. Neurosci.* 20: 136–144.
5. van de Beek, D., de Gans, J., Tunkel, A.R., and Wijdicks, E.F. (2006). *Community-acquired bacterial meningitis in adults. N. Engl. J. Med.* 354: 44–53.
6. Wang, Y.Y. and Xie, B.D. (2018). *Progress on diagnosis of Tuberculous Meningitis. Methods Mol. Biol.* 1754: 375–386.
7. Chun, C.H., Johnson, J.D., Hofstetter, M., and Raff, M.J. (1986). *Brain abscess. A study of 45 consecutive cases. Medicine (Baltimore)* 65: 415–431.
8. Heusner, A.P. (1948). *Nontuberculous spinal epidural infections. N. Engl. J. Med.* 239: 845–854.
9. Brandt, C.T., Holm, D., Liptrot, M. et al. (2008). *Impact of bacteremia on the pathogenesis of experimental pneumococcal meningitis. J. Infect. Dis.* 197: 235–244.
10. Smith, A.L., Scheifele, D., Syriopoulou, V. et al. (1982). Haemophilus Influenzae, Epidemiology, Immunology and Prevention of the Disease. In: *Pathogenesis of Haemophilus influenzae meningitis* (eds. S.H. Sell and P.F. Wright), 89–109. New-York: Elsevier Sciences Publishing Co. Inc.
11. Mairey, E., Genovesio, A., Donnadieu, E. et al. (2006). *Cerebral microcirculation shear stress levels determine*

Neisseria meningitidis attachment sites along the blood-brain barrier. J. Exp. Med. 203: 1939–1950.

12. Cundell, D.R., Gerard, C., Idanpaan-Heikkila, I. et al. (1996). *PAf receptor anchors Streptococcus pneumoniae to activated human endothelial cells.* Adv. Exp. Med. Biol. 416: 89–94.

13. Bernard, S.C., Simpson, N., Join-Lambert, O. et al. (2014). *Pathogenic Neisseria utilizes CD147 for vascular colonization.* Nat. Med. 20: 725–731.

14. Ring, A., Weiser, J.N., and Tuomanen, E.I. (1998). *Pneumococcal trafficking across the blood-brain barrier. Molecular analysis of a novel bidirectional pathway.* J. Clin. Invest. 102: 347–360.

15. Stins, M.F., Badger, J., and Sik Kim, K. (2001). *Bacterial invasion and transcytosis in transfected human brain microvascular endothelial cells.* Microb. Pathog. 30: 19–28.

16. Nizet, V., Kim, K.S., Stins, M. et al. (1997). *Invasion of brain microvascular endothelial cells by group B streptococci.* Infect. Immun. 65: 5074–5081.

17. Virji, M., Kayhty, H., Ferguson, D.J. et al. (1992). *Interactions of Haemophilus influenzae with human endothelial cells in vitro.* J. Infect. Dis. 165 (Suppl 1): S115–S116.

18. Nikulin, J., Panzner, U., Frosch, M., and Schubert-Unkmeir, A. (2006). *Intracellular survival and replication of Neisseria meningitidis in human brain microvascular endothelial cells.* Int. J. Med. Microbiol. 296: 553–558.

19. Koedel, U., Scheld, W.M., and Pfister, H.W. (2002). *Pathogenesis and pathophysiology of pneumococcal meningitis.* Lancet Infect. Dis. 2: 721–736.

20. Mook-Kanamori, B.B., Geldhoff, M., van der Poll, T., and van de Beek, D. (2011). *Pathogenesis and pathophysiology of pneumococcal meningitis.* Clin. Microbiol. Rev. 24: 557–591.

21. Zysk, G., Schneider-Wald, B.K., Hwang, J.H. et al. (2001). *Pneumolysin is the main inducer of cytotoxicity to brain microvascular endothelial cells caused by Streptococcus pneumoniae.* Infect. Immun. 69: 845–852.

22. Mann, B., Thornton, J., Heath, R. et al. (2014). *Broadly protective protein-based pneumococcal vaccine composed of pneumolysin toxoid-CbpA peptide recombinant fusion protein.* J. Infect. Dis. 209: 1116–1125.

23. van Ginkel, F.W., McGhee, J.R., Watt, J.M. et al. (2003). *Pneumococcal carriage results in ganglioside-mediated olfactory tissue infection.* Proc. Natl. Acad. Sci. U. S. A. 100: 14363–14367.

24. Pace, D. and Pollard, A.J. (2012). *Meningococcal disease: clinical presentation and sequelae.* Vaccine 30 (Suppl 2): B3–B9.

25. Coureuil, M., Bourdoulous, S., Marullo, S., and Nassif, X. (2014). *Invasive meningococcal disease: a disease of the endothelial cells.* Trends Mol. Med. 20: 571–578.

26. Bille, E., Ure, R., Gray, S.J. et al. (2008). *Association of a bacteriophage with meningococcal disease in young adults.* PLoS One 3: e3885.

27. Join-Lambert, O., Lecuyer, H., Miller, F. et al. (2013). *Meningococcal interaction to microvasculature triggers the tissular lesions of purpura fulminans.* J. Infect. Dis. 208: 1590–1597.

28. Schubert-Unkmeir, A., Sokolova, O., Panzner, U. et al. (2007). *Gene expression pattern in human brain endothelial cells in response to Neisseria meningitidis.* Infect. Immun. 75: 899–914.

29. Maissa, N., Covarelli, V., Janel, S. et al. (2017). *Strength of Neisseria meningitidis binding to endothelial cells requires highly-ordered CD147/beta2-adrenoceptor clusters assembled by alpha-actinin-4.* Nat. Commun. 8: 15764.

30. Coureuil, M., Lecuyer, H., Bourdoulous, S., and Nassif, X. (2017). *A journey into the brain: insight into how bacterial pathogens cross blood-brain barriers.* Nat. Rev. Microbiol. 15: 149–159.

31. Tazi, A., Bellais, S., Tardieux, I. et al. (2012). *Group B Streptococcus surface proteins as major determinants for meningeal tropism.* Curr. Opin. Microbiol. 15: 44–49.

32. Six, A., Bellais, S., Bouaboud, A. et al. (2015). *Srr2, a multifaceted adhesin expressed by ST-17 hypervirulent Group B Streptococcus involved in binding to both fibrinogen and plasminogen.* Mol. Microbiol. 97: 1209–1222.

33. Kim, B.J., Hancock, B.M., Bermudez, A. et al. (2015). *Bacterial induction of Snail1 contributes to blood-brain barrier disruption.* J. Clin. Invest. 125: 2473–2483.

34. Ouchenir, L., Renaud, C., Khan, S. et al. (2017). *The epidemiology, management, and outcomes of bacterial meningitis in infants.* Pediatrics 140 (pii): e20170476.

35. Xie, Y., Kim, K.J., and Kim, K.S. (2004). *Current concepts on Escherichia coli K1 translocation of the blood-brain barrier.* FEMS Immunol. Med. Microbiol. 42: 271–279.

36. Disson, O. and Lecuit, M. (2013). *In vitro and in vivo models to study human listeriosis: mind the gap.* Microbes Infect. 15: 971–980.

37. Antal, E.A., Løberg, E.M., Bracht, P. et al. (2001). *Evidence for intraaxonal spread of Listeria monocytogenes from the periphery to the central nervous system.* Brain Pathol. 11: 432–438.

38. Sellner, J. and Leib, S.L. (2006). *In bacterial meningitis cortical brain damage is associated with changes in parenchymal MMP-9/TIMP-1 ratio and increased collagen type IV degradation.* Neurobiol. Dis. 21: 647–656.

39. Greenwood, J., Etienne-Manneville, S., Adamson, P., and Couraud, P.O. (2002). *Lymphocyte migration into the central nervous system: implication of ICAM-1 signalling at the blood-brain barrier. Vasc. Pharmacol.* 38: 315–322.

40. Eisenhut, M. (2014). *Vasospasm in cerebral inflammation. Int. J. Inflamm.* 2014: 509707.

41. Schaper, M., Gergely, S., Lykkesfeldt, J. et al. (2002). *Cerebral vasculature is the major target of oxidative protein alterations in bacterial meningitis. J. Neuropathol. Exp. Neurol.* 61: 605–613.

30 Pyogenic Infections of the CNS 1: Acute Bacterial Meningitis

Loic Le Guennec[1,2] and Sandrine Bourdoulous[1]

[1] Inserm, U1016, Institut Cochin, CNRS, UMR8104, Paris University, Paris, France
[2] La Pitie-Salpetriere Hospital, APHP, Paris, France

Abbreviations

BBB	blood-brain barrier
BM	bacterial meningitis
CNS	central nervous system
CSF	cerebrospinal fluid
DIC	disseminated intravascular coagulation
E. coli	Escherichia coli
EEG	electroencephalography
EoD	early-onset disease
GBS	group B Streptococcus
Hib	Haemophilus influenzae type b:
L. monocytogenes	Listeria monocytogenes
LoD	late-onset disease
LP	Lumbar puncture
MRI	magnetic resonance imaging
M. tuberculosis	Mycobacterium tuberculosis
NCAM	neural cell adhesion molecule
N. meningitidis	Neisseria meningitidis
PCR	polymerase chain reaction
PCV13	13-valent pneumococcal conjugate vaccine
PMNL	polymorphonuclear leukocytes
PPV23	23-valent pneumococcal polysaccharide vaccine

Introduction, definition, and historical perspective

Bacterial meningitis (BM) is an acute purulent infection of the meninges. It is the most common bacterial infection of the CNS and is a medical emergency that still has a high mortality and morbidity despite the overall improvements in its diagnosis and management. BM is one of the top 10 causes of infection-related deaths worldwide, and about 40% of the survivors suffer neurological sequelae [1]. Hippocrates described meningitis 25 centuries ago [2], but the first described meningitis outbreak was in Geneva in 1805. An African outbreak was reported in 1840. One of the main causative bacteria, *Neisseria meningitidis,* was described by Anton Weichselbaum, an Austrian pathologist in 1887 (which he named "*Diplococcus intracellularis meningitidis*") [3]. The clinical features were described by Kernig, a Russian neurologist in 1884, and later by Brudinski, a Polish physician. Both their names are associated with the classical signs of testing resistance to stretching of the inflamed meninges [4]. Meningococcal vaccine was developed in the 1970s and since then, vaccines have been introduced for several serotypes

---

Infections of the Central Nervous System: Pathology and Genetics, First Edition. Edited by Fabrice Chrétien,
Kum Thong Wong, Leroy R. Sharer, Catherine (Katy) Keohane and Françoise Gray.
© 2020 John Wiley & Sons Ltd. Published 2020 by John Wiley & Sons Ltd.

of meningococcus, pneumococcus, and other causes of BM (e.g. *Haemophilus influenzae b* [Hib]).

Epidemiology

The incidence and types of BM are markedly different depending on the geographic region and the patient's age. In Western Europe, the incidence is more than 1 per 100 000 population per year, whereas it reaches 1000 per 100 000 people per year in sub-Saharan Africa, which is known as the "African meningitis belt," mainly due to *N. meningitidis* epidemics [5]. The pathogens also vary according to host age and risk factors.

The incidence of BM is highest during the neonatal period. In industrialized countries, the incidence of culture-proven neonatal meningitis is estimated at 0.3 per 1000 live births and mortality ranges from 10 to 15% [6]. Long-term morbidity is observed in 50% of infants, with 25% having severe disability [7]. In a study conducted in 2011 [8], Group B Streptococci (GBS) and *Escherichia coli* were responsible for 59% and 28% of neonatal BM cases, respectively, followed by Gram-negative bacilli other than *E. coli* (4%), other streptococci (4%), *N. meningitidis* (3%), and *Listeria monocytogenes* (1.5%). GBS was the most common pathogen both in early-onset disease (EoD) (77% GBS vs. 18% for *E. coli*) and in late-onset disease (LoD) (50% GBS vs. 33% for *E. coli*). EoD is defined as within 48 hours of birth, the pathogen is usually acquired from the mother before or during birth, whereas LoD is more than 48 hours after birth, and the pathogen may be acquired in the community. In more recent studies, *E. coli* was the primary cause of meningitis in preterm neonates and also the primary cause of LoD, followed by GBS [9].

Microbiological characteristics

Acute BM is mainly caused by *Streptococcus pneumoniae*, *N. meningitidis*, and Hib in children and adults. Older than the age of three months, *S. pneumoniae* and *N. meningitidis* are the two main bacteria responsible for community-acquired BM. Hib meningitis has almost disappeared in Europe and North America following widespread immunization campaigns, but it remains an important cause of death in some countries. Before the age of two months, BM is mainly caused by GBS and *E. coli*). *L. monocytogenes* affects both neonates and patients who are immunocompromised or older.

Less common bacteria causing acute meningitis include nontyphoidal *Salmonella*, *Klebsiella* spp., *Staphylococcus aureus*, and the porcine zoonotic pathogen *Streptococcus suis*. These will not be addressed in this chapter.

S. pneumoniae

S. pneumoniae (also called pneumococcus) is an alpha-hemolytic Gram-positive extracellular diplococcus. It is the most frequent organism responsible for community-acquired BM worldwide, affecting young children and older people. Between the ages of 2 and 12 months, it causes 48% of BM [10]. Pneumococcus is an asymptomatic colonizer of the nasopharyngeal mucosa, responsible for otitis media, sinusitis, and also for severe invasive infections such as pneumonia, bacteremia, and acute meningitis. The mortality rate for pneumococcal meningitis is high, (up to 11% of deaths in children) [10]. Splenectomy or functional hyposplenism is an important risk factor for pneumococcal invasive infections, with a higher rate of mortality and unfavorable outcome [11].

N. meningitidis

N. meningitidis (also called meningococcus) is an extracellular Gram-negative diplococcus. In industrialized countries it accounts for about 10% of all adult, and up to 25% of pediatric BM cases. It is a major cause of epidemics in the "meningitis belt" of sub-Saharan Africa [12]. It is also highly virulent, responsible for 10% of meningitis deaths. It is restricted to humans and is a frequent nasopharyngeal commensal. Asymptomatic carriage in healthy individuals occurs in 8–20% of the population but is up to 25% in children. Meningococci are transmitted by respiratory secretions, saliva, or by inhalation of aerosolized bacteria within droplets.

Nasopharyngeal acquisition may be transient, lead to colonization, or result in invasive disease. Mucosal colonization and crossing mechanisms are discussed in Chapter 29, but remain largely unexplained. Meningococcal carriage and acquisition are influenced by age, close contact, and cofactors such as smoking and coinfections. Disease occurrence is influenced by the pathogenicity of the strain and human host susceptibility [13]. Deficiencies in alternative and terminal complement pathways are major risk factors for meningococcal meningitis, particularly with uncommon pathogenic serogroups, such as serotypes Y and W135 [14]. A high risk for invasive meningococcal disease has been observed in patients receiving eculizumab (a monoclonal antibody, directed against complement effectors) used in the treatment of paroxysmal nocturnal hemoglobinuria and atypical hemolytic uremic syndrome or for solid organ transplantation [15].

H. influenzae Type b

Hib is a small Gram-negative rod-shaped bacterium, residing in the upper respiratory tract, especially in childhood. In Europe and America, Hib meningitis was the most important cause of acute childhood meningitis, but its incidence has greatly decreased since the early 1990s, following mass vaccination campaigns with conjugate vaccines. It remains a major health problem in areas where vaccination is not available. Southeast Asia, Africa, the western Pacific, and the eastern Mediterranean regions still have the largest numbers of cases and deaths [16].

GBS

GBS (*Streptococcus agalactiae*) is a Gram-positive extracellular coccus that often forms chains of organisms. Although all GBS serotypes can cause invasive infections, five serotypes, classified by cell wall polysaccharides (i.e. Ia, Ib, II, III, and V) account for the majority of diseases in neonates. Five major clonal complexes have been identified: CC1, CC12, CC19, CC17, and CC23. CC17 represent 70% of GBS isolates responsible for neonatal meningitis [17]. The prevalence of GBS carriage in the anogenital area in women who are pregnant varies from 10 to 20% depending on the country. Fifty percent of neonates born to these women are colonized with GBS, and 1% will develop invasive infection [16]. GBS meningitis accounts for 14% of meningitis mortality [10]. Premature rupture of membranes during pregnancy is the main risk factor. For these women, intrapartum antibiotic prophylaxis with penicillin is recommended for prevention of GBS disease. GBS is mostly responsible for early-onset disease (EoD), which typically occurs within the first week of life, manifesting as pneumonia and severe sepsis and for late-onset disease (LoD), occurring in infants up to 2 months of age, with fewer symptoms related to bacteremia and a higher incidence of meningitis. LoD as a result of GBS accounts for 30% of all cases, and the source of infection may be through contaminated breast milk or nosocomial or community transmission. Prematurity is the main risk factor for GBS LoD, and 84% are caused by Serotype III [18]. Recommended guidelines include screening pregnant women for GBS carriage and using antibiotics during delivery. Although antibiotic prophylaxis significantly reduced EoD, it had no effect on LoD.

E. coli

E. coli is an extracellular Gram-negative bacillus. It is the second-leading cause of meningitis in neonates and the leading cause in premature infants [9, 19]. Rectal carriage of *E. coli* in women of childbearing age is as high as 50% and maternal-fetal colonization occurs in about 70% of newborns in these women, without necessarily causing disease. In about 80% of cases, *E. coli* strains with K1 capsular polysaccharides are isolated [20]. This capsular polysaccharide enables bacterial survival within the blood, protecting bacteria against complement activation [21]. Preterm birth, severe reduction in cerebrospinal fluid (CSF) glucose (hypoglycorrhachia) with CSF-to-blood glucose ratio 1:10, and serogroups O are independent risk factors for severe disease or death [22].

Special features of *L. monocytogenes*

L. monocytogenes is a facultative intracellular Gram-positive bacillus. It can survive at freezing temperatures and proliferate at low temperatures such as those used in refrigeration, so it is associated with foodborne illness, particularly from soft cheeses. *Listeria* is the third leading cause of BM in adults (5% of cases [23]) but justifies separate mention because of its association with brainstem microabscesses. It is responsible for meningitis in neonates (both EoD and LoD) and adults, but particularly affects adult patients with underlying immunosuppression and solid organ cancer [24]. The three-month mortality in adults is high (30%) despite antibiotic treatment; outcome is dependent on timely antibiotic therapy [24]. *L. monocytogenes* is naturally resistant to third-generation cephalosporins. Amoxicillin should be introduced in the empirical antibiotic regimens as soon as the diagnosis is suspected. Carriage in the digestive tract is observed in several animals, and the bacteria are widespread in soil and the environment. A Japanese study showed asymptomatic fecal carriage of *L. monocytogenes* in more than 1% of patients [25]. At an individual level, fecal carriage varies over time [26]. In pregnancy, the bacteria can cross the placenta and cause congenital infection.

Clinical features

Clinical presentation

BM should be suspected in a patient with fever, associated meningism (i.e. headache, neck stiffness, Kernig and Brudzinski signs, nausea and vomiting, and phono- and photophobia) or neurological impairment (alteration of consciousness, coma, focal neurologic signs, and seizures [27]). Some extraneurological signs help suggest the causative agent.
- Cerebral vasculitis is often a feature of pneumococcal meningitis and may be responsible for multiple strokes (Figure 30.1a and b).
- Meningococcal meningitis presents with skin purpuric lesions in 50% of patients (Figure 30.2). Adrenal hemorrhage with circulatory collapse (Waterhouse–Friderichsen syndrome) may develop rapidly after disease onset in a small proportion of children. Systemic complications, such as septic shock and disseminated intravascular coagulation (DIC), contribute to unfavorable outcomes. Magnetic resonance imaging (MRI) with contrast may show abnormal leptomeningeal and cortical enhancement (Figure 30.3).

The symptoms and signs of BM in infants and neonates are rather non-specific, with behavioral changes (irritability), gastrointestinal features (i.e. poor feeding, vomiting, and diarrhea), cardiovascular symptoms (i.e. tachycardia, long capillary refill time, and cyanosis). If present, neurological features (i.e. bulging fontanelle, nuchal rigidity, muscle hypotonia, seizures lethargy, and coma) signal a poor prognosis. Grave signs include cutaneous purpura, focal neurologic signs, respiratory problems, altered consciousness, or coma. Signs of intracranial hypertension may indicate CSF obstruction because of hydrocephalus.
- GBS meningitis in infants is associated with multiple cerebral complications, including cerebral phlebitis (Figure 30.4) and hydrocephalus (Figure 30.5).

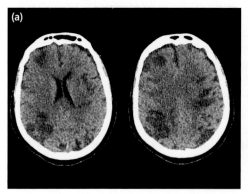 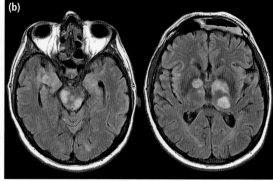

Figure 30.1 Multiple strokes due to cerebral vasculitis associated with pneumococcal meningitis. (a) Computed tomography (CT) brain scan (axial plane). (b) Brain magnetic resonance imaging (MRI) (axial plane), T2 fluid attenuated inversion recovery (FLAIR) sequence.

Pyogenic Infections of the CNS 1: Acute Bacterial Meningitis Chapter 30

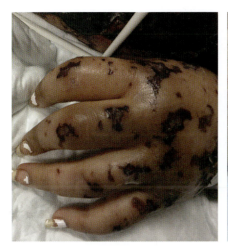
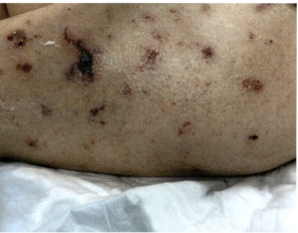

Figure 30.2 Skin purpuric lesions in a young adult with meningococcal septicemia (serogroup C) associated with disseminated intravascular coagulation.

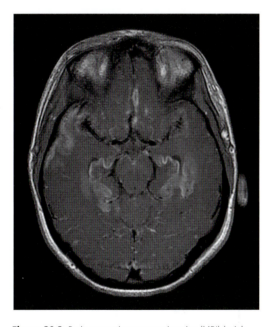

Figure 30.3 Brain magnetic resonance imaging (MRI) (axial plane), T1 sequence showing leptomeningeal and cortical enhancement in meningococcal meningitis.

- Focal neurological signs with cranial nerve palsy are suggestive of *L. monocytogenes* infection [22] and brain MRI can be normal, or show rhomboencephalitis (Figure 30.6a) with meningeal contrast and focal parenchymal lesions, with or without hydrocephalus [28].

Laboratory investigations

Clinical signs and symptoms alone are not sufficient to diagnose meningitis. CSF examination is the cornerstone of diagnosis. However, lumbar puncture (LP) should never delay starting appropriate antibiotic treatment, particularly if meningococcal septicemia (purpura fulminans) is suspected. In patients with coagulopathy (e.g. during meningococcal septicemia associated with DIC or with significant raised intracranial pressure), LP is contraindicated. Brain imaging must be performed before LP if the patient shows focal neurologic signs. CSF examination includes direct microscopy, biochemical, bacterial, and viral analysis. In BM, the CSF is cloudy and turbid, white blood cells are increased >10 cells/mm^3 (> 50% polymorphonuclear leukocytes [PMNL]), there is a low glucose (<40% of serum glucose) and elevated protein (>50 mg/dl) [27]. Gram stain is routinely performed for direct microscopic examination. Bacterial identification is made on CSF culture; its sensitivity ranges from 60 to 90% depending on the organism and whether antibiotic treatment has already been started [29]. Antibiotic sensitivity should be determined, but antibiotic treatment before LP may decrease the yield of culture.

Highly sensitive and specific dipstick rapid diagnostic tests based on immunochromatography have been developed to detect *S. pneumoniae* and *N. meningitidis* antigens, although their performance is

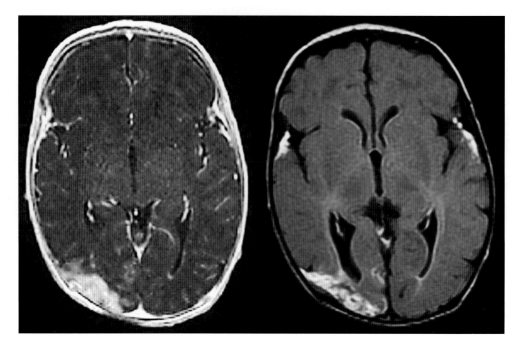

Figure 30.4 Brain magnetic resonance imaging (MRI; axial plane). Group B streptococcal meningitis in an 18-day-old infant, associated with cerebral phlebitis. Left panel: T1 sequence showing phlebitis within the right transverse sinus. Right panel: T2 fluid attenuated inversion recovery (FLAIR) sequence showing a venous infarct in the right occipital lobe.

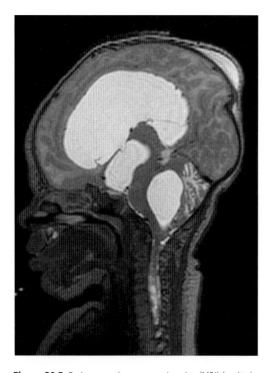

Figure 30.5 Brain magnetic resonance imaging (MRI) (sagittal plane) T2 sequence from a 20-day-old infant with group B streptococcal meningitis complicated by hydrocephalus. Note the bulging fontanelle.

variable for *N. meningitidis* [30]. Molecular diagnostic tests, including multiplex polymerase chain reaction (PCR) are sensitive and improve the diagnosis by rapid detection of microbial nucleic acids, including from nonviable organisms [31]. Currently, microorganisms are best identified using 16S rRNA and 18S rRNA gene sequencing. New-generation sequencing tools should improve this in the future, but their cost-effectiveness should be assessed. Recently, matrix-assisted laser desorption ionization-time-of-flight mass spectrometry has emerged as a tool for microbial identification and diagnosis, using either intact microorganisms or microbial extracts [32]. The process is rapid, sensitive, and economical in terms of costs. In suspected meningococcal infection, culture and PCR analysis can also be performed on skin biopsy of purpuric lesions (if present) as meningococci remain for approximately 24 hours in skin lesions after antibiotics have been started.

Differential diagnosis

The main differential diagnosis of acute BM is herpes simplex 1 encephalitis because both infections have substantial clinical overlap. Electroencephalography (EEG), MRI, and LP can help in making the distinction (see Chapter 5).

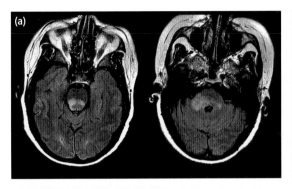
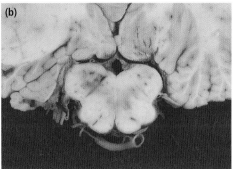

Figure 30.6 *Listeria* meningitis with involvement of the brainstem. (a) Brain magnetic resonance imaging (MRI) (axial plane), T2 fluid attenuated inversion recovery (FLAIR) sequence. Listeriosis showing rhomboencephalitis. (b) Horizontal section of the medulla showing congestion and necrosis in the left part of the floor of the fourth ventricle (Source: courtesy of Pr. F. Gray).

Prognostic factors

The mortality rate is above 9% at any age and reaches 15% in neonates. It depends on the pathogen and on the clinical history and situation of the patient. Thirty percent of survivors have functional sequelae, mainly neurologic deficits and hearing loss (the latter particularly with S. *pneumoniae*).

Early antibiotic treatment is crucial, but several other factors also impact survival. These include the severity of infection which is reflected by: (i) neurological symptoms (i.e. coma, focal neurologic signs, seizures, and intracranial hypertension); (ii) respiratory symptoms (i.e. Cheyne-Stokes respiration, cyanosis, signs of hypercapnia); (iii) autonomic dysfunction; (iv) extensive purpura; and (v) underlying host risk factors such as prematurity or advanced age, immunodeficiency, or splenectomy [27].

Pathology

The neuropathological features in patients who have died from BM are largely similar, irrespective of the bacterial cause [33].

In rapidly fatal (hyperacute) disease, when death occurs within 24 hours, postmortem examination may disclose adrenal hemorrhage, centrilobular liver necrosis, or DIC. A local source of infection may be evident in the scalp, cranium, air sinuses, or middle ear. In blood-borne infection, the source may be impossible to trace, but the initial infection in pneumococcal meningitis is usually in the respiratory tract.

In the hyperacute stage, there may be no visible exudate, but organisms are numerous; margination of PMNL may be obvious in the leptomeningeal arterioles (Figure 30.7). There is no pus in the meninges, but they are severely congested. The congestion and associated brain edema resembles nonperfused brain ("respirator brain") seen following prolonged assisted ventilation. Death in hyperacute meningitis may be the result of meningococcus, pneumococcus and Hib, or to rarer pathogens such as *Bacillis anthracis*.

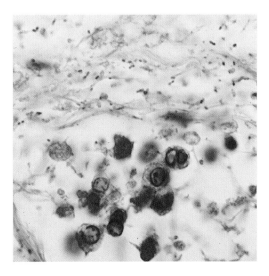

Figure 30.7 Microscopy of leptomeninges in fatal hyperacute bacterial meningitis (BM) shows polymorphonuclear leukocytes and numerous organisms (hematoxylin and eosin [H&E]) (Source: courtesy of Pr. F. Gray).

In acute meningitis, if survival is for two days or longer, a meningeal exudate is visible. Pus is first detectable macroscopically only as cloudiness in the basal cisterns and as thin creamy lines alongside meningeal veins, so-called "tramtracking" (Figure 30.8a). In patients who die within three to seven days (usually patients who were untreated or debilitated), the entire brain, vertex and base can be enveloped by pus, which is creamy, yellow, or green depending on the responsible organism. Microscopy and culture should always be performed. At this stage, the meningeal cellular exudate is composed almost entirely of PMNL (Figure 30.8b), and both intracellular and extracellular bacteria are visible. Involvement of small meningeal arteries or veins is rare initially, but the exudate is often accompanied by wisps of fibrin. The contrast between the inflamed meninges and that of the underlying cortex is remarkable; few PMNLs enter the cortical perivascular spaces. The cortex is edematous and neurons frequently show ischemic change.

In cases with a subacute course (in patients with delayed or ineffective treatment or with drug-resistant microorganisms), death may occur after one week; PMNLs are less numerous in the exudate, and lymphocytes, a few plasma cells, fibrin, and macrophages are also present, the latter becoming more prominent. A small number of blood vessels surrounded by exudate may show fibrinoid necrosis and thrombosis, (especially in pneumococcal meningitis), resulting in focal cortical or even larger areas of infarction (Figure 30.9a). Inflammatory cells enter the outer cortical perivascular spaces and there is proliferation of subpial microglia and astrocytes, the latter particularly prominent in pneumococcal meningitis. Infection extends to the ventricular system by reverse flow from the subarachnoid space into the ventricular space: the ventricular CSF is purulent, and the ependyma and subependymal region are deeply congested and often covered by flakes of pus (Figure 30.9b). The choroid plexus is similarly affected. In pneumococcal meningitis, hemorrhagic ependymitis may also be seen. Exudate covering the ventricular wall denudes the ependyma, and mild subependymal perivascular infiltration occurs. The brain shows edema, yet the ventricles may be slightly enlarged rather than compressed, as hydrocephalus is an almost constant feature at this stage. Obstructive hydrocephalus or even pyocephalus may be the result of thick pus in the aqueduct and fourth ventricle or to its organization in the aqueduct or at the exit foramina of the fourth ventricle. Communicating hydrocephalus may also occur as a consequence of impaired CSF resorption because of an extensive meningeal exudate. The infection may extend to the cranial nerves (particularly the ophthalmic and auditory nerves) and spinal roots, which show cellular infiltration with eventual demyelination.

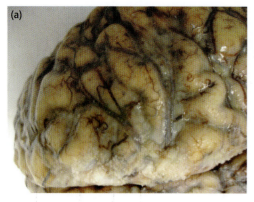 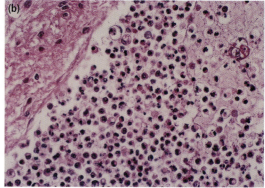

Figure 30.8 Meningeal exudate in acute meningitis. (a) Thin creamy lines of exudate alongside meningeal vessels: so-called "tramtracking" (Source: courtesy of Pr. K. Keohane). (b) At this acute stage, the meningeal cellular exudate is composed almost entirely of polymorphs and bacteria are both intracellular and extracellular. The exudate is often accompanied by wisps of fibrin (Source: courtesy of Pr. K. Keohane).

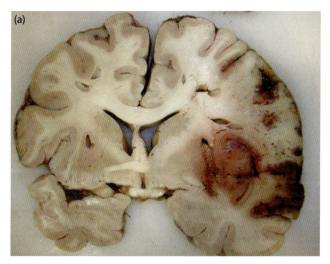
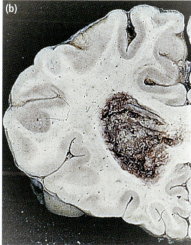

Figure 30.9 Complications of purulent meningitis with a subacute course. (a) Hemorrhagic wedge-shaped infarction in the right hemisphere with associated greenish discoloration of the cortex and meninges because of venous thrombosis in a patient with delayed treatment and prolonged purulent meningitis (Source: courtesy of Pr. K. Keohane). (b) Coronal section of the right cerebral hemisphere at the level of the rostrum of corpus callosum showing purulent ventriculitis (Source: courtesy of Pr. F. Gray).

Chronic changes in those who survive after weeks or months (possibly following initial cryptic infection) are inevitably accompanied by complications and accompanying neurological deficits. Meningeal thickening or fibrosis will produce hydrocephalus by blocking the basal cisterns. Fibrous organization around the spinal cord can cause infarction due to thrombosis or venous occlusion by compression. The meningeal thickening around the cord is similar to progressive spinal arachnoiditis. Encysted collections of fluid may develop over the surface of the cerebral hemispheres (cystic arachnoiditis) and can cause significant compression if they are numerous or large.

Clear or blood-stained subdural effusions (hygromas) are frequent complications, especially in infants and may be large enough to require surgical intervention. The suggested etiology is that a valvular tear forms in the arachnoid, although it is not clear how the tear occurs. Subdural empyemas rarely complicate meningitis.

Because the pia is an efficient barrier, brain abscess is a rare complication of BM in adults. In contrast, cerebral abscesses are frequent in neonates with BM caused by *Citrobacter* spp. Extensive hemorrhagic necrosis of the cerebral white matter with vasculitis and abundant organisms has been described as a complication in neonatal meningitis (particularly in premature neonates) caused by *E. coli*, *Proteus* spp., and *Citrobacter* spp. *L. monocytogenes* meningitis is frequently associated with rhombencephalitis (Figure 30.6b). Brainstem abscesses caused by *L. monocytogenes* may occur in the absence of clinical meningitis, and spinal intramedullary abscess and chronic spinal arachnoiditis have been described occasionally.

Treatment

In suspected BM, empiric therapy with antibiotics should not be delayed for more than an hour while awaiting diagnostic testing [34]. Recommended therapy is based on the patient's age, risk factors, and clinical features. Therapy includes cefotaxime or ceftriaxone to cover potential infection by *S. pneumoniae* with reduced susceptibility to penicillin, until susceptibility is known. Amoxicillin must be added in suspected listeriosis because *L. monocytogenes* is often naturally resistant to cephalosporins. Antibiotic therapy is modified when the culture sensitivity is known, and treatment duration is seven days [35].

Adjuvant corticosteroid therapy can improve adult mortality and reduce neurological sequelae, including deafness, in adults and children [36]. Dexamethasone is recommended in suspected pneumococcal or meningococcal meningitis in adults and if pneumococcal or Hib meningitis is suspected in children and infants (administered just before or concomitantly with antibiotic therapy). Dexamethasone is not recommended if meningitis occurs in patients who are immunocompromised or in meningococcal disease in children and infants. If BM is excluded, dexamethasone should be discontinued.

To improve outcomes, external ventricular drainage of CSF can be performed in patients with intracranial hypertension [37]. A clinical trial of induced therapeutic hypothermia to reduce neuronal damage in severe BM was discontinued because of a higher mortality in the hypothermia group [38]. A trial with daptomycin, a nonlytic antimicrobial, is ongoing in Gram-positive meningitis (NCT01522105) to try to decrease bacterial lysis and its associated systemic inflammation [39].

Mass vaccination remains the best way to reduce the incidence of BM. Vaccination against serogroup A *N. meningitidis* in the African meningitis belt dramatically reduced the number of cases [40]. Different strategies have been developed, depending on the infectious agent.

S. pneumoniae: [41] More than 90 distinct polysaccharide capsular types of *S. pneumoniae* make vaccine development challenging. The 23-valent pneumococcal polysaccharide vaccine (PPV23) and the 13-valent pneumococcal conjugate vaccine (PCV13), covering 23 and 13 serotypes, respectively, are the most widely used. Recommendations differ from country to country and change over time. Usually, PCV13 is recommended for children <2 years, for older children with splenectomy or hyposplenism, and all individuals ≥5 years infected with HIV or who have a stem cell transplant; it is also recommended for CSF leakage and in infants with cochlear implants. Patients >65 years also had good protection from invasive pneumococcal infections. PPV23 is recommended in subjects ≥2 years with an increased risk of pneumococcal infections. Mass immunization reduces disease from vaccine-preventable serotypes, which is important for community protection. In Spain, since PCV 13 was introduced, pneumococcal meningitis incidence fell from 2.3 per 100 000 to 0.5 per 100 000 [42]. Increasing incidence of infections by nonvaccine serotypes now necessitates a vaccine against all serogroups [43]. Clinical trials are already underway to evaluate *S. pneumoniae* whole cell vaccine (NCT01537185).

N. meningitidis: Thirteen *N. meningitidis* serogroups have been described based on capsular serologic differences; six (i.e. A, B, C, W, X, Y) cause invasive disease. The polysaccharide capsule is a key virulence determinant. For serogroups A, C, W, and Y, it forms the basis of polysaccharide conjugate vaccines (PCVs). In industrialized countries, serogroups B, C, W135, and Y are responsible for invasive diseases. Serogroup A is mainly found in sub-Saharan Africa; its incidence has dramatically decreased recently because of vaccination [44]. Serogroup C disease first appeared in 2015 in the Sahel region of Africa [45]. Serogroup W135 is found in Mecca and Africa. Serogroup B is prevalent in European countries, which use multivalent vaccines against A, C, W-135, and Y serogroups. The Centers for Disease Control and Prevention (CDC) has reported all-time low rates of meningococcal disease in the United States (375 total cases in 2015). In France, vaccination against serogroup C for children aged <2 years is mandatory, serogroup B accounts for approximately 60% of cases in those aged <5 years; vaccine-preventable serogroups C, Y, or W cause approximately two-thirds of meningococcal disease in those aged >11 years.

Serogroup W135 is increasing in the United Kingdom because of an emergent South American clone (the hyperinvasive ST-11 clonal complex [cc11] associated with higher mortality). Another strain containing cc11, responsible for outbreaks of invasive meningococcal disease, has emerged as a cause of urethritis [46].

The α (2–8) linked sialic acid homopolymer of serogroup B is identical to a modification of the mammalian neural cell adhesion molecule (NCAM), consequently serogroup B polysaccharide is poorly immunogenic. MenB-FHbp and MenB-4C vaccines against noncapsular antigens have been licensed but are unlikely to provide herd protection in an outbreak [47]. Immunization with MenB vaccine in a young adult receiving eculizumab for atypical hemolytic uremic syndrome failed to protect against invasive meningococcal disease [48]. Trials are ongoing (ISRCTN46336916) for serogroup B vaccination using adenovirus as a vector [49].

Hib. Virulence factors of Hib consist of a capsule, adhesion proteins, pili, the IgA1 protease, and the lipooligosaccharide [50]. Current vaccines target the capsular polysaccharide.

GBS: Currently, there is no licensed GBS vaccine available. In 2014, the World Health Organization (WHO) summoned the first meeting to develop GBS vaccines [51]. Novartis has developed a trivalent PCV, and performed a phase Ib/2 clinical trial (NCT01193920) in neonates born to vaccinated women [52], which showed that maternal immunization could be protective. In 2017, Pfizer started a phase 1/2 clinical trial evaluating their pentavalent PCV (NCT03170609).

E. coli: There is no currently available licensed vaccine.

L. monocytogenes: Although research is ongoing [53], there is no vaccine available to prevent listeriosis.

Conclusions

Despite improvements in vaccination and antibiotic therapy, acute BM is still an important cause of death and morbidity. The lack of effective vaccines and development of antimicrobial-resistant strains necessitate adjuvant preventive therapy to reduce both its incidence and neurological sequelae. Despite advances in understanding host-pathogen interactions responsible for bacterial invasion of the CNS, further research with a multidisciplinary approach is required to design new therapies to block bacterial invasion, and to develop new vaccines.

References

1. van de Beek, D., de Gans, J., Tunkel, A.R., and Wijdicks, E.F. (2006). Community-acquired bacterial meningitis in adults. *N Engl J Med* 354: 44–53.
2. Pappas, G., Kiriaze, I.J., and, Falagas, M.F. (2008). Insight into infectious disease in the era of Hippocrates. *Int J Infect Dis* 12: 347–350.
3. Yazdankhah, S.P. and Caugant, D.A. (2004). *Neisseria meningitidis*: an overview of the carriage state. *J Med Microbiol* 53: 821–832.
4. Tyler, K.L. (2010). Chapter 28: a history of bacterial meningitis. *Handb Clin Neurol* 95: 417–433.
5. Heath, P.T., Okike, I.O., and Oeser, C. (2011). Neonatal meningitis: can we do better? *Adv Exp Med Biol* 719: 11–24.
6. Harrison, L.H., Trotter, C.L., and Ramsay, M.E. (2009). Global epidemiology of meningococcal disease. *Vaccine* 27 (Suppl 2): B51–B63.
7. Galiza, E.P. and Heath, P.T. (2009). Improving the outcome of neonatal meningitis. *Curr Opin Infect Dis* 22: 229–234.
8. Gaschignard, J., Levy, C., Romain, O. et al. (2011). Neonatal bacterial meningitis: 444 cases in 7 years. *Pediatr Infect Dis J* 30: 212–217.
9. Ouchenir, L., Renaud, C., Khan, S. et al. (2017). The epidemiology, management, and outcomes of bacterial meningitis in infants. *Pediatrics* 140 (1).
10. Levy, C., Bingen, E., Aujard, Y. et al. (2008). Surveillance network of bacterial meningitis in children, 7 years of survey in France. *Arch Pediatr* 15 (Suppl 3): S99–S104.
11. Adriani, K.S., Brouwer, M.C., van der Ende, A., and van de Beek, D. (2013). Bacterial meningitis in adults after splenectomy and hyposplenic states. *Mayo Clin Proc* 88: 571–578.
12. Lapeyssonnie, L. (1963). Cerebrospinal meningitis in Africa. *Bull World Health Organ* 28 (Suppl): 1–114.
13. Stephens, D.S., Greenwood, B., and Brandtzaeg, P. (2007). Epidemic meningitis, meningococcaemia, and *Neisseria meningitidis*. *Lancet* 369: 2196–2210.
14. Rameix-Welti, M.A., Chedani, H., Blouin, J. et al. (2005). *Neisseria meningitidis* infection. Clinical criteria orienting towards a deficiency in the proteins of the complement. *Presse Med* 34: 425–430.
15. Benamu, E. and Montoya, J.G. (2016). Infections associated with the use of eculizumab: recommendations for prevention and prophylaxis. *Curr Opin Infect Dis* 29: 319–329.
16. Watt, J.P., Wolfson, L.J., O'Brien, K.L. et al. (2009). Burden of disease caused by *Haemophilus influenzae* type b in children younger than 5 years: global estimates. *Lancet* 374 (9693): 903–911.
17. Manning, S.D., Springman, A.C., Lehotzky, E. et al. (2009). Multilocus sequence types associated with neonatal group B streptococcal sepsis and meningitis in Canada. *J Clin Microbiol* 47: 1143–1148.

18. Edmond, K.M., Kortsalioudaki, C., Scott, S. et al. (2012). Group B streptococcal disease in infants aged younger than 3 months: systematic review and meta-analysis. *Lancet* 379: 547–556.
19. Gaschignard, J., Levy, C., Bingen, E., and Cohen, R. (2012). Epidemiology of *Escherichia coli* neonatal meningitis. *Arch Pediatr* 19 (Suppl 3): S129–S134.
20. Glode, M.P., Sutton, A., Robbins, J.B. et al. (1977). Neonatal meningitis due of *Escherichia coli* K1. *J Infect Dis* 136 (Suppl): S93–S97.
21. Kim, K.S., Itabashi, H., Gemski, P. et al. (1992). The K1 capsule is the critical determinant in the development of *Escherichia coli* meningitis in the rat. *J Clin Invest* 90: 897–905.
22. Basmaci, R., Bonacorsi, S., Bidet, P. et al. (2015). *Escherichia Coli* meningitis features in 325 children from 2001 to 2013 in France. *Clin Infect Dis* 61: 779–786.
23. Bijlsma, M.W., Brouwer, M.C., Kasanmoentalib, E.S. et al. (2016). Community-acquired bacterial meningitis in adults in the Netherlands, 2006–14: a prospective cohort study. *Lancet Infect Dis* 16: 339–347.
24. Charlier, C., Perrodeau, E., Leclercq, A. et al. (2017). Clinical features and prognostic factors of listeriosis: the MONALISA national prospective cohort study. *Lancet Infect Dis* 17: 510–519.
25. Iida, T., Kanzaki, M., Nakama, A. et al. (1998). Detection of *Listeria monocytogenes* in humans, animals and foods. *J Vet Med Sci* 60: 1341–1343.
26. Grif, K., Patscheider, G., Dierich, M.P., and Allerberger, F. (2003). Incidence of fecal carriage of *Listeria monocytogenes* in three healthy volunteers: a one-year prospective stool survey. *Eur J Clin Microbiol Infect Dis* 22: 16–20.
27. Moisi, J.C., Saha, S.K., Falade, A.G. et al. (2009). Enhanced diagnosis of pneumococcal meningitis with use of the Binax NOW immunochromatographic test of *Streptococcus pneumoniae* antigen: a multisite study. *Clin Infect Dis* 48 (Suppl 2): S49–S56.
28. Mylonakis, E., Hohmann, E.L., and Calderwood, S.B. (1998). Central nervous system infection with *Listeria monocytogenes*. 33 years' experience at a general hospital and review of 776 episodes from the literature. *Medicine (Baltimore)* 77: 313–336.
29. Brouwer, M.C., Tunkel, A.R., and van de Beek, D. (2010). Epidemiology, diagnosis, and antimicrobial treatment of acute bacterial meningitis. *Clin Microbiol Rev* 23: 467–492.
30. Rose, A.M., Mueller, J.E., Gerstl, S. et al. (2010). Meningitis dipstick rapid test: evaluating diagnostic performance during an urban *Neisseria meningitidis* serogroup A outbreak, Burkina Faso, 2007. *PLoS One* 5: e11086.
31. Seth, R., Murthy, P.S.R., Sistla, S. et al. (2017). Rapid and accurate diagnosis of acute pyogenic meningitis due to *Streptococcus Pneumoniae, Haemophilus influenzae* type b and *Neisseria meningitidis* using a multiplex PCR assay. *J Clin Diagn Res* 11: FC01–FC04.
32. Singhal, N., Kumar, M., Kanaujia, P.K., and Virdi, J.S. (2015). MALDI-TOF mass spectrometry: an emerging technology for microbial identification and diagnosis. *Front Microbiol* 6: 791.
33. Deckert, M. (2015). Bacterial infections. In: *Greenfield's Neuropathology*, 9e (eds. S. Love, H. Budka, J.W. Ironside and A. Perry), 119. New York, NY: CRC Press.
34. Koster-Rasmussen, R., Korshin, A., and Meyer, C.N. (2008). Antibiotic treatment delay and outcome in acute bacterial meningitis. *J Infect* 57: 449–454.
35. Boisier, P., Mahamane, A.E., Hamidou, A.A. et al. (2009). Field evaluation of rapid diagnostic tests for meningococcal meningitis in Niger. *Trop Med Int Health* 14: 111–117.
36. de Gans, J. and van de Beek, D. (2002). Dexamethasone in adults with bacterial meningitis. *N Engl J Med* 347: 1549–1556.
37. Glimaker, M., Johansson, B., Halldorsdottir, H. et al. (2014). Neuro-intensive treatment targeting intracranial hypertension improves outcome in severe bacterial meningitis: an intervention-control study. *PLoS One* 9: e91976.
38. Mourvillier, B., Tubach, F., van de Beek, D. et al. (2013). Induced hypothermia in severe bacterial meningitis: a randomized clinical trial. *JAMA* 310: 2174–2183.
39. Grandgirard, D., Oberson, K., Buhlmann, A. et al. (2010). Attenuation of cerebrospinal fluid inflammation by the nonbacteriolytic antibiotic daptomycin versus that by ceftriaxone in experimental pneumococcal meningitis. *Antimicrob Agents Chemother* 54: 1323–1326.
40. Trotter, C.L., Lingani, C., Fernandez, K. et al. (2017). Impact of MenAfriVac in nine countries of the African meningitis belt, 2010–15: an analysis of surveillance data. *Lancet Infect Dis* 17: 867–872.
41. Moreira, M., Castro, O., Palmieri, M. et al. (2017). A reflection on invasive pneumococcal disease and pneumococcal conjugate vaccination coverage in children in Southern Europe (2009–2016). *Hum Vaccin Immunother* 13: 1–12.
42. Gonzalez-Escartin, E., Angulo Lopez, I., Ots Ruiz, E. et al. (2017). Pneumococcal meningitis in Cantabria

(Spain) in the pneumococcal conjugate vaccine era (2001–2015). *Arch Argent Pediatr* 115: 160–164.
43. Pichichero, M.E. (2017). Pneumococcal whole-cell and protein-based vaccines: changing the paradigm. *Expert Rev Vaccines* 16: 1181–1190.
44. Daugla, D.M., Gami, J.P., Gamougam, K. et al. (2014). Effect of a serogroup A meningococcal conjugate vaccine (PsA-TT) on serogroup A meningococcal meningitis and carriage in Chad: a community study [corrected]. *Lancet* 383: 40–47.
45. Mainassara, H.B., Oumarou, G.I., Issaka, B. et al. (2017). Evaluation of response strategies against epidemics due to *Neisseria meningitidis* C in Niger. *Trop Med Int Health* 22: 196–204.
46. Tzeng, Y.L., Bazan, J.A., Turner, A.N. et al. (2017). Emergence of a new *Neisseria meningitidis* clonal complex 11 lineage 11.2 clade as an effective urogenital pathogen. *Proc Natl Acad Sci USA* 114: 4237–4242.
47. McNamara, L.A., Thomas, J.D., MacNeil, J. et al. (2017). Meningococcal carriage following a vaccination campaign With MenB-4C and MenB-FHbp in response to a University Serogroup B Meningococcal Disease Outbreak-Oregon, 2015–2016. *J Infect Dis* 216: 1130–1140.
48. Parikh, S.R., Lucidarme, J., Bingham, C. et al. (2017). Meningococcal B vaccine failure with a penicillin-resistant strain in a young adult on long-term Eculizumab. *Pediatrics* 140.
49. Morris, S.J., Sebastian, S., Spencer, A.J., and Gilbert, S.C. (2016). Simian adenoviruses as vaccine vectors. *Future Virol* 11: 649–659.
50. Kostyanev, T.S. and Sechanova, L.P. (2012). Virulence factors and mechanisms of antibiotic resistance of *Haemophilus influenzae*. *Folia Med (Plovdiv)* 54: 19–23.
51. Giersing, B.K., Modjarrad, K., Kaslow, D.C., and Moorthy, V.S. (2016). Report from the World Health Organization's product development for vaccines advisory committee (PDVAC) meeting, Geneva, 7-9th Sep 2015. *Vaccine* 34: 2865–2869.
52. Madhi, S.A., Koen, A., Cutland, C.L. et al. (2017). Antibody kinetics and response to routine vaccinations in infants born to women who received an investigational trivalent group B streptococcus polysaccharide CRM197-conjugate vaccine during pregnancy. *Clin Infect Dis* 65: 1897–1904.
53. Rodriguez-Del Rio, E., Marradi, M., Calderon-Gonzalez, R. et al. (2015). A gold glyco-nanoparticle carrying a Listeriolysin O peptide and formulated with Advax delta inulin adjuvant induces robust T-cell protection against listeria infection. *Vaccine* 33: 1465–1473.

31

Pyogenic Infections of the CNS 2: (Brain Abscess, Subdural Abscess or Empyema, Epidural Abscess, Septic Embolism, and Suppurative Intracranial Phlebitis)

Arnault Tauziede-Espariat[1,2], Alexandre Roux[2,3,4], Megan Still[3,5], Marc Zanello[2,3,4], Gilles Zah-Bi[3], Ghazi Hmeydia[1], Catherine Oppenheim[2,4,6], Michel Wolff[7,8], Johan Pallud[2,3,4], and Fabrice Chrétien[1,2,9]

[1] Department of Neuropathology, Sainte Anne Hospital, Paris, France
[2] Paris University, Paris, France
[3] Department of Neurosurgery, Sainte-Anne Hospital, Paris, France
[4] Inserm U894, IMA-Brain, Psychiatry and Neurosciences Center, Paris, France
[5] University of Texas Southwestern Medical Center, Dallas, TX, USA
[6] Department of Neuroradiology, Sainte-Anne Hospital, Paris, France
[7] Department of Anesthesiology and Neurological Intensive Care, Sainte Anne Hospital, Paris, France
[8] Department of Intensive Care Medicine and Infectious Diseases, Bichat-Claude-Bernard Hospital, APHP, Paris, France
[9] Experimental Neuropathology Unit, Pasteur Institute, Paris, France

Abbreviations

BBB   blood-brain barrier
CNS   central nervous system
CSF   cerebrospinal fluid
CT scan   computed tomography scan
FLAIR   fluid attenuated inversion recovery
IE   infective endocarditis
MA   mycotic aneurysm
MRI   magnetic resonance imaging
PMNLs   polymorphonuclear leukocytes

Infections of the Central Nervous System: Pathology and Genetics, First Edition. Edited by Fabrice Chrétien, Kum Thong Wong, Leroy R. Sharer, Catherine (Katy) Keohane and Françoise Gray.
© 2020 John Wiley & Sons Ltd. Published 2020 by John Wiley & Sons Ltd.

Introduction

The brain and spinal cord are remarkably resistant to infection caused by bacterial pathogens. This is because of the combined protective effects of the skull and vertebral column, the meninges, the dura, the brain's abundant blood supply, and the blood-brain barrier (BBB) (cf. Chapter 29). However, the CNS differs from other anatomical sites in that, once infection has been initiated, host defense mechanisms are inadequate to prevent replication of the pathogens and progression of disease. In the last few decades, the marked increase in immunodeficiencies along with developments in modern medical practice have resulted in increased susceptibility of patients who are hospitalized to bacterial infections, including those of the CNS. This may account for their continuing high morbidity and mortality rates, despite advances in diagnostic techniques and therapy. Moreover, post-operative complications have been observed with increasing frequency (see Chapter 32).

Acute meningitis represents the most frequent and life-threatening CNS bacterial infection (see Chapters 29 and 30), but other frequently encountered or challenging infections include brain abscess, epidural abscess, subdural abscess or empyema, septic embolism, and suppurative intracranial phlebitis.

The pathogenesis of brain abscesses, epidural abscess, and subdural abscess or empyema have been described in Chapter 29. In this chapter, we describe their clinicopathological features and those of septic embolism and suppurative intracranial phlebitis.

Brain abscesses

Definition

An abscess is a focal suppurative parenchymal infection, which when formed, has a surrounding granulation tissue capsule. There are two stages in its formation: (i) during the first two weeks there is poorly demarcated focal cerebritis with acute inflammatory changes such as vascular congestion and localized edema; and (ii) later, an abscess cavity with a distinct capsule forms, which occurs after the necrosis and liquefaction processes [1]. Intracranial abscesses require prompt recognition and treatment to avoid high mortality rates (10%) and poor neurological outcomes [2].

The epidemiology, microbiology, pathogenesis, clinical features, diagnostic approach, and treatment of community-acquired brain abscesses were described in Chapter 4.

Pathology

The topography of abscesses depends on their etiology. Abscesses resulting from direct spread from an adjacent suppurative focus such as otitis media or mastoiditis are usually in the temporal lobe or cerebellum or in the frontal lobe following sinusitis (Figure 31.1a). Abscesses of hematogenous origin are often multiple and are frequently located in the territory of the middle cerebral artery. They are secondary to septic emboli from bacterial endocarditis or chronic suppurative intrathoracic infection. Paradoxical cerebral septic emboli may occur in congenital cyanotic heart disease. Post-traumatic abscesses develop at sites of craniocerebral wounds or neurosurgery. These abscesses tend to occur at gray and white matter junctions and within the white matter.

In animal models, bacterial brain abscesses go through five stages in their development; these correlate well with the evolution of brain abscess in man [3–5].

- The initial stage of focal cerebritis (days 1–3 after inoculation) appears macroscopically as an ill-defined region of hyperemia surrounded by edema. Microscopically, there is early parenchymal necrosis with vascular congestion, petechial hemorrhage, microthrombosis, perivascular fibrinous exudate, and infiltration by polymorponuclear leukocytes (PMNLs). Surrounding edema is invariable and adds to the mass effect of the abscess.
- Late cerebritis (days 4–9) is characterized by a necrotic purulent center resulting from confluence of adjacent necrotic foci. The pus is surrounded by a narrow irregular layer of inflammatory granulation tissue infiltrated by PMNLs, lymphocytes, and some macrophages (Figure 31.1b). Perivascular spaces in the vicinity are cuffed with PMNLs and lymphocytes.
- The early abscess capsule develops at days 10–13 and is made up of granulation tissue, which

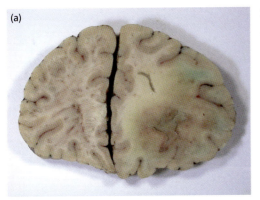

Figure 31.1 Recent right frontal abscess secondary to sinusitis. (a) Macroscopic appearance: Focal necrotic lesion containing pus in its center in the white matter of the right frontal lobe, at the gray and white matter junction, surrounded by congestion. Note marked edema with light green tint of the cerebral hemisphere. (b) Microscopic appearance: Necrotic center on the left, surrounded by inflammatory granulation tissue (on the right) infiltrated by polymorphonuclear leukocytes (PMNLs), lymphocytes, and some macrophages (hematoxylin and eosin [H&E]).

includes lymphocytes, plasma cells, monocytes and macrophages, numerous newly formed blood vessels, and scattered fibroblasts. The developing capsule is at first poorly defined; it is thickest on its cortical surface and often very thin or deficient on its ventricular surface. For this reason, abscesses tend to expand inward and rupture into the ventricular system, resulting in purulent ependymitis, pyoventricle, or pyocephalus. Purulent leptomeningitis resulting from abscess extension onto the cortical surface is less common.

- As time passes (day 14 and later), the capsule becomes firmer and can be stripped easily from the surrounding edematous white matter. Microscopically, more fibroblasts appear, so that a well-encapsulated abscess consists of five layers [6]: (Figure 31.2a).
- (i) The central portion is pus (Figure 31.2b) forming an eosinophilic area with PMNLs in different stages of disintegration and necrotic tissue with debris and macrophages. The pus may contain clusters of bacteria, (if Gram-positive they suggest *Staphylococcus* species) (Figure 31.3a and b) or chains of Gram-positive cocci (suggestive of *Streptococcus* species) (Figure 31.3c).
- A surrounding rim of granulation tissue has two layers: (ii) Granulation tissue with proliferating fibroblasts and capillaries, and long radially oriented blood vessels and (iii) a zone of lymphocytes and plasma cells in granulomatous tissue.
- (iv) A dense fibrous peripheral "capsule" with embedded astrocytes (Figure 31.2c). Fibrosis with collagen formation is unusual within the CNS, but brain abscess is an important exception.
- (v) A surrounding edematous zone. This edema is often widespread, giving the white matter a delicate light green tint (Figure 31.1). Microscopically, there is chronic edema with cavitation and myelin pallor, reactive gemistocytic astrocytes (Figure 31.3d) and diffuse inflammatory cells.

The two most serious complications of brain abscesses are raised intracranial pressure with the risk of cerebral herniation and rupture into a ventricle, resulting in ventricular empyema. Cortical thrombophlebitis, tension pneumocephalus, and noncommunicating hydrocephalus may also occur.

Subdural empyema

Definition

A subdural empyema is a spinal or intracranial collection of pus in the virtual space between the dura mater and the arachnoid membrane. Subdural space infection may occasionally be localized by adhesions forming an abscess, but the wide extent of this potential space and the relative avascularity of its walls are such that pus, once formed, normally spreads too rapidly for effective adhesions to

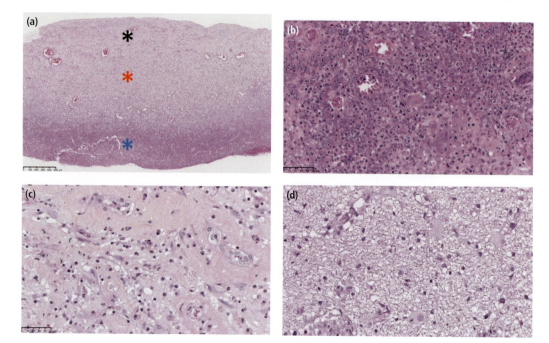

Figure 31.2 Histopathologic features of a formed brain abscess. (a) Low magnification showing different parts of the abscess: the central portion (pus formation, blue asterisk), the peripheral portion (granulation tissue, red asterisk), and an outer zone (the adjacent brain parenchyma, black asterisk) (hematoxylin phloxin safran [HPS]). (b) Central portion with numerous polymorphonuclear leukocytes (PMNLs) and tissue debris (HPS). (c) Surrounding inflammatory granulation tissue with vascular and fibroblastic proliferation and more chronic inflammatory cells (HPS). (d) Outer zone of gliosis with reactive astrocytes and edema (HPS).

develop. It is then a subdural empyema. This rare condition is a neurosurgical emergency and can result in life-threatening complications such as thrombophlebitis, edema, or infarction [7–9].

Epidemiology

Subdural empyema is less common than brain abscess and accounts for approximately 20% of all intracranial infections. Although all ages are affected, 76% of cases occur in the second and third decades. There is a male preponderance, the male-to-female ratio is 4:1 [10].

Pathogenesis

Subdural empyemas are mainly intracranial. Infection most often extends from adjacent sinusitis, otitis, or osteomyelitis, or in infants from purulent leptomeningitis. Spinal examples are rare and are usually the result of spread from infected cerebrospinal fluid (CSF) following spinal surgery or local intervention (cf. Chapter 32).

Microbiology

The organisms causing subdural empyema closely mirror those causing brain abscesses although, unlike brain abscess, the majority of infections are monomicrobial. *Streptococci* (i.e. aerobic, anaerobic, and microaerophilic) are the predominant pathogens, being isolated from 50 to 75% of patients. The organisms in infants are the same as those causing leptomeningitis. In approximately one-third of cases, no pathogens are isolated, either because patients were receiving antibiotics when the specimens were obtained or due to suboptimal culture techniques [10].

Clinical features

Acute subdural empyema has been described as the most imperative surgical emergency and its course is rapid and fulminating. The presenting clinical features of cranial subdural empyema are varied and nonspecific; the most common are headache, fever, meningism, nausea or vomiting, impaired

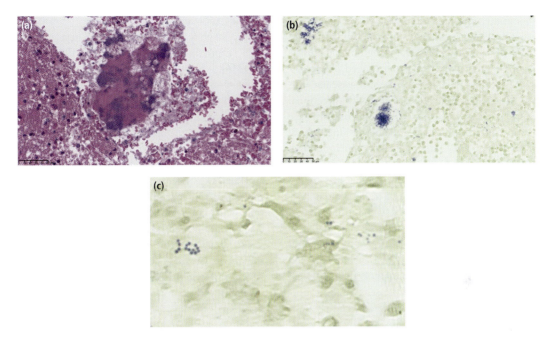

Figure 31.3 Microscopic appearance of microorganisms which may be seen within brain abscesses. (a) Cluster of bacterial elements (hematoxylin phloxin safran [HPS]). (b) Gram-positive bacilli single and grouped in clusters corresponding to *Corynebacterium* species proved by bacteriological studies (Gram). (c) Gram-positive cocci grouped in clusters corresponding to *Staphylococcus* species (Gram).

consciousness, focal neurological deficits (i.e. including hemiparesis, hemiplegia, and dysphasia), and focal or generalized seizures [2, 10, 11, 12]. Because of the rapid course, papilledema develops in <50% of patients. Concurrent sinusitis or otitis media have been reported in 60–90% of cases.

Infants develop high fever, seizures, vomiting, lethargy, irritability, bulging fontanelle, neck stiffness, and coma.

CSF analysis is not helpful in establishing the diagnosis and lumbar puncture is contraindicated, particularly in patients with increased intracranial pressure. magnetic resonance imaging (MRI) with contrast enhancement is the diagnostic procedure of choice [2, 9, 10].

Pathology

In most cases, the subdural infection tends to spread over the cerebral convexities but is prevented from crossing the midline by the falx. Empyema is less common in the posterior fossa and rare in the spinal canal. As there is virtually no capillary bed in the arachnoid, pus in the subdural space produces inflammation and granulation tissue in the subarachnoid space where capillaries are numerous. In chronic infections, adhesions develop, which pass through the pia-arachnoid to the cortical surface, and occasionally small perforating arteries undergo thrombosis to produce small cortical infarcts [10].

Epidural abscess

An epidural abscess is a circumscribed collection of pus in the cranial epidural space between the calvaria and the dura mater or in the spinal epidural space between the vertebra and the dura mater [13].

Intracranial epidural abscess

Localized infection of the intracranial epidural space is rare. It usually spreads from a frontal sinus or mastoid infection, often accompanied by focal osteomyelitis. Invasion through the cranial dura along emissary veins may lead to associated subdural empyema. An epidural abscess may follow neurosurgery, and a history of trauma is found in 15–35% of cases. Intracranial epidural abscess is more frequent in young patients aged between 7 and 20 years. They are likely to have vascular diploic bone, which increases valveless bidirectional flow between the frontal sinus mucosa and the dural veins emptying into the superior longitudinal sinus [14]. They are frequently polymicrobial including anaerobic cocci, *Staphylococcus* and *Streptococcus* spp.

The strong adhesion of dura to the cranial periosteum confines the infection, which usually takes the form of a small, flattened abscess. The CSF is usually normal. Radiology shows an extracerebral biconvex collection (Figure 32.3), which may be adjacent to an infected sinus or neurosurgical focus. The inflammatory response is similar to spinal epidural abscess (see below); its composition depends on the age of the lesion. Characteristically, the underlying brain parenchyma is not involved.

Spinal epidural (extradural) abscess
Epidemiology
The incidence of spinal epidural abscesses has increased in the last decades accounting for 2.5–3 cases per 10 000 hospital admissions [15], likely due to an aging population in developed countries with increasing numbers of patients at risk. Although all ages are affected, it is rare in infants and young children; the mean age is 50–60 years with a male predominance.

Etiology
Spinal epidural abscesses almost always originate from foci of infection elsewhere in the body (most commonly from the skin and soft tissue) and spread to the epidural space via the bloodstream or lymphatics. Direct spread also occurs from a contiguous focus of infection, such as vertebral osteomyelitis, perinephric, retropharyngeal, or psoas abscesses, decubitus ulcers, or persistent or congenital dermal sinus. Iatrogenic inoculation following penetrating injury, lumbar puncture, spinal surgery, epidural anesthesia, or use of epidural catheters may account for 15% of cases [15].

The responsible organisms are those that caused the primary infection, predominantly *Staphylococcus aureus* (60–90% of infections), *streptococci* (approximately 20%), aerobic Gram-negative bacteria (approximately 15%), and anaerobes (up to 7%) [16].

Clinical features and diagnosis
The symptoms of spinal epidural abscesses and subdural empyema appear in the following order: (i) back pain at the level of the affected spine (more painful in spinal epidural abscesses); (ii) pain radiating in the distribution of the regional spinal nerve roots; (iii) spinal cord or cauda equina compression with motor weakness, sensory deficits, and bladder and bowel dysfunction; and (iv) paralysis progressing to paraplegia after prolonged or major spinal cord or cauda equina compression [13, 16]. Fever is present in 50% of patients [13]. The classic triad of fever, axial pain, and neurological deficits occurs in less than 15% of patients [13, 17].

Rapid diagnosis and treatment are of utmost importance in minimizing neurological sequelae. The most important prognostic parameter is the patient's neurological status immediately before surgery [16]. The likelihood of complete recovery is high if intervention precedes significant neurological deficit, but the prognosis worsens rapidly once weakness develops. There is little likelihood of full recovery if surgery for decompression and drainage is delayed by more than 24 hours after the onset of paralysis, and no chance if the delay is more than 48 hours. The abscess site is also important; a noncervical location has a better prognosis. Mortality is approximately 5% with a range of 2–20% [16] mostly because of sepsis, meningitis, or other underlying disorder [13]. Patients with concomitant sepsis have a particularly poor prognosis.

Pathogens may be isolated from blood cultures in approximately 60% of cases. CSF analysis is of limited value and lumbar puncture is not recommended because it may induce meningitis or subdural empyema. Spinal MRI has a high degree of sensitivity and is the diagnostic tool of choice [13].

Pathology
Due to the lack of resistance to longitudinal spread of infection through the epidural space, several vertebral segments (average 3–6) are affected,

although the entire length of the spinal cord can be involved; whether the abscess is localized or diffuse depends on the development of fibrous adhesions. The abscess is thoracic in 50–80% of cases, lumbar in 17–38%, and cervical in 10–25%; in children, infection usually affects the cervical and lumbar regions. Abscesses are located posterior to the cord in more than 70% of patients but may also be anterior or circumferential. Perhaps because of the small volume of the lateral extradural space, most abscesses are dorsal or dorsolateral [10].

Acute abscesses consist of granulation tissue containing pus that is loculated or collected in a number of communicating pockets, whereas chronic abscesses consist of both granulation and fibrous tissue. As the abscess enlarges, it may compress the spinal cord. Thrombosis of spinal blood vessels may ensue, particularly in one of the radicular arteries, leading to spinal cord infarction and permanent paraplegia. Subacute and chronic infections produce widespread inflammation, with granulation tissue involving the dura extending over many spinal segments. The infection may be so protracted before it compresses the cord that the original focus is no longer obvious [10].

The resistance of the dura mater to infection usually limits the inflammation to the epidural space. Occasionally, infection spreads within the dural layers, causing pachymeningitis, which may subsequently spread into the subdural space [10].

Septic embolism and mycotic aneurysm

Septic emboli are made up of infected matter that travels in the bloodstream, arising from a distal site of infection and usually caused by pyogenic bacteria. They are most commonly associated with infective endocarditis (IE) [18, 19].

Septic emboli may cause multiple cerebral infarcts, hemorrhages, and abscesses. The neuroimaging findings reflect this heterogeneity. On computed tomography (CT) scan, loss of gray–white differentiation or hypoattenuation correspond to acute strokes. MRI may reveal multifocal fluid attenuated inversion recovery (FLAIR) signal hyperintensity areas or restricted diffusion at the gray-white interface. These abnormalities are often concomitant with small areas of abnormal susceptibility on gradient-echo images. Contrast-enhanced images reveal multiple peripheral-enhancing lesions at the gray and white interface. In early disease, this pattern can be absent. Multifocal subarachnoid hemorrhages of the cerebral convexities can also occur, with peripheral hyperdensity within the cerebral sulci on CT scan or subarachnoid space FLAIR signal hyperintensity on MRI [18, 19].

Implantation of a septic embolus in a cerebral artery may result in a mycotic aneurysm (MA) because of local infection and weakening of the arterial wall. Despite the name, MAs are usually the result of pyogenic bacteria rather than to fungi. *Streptococci* and *staphylococci* account for the majority of bacteria that cause intracranial MAs, similar to IE. MAs complicating IE may occur anywhere in any artery. They tend to be small, either saccular or fusiform, and characteristically develop at cerebral arterial peripheral bifurcations or branching points, most frequently the middle cerebral artery. On histology, there is destruction of the arterial wall architecture, focal necrosis, and infiltration by inflammatory cells (PMNLs in acute lesions, and mixed PMNLs, lymphocytes, and plasma cells in fibroblastic granulation tissue in chronic lesions). Adhesions may form between the arachnoid and the brain parenchyma in proximity to the aneurysm [10]. Rupture of a mycotic aneurysm causes hemorrhage into the brain or subarachnoid space.

MAs are often clinically silent. Neurological warning signs, including focal deficits, seizures, cranial nerve abnormalities, and severe, unremitting localized headache in patients with IE, may precede rupture by several days but can also be present in patients with IE without MAs. Nonetheless, these symptoms should prompt further investigation. MA rupture usually presents as a sudden, often fatal, subarachnoid or intracerebral hemorrhage with sudden onset of severe headache and rapid deterioration in the level of consciousness. Other patients present with infarction or hemorrhagic transformation of an embolic stroke. Some patients may not exhibit symptoms at any stage, or only after initiation or completion of antibiotic therapy for IE.

Diagnosis of MA is best established by MRI combined with magnetic resonance angiography (MRA), especially when there is no bleeding. CT scan, with or without contrast enhancement, is not sufficiently sensitive to detect MA (although MA is unlikely if the CT scan is normal) but is the optimal diagnostic procedure when subarachnoid or intracerebral hemorrhage is suspected. Once hemorrhage is confirmed, conventional angiography is the method of choice to outline the aneurysm and its relationship to the parent vessel prior to surgery [10].

Treatment includes primary prevention of embolization and prevention of further episodes, optimal treatment for existing lesions, and detection of secondary complications. Arterial blood pressure should be controlled and supportive care provided. Close clinical monitoring is mandatory to detect secondary hemorrhages. If the patient's condition worsens, repeat CT scan should be performed promptly. Quick initiation of antibiotic treatment has an impact on the incidence of stroke in septic emboli. Thrombolysis and other antithrombotic therapies are not recommended for embolic strokes in patients with IE because of the high risk of intracranial hemorrhage [20].

Suppurative intracranial phlebitis

Suppurative intracranial phlebitis occurs from thrombosis of a cerebral vein due to infection, mostly following infection of paranasal sinuses, middle ear, mastoid, face, or oropharynx. The infection spreads centrally along the emissary vein. Septic thrombophlebitis may also occur in association with epidural abscess, subdural empyema, or meningitis. Any dural venous sinus can be affected; the most common are the cavernous, lateral, or superior sagittal sinuses [21, 22].

Septic intracranial phlebitis may cause hemorrhagic infarction, and local suppuration may produce venous hemorrhage, venous necrosis, epidural abscess, subdural empyema, meningitis, and brain abscess.

The clinical manifestations depend on the primary infection site. For example, when a venous sinus is involved, adjacent anatomic structures may be affected because of their proximity to the affected sinus [23–26]. These are summarized in Table 31.1. The most common symptoms are fever and headache, but altered mental status and focal neurological deficits related to a venous system are also frequent. Seizures occur in up to 20% of cases [22].

- Cavernous sinus phlebitis can induce fever (>90%), periorbital edema (73%), changes in mental status (55%), headache (52%), meningism (40%), diplopia, eye tearing, photophobia, ptosis, proptosis, chemosis, weakness of extraocular eye muscles, papilledema (65%), cranial nerve palsies (cranial nerves II, III, IV, VI, and maxillary branches of V), or cortical vein thrombophlebitis [23–26].
- Lateral sinus phlebitis can induce headache (>80%), fever (79%), abnormal ear findings (98%), photophobia, vomiting, vertigo, cranial nerve VI palsy, facial pain or altered sensation, papilledema, mastoid tenderness, nuchal rigidity, Griesinger sign (posterior auricular swelling and pain), or otitic hydrocephalus [23–26].
- Superior sagittal sinus phlebitis can induce altered mental status, motor deficits, nuchal rigidity, papilledema, or seizures (>50%) [23–26].
- Inferior petrosal sinus phlebitis can induce ipsilateral facial pain and lateral rectus muscle involvement [23–26]

Laboratory investigations may be non-specific. Sometimes, septic thrombosis of the superior sagittal sinus leads to frank meningitis, and blood cultures may be positive. Radiologic imaging is mandatory. MRI, with MR angiogram and venogram, has become the imaging modality of choice. Radiologic signs include a hyperdense venous sinus on CT, abnormal flow voids on MRI, absence of the normal flow-related signal on MR venogram, and filling defects on contrast-enhanced CT venography or MR venogram. An expanded contour of the cavernous sinus is a classical finding [27]. Radiological signs can be subtle in cases of incomplete thrombosis or following partial recanalization. Secondary complications of venous hypertension and venous infarction may be visible on CT or MRI as vasogenic edema, parenchymal hemorrhages, ischemic or hemorrhagic infarcts, or sometimes as isolated subarachnoid hemorrhage

Table 31.1 Suppurative intracranial phlebitis: major sites and related clinical manifestations.

Dural Venous Sinus Involved	Predisposing Infection	Clinical Presentation	Miscellaneous
Cavernous sinus	1/ Sphenoid and ethmoid sinusitis 2/ Facial infections 3/ Middle ear infections 4/ Dental infection 5/ Mastoiditis	Fever Periorbital edema Change in mental status Headache Meningism Diplopia, eye tearing, photophobia, ptosis, proptosis, chemosis, weakness of extraocular eye muscles, papilledema Cranial nerve palsies (cranial nerves II, III, IV, VI, and maxillary branches of V) Cortical vein thrombophlebitis	1/ Usually acute 2/ Most common site of suppurative phlebitis – 30% mortality – Less than 50% full recovery
Superior sagittal sinus	1/ Bacterial meningitis 2/ Frontal and maxillary sinusitis 3/ Subdural or epidural empyema	Altered mental status Motor deficits Nuchal rigidity Papilledema Seizures	1/ Largest venous sinus 2/ High mortality
Lateral sinuses	Acute or chronic otitis media Mastoiditis Pharyngitis	Headache Fever Abnormal ear findings Photophobia, vomiting, vertigo Cranial nerve VI palsy Facial pain/altered sensation Papilledema Mastoid tenderness Nuchal rigidity Griesinger sign (posterior auricular swelling and pain) Otitic hydrocephalus	1/ Subacute presentation 2/ Less than 5% mortality

located at the convexity. Multiple infarcts or hemorrhages in a nonarterial distribution are suggestive of the diagnosis. Unlike the restricted diffusion in arterial infarcts, in venous infarcts the findings on diffusion-weighted imaging are variable. Cortical vein thrombosis demonstrates the "cord sign" wherein the thrombosed vein appears as a hyperdense serpiginous cortical structure [28].

Suppurative intracranial thrombophlebitis necessitates appropriate high-dose antibiotics with good BBB penetration. Sinus drainage or surgical evacuation of subdural collections are often required. Antimicrobial therapy is continued usually for at least three to four weeks. Complementary treatment with anticoagulants remains controversial [29, 30].

References

1. Brouwer, M.C., Tunkel, A.R., and van de Beek, D. (2014). Brain abscess. *N Engl J Med* 371: 1758.
2. Brouwer, M.C., Coutinho, J.M., and van de Beek, D. (2014). Clinical characteristics and outcome of brain abscess: systematic review and meta-analysis. *Neurology* 82: 806–813.
3. Britt, R.H. and Enzmann, D.R. (1983). Clinical stages of human brain abscesses on serial CT scans after contrast infusion. *J Neurosurg* 59: 972–989.
4. Britt, R.H., Enzmann, D.R., and Yeager, A.S. (1981). Neuropathological and computerized tomographic findings in experimental brain abscess. *J Neurosurg* 55: 590–603.
5. Chrétien, F., Jouvion, G., Wong, K.T., and Sharer, L.R. (2018). Infections of the central nervous system.

In: *Escourolle & Poirier's Manual of Basic Neuropathology*, 6e (eds. F. Gray, C. Duyckaerts and U. DeGirolami), 114–138. Oxford University Pres.
6. Weller, R.O. and Steart, P. (1984). Cytology of cerebral abscesses. An immunocytochemical and ultrastructural study. *Neuropathol Appl Neurobiol* 10: 305–306.
7. Bartt, R.E. (2010). Cranial epidural abscess and subdural empyema. *Handb Clin Neurol* 96: 75–89.
8. De Bonis, P., Anile, C., Pompucci, A. et al. (2009). Cranial and spinal subdural empyema. *Br J Neurosurg* 23: 335–340.
9. Greenlee, J.E. (2003). Subdural empyema. *Curr Treat Options Neurol* 5: 13–22.
10. Brown, E. and Gray, F. (2008). Bacterial infections. In: *Greenfield's Neuropathology*, 8e, vol. 2 (eds. S. Love, D. Louis and D. Ellison), 1391–1445. London: Hodder Arnold.
11. Roche, M., Humphreys, H., Smyth, E. et al. (2003). A twelve-year review of central nervous system bacterial abscesses; presentation and aetiology. *Clin Microbiol Infect* 9: 803–809.
12. Kombogiorgas, D., Seth, R., Athwal, R. et al. (2007). Suppurative intracranial complications of sinusitis in adolescence. Single institute experience and review of literature. *Br J Neurosurg* 21: 603–609.
13. Darouiche, R.O. (2006). Spinal epidural abscess. *N Engl J Med* 355: 2012–2020.
14. Pradilla, G., Ardila, G.P., Hsu, W., and Rigamonti, D. (2009). Epidural abscess of the CNS. *Lancet Neurol* 8: 292–300.
15. Sendi, P., Bregenzer, T., and Zimmerli, W. (2008). Spinal epidural abscess in clinical practice. *QJM* 101: 1–12.
16. Darouiche, R.O. (2010). Spinal epidural abscess and subdural empyema. *Handb Clin Neurol* 96: 91–99.
17. DeFroda, S.F., DePasse, J.M., Eltorai, A.E.M. et al. (2016). Evaluation and management of spinal epidural abscess. *J Hosp Med* 11: 130–135.
18. Murdoch, D.R., Corey, G.R., Hoen, B. et al. (2009). Clinical presentation, etiology, and outcome of infective endocarditis in the 21st century: the international collaboration on endocarditis-prospective cohort study. *Arch Intern Med* 169: 463–473.
19. Pujadas Capmany, R., Arboix, A., Casañas-Muñoz, R., and Anguera-Ferrando, N. (2004). Specific cardiac disorders in 402 consecutive patients with ischaemic cardioembolic stroke. *Int J Cardiol* 95: 129–134.
20. Bhuva, P., Kuo, S.-H., Claude Hemphill, J., and Lopez, G.A. (2010). Intracranial hemorrhage following thrombolytic use for stroke caused by infective endocarditis. *Neurocrit Care* 12: 79–82.
21. Kojan, S. and Al-Jumah, M. (2006). Infection related cerebral venous thrombosis. *J Pak Med Assoc* 56: 494–497.
22. Osborn, M.K. and Steinberg, J.P. (2007). Subdural empyema and other suppurative complications of paranasal sinusitis. *Lancet Infect Dis* 7: 62–67.
23. Southwick, F.S., Richardson, E.P., and Swartz, M.N. (1986). Septic thrombosis of the dural venous sinuses. *Medicine (Baltimore)* 65: 82–106.
24. Tovi, F. and Hirsch, M. (1991). Posttraumatic septic superior sagittal sinus thrombosis: report of a case. *J Oral Maxillofac Surg* 49: 303–305.
25. Au, J.K., Adam, S.I., and Michaelides, E.M. (2013). Contemporary management of pediatric lateral sinus thrombosis: a twenty year review. *Am J Otolaryngol* 34: 145–150.
26. Khatri, I.A. and Wasay, M. (2016). Septic cerebral venous sinus thrombosis. *J Neurol Sci* 362: 221–227.
27. Lee, J.H., Lee, H.K., Park, J.K. et al. (2003). Cavernous sinus syndrome: clinical features and differential diagnosis with MR imaging. *Am J Roentgenol* 181: 583–590.
28. Scheld, W.M., Whitley, R.J., Marra, C.M. et al. (2014). *Infections of the Central Nervous System*, 928 p, 4e. Philadelphia: LWW.
29. Bhatia, K. and Jones, N.S. (2002). Septic cavernous sinus thrombosis secondary to sinusitis: are anticoagulants indicated? A review of the literature. *J Laryngol Otol* 116: 667–676.
30. Saposnik, G., Barinagarrementeria, F., Brown, R.D. et al. (2011). Diagnosis and management of cerebral venous thrombosis: a statement for healthcare professionals from the American Heart Association/American Stroke Association. *Stroke* 42: 1158–1192.

32

Pyogenic Infections of the CNS 3: Following Neurosurgical Procedures

Alexandre Roux[1,2,4]**, Megan Still**[1,3]**, Marc Zanello**[1,2,4]**, Gilles Zah-Bi**[1]**, Arnault Tauziede-Espariat**[4,5]**, Ghazi Hmeydia**[5]**, Catherine Oppenheim**[2,4,6]**, Michel Wolff**[7,8]**, Fabrice Chrétien**[4,5,9]**, and Johan Pallud**[1,2,4]

[1] Department of Neurosurgery, Sainte-Anne Hospital, Paris, France
[2] Inserm U894, IMA-Brain, Psychiatry and Neurosciences Center, Paris, France
[3] University of Texas Southwestern Medical Center, Dallas, TX, USA
[4] Paris University, Paris, France
[5] Department of Neuropathology, Sainte-Anne Hospital, Paris, France
[6] Department of Neuroradiology, Sainte-Anne Hospital, Paris, France
[7] Department of Anesthesiology and Neurological Intensive Care, Sainte Anne Hospital, Paris, France
[8] Department of Intensive Care Medicine and Infectious Diseases, Bichat-Claude-Bernard Hospital, APHP, Paris, France
[9] Experimental Neuropathology Unit, Pasteur Institute, Paris, France

Abbreviations

CNS	central nervous system
CT	computed tomography
FLAIR	fluid attenuated inversion recovery
MRI	magnetic resonance imaging
SSI	surgical site infection

Introduction

Of all postoperative neurosurgical complications, surgical site infections (SSIs) are the most common, occurring in low- and high-risk patients undergoing craniotomy and spinal surgery [1–5]. SSIs lead to increased morbidity, mortality, cost,

Infections of the Central Nervous System: Pathology and Genetics, First Edition. Edited by Fabrice Chrétien, Kum Thong Wong, Leroy R. Sharer, Catherine (Katy) Keohane and Françoise Gray.
© 2020 John Wiley & Sons Ltd. Published 2020 by John Wiley & Sons Ltd.

Infections of the Central Nervous System

unplanned readmissions, reoperation, prolonged length of stay after neurological surgery, and decreased patient satisfaction. Early recognition and treatment are crucial to reduce adverse outcomes and long-term complications. This chapter describes the different types of intracranial and spinal infections following neurosurgical procedures, the differential diagnoses, clinical presentation, and treatment options.

Definitions

SSI is defined in neurosurgical practice as any bacterial infection occurring at a cranial or spinal surgical site. For cranial surgery, this encompasses wound infections with or without osteitis, meningitis, ventriculitis, extradural empyema, subdural empyema, brain abscess, and encephalitis. For spinal surgery this encompasses wound infections, subcutaneous abscess, meningitis, epidural abscess, subdural empyema, and spondylodiscitis.

Brain abscess

A brain abscess is a focal area of suppurative necrosis with a surrounding membrane within the brain parenchyma (Figure 32.1) (see Chapters 29 and 30). There are two stages in its formation: (i) in the first two weeks there is a poorly demarcated focal cerebritis, with acute inflammatory changes, vascular congestion and localized edema, (ii) following necrosis and liquefaction a distinct peripheral collagenous capsule is formed [6]. Postoperative intracranial abscesses require prompt recognition and treatment to avoid high mortality rates (15%) and poor neurological outcomes [7]. Carmustine wafer implantation may increase postoperative infections especially brain abscess, but the risk depends on the experience of centers using this device [8–11].

Subdural empyema

A subdural empyema is a spinal or intracranial collection of pus in the virtual space between the dura mater and the arachnoid membrane (Figure 32.2). This rare condition can result in life-threatening complications such as thrombophlebitis, edema, or infarction and is a neurosurgical emergency [12–14].

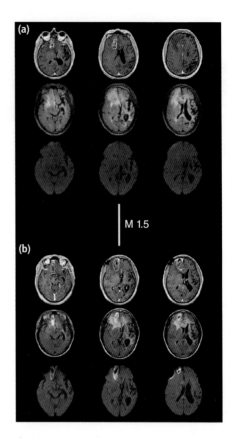

Figure 32.1 Brain abscess magnetic resonance imaging (MRI) appearance. (a) Spontaneous abscess: A 70-year-old man presented with headaches and behavior disorder. Brain MRI (contrast-enhanced T1-weighted images) (superior) demonstrated a right frontal enhancing mass with a central necrotic core and mass effect on the lateral ventricles. Fluid attenuated inversion recovery (FLAIR) images (middle) showed perilesional brain edema extending to the corpus callosum and periventricular spaces. Diffusion-weighted imaging (inferior) showed a high signal in the enhancing component and low signal in the necrotic core. Total surgical removal was performed. Postoperative course was unremarkable. (b) Postoperative abscess: Right frontal abscess developing six weeks after surgery and before standard chemoradiation protocol. The patient presented with headaches, drowsiness, fever, and had a generalized onset tonic-clonic epileptic seizure. New brain MRI (contrast-enhanced T1-weighted images) (superior) demonstrated a new right frontal enhancing mass in the surgical site and contrast-enhancement of the dura. FLAIR images (middle) showed perilesional brain edema involving the corpus callosum and periventricular spaces. Diffusion-weighted imaging (inferior) showed a high signal in the whole mass compatible with a postoperative brain abscess. The abscess was surgically evacuated and multiple organisms including *Staphylococcus aureus* were identified.

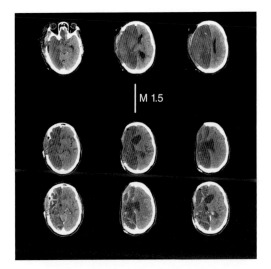

Figure 32.2 Subdural empyema magnetic resonance imaging (MRI) appearance. A 55-year-old man presented to the neurovascular unit with sudden left hemiplegia, hemineglect, and drowsiness. Internal carotid artery infarction was diagnosed on brain MRI. After medical management, a right decompressive hemicraniectomy with intracranial pressure monitoring was performed. Postoperative computed tomography (CT) scan (superior) showed massive brain herniation through the craniectomy site with no hemorrhagic complications. Six weeks later, the patient presented with a purulent wound infection. On repeat CT scan the noncontrast sequences (middle) showed an atrophic brain parenchyma with subdural collections. Contrast-enhanced sequences (inferior) showed bi-convex collection "pockets" with surrounding enhancing membranes. At a second surgical procedure the subdural empyema was evacuated. The responsible organism was *Propionibacterium acnes*.

Epidural abscess

An epidural abscess is a circumscribed collection of pus occurring in the cranial epidural space between the calvaria and the dura mater (Figure 32.3) or in the spinal epidural space between the vertebra and the dura mater [15] (Figure 32.4) (see Chapter 30).

Postoperative meningitis

Postoperative meningitis is an acute inflammation of the protective membranes covering the brain and spinal cord following a cranial or spinal intradural surgical procedure or incidental durotomy [16–18]. It is a severe complication with varying clinicopathological definitions and multiple pathogenic mechanisms [18]. Isolated postoperative meningitis should be differentiated from meningitis associated with implantable material, such as ventricular catheters [18] or carmustine wafers [11, 19–21].

Suppurative intracranial phlebitis

Suppurative intracranial phlebitis occurs from thrombosis of a cerebral vein resulting from infection. Any dural venous sinus can be involved but the cavernous sinus, lateral sinus, or superior sagittal sinus are most commonly affected [22, 23]. To date, only one published report described postoperative suppurative intracranial phlebitis. This was a cavernous sinus thrombosis and bacterial abscess due to multiple organisms (*Streptococcus* spp., coagulase-negative *Staphylococcus*, and *Haemophilus influenzae*), following transsphenoidal surgery for a pituitary macroadenoma [24]. The clinical features, diagnostic methods and treatment of suppurative intracranial phlebitis are described in Chapter 30.

Risk factors

The known risk factors for postoperative infections are detailed in Table 32.1. Several studies have identified risk factors for surgical site infections in neurosurgery [1, 2, 4, 5, 25–35]. These should be identified to avoid potentially devastating consequences of SSI and to plan preventive strategies. Many, such as gender, older age, ventilator dependence, preoperative steroid use, hyponatremia, anemia, and emergent (urgent) status are not easily modified and require improved perioperative anesthetic and surgical care [27, 36, 37]. Using evidence-based guidelines, up to 60% of SSIs are estimated to be preventable [36]. Perioperative antibiotic prophylaxis is considered as standard care in the management of patients undergoing cranial or spinal surgery and reduces the rate of SSI [38–40]. Carmustine wafer implantation should be reserved for centers specializing in neurosurgical oncology [8–11] because data vary regarding the associated infectious risk.

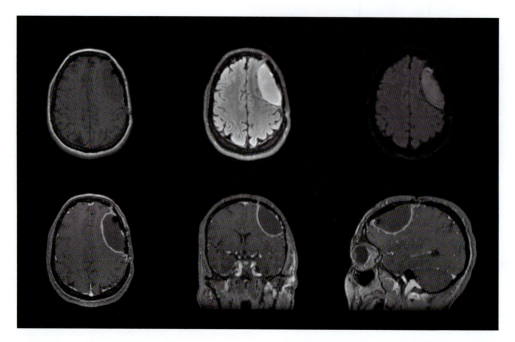

Figure 32.3 Cranial epidural abscess magnetic resonance (MR) appearance. A 43-year-old woman presented to the neurosurgical unit for headaches and asthenia five weeks after the surgical resection of a left frontal meningioma. Brain magnetic resonance imaging (MRI) was performed: the nonenhanced T1-weighted images (superior, left) demonstrated a biconvex hypointense collection, which was hyperintense in fluid attenuated inversion recovery (FLAIR) sequences (superior, middle). Diffusion-weighted imaging (superior, right) showed an elevated signal on the whole collection compatible with a postoperative epidural abscess. The contrast-enhanced T1-weighted images (inferior) showed ringlike enhancement of the collection. A new surgical procedure was performed consisting of the evacuation of the epidural abscess and the removal of the infected bone flap. The responsible organism was *Propionibacterium acnes*.

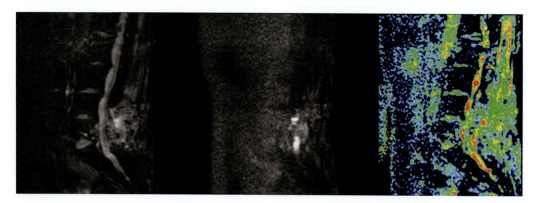

Figure 32.4 Spinal epidural abscess. A 51-year-old woman presented to the neurosurgical unit for low back pain, fever, and wound infection two weeks after a lumbar laminectomy and foraminotomy for L4-L5, L5-S1 spinal stenosis. A lumbar magnetic resonance imaging (MRI) was performed: the b0 (left) and the b1000 (middle) diffusion-weighted imaging sequences demonstrated a heterogeneous hyperintense collection through the surgical site, which reached the anterior epidural space. Apparent diffusion coefficient cartography (right) showed restriction on the whole collection compatible with a postoperative epidural abscess. A new surgical procedure was performed consisting of the evacuation of the whole collection of pus. The responsible organism was *Staphylococcus aureus*.

Table 32.1 Risk factors for postoperative surgical site infections for cranial and spinal procedures.

Parameters	References
Patient-related factors	
Male	31, 32
Older age	1, 5, 55, 56
BMI > 30 kg/m²	1, 34, 40, 46, 48, 51, 52, 54, 56
Diabetes	1, 5, 34, 35, 46, 48, 51, 54, 55, 56, 58
ASA Class 3–5	1, 29, 34, 48, 49, 56
Preoperative quality of wound	1, 32
External factors	
Current smoking status	1, 34, 46, 51, 56
Preoperative steroid use	1, 48, 59
Emergent case status	1, 5, 29
Absence of antibiotic prophylaxis	39, 59
Transfusion	34
Inpatient disposition	1, 2, 27, 29, 48,
Previous irradiation	29
Biological	
Anemia	1
Preoperative infection	27, 28, 34
Surgical	
Operative duration	1, 2, 25, 29, 31, 32, 46, 47, 48, 49, 51, 56
Surgical implants	5, 55, 60
Surgical drainage	29, 46
Duration of drainage	27
CSF drainage	33, 56, 58, 59, 60
CSF leak	27, 29, 31, 34, 35, 56, 60
Repeated surgery	29, 35, 51, 55, 60
Operating room personnel turnover	30
Carmustine wafer implantation	19, 61, 62

ASA, American Society of Anesthesiologists Physical Status score; BMI, body mass index; CSF, cerebrospinal fluid.

Epidemiology and microbiological characteristics

The epidemiology of SSIs in neurosurgery varies according to the type of procedure, with variable prevalence between cranial (1–8%) and spinal surgeries (0.5–18%) [1–5, 16, 19–21, 27, 31, 39–62]. The prevalence is detailed in Tables 32.2 and 32.3.

For cranial and spinal procedures, the most common reported organisms are *Staphylococcus aureus* and *Staphylococcus epidermidis* (approximately 50% of infections) [2–5, 16, 21, 27, 31, 39, 40, 42, 44, 49, 50, 53, 55–57]. The less virulent Gram-positive *Propionibacterium acnes* also plays a significant role in many series (approximately 25% of infections) and can be involved in long-delayed postoperative infections [4, 31, 39]. However, a large variety of organisms may be responsible, including Gram-negative organisms (*Acinetobacter baumannii, Pseudomonas, Enterobacter, Klebsiella pneumoniae,* and *Escherichia coli*) and rare Gram-positive organisms (*Micrococcus, Enterococcus faecium*) (Table 32.2 and 32.3). Additionally, multiple organisms may be found concomitantly in a single infection site, complicating the interpretation of results and therapeutic management [4].

Clinical features

Presenting symptoms

The presenting symptoms depend on the nature of the underlying infectious pathology (see Chapter 31) and of the offending pathogen.

Presenting symptoms of brain abscesses, cranial subdural empyema, cranial epidural abscesses, and postoperative meningitis are heterogeneous, non-specific, and do not depend on the presence of implantable material. The most common clinical feature is headache, found in about 70% of cases [7], followed by fever, focal neurological deficits, seizures, and disorders of higher neurological and cognitive function [7, 63]. The classic triad of fever, headache, and neurological deficit is found in only 20% of cases [7]. Fever and decreased level of consciousness are the most consistent signs for isolated postoperative meningitis [18]. Lethargy, nuchal rigidity, nausea, vomiting, and new-onset epileptic seizures also often accompany the development of brain abscesses, cranial subdural empyema, postoperative meningitis, and to a lesser degree, cranial epidural abscesses [7, 18, 64].

The symptoms of spinal epidural abscesses and subdural empyema include: back pain at the level

Table 32.2 Characteristics of surgical site infections after cranial surgery.

Studies, Year	Study design	Country	Patients (n)	Surgical site infection rate	First offending organism	Second offending organism
Savin et al. [60]	Unicenter retrospective study	RUS	2286	n = 216–9.4%	n/a	n/a
Chen et al.[a] [59]	Unicenter retrospective study	CHI	1016	n = 84–8.27%	n/a	n/a
Karhade et al. [1]	Multicenter prospective study	USA	132.063	n = 2377–1.8%	n/a	n/a
Lieber et al. [41]	Multicenter prospective study	USA	8215	n = 158–1.92%	n/a	n/a
Cassir et al. [27]	Unicenter prospective study	FR	526	n = 25–4.7%	Staphylococcus aureus n = 6–24.0%	Propionibacterium acnes n = 4–16.0%
Zhan et al. [42]	Unicenter retrospective study	CHI	1470	n = 109–7.4%	Staphylococcus aureus n = 13–11.9%	Acinetobacter baumannii n = 4–3.7%
Chen et al.[a] [58]	Unicenter retrospective study	CHI	775	n = 65–8.4%	Acinetobacter baumannii n = 2–3.0%	Klebsiella n = 1–1.5%
Abu Hamdeh et al. [2]	Unicenter retrospective study	SWE	448	n = 23–5.1%	Staphylococcus epidermidis n = 8–34.8%	Propionibacterium acnes n = 6–26.1%
O'Keeffe et al. [3]	Unicenter retrospective study	UK	245	n = 20–8.2%	Staphylococcus epidermidis n = 8–38%	Staphylococcus aureus n = 4–22%
McClelland et al. [4]	Unicenter retrospective study	USA	1587	n = 14–0.8%	Staphylococcus aureus n = 8–50.0%	Propionibacterium acnes n = 4–25.0%
Korinek et al.[a] [39]	Unicenter prospective study	FR	6243	n = 95–1.5%	Enterobacteriaceae n = 28–29.5%	Staphylococcus epidermidis n = 20–21.0%
Erman et al. [5]	Unicenter prospective study	TUR	503	n = 31–6.2%	Staphylococcus aureus n = 22–71.0%	Acinetobacter baumannii n = 5–16.1%
NNIS report. [43]	Multicenter retrospective study	USA	4312	n = 37–0.9%	n/a	n/a
Maurice-Williams et al.[b] [44]	Unicenter retrospective study	UK	1476	n = 17–1.2%	Staphylococcus epidermidis n = 3–17.6%	Klebsiella n = 1–5.9%
Dettenkofer et al. [45]	Unicenter retrospective study	GER	545	n = 19–3.5%	n/a	n/a
Korinek. [31]	Multicenter prospective study	FR	2944	n = 117–4.0%	n/a	n/a

BRA, Brazil; CHI, China; FR, France; GER, Germany; n/a, not available; RUS, Russia; SWE, Sweden; TUR, Turkey; UK, United Kingdom; USA, United States of America.
[a] These studies focused on postoperative meningitis.
[b] this study assessed the prevalence of surgical site infections comparing two groups with different antibiotic prophylaxis procedures.

Table 32.3 Characteristics of surgical site infections after spinal surgery.

Studies, Year	Study design	Country	Patients (n)	Surgical site infection rate	First offending organism	Second offending organism
Lai et al. [46]	Unicenter retrospective study	CHI	923	n = 40–2.8%	n/a	n/a
Habiba et al [47]	Multicenter retrospective study	NOR	1.772	n = 40–2.3%	n/a	n/a
Lieber et al. 2016 [48]	Multicenter prospective study	USA	60.179	n = 1110–1.8%	n/a	n/a
Tominaga et al. [49]	Unicenter retrospective study	JAP	825	n = 14–1.7%	*Staphylococcus aureus* n = 5–35.7%	*Staphylococcus epidermidis* n = 5–35.7%
Cassir et al. [27]	Unicenter prospective study	FR	423	n = 18–4.2%	*Enterobacteriaceae* n = 6–33.3%	*Staphylococcus aureus* n = 4–22.2%
Lin et al. [16]	Unicenter retrospective study	TAI	20.178	n = 21–0.1%	*Staphylococcus aureus* n = 3–14.3%	*Staphylococcus epidermidis* n = 3–14.3%
Abdul-Jabbar 2013 [50]	Unicenter retrospective study	USA	7529	n = 239–3.2%	*Staphylococcus aureus* n = 108–45.2%	*Staphylococcus epidermidis* n = 75–31.4%
Xing et al. [51]	Systematic review	CHI	24.774	n = 2.439–9.8%	n/a	n/a
Kurtz et al.[a] [52]	Multicenter retrospective study	USA	15.069	n = 1.281–8.5%	n/a	n/a
Pull ter Gunne et al. [53]	Unicenter retrospective study	USA	3174	n = 132–4.2%	*Staphylococcus aureus* n = 54–65.1%	*Enterococcus faecalis* n = 12–14.5%
Olsen et al. [54]	Unicenter retrospective study	USA	2316	n = 46–2.0%	n/a	n/a
Kanafani et al. [55]	Unicenter retrospective study	LEB	997	n = 27–2.7%	*Staphylococcus epidermidis* n = 12–44.4%	*Proteus mirabilis* n = 3–11.1%
Fang et al.[b] [56]	Unicenter retrospective study	USA	1629	n = 48–4.4%	*Staphylococcus aureus* n = 27–56.3%	*Staphylococcus epidermidis* n = 18–37.5%
Olsen et al. [40][c]	Unicenter retrospective study	USA	1918	n = 53–2.8%	*Staphylococcus aureus* n = 9–17.0%	*Staphylococcus epidermidis* n = 2–3.8%
Picada et al. [57]	Unicenter retrospective study	USA	817	n = 26–3.2%	*Staphylococcus epidermidis* n = 8–30.8%	*Escherichia coli* n = 8–30.8%

CHI, China; JAP, Japan; LEB, Lebanon; n/a not available; NOR, Norway; TAI, Taiwan; USA, United States of America.

[a] This study focused on instrumented lumbar fusion procedures with a 10-year follow-up period.
[b] This study included surgical site infections with multiple infecting organisms.
[c] This study focused on postoperative meningitis.

of the affected spine; pain in the distribution of the spinal nerve roots in the area, and spinal cord or cauda equina compression with motor weakness, sensory deficits, and bladder and bowel dysfunction. Paralysis may occur after prolonged or major compression of the spinal cord or cauda equina [15, 65]. The classic triad of fever, axial pain, and neurological deficits occurs in less than 15% of patients, highlighting their diagnostic challenges [15, 66].

Investigations

The initial assessment should include: (i) a blood workup to determine an inflammatory syndrome; (ii) blood cultures to identify a specific organism; (iii) samples from the suspected primary infectious site; and (iv) cranial or spinal imaging (magnetic resonance imaging [MRI] with contrast enhancement when available is preferable to computed tomography [CT] scan with contrast enhancement) [7, 13, 15]. Special care is needed with brain MRI performed for suspected infection following carmustine wafer implantation because this can induce changes that may be misinterpreted as an SSI [67–70]. Wounds should be systematically checked because intracranial or intraspinal suppuration is frequently associated with a healing defect.

With the exception of postoperative meningitis, lumbar puncture to obtain cerebrospinal fluid (CSF) is never recommended, and may be completely contraindicated [7, 13, 15, 71]. It does not help the diagnosis and may increase the chances of herniation because of mass effect from the infected site with consequent clinical deterioration [7, 71]. In spinal infections, it increases the risk of CSF contamination [13, 15]. For these cases, surgical intervention serves two important purposes: microbiological investigation and primary treatment.

Treatment, future perspective, and conclusions

Treatment
Medical treatment
Medical and neurosurgical treatment must be given in parallel. Initial empirical antimicrobial therapy can include a combination of intravenous antibiotics, selected according to whether the postoperative infection is cranial or spinal. Recommendations and regular supervision from an infectious disease specialist is mandatory. Between three and five days later, treatment can be adapted if necessary, based on the results of susceptibility testing. Intravenous antibiotic therapy should continue for 4–12 weeks, depending on the type of SSI, adjusted by the therapeutic response and neuroimaging findings. Staphylococcal infections can be treated with a combination of a fluoroquinolone and rifampin; both have good penetration in brain. *Propionibacterium acnes* is usually susceptible to amoxicillin and rifampin. The treatment of Gram-negative infections should include a combination of a third-generation cephalosporin and a fluoroquinolone.

For brain abscesses, low-dose corticosteroids may be used to manage perilesional edema in cases with significant mass effect but must be discontinued as soon as possible [6, 72]. For brain abscesses and subdural empyema, epilepsy prophylaxis is also necessary and may be continued for extended periods of time [13, 72].

Neurosurgical management
Neurosurgical operations are mandatory (i) to identify the causative pathogen if not otherwise determined, (ii) to treat the infection or (iii) to improve neurologic deficits. For cranial brain abscesses, subdural empyema and epidural abscesses, craniotomy is required to enable surgical drainage of the pus collection and vigorous washing of the surgical site. If applicable, carmustine wafers or ventricular shunts should be removed [18], and if necessary, a temporary external ventricular drain can be placed [18]. For spinal subdural empyema, antimicrobial therapy alone is usually not sufficient, and a surgical laminectomy, durotomy, and aspiration of the collection is often necessary to preserve neurological function and prevent sepsis [65]. Neurosurgery is not necessary for isolated postoperative meningitis [18]. For spinal epidural abscesses, the best option, when feasible, is to perform a decompressive laminectomy to drain the collection to preserve neurological function, to identify the causative pathogen, and to control sepsis [15, 65, 66, 73–78].

Conclusions

The outcome for patients with SSIs has improved over the past 50 years, following improvements in neuroimaging, neurosurgery, and antimicrobial treatment. Mortality has declined in the past decade and patients now have better outcomes, with minimal or no neurological sequelae, although functional and neuropsychological evaluations are lacking. Future studies will include better cognitive assessment of patients and quality of life scores on long-term follow-up.

References

1. Karhade, A.V., Cote, D.J., Larsen, A.M.G., and Smith, T.R. (2017). Neurosurgical infection rates and risk factors: a national surgical quality improvement program analysis of 132,000 patients, 2006-2014. *World Neurosurg.* 97: 205–212.
2. Abu Hamdeh, S., Lytsy, B., and Ronne-Engström, E. (2014). Surgical site infections in standard neurosurgery procedures- a study of incidence, impact and potential risk factors. *Br. J. Neurosurg.* 28: 270–275.
3. O'Keeffe, A.B., Lawrence, T., and Bojanic, S. (2012). Oxford craniotomy infections database: a cost analysis of craniotomy infection. *Br. J. Neurosurg.* 26: 265–291.
4. McClelland, S. and Hall, W.A. (2007). Postoperative central nervous system infection: incidence and associated factors in 2111 neurosurgical procedures. *Clin. Infect. Dis.* 45: 55–59.
5. Erman, T., Demirhindi, H., Göçer, A.I. et al. (2005). Risk factors for surgical site infections in neurosurgery patients with antibiotic prophylaxis. *Surg. Neurol.* 63: 107–112, discussion 112-113.
6. Brouwer, M.C., Tunkel, A.R., and van de Beek, D. (2014). Brain abscess. *N. Engl. J. Med.* 371: 1758.
7. Brouwer, M.C., Coutinho, J.M., and van de Beek, D. (2014). Clinical characteristics and outcome of brain abscess: systematic review and meta-analysis. *Neurology* 82: 806–813.
8. National Institute for Care and Health Excellence (NICE) (2007). Carmustine implants and temozolomide for the treatment of newly diagnosed high-grade glioma | Guidance and guidelines. http://www.nice.org.uk/guidance/ta121?unlid=889143998201612164542 (accessed 19 March 2017).
9. Hart, M.G., Grant, R., Garside, R. et al. (2008). Chemotherapeutic wafers for high grade glioma. *Cochrane Database Syst. Rev.* (3): CD007294.
10. Hart, M.G., Grant, R., Garside, R. et al. (2011). Chemotherapy wafers for high grade glioma. *Cochrane Database Syst. Rev.* 2011 (3): CD007294. https://doi.org/10.1002/14651858.CD007294.pub2.
11. Roux, A., Caire, F., Guyotat, J. et al. (2017). Carmustine wafer implantation for high-grade gliomas: evidence-based safety efficacy and practical recommendations from the neuro-oncology club of the French society of neurosurgery. *Neurochirurgie* 63: 433–443.
12. Bartt, R.E. (2010). Cranial epidural abscess and subdural empyema. *Handb. Clin. Neurol.* 96: 75–89.
13. De Bonis, P., Anile, C., Pompucci, A. et al. (2009). Cranial and spinal subdural empyema. *Br. J. Neurosurg.* 23: 335–340.
14. Greenlee, J.E. (2003). Subdural Empyema. *Curr. Treat. Options Neurol.* 5: 13–22.
15. Darouiche, R.O. (2006). Spinal epidural abscess. *N. Engl. J. Med.* 355: 2012–2020.
16. Lin, T.-Y., Chen, W.-J., Hsieh, M.-K. et al. (2014). Postoperative meningitis after spinal surgery: a review of 21 cases from 20,178 patients. *BMC Infect. Dis.* 14: 220.
17. Korinek, A.-M., Baugnon, T., Golmard, J.-L. et al. (2008). Risk factors for adult nosocomial meningitis after craniotomy: role of antibiotic prophylaxis. *Neurosurgery* 62 (Suppl 2): 532–539.
18. van de Beek, D., Drake, J.M., and Tunkel, A.R. (2010). Nosocomial bacterial meningitis. *N. Engl. J. Med.* 362: 146–154.
19. Pallud, J., Audureau, E., Noel, G. et al. (2015). Long-term results of carmustine wafer implantation for newly diagnosed glioblastomas: a controlled propensity-matched analysis of a French multicenter cohort. *Neuro-Oncol.* 17: 1609–1619.
20. Pavlov, V., Page, P., Abi-Lahoud, G. et al. (2015). Combining intraoperative carmustine wafers and Stupp regimen in multimodal first-line treatment of primary glioblastomas. *Br. J. Neurosurg.* 29: 524–531.
21. Roux, A., Peeters, S., Zanello, M. et al. (2017). Extent of resection and Carmustine wafer implantation safely improve survival in patients with a newly diagnosed glioblastoma: a single center experience of the current practice. *J. Neuro-Oncol.* 135: 83–92.
22. Osborn, M.K. and Steinberg, J.P. (2007). Subdural empyema and other suppurative complications of paranasal sinusitis. *Lancet Infect. Dis.* 7: 62–67.
23. Kojan, S. and Al-Jumah, M. (2006). Infection related cerebral venous thrombosis. *J. Pak. Med. Assoc.* 56: 494–497.

24. Sadun, F., Feldon, S.E., Weiss, M.H., and Krieger, M.D. (1996). Septic cavernous sinus thrombosis following transsphenoidal craniotomy. Case report. *J. Neurosurg.* 85: 949–592.
25. Bekelis, K., Coy, S., and Simmons, N. (2016). Operative duration and risk of surgical site infection in neurosurgery. *World Neurosurg.* 94: 551–555.e6.
26. Buffet-Bataillon, S., Saunders, L., Campillo-Gimenez, B., and Haegelen, C. (2013). Risk factors for neurosurgical site infection after neurosurgery in Rennes, France: comparison of logistic and cox models. *Am. J. Infect. Control* 41: 1290–1292.
27. Cassir, N., De La Rosa, S., Melot, A. et al. (2015). Risk factors for surgical site infections after neurosurgery: a focus on the postoperative period. *Am. J. Infect. Control* 43: 1288–1291.
28. Fang, C., Zhu, T., Zhang, P. et al. (2017). Risk factors of neurosurgical site infection after craniotomy: a systematic review and meta-analysis. *Am. J. Infect. Control* 45: e123–e134.
29. Schipmann, S., Akalin, E., Doods, J. et al. (2016). When the infection hits the wound: matched case-control study in a neurosurgical patient collective including systematic literature review and risk factors analysis. *World Neurosurg.* 95: 178–189.
30. Wathen, C., Kshettry, V.R., Krishnaney, A. et al. (2016). The association between operating room personnel and turnover with surgical site infection in more than 12 000 neurosurgical cases. *Neurosurgery* 79: 889–894.
31. Korinek, A.M. (1997). Risk factors for neurosurgical site infections after craniotomy: a prospective multicenter study of 2944 patients. The French study group of neurosurgical infections, the SEHP, and the C-CLIN Paris-Nord. Service Épidémiologie Hygiène et Prévention. *Neurosurgery* 41: 1073–1079, discussion 1079-1081.
32. McCutcheon, B.A., Ubl, D.S., Babu, M. et al. (2016). Predictors of surgical site infection following craniotomy for intracranial neoplasms: an analysis of prospectively collected data in the American college of surgeons national surgical quality improvement program database. *World Neurosurg.* 88: 350–358.
33. Sneh-Arbib, O., Shiferstein, A., Dagan, N. et al. (2013). Surgical site infections following craniotomy focusing on possible post-operative acquisition of infection: prospective cohort study. *Eur. J. Clin. Microbiol. Infect. Dis.* 32: 1511–1156.
34. Meng, F., Cao, J., and Meng, X. (2015). Risk factors for surgical site infections following spinal surgery. *J. Clin. Neurosci.* 22: 1862–1866.
35. Jin, Y., Liu, X., Gao, L. et al. (2018). Risk factors and microbiology of meningitis and/or bacteremia after transsphenoidal surgery for pituitary adenoma. *World Neurosurg.* 110: e851–e863.
36. Umscheid, C.A., Mitchell, M.D., Doshi, J.A. et al. (2011). Estimating the proportion of healthcare-associated infections that are reasonably preventable and the related mortality and costs. *Infect. Control Hosp. Epidemiol.* 32: 101–114.
37. Anderson, P.A., Savage, J.W., Vaccaro, A.R. et al. (2017). Prevention of surgical site infection in spine surgery. *Neurosurgery* 80: S114–S123.
38. Abraham, P., Lamba, N., Acosta, M. et al. (2017). Antibacterial prophylaxis for gram-positive and gram-negative infections in cranial surgery: a meta-analysis. *J. Clin. Neurosci.* 45: 24–32.
39. Korinek, A.-M., Baugnon, T., Golmard, J.-L. et al. (2006). Risk factors for adult nosocomial meningitis after craniotomy: role of antibiotic prophylaxis. *Neurosurgery* 59: 126–133.
40. Olsen, M.A., Mayfield, J., Lauryssen, C. et al. (2003). Risk factors for surgical site infection in spinal surgery. *J. Neurosurg.* 98 (2 Suppl): 149–155.
41. Lieber, B.A., Appelboom, G., Taylor, B.E. et al. (2016). Preoperative chemotherapy and corticosteroids: independent predictors of cranial surgical-site infections. *J. Neurosurg.* 125: 187–195.
42. Zhan, R., Zhu, Y., Shen, Y. et al. (2014). Post-operative central nervous system infections after cranial surgery in China: incidence, causative agents, and risk factors in 1,470 patients. *Eur. J. Clin. Microbiol. Infect. Dis.* 33: 861–866.
43. NNIS System (2003). National Nosocomial Infections Surveillance (NNIS) system report, data summary from January 1992 through June 2003, issued august 2003. *Am. J. Infect. Control* 31: 481–498.
44. Maurice-Williams, R.S. and Pollock, J. (1999). Topical antibiotics in neurosurgery: a re-evaluation of the Malis technique. *Br. J. Neurosurg.* 13: 312–315.
45. Dettenkofer, M., Ebner, W., Hans, F.J. et al. (1999). Nosocomial infections in a neurosurgery intensive care unit. *Acta Neurochir.* 141: 1303–1308.
46. Lai, Q., Song, Q., Guo, R. et al. (2017). Risk factors for acute surgical site infections after lumbar surgery: a retrospective study. *J. Orthop. Surg.* 12: 116.
47. Habiba, S., Nygaard, Ø.P., Brox, J.I. et al. (2017). Risk factors for surgical site infections among 1,772 patients operated on for lumbar disc herniation: a multicentre observational registry-based study. *Acta Neurochir.* 159: 1113–1118.

48. Lieber, B., Han, B., Strom, R.G. et al. (2016). Preoperative predictors of spinal infection within the national surgical quality inpatient database. *World Neurosurg.* 89: 517–524.
49. Tominaga, H., Setoguchi, T., Ishidou, Y. et al. (2016). Risk factors for surgical site infection and urinary tract infection after spine surgery. *Eur. Spine J.* 25: 3908–3915.
50. Abdul-Jabbar, A., Berven, S.H., Hu, S.S. et al. (2013). Surgical site infections in spine surgery: identification of microbiologic and surgical characteristics in 239 cases. *Spine* 38: E1425–E1431.
51. Xing, D., Ma, J.-X., Ma, X.-L. et al. (2013). A methodological, systematic review of evidence-based independent risk factors for surgical site infections after spinal surgery. *Eur. Spine J.* 22: 605–615.
52. Kurtz, S.M., Lau, E., Ong, K.L. et al. (2012). Infection risk for primary and revision instrumented lumbar spine fusion in the medicare population. *J. Neurosurg. Spine* 17: 342–347.
53. Pull ter Gunne, A.F., Mohamed, A.S., Skolasky, R.L. et al. (2010). The presentation, incidence, etiology, and treatment of surgical site infections after spinal surgery. *Spine* 35: 1323–1328.
54. Olsen, M.A., Nepple, J.J., Riew, K.D. et al. (2008). Risk factors for surgical site infection following orthopaedic spinal operations. *J. Bone Joint Surg. Am.* 90: 62–69.
55. Kanafani, Z.A., Dakdouki, G.K., El-Dbouni, O. et al. (2006). Surgical site infections following spinal surgery at a tertiary care center in Lebanon: incidence, microbiology, and risk factors. *Scand. J. Infect. Dis.* 38: 589–592.
56. Fang, A., Hu, S.S., Endres, N., and Bradford, D.S. (2005). Risk factors for infection after spinal surgery. *Spine* 30: 1460–1465.
57. Picada, R., Winter, R.B., Lonstein, J.E. et al. (2000). Postoperative deep wound infection in adults after posterior lumbosacral spine fusion with instrumentation: incidence and management. *J. Spinal Disord.* 13: 42–45.
58. Chen, C., Zhang, B., Yu, S. et al. (2014). The incidence and risk factors of meningitis after major craniotomy in China: a retrospective cohort study. *PLoS One* 9: e101961.
59. Chen, S., Cui, A., Yu, K. et al. (2018). Risk factors associated with meningitis after neurosurgery: a retrospective cohort study in a Chinese hospital. *World Neurosurg.* 111: e546–e563.
60. Savin, I., Ershova, K., Kurdyumova, N. et al. (2018). Healthcare-associated ventriculitis and meningitis in a neuro-ICU: incidence and risk factors selected by machine learning approach. *J. Crit. Care* 45: 95–104.
61. Subach, B.R., Witham, T.F., Kondziolka, D. et al. (1999). Morbidity and survival after 1,3-bis(2-chloroethyl)-1-nitrosourea wafer implantation for recurrent glioblastoma: a retrospective case-matched cohort series. *Neurosurgery* 45: 17–22; discussion 22-23.
62. De Bonis, P., Anile, C., Pompucci, A. et al. (2012). Safety and efficacy of Gliadel wafers for newly diagnosed and recurrent glioblastoma. *Acta Neurochir.* 154: 1371–1378.
63. Roche, M., Humphreys, H., Smyth, E. et al. (2003). A twelve-year review of central nervous system bacterial abscesses; presentation and aetiology. *Clin. Microbiol. Infect.* 9: 803–809.
64. Kombogiorgas, D., Seth, R., Athwal, R. et al. (2007). Suppurative intracranial complications of sinusitis in adolescence. Single institute experience and review of literature. *Br. J. Neurosurg.* 21: 603–609.
65. Darouiche, R.O. (2010). Spinal epidural abscess and subdural empyema. *Handb. Clin. Neurol.* 96: 91–99.
66. DeFroda, S.F., DePasse, J.M., Eltorai, A.E.M. et al. (2016). Evaluation and management of spinal epidural abscess. *J. Hosp. Med.* 11: 130–135.
67. Dyke, J.P., Sanelli, P.C., Voss, H.U. et al. (2007). Monitoring the effects of BCNU chemotherapy wafers (Gliadel) in glioblastoma multiforme with proton magnetic resonance spectroscopic imaging at 3.0 Tesla. *J. Neuro-Oncol.* 82: 103–110.
68. Colen, R.R., Zinn, P.O., Hazany, S. et al. (2011). Magnetic resonance imaging appearance and changes on intracavitary Gliadel wafer placement: a pilot study. *World J. Radiol.* 3: 266–272.
69. Doishita, S., Shimono, T., Yoneda, T. et al. (2018). In vitro study of serial changes to Carmustine wafers (Gliadel) with MR imaging and computed tomography. *Magn. Reson. Med. Sci.* 17: 58–66.
70. Masuda, Y., Ishikawa, E., Yamamoto, T. et al. (2016). Early postoperative expansion of parenchymal high-intensity areas on T2-weighted imaging predicts delayed cerebral Edema caused by Carmustine wafer implantation in patients with high-grade Glioma. *Magn. Reson. Med. Sci.* 15: 299–307.
71. Alvis Miranda, H., Castellar-Leones, S.M., Elzain, M.A., and Moscote-Salazar, L.R. (2013). Brain abscess: current management. *J. Neurosci. Rural Pract.* 4 (Suppl 1): S67–S81.
72. Zhang, C., Hu, L., Wu, X. et al. (2014). A retrospective study on the aetiology, management, and outcome of brain abscess in an 11-year, single-Centre study from China. *BMC Infect. Dis.* 14: 311.

73. Pereira, C.E. and Lynch, J.C. (2005). Spinal epidural abscess: an analysis of 24 cases. *Surg. Neurol.* 63 (Suppl 1): S26–S29.
74. Patel, A.R., Alton, T.B., Bransford, R.J. et al. (2014). Spinal epidural abscesses: risk factors, medical versus surgical management, a retrospective review of 128 cases. *Spine J.* 14: 326–330.
75. Pradilla, G., Ardila, G.P., Hsu, W., and Rigamonti, D. (2009). Epidural abscess of the CNS. *Lancet Neurol.* 8: 292–300.
76. Tompkins, M., Panuncialman, I., Lucas, P., and Palumbo, M. (2010). Spinal epidural abscess. *J. Emerg. Med.* 39: 384–390.
77. Shweikeh, F., Saeed, K., Bukavina, L. et al. (2014). An institutional series and contemporary review of bacterial spinal epidural abscess: current status and future directions. *Neurosurg. Focus.* 37: E9.
78. Johnson, K.G. (2013). Spinal epidural abscess. *Crit. Care Nurs. Clin. North Am.* 25: 389–397.

33 CNS Involvement in *Tropheryma whipplei* Infection

Emmanuèle Lechapt-Zalcman
Department of Neuropathology, Sainte Anne Hospital, Paris, France

Abbreviations

CNS	central nervous system
CSF	cerebrospinal fluid
18 FDG-PET	^{18}Fluorodeoxyglucose-positron emission tomography
FLAIR	fluid attenuated inversion recovery
HLA	human leukocyte antigens
IRIS	immune reconstitution inflammatory syndrome
MRI	magnetic resonance imaging
OFSM	oculofacial-skeletal myorhythmia
OMM	oculomasticatory myorhythmia
PAS	periodic acid-Schiff
PCR	polymerase chain reaction
qPCR	quantitative PCR
T. whipplei	*Tropheryma whipplei*
WD	Whipple disease

Definition of the disorder and historical perspective

Whipple disease (WD) is an uncommon chronic systemic infection caused by *Tropheryma whipplei*. The first case was described in 1907 as an intestinal lipodystrophy by George Whipple, a pathologist at Johns Hopkins in Baltimore, Maryland [1], but the illness remained little known until the classic paper by Maizel and colleagues in 1970 [2]. A bacterial cause was suspected, supported by the success of antibiotic therapy, and then confirmed by electron microscopy (EM). Although the causative bacillus had remained uncultured, in 1992 it was identified with the aid of polymerase chain reaction (PCR) [3]. In the 2000s, stable culture of *T. whipplei* was achieved [4], and its genome was sequenced [5]. Subsequently, the spectrum of *T. whipplei* diseases broadened and now encompasses (i) acute infections (i.e. pneumonia, gastroenteritis), (ii) classic WD characterized by weight loss, fever, chronic diarrhea, and arthralgia, and (iii) localized chronic WD in extra-intestinal organs (e.g. endocarditis or encephalitis without any intestinal involvement) [6, 7].

T. whipplei is an Actinobacteria, taxonomically located between the subdivision of Gram-positive Actinomycetes and the Cellulomonadaceae.

Epidemiology

T. whipplei is ubiquitous and can be detected in 1–11% of samples (i.e. feces, saliva) in the general population in developed countries [8, 9], but the prevalence is higher in Africa. *T. whipplei* is

---

Infections of the Central Nervous System: Pathology and Genetics, First Edition. Edited by Fabrice Chrétien, Kum Thong Wong, Leroy R. Sharer, Catherine (Katy) Keohane and Françoise Gray.
© 2020 John Wiley & Sons Ltd. Published 2020 by John Wiley & Sons Ltd.

probably transmitted between humans via oro-oral or feco-oral routes. Close contacts of carriers of the organism, family members of patients with WD, and poor living conditions all increase the risk of colonization. Although the pathogen is distributed universally, very few carriers develop WD (<0.01%) [9]; its incidence is estimated as 1 per million population [7]. Patients are typically men who are Caucasian and middle-aged. This suggests that both host genetic and immune factors determine susceptibility. WD has also been reported in association with acquired immunodeficiency syndrome (AIDS) [10].

Neurologic symptoms have been reported in 6–63% of patients with classic WD [11]. However, CNS involvement is probably more common because *T. whipplei* can be identified by PCR in cerebrospinal fluid (CSF) from patients with WD without CNS manifestations [12]. CNS involvement is the most serious complication of WD and without early treatment can be fatal or result in disabling sequelae [7, 13–15]. It may occur during the systemic stage of untreated classic WD or at relapse of previously treated WD. Very rarely, the bacterium may also be responsible for a primary CNS disease (i.e. isolated encephalitis without gastrointestinal or rheumatological features).

Clinical features

Clinical presentation
Neurologic manifestations are protean [13–16], but cognitive changes (such as in dementia) are the most common neurological symptoms. They tend to progress insidiously and are associated with psychiatric signs (i.e. depression, changes in personality, and behavioral abnormalities). Oculofacial-skeletal myorhythmia (OFSM) or oculomasticatory myorhythmia (OMM) are rare but are typically associated with WD. Other neurologic involvement includes ophthalmoplegia, upper motor neuron signs, hypothalamic manifestations, cerebellar ataxia, frontal lobe syndrome, headache, seizures, and coma. Meningitis, cranial and peripheral neuropathies, spinal cord involvement, ischemic lesions, or strokelike symptoms have also been reported. The combination of cognitive impairment with ataxia or obesity is highly suggestive of isolated encephalitis [17].

Investigations
Brain magnetic resonance imaging (MRI) findings are nonspecific and may be normal even in symptomatic patients. Multifocal, uni- or bilateral T2 and fluid attenuated inversion recovery (FLAIR) hyperintensities in the medial temporal lobe, midbrain, hypothalamus, and thalamus can be detected. Enhancement is usually minimal and WD lesions do not typically produce restricted diffusion [18]. Solitary tumor-like lesions producing mass effect, periventricular diffuse leukoencephalopathy, corticospinal tract lesions, cortical atrophy, and pachymeningitis have all been reported [7, 18]. 18Fluorodeoxyglucose-positron emission tomography (^{18}FDG-PET) may be useful for diagnosis and follow-up of patients with neurological involvement [19].

CSF cytology is normal in more than 50% of cases but can show modest pleocytosis. Rarely, PAS-positive cells may be detected in the CSF of patients with WD[15].

Diagnosis
Depending on the neurologic signs, the differential diagnosis includes neurodegenerative disorders, systemic infections or inflammatory diseases, vasculitis, and even tumors.

Serology is not routinely used for the diagnosis.

It is widely recommended to use at least two independent tests (i.e. histopathology and PCR) on different tissues and fluids to reliably identify *T. whipplei*. Multiple gastrointestinal biopsies enable a diagnosis of classic WD, but they are negative in most localized extra-intestinal WD. The diagnosis of CNS WD may require cerebral biopsy.

PCR is the most specific and sensitive technique for establishing the diagnosis, especially for chronic localized WD, and has become the diagnostic method of choice [15]. The gold standard is quantitative PCR (qPCR) targeting repeated *T. whipplei* sequences. CSF qPCR analysis is recommended to diagnose CNS infection in all WD forms and can detect *T. whipplei* DNA in 92% of patients, irrespective of CSF cytology [15]. However, because bacteria are scarce in CSF, negative CSF qPCR does not exclude encephalitis

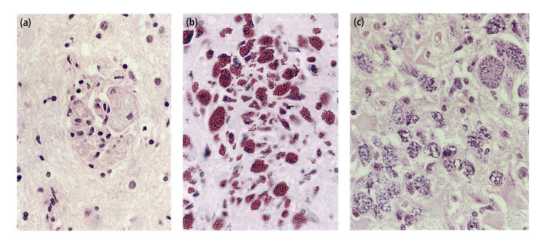

Figure 33.1 Cerebral biopsy from a patient with Whipple disease (WD), microscopic appearance. (a) Perivascular accumulation of foamy macrophages. Note the reactive astrocytes in the surrounding brain parenchyma (hematoxylin and eosin [H&E]). (b) The macrophages contain periodic acid-Schiff (PAS)-positive, sickle-shaped inclusions (PAS). (c) The inclusions are Gram positive (Gram stain).

caused by *T. whipplei* [16]. Culture of the bacterium from CSF is only carried out in specialized laboratories [7]. In this setting, qPCR tests should be performed in any available samples to avoid brain biopsy, but qPCR on saliva or stools has poor predictive value for isolated WD. In the near future, PCR of urine may become an additional useful noninvasive test to identify *T. whipplei* [8].

In some strongly suspected cases with negative CSF qPCR, antimicrobial treatment may be started.

On follow-up of patients with improved CNS disease, without evidence of ongoing infection, CSF analysis may indicate persistent or de novo mild meningitis. In the early months of treatment this is suggestive of immune reconstitution inflammatory syndrome (IRIS) [20].

Pathology

Macroscopy

Macroscopically, small yellow-grayish nodules, 1–2 mm in diameter are disseminated throughout the entire CNS. They are particularly abundant in gray matter, with a predilection for the subpial regions, basal ganglia, hypothalamic nuclei, periaqueductal gray matter, brainstem nuclei, and cerebellar dentate nuclei. The lesions may coalesce to form larger foci. Solitary space-occupying lesions mimicking a tumor are not uncommon. Cystic noninflammatory residual lesions, devoid of bacteria may be found following successful treatment [21].

Microscopy

Brain biopsy usually shows accumulation of foamy macrophages (Figure 33.1a) often forming perivascular clusters associated with reactive changes, including edema, lymphocyte infiltration, astrocytosis, and microglial activation. The macrophages contain tiny, sickle-shaped inclusions, positive with PAS (Figure 33.1b), Gram (Figure 33.1c), and methenamine silver stains and negative on Ziehl-Neelsen stain. Extracellular bacteria are also present. On electron microscopy, lamellar partially degraded bacterial cell walls (Figure 33.2a) and better-preserved bacilli with a trilaminar plasma membrane (Figure 33.2b) are found in macrophages, astrocytes, and pericytes.

Histological detection of *T. whipplei* on PAS stains leads to a presumptive diagnosis of WD [6], but although highly characteristic, this finding is not specific. In doubtful or negative cases, immunohistochemistry (IHC) can improve the histological diagnosis, but specific antibodies against *T. whipplei* are not commercially available [22]. Fluorescence in situ hybridization to identify *Tropheryma* species in formalin-fixed paraffin-embedded tissues has been developed in specialized laboratories. PCR analysis

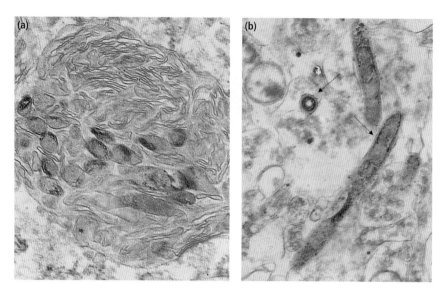

Figure 33.2 Cerebral biopsy from a patient with Whipple disease (WD), electron microscopy (EM). (a) The inclusions are composed of lamellar, partially degraded bacterial cell walls. (b) Better-preserved bacilli with a trilaminar plasma membrane (arrows) are less numerous.

of formalin-fixed paraffin-embedded tissue can be employed but is not recommended as a screening method and should be reserved for patients with clinically suspected WD.

Genetics and pathogenesis

The pathogenesis of WD is still uncertain and relies on observations in humans because animal models are not currently available.

Despite the presumed widespread presence of *T. whipplei*, very few carriers, mostly Caucasian males, develop WD, suggesting some specific immunological host susceptibility. Human leukocyte antigens (HLA) alleles (HLA-B27, HLA-DRB1*13, and HLA-BDQ*01) are reportedly more frequent in patients with WD but not confirmed by all studies [6, 12]. The disease is mostly sporadic, but multiple members in a few families have developed WD. A single very rare nonsynonymous mutation in IRF4, a transcription factor involved in immunity, was found in a multiplex kindred with four patients with WD [23].

Dysfunction of the mononuclear-phagocytic system is another possible factor involved in WD pathogenesis and is suggested by the large number of macrophages apparently unable to degrade the bacteria. Studies on systemic (mucosa and peripheral blood) immune reactions of patients with WD showed impaired ability to mount a Th1 immune response against *T. whipplei*, indicating a host immune defect at the T-cell and macrophage levels [24]. In WD, peripheral Th1 responses of CD4-Tcells are significantly reduced, and a high production of interleukin (IL)-4 contrasts with low interferon gamma (IFN-γ) production. Reduced IL-12 levels also result in reduced IFN-γ levels, which contribute to impaired macrophage activation and function [25]. Macrophage dysfunction is evidenced by their impaired microbicidal function with an impaired oxidative burst.

In WD, macrophages are able to phagocytose *T. whipplei*, but bacterial degradation is impaired, allowing further immunomodulation and *T. whipplei* replication. Interestingly, the pathogen itself contributes to its multiplication by triggering alternatively activated macrophages. This favors Th2 responses, which ultimately reduce the capacity to digest bacteria and also favors macrophage apoptosis, thereby facilitating bacterial dissemination [26].

In summary, impaired local immune response, and the alternative activation of macrophages, triggered in part by the agent *T. whipplei* itself, may explain the hallmark of WD: invasion of the intestinal mucosa with macrophages incapable of degrading *T. whipplei* [26]. The mechanisms and molecular pathways responsible for non-eradication of *T. whipplei* are still not clear.

Treatment, future perspective, and conclusions

Although the diagnosis of WD is challenging, if diagnosed early, it can be successfully treated by antibiotic therapy. Several antibiotic combinations have been proposed, albeit based on studies with small patient numbers. In vitro data support treatment with the combination of doxycycline (200 mg/d) and hydrochloroquinine (600 mg/d) for one year, followed by lifelong treatment with doxycycline to avoid reinfection [6, 16]. Clinicians should be aware of IRIS, which can be fatal [20]. Long-term follow-up with repeated PCR on CSF is mandatory to monitor treatment [6, 16].

Much knowledge on WD has been gained thanks to the development of specific molecular tools and multidisciplinary approaches. However, WD, particularly chronic isolated encephalitis, remains a diagnostic challenge and has significant morbidity and mortality. Many questions regarding pathogenesis, various clinical manifestations and treatment options remain unsolved.

References

1. Whipple, G.H. (1907). A hitherto undescribed disease characterized anatomically by deposits of fat and fatty acids in the intestinal and myenteric lymphatic tissues. *Bull. Johns Hopkins Hosp.* 18: 382–391.
2. Maizel, H., Ruffin, J.M., and Dobbins, W.O. III (1970). Whipple's disease: a review of 19 patients from one hospital and a review of the literature since 1950. *Medicine* 49: 175–205.
3. Relman, D.A., Schmidt, T.M., MacDermott, R.P., and Falkow, S. (1992). Identification of the uncultured bacillus of Whipple's disease. *N. Engl. J. Med.* 327: 293–301.
4. Raoult, D., Birg, M.L., La Scola, B. et al. (2000). Cultivation of the bacillus of Whipple's disease. *N. Engl. J. Med.* 342 (9): 620–625.
5. Bentley, S.D., Maiwald, M., Murphy, L.D. et al. (2003). Sequencing and analysis of the genome of the Whipple's disease bacterium Tropheryma whipplei. *Lancet* 361 (9358): 637–644.
6. Dolmans, R.A., Boel, C.H., Lacle, M.M., and Kusters, J.G. (2017). Clinical manifestations, treatment, and diagnosis of Tropheryma whipplei infections. *Clin. Microbiol. Rev.* 30 (2): 529–555. Review.
7. El-Abassi, R., Soliman, M.Y., Williams, F., and England, J.D. (2017). Whipple's disease. *J. Neurol. Sci.* 377: 197–206.
8. Amsler, L., Bauernfeind, P., Nigg, C. et al. (2003). Prevalence of Tropheryma whipplei DNA in patients with various gastrointestinal diseases and in healthy controls. *Infection* 31: 81–85.
9. Fenollar, F., Trani, M., Davoust, B. et al. (2008). Prevalence of asymptomatic Tropheryma whipplei carriage among humans and nonhuman primates. *J. Infect. Dis.* 197: 880–887.
10. Autran, B., Gorin, I., Leibowitch, M. et al. (1983). AIDS in a Haitian woman with cardiac Kaposi's sarcoma and Whipple's disease (Letter). *Lancet* i: 767–768.
11. Fenollar, F., Puechal, X., and Raoult, D. (2007). Whipple's disease. *N. Engl. J. Med.* 356: 55–66.
12. von Herbay, A., Ditton, H.J., Schuhmacher, F., and Maiwald, M. (1997). Whipple's disease: staging and monitoring by cytology and polymerase chain reaction analysis of cerebrospinal fluid. *Gastroenterology* 113: 434–441.
13. Louis, E.D., Lynch, T., Kaufmann, P. et al. (1996). Diagnostic guidelines in central nervous system Whipple's disease. *Ann. Neurol.* 40: 561–568.
14. Gerard, A., Sarrot-Reynauld, F., Liozon, E. et al. (2002). Neurologic presentation of Whipple disease: report of 12 cases and review of the literature. *Medicine* 81: 443–457.
15. Compain, C., Sacre, K., Puéchal, X. et al. (2013). Central nervous system involvement in Whipple disease: clinical study of 18 patients and long-term follow-up. *Medicine* 92: 324–330.
16. Lagier, J.C. and Raoult, D. (2018). Whipple's disease and Tropheryma whipplei infections: when to suspect them and how to diagnose and treat them. *Curr. Opin. Infect. Dis.* 31: 463–470.
17. Fenollar, F., Nicoli, F., Paquet, C. et al. (2011). Progressive dementia associated with ataxia or obesity in patients with Tropheryma whipplei encephalitis. *BMC Infect. Dis.* 15 (11): 171.
18. Black, D.F., Aksamit, A.J., and Morris, J.M. (2010). MR imaging of central nervous system Whipple disease: a 15-year review. *AJNR Am. J. Neuroradiol.* 31 (8): 1493–1497.

19. Lagier, J.C., Cammilleri, S., and Raoult, D. (2016). Classic Whipple's disease diagnosed by (18)F-fluorodeoxyglucose PET. *Lancet Infect. Dis.* 16: 130.
20. Lagier, J.C., Fenollar, F., Lepidi, H. et al. (2010). Successful treatment of immune reconstitution inflammatory syndrome in Whipple's disease using thalidomide. *J. Infect.* 60: 79–82.
21. Balasa, M., Gelpi, E., Rey, M.J. et al. (2014). Clinical and neuropathological variability in clinically isolated central nervous system Whipple's disease. *Brain Pathol.* 24: 230–238.
22. Lepidi, H., Fenollar, F., Gerolami, R. et al. (2003). Whipple's disease: immunospecific and quantitative immunohistochemical study of intestinal biopsy specimens. *Hum. Pathol.* 34: 589–596.
23. Guérin, A., Kerner, G., Marr, N. et al. (2018). IRF4 haploinsufficiency in a family with Whipple's disease. *elife* 7: e32340.
24. Marth, T. and Schneider, T. (2008). Whipple disease. *Curr. Opin. Gastroenterol.* 24: 141–148.
25. Marth, T., Neurath, M., Cuccherini, B.A., and Strober, W. (1997). Defects of monocyte interleukin 12 production and humoral immunity in Whipple's disease. *Gastroenterology* 113: 442–448.
26. Moos, V., Schmidt, C., Geelhaar, A. et al. (2010). Impaired immune functions of monocytes and macrophages in Whipple's disease. *Gastroenterology* 138: 210–220.

34 Cerebral Actinomycosis

Arnault Tauziede-Espariat[1,2]

[1] Department of Neuropathology, Sainte Anne Hospital, Paris, France
[2] Paris University, Paris, France

Abbreviations

ADC	apparent diffusion coefficient
CNS	central nervous system
CSF	cerebrospinal fluid
MRI	magnetic resonance imaging
spp.	species

Definition of the disorder and historical perspective

Actinomyces are small, anaerobic, Gram-positive organisms whose appearance as thin, branching filaments formerly led to their inclusion (with *Nocardia*) among fungi.

Actinomycosis was first described in the nineteenth century as a disease in bovine animals. In 1876, Bollinger described Actinomyces as a specific parasitic disease after finding mycelia in purulent specimens taken from the mandibles of cattle. In 1877, the microbiologist Hartz, using material collected by Bollinger, named the radial microorganisms *Actinomyces bovis* (*Actino* for radial discharge of sulfur granules and *Mycos* for mycelia). Human actinomycosis was first described in 1878 by Israel and Wolff, who first isolated *Actinomyces* in culture and defined the organisms as anaerobic in culture [for historical review see [1]. Currently, *Actinomyces* are formally classified as bacteria.

Involvement of the CNS is rare. After the first reported case of infection of the nervous system [2], Sanford and Voelker [3] could only find 8 cases among 587 patients with actinomycosis. In 1937, Frideman and Levy reviewed CNS actinomycoses in 108 cases reported in the literature [4]. However, many of those cases were later considered to be nocardioses. Bolton and Ashenhurst [5] described 17 cases of CNS actinomycosis. Smego [6] performed a comprehensive analysis of 70 cases of newly reported CNS actinomycosis and described the main features.

Microbiological characteristics

Actinomyces species are Gram-positive, non-acid-fast, non-spore-forming bacilli that appear as filamentous thin branching rods. They are strictly anaerobic bacteria. The classification of *Actinomyces* spp., initially based on phenotypic characteristics, has been recently revised because of advances in microbiological taxonomy using genotypic methods such as comparative 16S ribosomal RNA (rRNA) gene sequencing. More than 30 species of *Actinomyces* have been described [7]. *Actinomyces israelii* is the most prevalent species isolated in human infections and is found in most clinical forms of actinomycosis [8]. *Actinomyces*

Infections of the Central Nervous System: Pathology and Genetics, First Edition. Edited by Fabrice Chrétien, Kum Thong Wong, Leroy R. Sharer, Catherine (Katy) Keohane and Françoise Gray.
© 2020 John Wiley & Sons Ltd. Published 2020 by John Wiley & Sons Ltd.

viscosus and *Actinomyces meyeri* are less commonly reported in typical actinomycosis. *A. meyeri* is considered to have a great propensity for dissemination [9]. Some species, including *Actinomyces naeslundii, Actinomyces odontolyticus, Actinomyces gerencseriae* (formerly *A. israelii* serotype 2), *Actinomyces neuii, Actinomyces turicensis,* and *Actinomyces radingae,* have been associated with particular clinical syndromes.

These bacteria belong to the endogenous flora and colonize the oral cavity, dental plaque, tonsillar lacunae, and the mucous membranes of the gastrointestinal tract, vagina, and other sites. They become pathogenic and cause a chronic inflammatory response if the integrity of mucosal barriers is compromised or if there is an accompanying bacterial infection. Pathogenic species do not exist freely in nature, and there has been no documented person-to-person transmission.

Actinomycosis is a diagnostic challenge. Culture is positive in only 50% of cases and the bacteria grow slowly (two to three weeks) in selective agar medium [10, 11].

Actinomyces-specific antigens induce a delayed hypersensitivity (tuberculin-type) reaction as well as generation of antibodies (complement binding, agglutinins, precipitins).

Epidemiology

Actinomyces have a worldwide distribution but occur predominantly in rural areas. There is no age, race, sex, or seasonal predilection. Actinomycosis is a chronic suppurative infectious disease. Fifty-percent of cases involve the cervicofacial region, 20% the lung and thoracic region, and 30% the abdomen and pelvis. In the majority of cases the disease onset involves the teeth or tonsils. From the buccal or pharyngeal mucous membranes, disease spreads directly to other areas, particularly the mandible [12].

CNS actinomycosis accounts for only 1–15% of actinomycotic infections [13–15]. It is usually secondary to a focus elsewhere in the body, spreading to the CNS either by direct extension from the cervicofacial region or hematogenously from primary infection in the lung, abdomen, pelvis, or oro-cervico-facial region [9]. It can also occur following neurosurgery or cranial trauma [8, 13]. The most frequent lesions are cerebral abscesses. Actinomycosis may also present as meningitis, meningoencephalitis, subdural empyema [16], actinomycetoma, and spinal epidural abscess [15].

Unlike nocardiosis, actinomycotic abscesses occur frequently in patients who are immunocompetent [8]. Poor oral hygiene, gingivitis, sinusitis and dental procedures, chronic mastoiditis, congenital heart disease, infected intrauterine devices, and alcoholism have all been described as risk factors [11].

Clinical features

Clinical presentation of CNS *Actinomyces* abscesses is highly variable and generally insidious and nonspecific. They present as slowly progressive mass lesions with neurologic findings related to the abscess location. Common clinical manifestations are focal neurologic signs, headache, seizure, and diplopia. High fever and intracranial hypertension are not usual. The mean duration of symptoms prior to diagnosis is >2 months, which is longer than most causes of pyogenic CNS infections. Abscesses are usually single but may be multifocal [17].

Magnetic resonance imaging (MRI) is the best diagnostic tool. Generally, it shows a lobulated mass with a necrotic center, surrounded by significant peripheral vasogenic edema. There is a hyperintensity on T2-weighted MRI and ring enhancement following gadolinium administration. Magnetic resonance spectroscopy features include the presence of lactates and increased choline peak and choline-to-N-acetylaspartate ratio in the enhancing areas. Restricted diffusion on apparent diffusion coefficient (ADC) is consistent with abscess, but necrotic brain metastases and primary brain tumors are uncommon differential diagnoses.

Leukocytosis and features of an inflammatory syndrome are often absent, and classically blood culture and cerebrospinal fluid (CSF) are sterile.

The diagnosis is mostly made by identifying *Actinomyces* spp. in cultures and sulfur granules in pathology specimens from stereotactic aspiration of pus [6, 13, 18–20].

A definite diagnosis of actinomycosis is established by isolating an actinomyces species in cultures. However, cultures are negative in up to 70% of cases. *Actinomyces* growth is slow; it takes at least 5 days and may take up to 15–20 days, so incubation is required for at least 10 days before concluding the culture is negative. The low yield of culture has been ascribed to various reasons, such as inappropriate culture conditions, short-term incubation, or previous antibiotic therapy [11]. Actinomycotic abscesses are often polymicrobial [6], and the multiple associated organisms include *Aggregatibacter*, *Capnocytophaga*, *Fusobacterium*, *Haemophilus*, *Staphylococcus*, and *Streptococcus* species. These pathogens are believed to facilitate actinomycotic infection by inhibiting host defenses and establishing a microaerophilic environment [21].

Serological assays have been developed but need improvement before they become clinically useful [7].

Pathology

The most frequent lesions are abscesses. These are most often single, but multifocal abscesses have been described [17]. They predominantly involve the frontal and temporal lobes [11]. They usually present as multiloculated lesions with a central necrotic inflammatory exudate containing polymorphs, necrotic debris, and colonies of branching organisms forming "sulfur granules" (Figure 34.1), so-named because of their macroscopic yellowish appearance. The surrounding granulation zone is usually thick and consists of highly cellular fibrous tissue containing collagen fibers, fibroblasts, capillaries, and inflammatory cells such as plasma cells, monocytes, and lymphocytes. Giant cells may also be found; however, true granulomas or "Actinomycomata" are most unusual [16]. Variable amounts of edema, vascular congestion, reactive gliosis, and fibrosis are observed in the adjacent parenchyma. When the abscess is near the brain surface, it may induce a meningitic reaction. Other intracranial lesions include meningitis or meningoencephalitis, subdural empyema, and epidural abscess [6].

Detecting the organisms on histology is pathognomonic. They appear as thin branching filaments about 1 μm in diameter, distinguishing them from filamentous fungi, which are typically 3 μm or greater in width. They often cannot be recognized in routinely stained preparations but are identified using Grocott methenamine-silver stain, applied for longer than usual (up to one hour). Sulfur granules are more characteristic of Actinomycosis. Histopathologically, these granules have an irregular central basophilic core surrounded by radially-arranged eosinophilic filaments with club-shaped outlines (Figure 34.1) [14, 22]. The granules may occur singly, or they may be multiple in loose aggregates. Ultrastructural studies demonstrate fimbriae and outer matrix material which help form cohesive colonies essential for survival within host tissues [23].

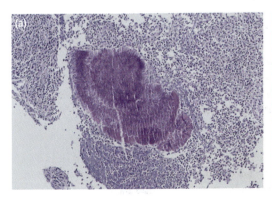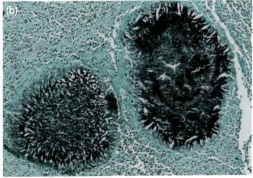

Figure 34.1 (a) Suppurative inflammation with actinomycotic colony surrounded by neutrophils and histiocytes (periodic acid-Schiff [PAS] staining, magnification 200×). (b) Colony of *Actinomyces* within purulent material, arranged in a radiating pattern with surface clubs (Grocott-Gomori staining, magnification 400×).

The differential diagnosis should include nocardiosis, which consists of comparable Gram-positive, filamentous branching bacteria, and can occasionally form sulfur granules and cause similar clinical syndromes involving the lungs, bones, joints, soft tissue, and the CNS. (cf. Chapter 35). It is critical to distinguish between these two types of organisms because they respond differently to antibiotics. Microbiologically, *Nocardia* species are Gram-positive, partially acid-fast organisms with aerobic requirements, whereas *Actinomycetes* are Gram-positive, non-acid-fast organisms with anaerobic or microaerophilic requirements [24]. However, a negative acid-fast stain does not exclude a diagnosis of nocardiosis.

Sequence analysis of the 16S rRNA gene constitutes a simple, reliable, efficient, and rapid method to identify *Nocardia* and *Actinomyces* isolates [25]. Besides 16S rRNA sequencing, 16S ribosomal DNA restriction analysis is a practical method of identification [26]. Polymerase chain reaction (PCR) with specific primers can also be used to directly detect *Actinomyces* in clinical material. Matrix-assisted laser desorption ionization time-of-flight should be a quicker and accurate tool for *Actinomyces* identification in the future [7].

Treatment

The mortality rate of *Actinomyces* abscesses (30%) is more than three times that of other bacterial brain abscesses [6]. The poor prognosis is the result of many factors including immunodeficiency, delayed diagnosis because of nonspecific clinical manifestations, and the presence of multiple abscesses.

Optimal management combines adequate surgical drainage (which additionally allows identification of the organism), with prolonged antibiotic therapy (mean duration five months). *Actinomyces* spp. are usually extremely susceptible to beta-lactams, and the drugs of choice are penicillin G or amoxicillin. As *Actinomyces* spp. do not produce beta-lactamases, combining amoxicillin with beta-lactam inhibitors such as clavulanic acid is not useful, unless there is coinfection with pathogens such as *Enterobacteriaceae*. Treatment duration is typically guided by the initial disease burden, as well as clinical and radiological improvement and should be individualized. Because of the indolent nature of these infections and the high rate of recurrence, prolonged treatment of at least six months is recommended [17].

Predictors of poor outcome include inappropriate antibiotic therapy, needle aspiration rather than open drainage or surgical excision, and delayed diagnosis and treatment (more than two months after disease onset) [6].

Conclusions

Cerebral actinomycosis is an uncommon, potentially life-threatening infection. Long delay in diagnosis is to the result of the difficulty of clinical diagnosis and detection of *Actinomyces* species. Pathologic examination of infective material is crucial and is a fast method to identify these pathogens because timely diagnosis impacts postoperative treatment and prognosis.

References

1. Plummer, P.J.G. (1946). Actinomycosis histological differentiation of actinomycosis and actinobacilliosis. *Can. J. Comp. Med. Vet. Sci.* 10: 331–371.
2. Ponfick, E. (1882). Die Aktinomycose des Menschen. In: *Die Actinomykose des Menschen eine neue Infectionskrankheit auf vergeiehend-pathologischer und experimenteller Grundlage geschildert*. Berlin: A Hirschwald.
3. Sanford, A. and Voelker, M. (1925). Actinomycosis in the United States. *Arch. Surg.* 11: 809–841.
4. Friedman, E.D. and Levy, H.H. (1937). Actinomycotic infection of the central nervous system: report of a case and review of the literature. *Int. Clin.* 2: 36–61.
5. Bolton, C.F. and Ashenhurst, E.M. (1964). Actinomycosis of the brain: case report and review of the literature. *Can. Med. Assoc. J.* 90: 922–928.
6. Smego, R.A. (1987). Actinomycosis of the central nervous system. *Rev. Infect. Dis.* 9: 855–865.
7. Valour, F., Sénéchal, A., Dupieux, C. et al. (2014). Actinomycosis: etiology, clinical features, diagnosis, treatment, and management. *Infect. Drug Resist.* 7: 183–197.

8. Liotier, J., Venet, C., Chambonnière, M.-L. et al. (2004). Multiple actinomycosis brain abscesses. *Presse Med.* 33: 318–320.
9. Clancy, U., Ronayne, A., Prentice, M.B., and Jackson, A. (2015). Actinomyces meyeri brain abscess following dental extraction. *BMJ Case Rep.* pii: bcr2014207548.
10. Louerat, C., Depagne, C., Nesme, P. et al. (2005). Disseminated actinomycosis. *Rev. Mal. Respir.* 22: 473–476.
11. Ravindra, N., Sadashiva, N., Mahadevan, A. et al. (2018). Central nervous system actinomycosis-A clinicoradiologic and histopathologic analysis. *World Neurosurg.* 116: e362–e370.
12. Bononi, F., Iazzetti, A.V., and Silva, N.S. (2001). Pediatric cervicofacial actinomycosis – case report and review of the literature. *J. Pediatr.* 77: 52–54.
13. Na, K.Y., Jang, J.H., Sung, J.Y. et al. (2013). Actinomycotic brain abscess developed 10 years after head trauma. *Korean J. Pathol.* 47: 82–85.
14. Winking, M., Deinsberger, W., Schindler, C. et al. (1996). Cerebral manifestation of an actinomycosis infection. A case report. *J. Neurosurg. Sci.* 40: 145–148.
15. Wang, S., Wolf, R.L., Woo, J.H. et al. (2006). Actinomycotic brain infection: registered diffusion, perfusion MR imaging and MR spectroscopy. *Neuroradiology* 48: 346–350.
16. Ismail, N.J., Bot, G.M., Sahabi, S. et al. (1987). Subdural actinomycoma presenting as recurrent chronic subdural hematoma. *Rev. Infect. Dis.* 9: 855–865.
17. Adeyemi, O.A., Gottardi-Littell, N., Muro, K. et al. (2008). Multiple brain abscesses due to Actinomyces species. *Clin. Neurol. Neurosurg.* 110: 847–849.
18. Wong, V.K., Turmezei, T.D., and Weston, V.C. (2011). Actinomycosis. *BMJ* 343: d6099.
19. Roth, J. and Ram, Z. (2010). Intracranial infections caused by Actinomyces species. *World Neurosurg.* 74: 261–262.
20. Haggerty, C.J. and Tender, G.C. (2012). Actinomycotic brain abscess and subdural empyema of odontogenic origin: case report and review of the literature. *J. Oral Maxillofac. Surg.* 70: e210–e213.
21. Akhaddar, A., Elouennass, M., Baallal, H., and Boucetta, M. (2010). Focal intracranial infections due to *Actinomyces* species in immunocompetent patients: diagnostic and therapeutic challenges. *World Neurosurg.* 74: 346–350.
22. Budenz, C.L., Tajudeen, B.A., and Roehm, P.C. (2010). Actinomycosis of the temporal bone and brain: case report and review of the literature. *Ann. Otol. Rhinol. Laryngol.* 119: 313–318.
23. Figdor, D. and Davies, J. (1997). Cell surface structures of Actinomyces israelii. *Aust. Dent. J.* 42: 125–128.
24. Sullivan, D.C. and Chapman, S.W. (2010). Bacteria that masquerade as fungi: actinomycosis/nocardia. *Proc. Am. Thorac. Soc.* 7: 216–221.
25. Clarridge, J.E. and Zhang, Q. (2002). Genotypic diversity of clinical *Actinomyces* species: phenotype, source, and disease correlation among genospecies. *J. Clin. Microbiol.* 40: 3442–3448.
26. Hall, V., Talbot, P.R., Stubbs, S.L., and Duerden, B.I. (2001). Identification of clinical isolates of Actinomyces species by amplified 16S ribosomal DNA restriction analysis. *J. Clin. Microbiol.* 39: 3555–3562.

35 Cerebral Nocardiosis

Arnault Tauziede-Espariat[1,2] and Leroy R. Sharer[3]

[1] Department of Neuropathology, Sainte Anne Hospital, Paris, France
[2] Paris University, Paris, France
[3] Division of Neuropathology, Department of Pathology, Immunology, and Laboratory Medicine, Rutgers New Jersey Medical School and University Hospital, Newark, NJ, USA

Abbreviations

16s rRNA	16s ribosomal ribonucleic acid
ADC	apparent diffusion coefficient
AIDS	acquired immunodeficiency syndrome
CNS	central nervous system
CSF	cerebrospinal fluid
HIV	human immunodeficiency virus
MRI	magnetic resonance imaging
PCR	polymerase chain reaction
spp.	species

Definition

The genus *Nocardia* was first isolated by a veterinarian, Edmond Nocard, in 1888 from a case of bovine farcy (lymphadenitis). One year later, Trevisan characterized the organism and named it *Nocardia farcinica*.

Microbiological characteristics

Nocardia spp. are ubiquitous in the environment, particularly in the soil but also in water and decaying organic matter. *Nocardia* primary infection results from inhalation or aspiration of the organism or direct post-traumatic cutaneous inoculation [1].

Nocardia spp. are members of the filamentous Gram-positive order Actinobacteria, which also includes the Actinomycetaceae family, including *Actinomyces israeli*, and the Nocardiaceae family, including the *Nocardia asteroides* complex and the *Nocardia brasiliensis* complex. The genus *Nocardia* consists of 87 species, of which 46 are considered to be medically relevant. Modern methods have separated *Nocardia cyriacigeorgica*, *N. farcinica*, and *N. nova* from the *N. asteroides* complex, whereas *Nocardia pseudobrasiliensis* has been separated from the *N. brasiliensis* complex [2].

Epidemiology

Nocardia spp. can cause cutaneous lesions because of direct exposure and, with inhalation, pulmonary disease. Disseminated *Nocardia* spp. infection has a high incidence of CNS involvement, particularly brain abscess but also meningitis with the primary source being pulmonary infection. Although dissemination and CNS involvement have been reported in patients who are immunocompetent [3, 4], they are more common in patients who are immune compromised, particularly with regard to

Infections of the Central Nervous System: Pathology and Genetics, First Edition. Edited by Fabrice Chrétien, Kum Thong Wong, Leroy R. Sharer, Catherine (Katy) Keohane and Françoise Gray.
© 2020 John Wiley & Sons Ltd. Published 2020 by John Wiley & Sons Ltd.

cell-mediated immunity. Surprisingly, relatively few cases have been described in patients who are seropositive for human immunodeficiency virus (HIV); (only around 5% of all patients with CNS *Nocardia*) [5–8]. This might be explained by a protective effect of trimethoprim-sulfamethoxazole used in prophylaxis against pneumocystis and toxoplasmosis in patients with HIV because this drug combination is the treatment of choice for nocardiosis. In general, bacterial brain abscesses are infrequent in patients with human immunodeficiency virus type 1 (HIV-1) infection and acquired immunodeficiency syndrome (AIDS), except in intravenous drug users. However, *Nocardia* spp. are one of the more frequently encountered bacteria in the CNS in this patient population. Transplantation, particularly renal transplantation, is a frequent risk factor of disseminated or CNS nocardiosis [7, 9], as is diabetes mellitus [10]. CNS *Nocardia* abscesses result from hematogenous dissemination, and in most reported cases, there is some evidence of concomitant primary pulmonary infection [9]. The incidence of CNS nocardiosis has been increasing in tandem with the number of patients undergoing transplantations, and with patients with AIDS.

Nocardiosis can be a diagnostic challenge. Some species are nonculturable, and others grow slowly, so that diagnosis by culture can take up to two weeks. Also, a contaminating organism can overgrow the culture before *Nocardia* grows [10]. *Nocardia* spp. are strictly aerobic bacteria (and very fragile in culture), nonmotile, and urease- and catalase-positive bacilli. Moreover, conventional phenotypic characterization of the strains is very time-consuming compared to genomic methods.

Clinical features

Neurological symptoms of *Nocardia* abscess are highly variable and generally insidious. Most often, there are signs of a slowly expanding mass lesion with neurologic findings related to the site of the CNS abscess. Classically, it is a single cerebral lesion, but exceptionally it may be located in the cerebellum [1, 11]. Multiple CNS abscesses may occur in cases of disseminated nocardiosis [12]. In brain, abscesses are most common in the cortical area, explaining seizures and neurological deficits, which are the most frequent clinical signs [7]. Fever or clinical signs of sepsis are lacking in most cases but may be present, particularly in disseminated nocardiosis [12].

Magnetic resonance imaging (MRI) is the best tool to diagnose CNS abscesses resulting from *Nocardia* spp. The appearance on imaging is similar to that of other brain abscesses. Generally, MRI demonstrates a lobulated mass with a necrotic center, surrounded by marked peripheral vasogenic edema. There is hyperintensity on T2-weighted MRI and rim enhancement following contrast. Spectroscopic features include the presence of lactate and an increase of the choline peak and choline-to-N-acetyl aspartate ratio in the enhancing areas. Restricted diffusion on apparent diffusion coefficient (ADC) is consistent with abscess, but necrotic brain metastases and primary brain tumors are possible differential diagnoses.

MRI criteria have been proposed to distinguish brain abscesses from neoplasms, but these signs have low specificity (the hypointense capsule and the absence of a smooth inner wall in abscesses) [13]. However, numerous cases mimicking brain metastases or primary tumors [13], have been reported. In exceptional cases, the clinical and radiological diagnosis was infarction [14].

Leukocytosis and signs of an inflammatory syndrome are frequently absent [1, 14]. Classically, blood culture has no growth, and the cerebrospinal fluid (CSF) is sterile [12, 13].

Pathology

The *N. asteroides* complex is the most common *Nocardia* species infecting the CNS. Diagnosis of a brain abscess resulting from *Nocardia* spp. is usually made by biopsy or excision of the lesion, with aerobic culture or identification by molecular techniques. On histology, the organism tends to be filamentous, beaded, branching, and weakly Gram-positive (Figure 35.1). The filaments are about 1 μm in diameter, distinguishing them from filamentous fungi (typically 3 μm or greater in width). The organisms can also be stained with the modified Kinyoun acid-fast stain, using 1% sulfuric acid

Cerebral Nocardiosis Chapter 35

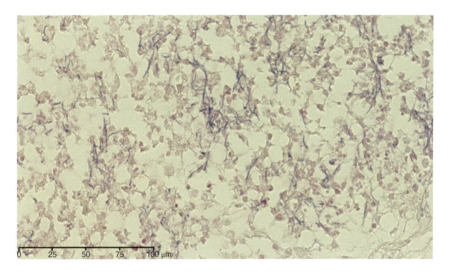

Figure 35.1 Typical beaded, filamentous appearance of *Nocardia farcinica*. (Brown-Brenn Gram stain, magnification 200×.)

(H_2SO_4), rather than the more acidic 5% hydrochloric acid (HCl), as part of the staining procedure [15]. In addition, they can be stained with either the Grocott or Gomori methenamine silver (GMS) stains for fungi (Figure 35.2), stained for longer than usual (up to one hour). A brain abscess resulting from *Nocardia* spp. is histologically similar to most bacterial abscesses, with necrosis and polymorphonuclear leukocytes (Figure 35.3), variable amounts of fibrosis, and reactive gliosis in the surrounding parenchyma. A granulomatous reaction is rarely observed and multinucleated giant cells are exceptional. The filamentous forms cannot be recognized with routine stains.

Genetics

Nocardia isolates are reliably and rapidly identified by sequence analysis of the 16S rRNA gene, and molecular diagnosis may become more important because of increasing resistance of *Nocardia* species to antibiotics, as well as the lengthy time for culture and the potential overgrowth by other

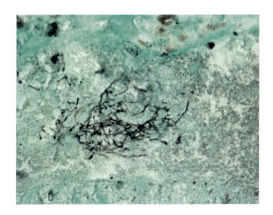

Figure 35.2 Filamentous, slender *Nocardia* organisms, stereotactic brain biopsy, 58-year-old woman with acquired immunodeficiency syndrome (AIDS). (Grocott methenamine silver stain, magnification 200×.)

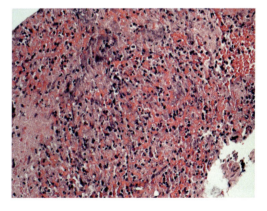

Figure 35.3 *Nocardia* abscess, 58-year-old woman with acquired immunodeficiency syndrome (AIDS), with necrosis, polymorphonuclear leukocytes and hemorrhage. (Hematoxylin and eosin [H&E] stain, magnification 50×.)

organisms. To avoid misinterpretation, molecular techniques should be used in combination with histopathologic features. One study showed almost 20% of *Nocardia* species isolated from clinical specimens were found not to be associated with clinical infection [16]. *Nocardia* species are not saprophytes of humans, so these false-positive cases result from transient colonization. Molecular diagnosis does not replace antimicrobial susceptibility patterns, and species identification is important due to species-specific differences [17]. The gold standard antibiotic in nocardiosis is trimethoprim-sulfamethoxazole, which penetrates the CSF [18]. However, *Nocardia otitidiscaviarum* is resistant to this drug [19].

Treatment

The mortality rate of patients with *Nocardia* brain abscesses is more than three times higher than those from other bacteria [7]. The poor prognosis is the result of multiple factors, including immunodeficiency, delayed diagnosis, and the presence of multiple abscesses.

Combination therapy with a carbapenem or a third-generation cephalosporin is generally recommended for severe disease or CNS involvement. Antibiotic susceptibility testing is essential because all species do not have the same sensitivity [20].

Because the abscesses form multilobulated thick-walled lesions, surgical excision is usually required in most cases. The type of surgery remains controversial. Craniotomy and total removal of the lesion is recommended for abscesses larger than 2.5 cm in diameter, for abscesses that enlarge after two weeks of antibiotic therapy, and for abscesses that fail to shrink after four weeks of antibiotics [3, 4, 11, 12, 21]. Stereotactic aspiration and drainage combined with antibiotics is also considered suitable and has the advantage of reduced risk and a lower prevalence of postoperative epilepsy.

Predictors of poor outcome include inappropriate antibiotic therapy, needle aspiration rather than open drainage or surgical excision, and delayed diagnosis and treatment (more than two months after disease onset).

Conclusions

Nocardiosis is rare and may infect the brain, particularly in patients who are immunodeficient. Pathologic examination of infective material is imperative and constitutes a fast method to identify the pathogen because a timely diagnosis can impact on postoperative treatment and prognosis. Newer techniques, such as next-generation sequencing, may help in identification of the organisms.

References

1. Arends, J.E., Stemerding, A.M., Vorst, S.P. et al. (2011). First report of a brain abscess caused by *Nocardia veterana*. *J. Clin. Microbiol.* 49: 4364–4365.
2. Bell, M., McNeil, M.M., Brown, J.M. (2014). *Nocardia* species (Nocardiosis). http://www.antimicrobe.org/b117.asp (accessed 31 October 2018).
3. Menkü, A., Kurtsoy, A., Tucer, B. et al. (2004). *Nocardia* brain abscess mimicking brain tumour in immunocompetent patients: report of two cases and review of the literature. *Acta Neurochir.* 146: 411–414. discussion 414.
4. Al Tawfiq, J.A., Mayman, T., and Memish, Z.A. (2013). *Nocardia abscessus* brain abscess in an immunocompetent host. *J. Infect. Public Health* 6: 158–161.
5. Barnaud, G., Deschamps, C., Manceron, V. et al. (2005). Brain abscess caused by *Nocardia cyriacigeorgica* in a patient with human immunodeficiency virus infection. *J. Clin. Microbiol.* 43: 4895–4897.
6. Diego, C., Ambrosioni, J.C., Abel, G. et al. (2005). Disseminated nocardiosis caused by *Nocardia abscessus* in an HIV-infected patient: first reported case. *AIDS* 19: 1330–1331.
7. Mamelak, A.N., Obana, W.G., Flaherty, J.F., and Rosenblum, M.L. (1994). Nocardial brain abscess: treatment strategies and factors influencing outcome. *Neurosurgery* 35: 622–631.
8. Godreuil, S., Didelot, M.-N., Perez, C. et al. (2003). *Nocardia veterana* isolated from ascitic fluid of a patient with human immunodeficiency virus infection. *J. Clin. Microbiol.* 41: 2768–2773.
9. Palomares, M., Martinez, T., Pastor, J. et al. (1999). Cerebral abscess caused by *Nocardia asteroides* in renal transplant recipient. *Nephrol. Dial. Transplant.* 14: 2950–2952.

10. Tatti, K.M., Shieh, W.-J., Phillips, S. et al. (2006). Molecular diagnosis of *Nocardia farcinica* from a cerebral abscess. *Hum. Pathol.* 37: 1117–1121.
11. Oktem, I.S., Akdemir, H., Sümerkan, B. et al. (1999). Cerebellar abscess due to *Nocardia asteroides*. *Acta Neurochir.* 141: 217–218.
12. Piau, C., Kerjouan, M., Le Mouel, M. et al. (2015). First case of disseminated infection with *Nocardia cerradoensis* in a human. *J. Clin. Microbiol.* 53: 1034–1037.
13. Cianfoni, A., Calandrelli, R., De Bonis, P. et al. (2010). *Nocardia* brain abscess mimicking high-grade necrotic tumour on perfusion MRI. *J. Clin. Neurosci.* 17: 1080–1082.
14. Börm, W. and Gleixner, M. (2003). *Nocardia* brain abscess misinterpreted as cerebral infarction. *J. Clin. Neurosci.* 10: 130–132.
15. Wilson, J.W. (2012). Nocardiosis: update and clinical review. *Mayo Clin. Proc.* 87: 403–407.
16. Georghiou, P.R. and Blacklock, Z.M. (1992). Infection with *Nocardia* species in Queensland. A review of 102 clinical isolates. *Med. J. Aust.* 156: 692–697.
17. Tanaka, Y., Yazawa, K., Dabbs, E.R. et al. (1996). Different rifampicin inactivation mechanisms in *Nocardia* and related taxa. *Microbiol. Immunol.* 40: 1–4.
18. Torres, O.H., Domingo, P., Pericas, R. et al. (2000). Infection caused by *Nocardia farcinica*: case report and review. *Eur. J. Clin. Microbiol. Infect. Dis.* 19: 205–212.
19. Ishihara, M., Takada, D., Sugimoto, K. et al. (2014). Primary brain abscess caused by *Nocardia otitidiscaviarum*. *Intern. Med. Tokyo Jpn.* 53: 2007–2012.
20. Yorke, R.F. and Rouah, E. (2003). Nocardiosis with brain abscess due to an unusual species, *Nocardia transvalensis*. *Arch. Pathol. Lab. Med.* 127: 224–226.
21. Hashimoto, M., Johkura, K., Ichikawa, T., and Shinonaga, M. (2008). Brain abscess caused by *Nocardia nova*. *J. Clin. Neurosci.* 15: 87–89.

36 CNS Tuberculosis

Michael A. Farrell[1], Eoin R. Feeney[2], and Jane B. Cryan[1]

[1] Department of Neuropathology, Beaumont Hospital, Dublin, Ireland
[2] Department of Infectious Diseases, St. Vincent's Hospital, Dublin, Ireland

Abbreviations

AFB	acid-fast bacilli
ART	antiretroviral therapy
CNS	central nervous system
CT	computed tomography
DNA	deoxyribonucleic acid
HIV	human immunodeficiency virus
IRIS	immune reconstitution inflammatory response
MDR	multidrug resistant
MRI	magnetic resonance imaging
MAC	*Mycobacterium avium* complex
MTB	*Mycobacterium tuberculosis*
MTBC	*Mycobacterium tuberculosis* complex
PCR	polymerase chain reaction
PDR	pan drug resistant
RIF	rifampicin
TB	tuberculosis
TBM	tuberculous meningitis
TNF	tumor necrosis factor
TST	tuberculin skin testing
XDR	extensively drug resistant

Introduction

Despite progress in diagnosis, treatment, and improved living standards, infection with the *Mycobacterium tuberculosis* complex (MTBC) results in over 10 million new cases of tuberculosis (TB) worldwide, with more than 1.5 million deaths annually [1]. A quarter of the world's population has latent TB infection. Although there are at least 10 species in the MTBC (there are at least 170 described species of the genus *Mycobacterium*), only *Mycobacterium tuberculosis* (MTB) affecting the CNS will be discussed here.

Definition of the disorder, major synonyms, and historical perspective

TB is an infectious granulomatous disease caused by the acid-fast, aerobic bacillus, MTB. TB primarily affects the distal airways but may involve the CNS through hematogenous dissemination arising from either primary pulmonary infection (i.e.

Infections of the Central Nervous System: Pathology and Genetics, First Edition. Edited by Fabrice Chrétien, Kum Thong Wong, Leroy R. Sharer, Catherine (Katy) Keohane and Françoise Gray.
© 2020 John Wiley & Sons Ltd. Published 2020 by John Wiley & Sons Ltd.

miliary TB) or through late reactivation of tuberculous infection elsewhere. TB is the leading single infectious cause of death worldwide. The emergence of drug-resistant (multidrug-resistant [MDR]; extensively drug-resistant [XDR] and pan drug-resistant ([PDR]) strains of MTB has necessitated an ongoing need for rapid laboratory determination of drug sensitivities.

TB was known as "consumption" and "phthisis" (from the Greek meaning "wasting"). Because of the pallor of many patients it was also called "the white plague".

Although it is suspected that TB dates from very ancient times, the first written descriptions come from India more than 3000 years ago. The disease has been recognized as contagious since the sixteenth century. The first illustrated pathological description was by Francis Sylvius in 1679. Vertebral collapse with paralysis due to spinal cord compression became known as Pott disease following the description by Sir Percival Pott in 1779, but spinal TB has been identified in the remains of individuals who were buried in South Siberia during the Iron Age [2]. The tubercle bacillus was isolated, cultured, and transmitted to laboratory animals by Robert Koch in 1882. Bacillus Calmette-Guérin (BCG) vaccine was developed by 1920, and streptomycin, the first effective drug treatment for TB, was discovered in 1943. In historic 1930s' experiments Arnold Rich and Howard McCordock showed that during a tuberculous bacteremia the brain is seeded with MTB, resulting in the formation of cerebral granulomas and tubercles. For more detailed history see [3].

Microbiological characteristics

MTB, an obligate aerobic and facultative intracellular bacterium is neither Gram positive nor Gram negative but is identified by Ziehl–Neelsen (ZN) or auramine fluorescent staining. Characterized by a lipid-rich envelope, it is extremely slow growing. In contrast to virtually all other bacteria, MTB is capable of adapting to hostile environments and of prolonged quiescent survival within macrophages (and granulomas) and neutrophils. Almost certainly, MTB represents the end result of an adapted environmental organism that, through multiple genetic events over thousands of years, has become an obligate human pathogen, spread by aerosol from human to human without any intervening animal or environmental reservoir. MTB has a single circular chromosome of approximately 4.4 Mb and shows low DNA sequence diversity [4]. There is very little evidence to support horizontal transfer of genes between MTB strains. Furthermore, it has not been possible to ascribe virulence and transmissibility to particular gene sequences. By contrast, antibiotic resistance, a devastating feature of MTB, reflects complex interactions over time between drug-resistant– and drug-sensitivity–conferring mutations [5].

Epidemiology

Each year since 1997, the World Health Organization (WHO) has reported its up-to-date assessment of the TB epidemic and its progress in prevention, diagnosis, and treatment at global, regional, and country levels [6]. The report highlights progress or lack of progress in reaching the goals of a 90% reduction in TB deaths and an 80% reduction in TB incidence by 2030, compared with 2015. As of 2018, the targets are unlikely to be met unless there are substantial improvements in global health care through improved social and economic conditions. In 2016, India, Pakistan, Philippines, China, and Indonesia accounted for 56% of the 10.4 million people who developed TB, and India, China, and the Russian Federation accounted for 47% of nearly 600 000 notified cases of drug-resistant TB. Children younger than age 15 accounted for 6.9% of new TB cases in 2016. Although TB mortality and incidence continue to decline (3 and 2%, respective yearly falls), the rate of fall is insufficient to reach the first targets set for 2020. Challenges to improving health care vary from region to region. Currently the fastest declines in TB mortality are in the WHO European and the WHO Western Pacific Regions. Coexistent human immunodeficiency virus (HIV) remains high at 57% of notified TB cases in 2016 worldwide, with rates of more than 80% in WHO African regions.

Clinicopathological presentations and diagnosis

CNS TB may present clinically with meningitis (subacute or chronic), an intracranial mass lesion (tuberculoma or abscess), or with spinal symptoms through involvement of spinal meninges, roots, ligaments, and vertebral bodies. An overriding problem for diagnosis is the pauci-bacillary nature of CNS TB. Additionally, the CNS may be profoundly compromised by an associated endarteritis obliterans with risk of infarction. Tuberculous meningitis (TBM) [7] is the most frequently encountered clinical form of neurological TB in low-prevalence countries. Where TB is widespread, all forms of neurological involvement occur with equal frequency. Even with adequate drug therapy, long-term neurological complications of resolving meningeal inflammation ensue in more than 50% of survivors and include shunt-dependent hydrocephalus, any cranial neuropathy, epilepsy, cognitive impairment, and hypothalamic-pituitary insufficiency.

Tuberculous meningitis
Diagnostic criteria

In the absence of acid-fast bacilli (AFB) in cerebrospinal fluid (CSF), it is difficult to establish a diagnosis of TBM. In the context of symptoms and signs of meningitis; that is, standard clinical entry criteria (CEC), a four-tiered classification system of diagnostic certainty has been proposed [8] based on points awarded for individual clinical criteria (6 points), CSF findings (4 points), and brain-imaging criteria (6 points), coupled with evidence of disease elsewhere (4 points) and exclusion of alternative diagnoses. Definite TBM is present when patients have CEC with evidence of AFB in CSF. Probable TBM is indicated if the total diagnostic score is ≥10 without, and 12 with, brain imaging, but at least 2 points must come from either the clinical or CSF criteria. Scores of 6–9 without and 6–11 with brain imaging indicate possible TBM (again CSF and imaging findings must be included). Remarkably, classic symptoms of meningitis (i.e. headache, drowsiness, photophobia, vomiting) may be minimal or even absent in the presence of a brisk basal meningeal exudate. Active disease elsewhere in the lungs or in other organs may not be evident, even at autopsy.

Pathology

Following seeding of the brain, enlarging coalescing and necrotic granulomas (Rich foci) impinge on the meninges or the ventricular ependymal lining with discharge of live mycobacteria into the subarachnoid space and CSF. The duration and degree of tuberculous bacillemia, coupled with the strain of MTB and the host's immune competence or otherwise to resolve developing cerebral granulomas, dictates the propensity for development of TBM. Having discharged into the subarachnoid space (or ventricle) a brisk-mixed polymorphonuclear, lymphocytic, histiocytic-inflammatory exudate develops, invariably over the base of the brain and involves cranial nerves, branches of the circle of Willis, and the foramina of Luschka [Figure 36.1a]. Tubercle bacilli are usually readily apparent in the exudate with ZN stain [Figure 36.1b]. Epithelioid and multinucleate giant cells accumulate; caseating granulomata with central necrosis can also be seen. Vessels including large vessels may show endarteritis obliterans leading to ischemic complications [Figure 36.1c and d]. The exudate becomes organized and fibrotic relatively quickly.

TB meningitis and diagnosis – Practical aspects of diagnosis

In a lymphocytic CSF, a very high protein >1 g/l, associated with a plasma glucose ratio of <50% or an absolute CSF glucose concentration <2.2 mmol/l is strongly suggestive of TBM and is highly unlikely to be found in any condition other than meningeal carcinomatosis and lymphomatosis. CSF cytology should assist in eliminating malignancy. It is unwise to rely on neuroimaging to separate TBM from malignant meningitis. CSF staining for AFB has low sensitivity and specificity but can be improved by large-volume CSF sampling (>6 ml) and by careful microscopy (at least 30 minutes) looking at both ZN- and auramine-stained cytospun CSF. A sensitivity of approximately 15% for microscopy contrasts with 50–70% sensitivity for CSF culture, but culture often requires up to six to eight weeks because of the slow growth rate of MTB.

Infections of the Central Nervous System

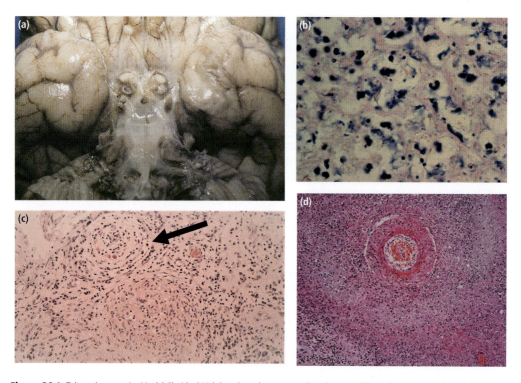

Figure 36.1 Tuberculous meningitis. (a) Florid whitish basal exudate surrounding the optic chiasm, brainstem, and cranial nerves in a child with tuberculous meningitis. (Source: Courtesy of Prof. C. Keohane). (b) Numerous acid-fast bacilli in basal meninges; Ziehl-Neelsen (ZN) stain. The organisms are stained pink and have a slightly curved shape. (c) Meningeal exudate showing central granuloma with small artery (arrowed) showing marked endarteritis. (d) Extensive fibrinoid necrosis in an artery, surrounded by a dense basal meningeal tuberculous exudate. Same case as Figure 35.1a. (Source: Courtesy of Prof. C Keohane).

The Xpert MTB/RIF, a polymerase chain reaction (PCR)-based automated nucleic acid amplification diagnostic test that can identify MTB DNA and resistance to rifampicin (RIF) was endorsed by the WHO in 2014 as the test of choice in suspected TBM cases. Its sensitivity when measured in a meta-analysis against clinical case definition and CSF culture positivity was 62.8% and 80.5%, respectively, meaning that the Xpert MTB/RIF could not be used to exclude TBM.

The newer Xpert MTB/RIF Ultra test appears to show greater sensitivity and specificity, even in HIV coinfection [9, 10]. This sensitivity may partly relate to its ability to detect dead tubercle bacilli. In the absence of a rapid test for viable tubercle bacilli, undoubtedly some patients will receive treatment for dead bacilli!

Although the Xpert/Ultra has also been endorsed by the WHO, it remains to be seen if it can yield similar sensitivities using lower CSF volumes. It is unlikely that any PCR-based CSF analysis of MTB can completely exclude TBM. Even with newer diagnostics, clinical judgment will remain paramount in deciding whether to initiate treatment in clinically suspected TBM [11]. Clinical expertise varies between regions of high and low TB prevalence; disease familiarity in the former probably surpasses all negative diagnostics in cases of suspected TB.

Finally, it is emphasized that patients suspected of having TBM should undergo an imaging-based search for TB outside the CNS. Invasive respiratory sampling may yield a positive culture with valuable information on drug sensitivity not otherwise available from CSF.

The differential diagnosis of persistent chronic, predominantly lymphocytic meningitis is discussed in Chapter 40. Dexamethasone adjunctive treatment is associated with reduced mortality in TBM,

CNS Tuberculosis Chapter 36

but reduced long-term morbidity and the role of steroids in HIV coinfection has not been conclusively demonstrated.

Spinal tuberculosis

Spinal TB results from hematogenous spread to the vertebral body vascular plexus from sites such as lung or kidney. Typically, there is spondylitis with vertebral body collapse and resultant kyphosis but with disc preservation, at least until late in the disease. Involvement of the posterior spinal elements is usually secondary to vertebral body involvement and rarely occurs in isolation [12, 13].

Before vertebral collapse, vertebral imaging may show signal abnormalities with contrast enhancement. With vertebral collapse, bony debris and pus is forced into the spinal canal with probable cord compression. Paraspinal pus may be present and reach an enormous size and, depending on cervical, thoracic or lumbar location, cause dysphagia, respiratory distress, or manifest as a groin or thigh swelling. Neurologic involvement as a compressive myelopathy or radiculomyelitis is common. It is important that radiculomyelitis may occur in the absence of bony destruction or TBM. An abscess or tuberculoma may form in the subdural and epidural spinal spaces. Intramedullary tuberculomas are very rare. Isolated tuberculous myelitis is rare and appears radiologically as longitudinally extensive myelitis. The differential diagnosis is broad, especially if a patient with systemic TB is immunocompromised or coinfected with HIV. Generally, confirmation that myelitis is tuberculous is only possible at postmortem examination.

Tuberculoma

Instead of rupturing into the subarachnoid space or ventricle, a Rich focus may continue to grow, becoming large enough to cause symptoms of a mass lesion (Figure 36.2a). Intracranial tuberculomas, either single or multiple, may occur with, or independently of, TBM.

As with any intracranial mass lesion, presentation is dictated by location, size, and rapidity of growth, though tuberculomas are usually slow

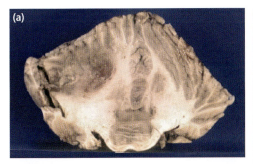
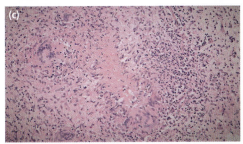
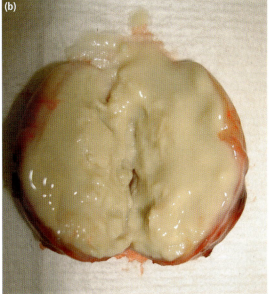

Figure 36.2 Tuberculoma. (a) Cerebellar tuberculous mass. lesion in a 56 year-old man with human immunodeficiency virus (HIV) with acutely raised intracranial pressure. (b) Intracerebral tuberculous abscess filled with caseous material resected from a five-year-old child. *Mycobacterium tuberculosis* was cultured from the caseous contents. (Source: Courtesy of Prof. C Keohane). (c) Cerebellar tuberculoma showing central caseous necrosis surrounded by multinucleate giant cells.

growing [14]. Clinical evidence of a tuberculoma may emerge during commencement of therapy for TB or occasionally during initiation of antiretroviral therapy (ART) for HIV infection. Computed tomography (CT) imaging is sensitive but not specific, and although MRI specificity is greater, CT has the added advantage of being able to demonstrate meningeal involvement and extracranial foci of TB. Radiologic expertise and diagnostic certainty, especially in regions of high TB prevalence, will obviate the need for biopsy in most cases.

Examination of ventricular CSF, even if supplemented by PCR, has a low diagnostic yield in patients with intracranial tuberculoma. Lumbar CSF should not be obtained if there is a suspicion of raised intracranial pressure. A tuberculous abscess [Figure 36.2b] is suggested by a fibrin-rich neutrophilic exudate surrounded by palisading epithelioid cells and sheets of foamy macrophages and is distinguished from tuberculoma by the presence of caseous necrosis in the latter [Figure 36.2c]. The pathologic differential diagnosis of a granulomatous intracranial mass lesion is discussed in Chapter 40. Imaging is vital for monitoring response to anti-TB medication and for early detection of complications such as paradoxical swelling of the tuberculoma with edema and hydrocephalus. Resource limitations may preclude regular image-based monitoring of response to treatment.

HIV/TB Co-infection

Individuals with HIV are at higher risk of TB/HIV coinfection. TB is the leading cause of death in HIV infection globally, with 400 000 deaths annually. Prevalence rates for HIV/TB coinfection show huge age and geographic variations, with up to 60% HIV prevalence in children with TB [15, 16].

In reducing the level of cellular immunity through targeting of CD4+ T lymphocytes, HIV infection increases the rate of TB infection and the likelihood of TB reactivation. In response to TB infection, HIV-infected CD4+ lymphocytes increase their replication rate with consequent increased viral production. Patients with HIV/TB also have higher incidences of both hepatitis C virus infection and infection with drug-resistant (i.e. isoniazid and rifampicin) strains of MTB.

Coexistent HIV/TB presents many diagnostic and therapeutic challenges and not least in the CNS. Overlap in symptoms and relative ease of making a HIV diagnosis, in contrast to the difficulty of MTB detection in suspected TBM, may lead to underdiagnosis of coexistent TBM [17].

Genetics

Population genetics

In MTBC infection, complex interactions exist between genetic variations in MTBC and disease distribution, together with drug resistance and genetic factors influencing the host's immune response. In patients coinfected with HIV, these associations are disrupted, reducing the relevance of the host genetic background. Application of whole-genome sequencing to the MTBC sourced from large, globally representative populations is generating important new data on the epidemiology of MTBC, especially on migration-related infection [18, 19]. The MTBC comprises seven phylogenetic lineages adapted to humans. Different MTBC sublineages vary in frequency between different geographic regions, suggesting adaptation to the local population; of these, lineage 4 (L4) is the most widely distributed. Within L4 there are at least 10 sublineages, some are geographically restricted, and others are more widely distributed. Whether these geographically restricted L4 sublineages represent founder effects with limited population mobility remains to be determined. Although the T-cell epitopes of MTBC are conserved with little antigenic variation, the more widely distributed L4 sublineages show a greater proportion of variable T-cell epitopes than geographically restricted L4 sublineages. This may simply mean a more diverse host population or possibly indicate escape of the particular L4 sublineage from the immune system.

Drug-resistance genetics

Only a few antibiotics are effective against MTBC. Apart from many extrinsic social, therapeutic, and patient-related factors contributing to MTBC antibiotic resistance, there is also evidence for a genetic contribution. MTBC is generally clonal with little horizontal gene transfer. The mutation rate in

MTBC is low, but the large numbers of bacteria (i.e. a large target size) in any individual infected means that resistant strains are destined to emerge, especially with poor compliance, subtherapeutic antibiotic dosages, and concurrent HIV infection. MTBC harboring resistance-conferring mutations were previously thought to have reduced transmissibility on the basis of poor attenuation in animal models. It is now accepted that different drug-resistant mutations result in different transmissibility rates, raising the concept of low or no-cost mutations for which there may be positive selection in terms of the bacteria's survival. Additionally, compensatory mutations may negate the effects of drug-resistant mutations. The prevalence and effects of competing mutations or epistasis in the various MTBC lineages will ultimately dictate the future survival or extinction of both drug-resistant and drug-sensitive strains of MTBC. Mutations can be detected in the 31 genetic regions known to be involved in resistance to 12 anti-TB drugs. For practical reasons, testing for new mutations will not be possible until whole-genome sequencing is deployed in large patient populations from all geographic regions, hence the continuing importance of conventional culture-based drug-sensitivity testing.

Host immune genetics

TB has an attached stigma, especially in migrants [20], and this could be used to imply an inherent genetic defect in the newly arrived, whether Irish people fleeing the Great Famine of the 1840s or South American refugees waiting today on the US-Mexican Border. Higher concordance rates for TB in monozygotic compared to dizygotic twins added to the idea of an intrinsic host genetic defect. Children with very rare primary immune-deficiency disorders are at great risk of MTB infection. It is difficult to analyze the genetic influences interacting with the host immune system in response to an MTBC infection, which varies widely in geographic sublineage prevalence and infectivity. Evolution of the pathogen and host in terms of co-evolved genes makes the task even more complex. MTB strains may be of relatively reduced infectivity and pathogenicity in some populations, but be highly infectious and devastating in others. Any potential single candidate gene for "TB susceptibility" must be shown to act independently of the MTB strain and not be population specific. In studies of weakly virulent nontuberculous mycobacteria species, germline mutations have been discovered in genes implicated in interferon gamma (IFN-γ) function. More attractive is the concept of "TB risk" related to perturbations in immune pathways uncompromised by concurrent HIV infection. A number of immune response pathways active in MTB infection have been uncovered by pathway analysis. However, although the pathways are altered by infection and treatment, primary disease-causing immune deficits have not yet been demonstrated. Identification of latent infection as determined by tuberculin skin testing (TST) and interferon-gamma is of itself heritable. Of interest is the finding of a TST locus (*TST1*), which may well be identical to the tumor necrosis factor locus (*TNF1*), raising the possibility that innate resistance to MTB might be partly mediated through a TNF-related mechanism [21].

Animal models

Small animals have been extensively used to study susceptibility to TB, with several loci mapped. Animal models of coinfection with HIV have also been developed by deploying genetically humanized mice, or Macaque monkeys infected with Simian immunodeficiency virus (SIV). Animal models of CNS TB infection have been particularly useful to evaluate vaccines and drugs used to prevent and manage CNS TB [22].

Treatment, future perspective, and conclusions

Generally, the drug treatment of TBM deploys the same drugs used in pulmonary TB. The management of raised intracranial pressure and hydrocephalus requires neurosurgical surveillance and support in TBM but especially in intracranial tuberculoma. Paradoxical increase in tuberculoma size may cause acute neurological deterioration. Hyponatremia is a particularly difficult problem to manage. Addition of corticosteroids has a survival benefit but no effect on long-term morbidity. Drug-drug interactions between combination ART and medications for TB are common. Treatment of HIV in advance of treating TB may, through an improved immune response lead to an immune reconstitution inflammatory response (IRIS), which can be fatal [15]. In contrast to HIV-naive TBM, dexamethasone adjunctive treatment is not associated with reduced mortality in HIV/TBM and the long-term morbidity of HIV/TBM is not reduced, but dexamethasone has a role in management of IRIS. Spinal TB is primarily managed medically. Surgery is required when there is a neurological deficit, a developing spinal deformity, or when biopsy is required for diagnosis. Insertion of metal into the spinal region is not contraindicated because MTB is not associated with biofilm formation. Development of biomarkers for separation of latent from active disease as well as for monitoring response to treatment will be of major importance in the fight against TB in the years ahead.

References

1. Floyd, K., Glaziou, P., Zumla, A., and Raviglione, M. (2018). The global tuberculosis epidemic and progress in care, prevention, and research: an overview in year 3 of the End TB era. *Lancet Respir. Med.* 6: 299–314.
2. Taylor, G.M., Murphy, E., Hopkins, R. et al. (2007). First report of Mycobacterium bovis DNA in human remains from the Iron Age. *Microbiology* 153: 1243–1249.
3. Barberis, I., Bragazzi, N.L., Galluzzo, L. et al. (2017). The history of tuberculosis: from the first historical records to the isolation of Koch's bacillus. *J. Prev. Med. Hyg.* 58 (1): E9–E12.
4. Gagneux, S. (2018). Ecology and evolution of Mycobacterium tuberculosis. *Nat. Rev. Microbiol.* 16: 202–213.
5. Muller, B., Borrell, S., Rose, G., and gagneux, S. (2012). The heterogenous evolution of multidrug – resistant Mycobacterium tuberculosis. *Trends Genet.* 29: 160–169.
6. World Health Organization (WHO) (2017). *Global tuberculosis report*. http://www.who.int/tb/publications/global_report/en (accessed 17 July 2019).
7. Marais, S., Thwaites, G., Schoeman, J.F. et al. (2010). Tuberculous meningitis: a uniform case definition for use in clinical research. *Lancet Infect. Dis.* 10: 803–812.
8. Marais, B.J., Heemskerk, A.D., Marais, S.S. et al. (2017). Tuberculous Meningitis International Research Consortium. Standardized methods for enhanced quality and comparability of tuberculous meningitis studies. *Clin. Infect. Dis.* 64: 501–509.
9. Walzl, G., McNerney, R., du Plessis, N. et al. (2018). Tuberculosis: advances and challenges in development of new diagnostics and biomarkers. *Lancet Infect. Dis.* 18: e199–e210.
10. Bahr, N.C., Nuwagira, E., Evans, E.E. et al. ASTRO-CM Trial Team. Diagnostic accuracy of Xpert MTB/RIF Ultra for tuberculous meningitis in HIV-infected adults: a prospective cohort study. *Lancet Infect. Dis.* 18: 68–75.
11. WHO Global Tuberculosis Report (2017). Treatment of Tuberculous Meningitis and its complications in adults. *Curr. Treat. Options Neurol.* 20: 1–15.
12. Dunn, R.N. and Ben, H.M. (2018). Spinal tuberculosis. *Bone Joint J.* 100-b: 425–431.
13. Marais, S., Roos, I., Mitha, A. et al. (2018). Spinal tuberculosis: clinicoradiological findings in 274 patients. *Clin. Infect. Dis.* 67: 89–98.
14. Ramachandran, R., Muniyandi, M., Iyer, V. et al. (2017). Dilemmas in the diagnosis and treatment of intracranial tuberculomas. *J. Neurol. Sci.* 381: 256–264.
15. Granich, R. and Gupta, S. (2018). Two diseases, same person: moving toward a combined HIV and tuberculosis continuum of care. *Int. J. STD AIDS* Epub ahead of print.
16. Scott, L., da Silva, P., Boehme, C.C. et al. (2017). Diagnosis of opportunistic infections: HIV co-infections - tuberculosis. *Curr. Opin. HIV AIDS* 12: 129–138.
17. Sulis, G., Amadasi, S., Odone, A. et al. (2018). Antiretroviral therapy in HIV-infected children with tuberculosis: a systematic review. *Pediatr. Infect. Dis. J.* 37: e117–e125.
18. Abel, L., Fellay, J., Haas, D.W. et al. (2018). Genetics of human susceptibility to active and latent tuberculosis: present knowledge and future perspectives. *Lancet Infect. Dis.* 18: e64–e75.
19. Stein, C.M., Sausville, L., Wejse, C. et al. (2017). Genomics of human pulmonary tuberculosis: from genes to pathways. *Curr. Genet. Med. Rep.* 5: 149–166.
20. Christodoulou, M. (2011). The stigma of tuberculosis. *Lancet Infect. Dis.* 11: 663–664.
21. Cobat, A., Hoal, E.G., Gallant, C.J. et al. (2013). Identification of a major locus, TNF1, that controls BCG-triggered tumor necrosis factor production by leukocytes in an area hyperendemic for tuberculosis. *Clin. Infect. Dis.* 57: 963–970.
22. Sánchez-Garibay, C., Hernández-Campos, M.E., Tena-Suck, M.L. et al. (2018). Experimental animal models of central nervous system tuberculosis: A historical review. *Tuberculosis* 110: 1–6.

37 Non-Tuberculous Mycobacterial Infections

Leroy R. Sharer
Division of Neuropathology, Department of Pathology, Immunology, and Laboratory Medicine, Rutgers New Jersey Medical School and University Hospital, Newark, NJ, USA

Abbreviations

16s rRNA	16s ribosomal ribonucleic acid
AIDS	acquired immunodeficiency syndrome
CDC	Centers for Disease Control and Prevention
CNS	central nervous system
HAART	highly active antiretroviral treatment
HIV-1	human immunodeficiency virus type 1
HIV-2	human immunodeficiency virus type 2
IRIS	immune reconstitution inflammatory syndrome
MAC	*Mycobacterium avium/intracellulare* complex
MOTT	Mycobacteria other than *Mycobacterium tuberculosis*
NTM	non-tuberculous mycobacteria
PCR	polymerase chain reaction

Introduction and definition

Non-tuberculous mycobacteria (NTM) also called "atypical mycobacteria," were traditionally often considered to be saprophytic organisms. With the increase in patients who are immunocompromised, especially those suffering from acquired immunodeficiency syndrome (AIDS), the role of atypical mycobacteria in opportunistic infections has become far more important. Cases of NTM, and Mycobacteria other than *Mycobacterium tuberculosis* (MOTT) in the United States are now more numerous than tuberculosis itself [1]. Many of these species cause pulmonary or cutaneous disease, but when disseminated, they can also involve the CNS, often as opportunistic pathogens.

Microbiological characteristics and classification

The NTM in the Runyon classification are divided into four groups based on their growth characteristics in the laboratory [2]:

Runyon Class I: Photochromogens
　Growth: Slow growing
　Pigment Production: Yellow-orange when exposed to light
　Species: *Mycobacterium kansasii, Mycobacterium marinum*
Runyon Class II: Scotochromogens
　Growth: Slow growing
　Pigment Production: Yellow-orange with or without light

Infections of the Central Nervous System: Pathology and Genetics, First Edition. Edited by Fabrice Chrétien, Kum Thong Wong, Leroy R. Sharer, Catherine (Katy) Keohane and Françoise Gray.
© 2020 John Wiley & Sons Ltd. Published 2020 by John Wiley & Sons Ltd.

Species: *Mycobacterium scrofulaceum, Mycobacterium gordonae, Mycobacterium szulgai*
Runyon Class III: Nonchromogens
 Growth: Slow growing
 Pigment Production: None
 Species: *Mycobacterium avium-intracellulare, Mycobacterium xenopi, Mycobacterium terrae*
Runyon Class IV: Rapid Growers
 Growth: Rapid (mature colonies in agar in seven days)
 Pigment Production: None
 Species: *Mycobacterium fortuitum, Mycobacterium peregrinum, Mycobacterium abscessus, Mycobacterium chelonae*
Several other species have been described in this group, most recently by molecular, phylogenetic analysis of 16S rRNA.

Clinicopathological presentation

The *Mycobacterium avium/intracellulare* complex

The *Mycobacterium avium/intracellulare* complex (MAC) is an important group of Mycobacteria species including *M. avium* and *M. intracellulare*, which are closely related nonchromogens. MAC species cause systemic disease in patients who are immunocompromised, especially those with AIDS. In these patients, disseminated infection may be found at postmortem in up to 53% of cases [3].

MAC infections of the CNS are rare, even in patients with AIDS and other immune-deficient states, compared with systemic infections in these same groups. These organisms appear to infect the CNS in a relatively noninvasive manner, and in most cases, with generalized *M. avium-intracellulare* infection, involvement of the CNS cannot be correlated with any clinical symptoms. Only a few symptomatic cases have been reported [4, 5], including one isolated cerebellar infection that occurred in the absence of systemic involvement [6]. Neurological symptoms included impaired cognitive function and psychomotor slowing associated with general (fever and weight loss) and systemic (mainly gastrointestinal) symptoms. Exceptionally, MAC-related immune reconstitution inflammatory syndrome (IRIS) following highly active antiretroviral therapy (HAART) institution in patients with AIDS has also been reported [7, 8].

Cerebrospinal fluid (CSF) analysis may reveal mild lymphocytosis with normal or slightly elevated protein and normal glucose. Cultures for NTM are positive. In occasional cases with cryptococcal meningitis [9] or cytomegalovirus (CMV) encephalitis [10], *M. intracellullare* has also been identified in the CSF, reinforcing the fact that multiple infectious agents are frequent in patients with AIDS [11].

Neuropathological examination may show mild to moderate meningeal inflammation. In the cerebral parenchyma, the most characteristic change is diffuse perivascular infiltration by macrophages containing clusters of acid-fast and periodic acid-Schiff (PAS)–positive [12] mycobacteria (Figure 37.1), often associated with microglial nodules and reactive astrocytosis.

Atypical mycobacterioses of the CNS are exceptional in individuals who are immunocompetent. Cerebral abscess resulting from *M. avium*, without evidence of systemic or pulmonary involvement, has been described in patients without immunosuppression and HIV [13, 14].

An unusual manifestation of MAC infection, spindle cell pseudotumor, in which histiocytic cells are filled with MAC organisms, has been described in patients with AIDS in the CNS and elsewhere [15]. A recent case was reported in the cerebellum of a patient who did not have either AIDS or immune suppression [16].

Other species are also included in the MAC group. One such, *M. chimaera*, has recently been recognized as a contaminant in heater-cooler units used in extracorporeal circulation during cardiac surgery [17]. A recent case was discovered in a 64-year-old man who had had an aortic graft with CNS dissemination (Figures 37.2).

Mycobacterium haemophilum

A non-MAC species, *M. haemophilum*, typically infects the skin, particularly in children. *M. haemophilum* is well-known to infect zebrafish [18], and it has also been isolated from a royal python [19]. *M. haemophilum* is a slowly-growing acid-fast bacillus

Non-Tuberculous Mycobacterial Infections Chapter 37

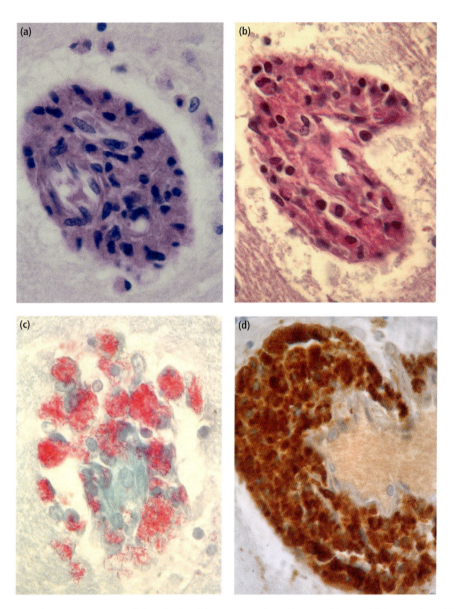

Figure 37.1 *Mycobacterium avium-intracellulare* infection of the CNS in a patient with acquired immunodeficiency syndrome (AIDS). (a) Perivascular macrophages containing granular eosinophilic material (hematoxylin and eosin [H&E]). (b) The material is positive on periodic acid-Schiff stain. (c) Ziehl-Neelsen stain shows numerous acid-fast bacilli. (d) Perivascular macrophages positively stained with CD 68 immunostain. Source: Courtesy of Professor F. Scaravilli.

that differs from all other identified *Mycobacterium* species in preferring a lower growth temperature and having a unique culture requirement for iron supplementation. Thus, the classification of NTM into several Runyon groups based on growth characteristics and pigment production may not be applicable to *M. haemophilum* [18]. Phylogenetic and gene sequence data indicate that *M. haemophilum* is more closely related to *M. leprae* than to other mycobacterial species [20]. *M. haemophilum* has recently been described as an opportunistic infection in the CNS in patients with AIDS [21–23].

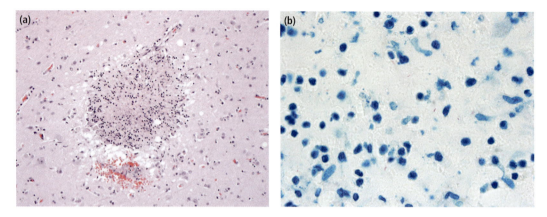

Figure 37.2 Infection by *Mycobacterium chimaera* in a 64-year-old man who had aortic replacement for aortic dissection five years before death. (a) Brain lesion with inflammation (hematoxylin and eosin [H&E]). (b) *Mycobacterium chimaera* bacilli in left frontal cortex (Kinyoun acid-fast stain). Source: Courtesy of Dr. Marco Hefti, University of Iowa Carver College of Medicine.

One report concerned a man with AIDS who had recent-onset seizures, with an intraventricular mass that was caused by *M. haemophilum* [22]. This man had a pet Burmese python, which was presumed to be the source for the infectious agent. When informed of this possibility, the patient gave the snake away before it could be cultured. On histological examination, the intraventricular mass was surrounded by a collagenous capsule containing granulomas. The interior was largely necrotic, with calcifications and extensive necrosis, as well as acid-fast bacilli (Figures 37.3). The organism was identified by polymerase chain reaction (PCR) done at the Centers for Disease Control and Prevention (the CDC) in Atlanta, Georgia. Other recent reports describe patients with AIDS who had ocular and infundibular involvement [21] and spinal cord abscesses [24] resulting from *M. haemophilum*; in both cases the organism was identified by PCR. A spindle cell tumor with combined infection with *M. haemophilum* and *M. simiae* was also reported in a patient with AIDS [25].

Involvement of the CNS by other NTB

Brain abscesses resulting from *M. kansasii* have been described in rare instances [26, 27]. *Rhodococcus equi*, a pulmonary pathogen in foals, and *Gordona terrae*, have also been reported in brain abscesses in AIDS.

Treatment

The British Thoracic Society has published an exhaustive analysis of treatment of NTM pulmonary disease, recommending three or more agents, depending on the severity of pulmonary disease and mycobacterial resistance to various agents [28].

The recommendations for severe MAC pulmonary disease can be extended for the treatment of NTM involving the CNS, using rifampicin 600 mg daily, ethambutol 15 mg/kg daily and either azithromycin 250 mg daily or clarithromycin 500 mg twice daily for a minimum of 12 months, also considering intravenous amikacin for up to 3 months. For clarithromycin-resistant MAC pulmonary disease, the British group has recommended rifampicin 600 mg daily, ethambutol 15 mg/kg daily and either isoniazid 300 mg (given with pyridoxine 10 mg) daily or moxifloxacin 400 mg daily for 12 months, also considering intravenous amikacin for up to 3 months.

The treatment regimen used for the patient with *M. haemophilum* in the right lateral ventricle, described previously, was clarithromycin, rifabutin, and ciprofloxacin. His antiretroviral regimen, which had been darunavir with ritonavir boosting, raltegravir, tenofovir, and emtricitabine, was modified to raltegravir and elvitegravir-emtricitabine to

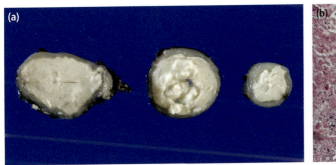
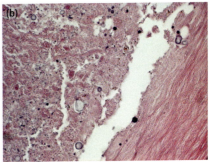
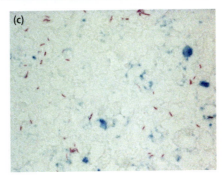

Figure 37.3 Intraventricular mass due to infection by *Mycobacterium haemophilum* bacilli in a 41-year-old man with human immunodeficiency virus type 1 (HIV-1) infection [10]. (a) Sections of intraventricular mass, resected from the right lateral ventricle. (b) Fibrous wall of intraventricular mass, with necrosis and calcifications in the interior of the mass (hematoxylin and eosin [H&E]). (c) *M. haemophilum* bacilli within the necrotic material of the intraventricular mass (Kinyoun acid-fast stain).

avoid drug interactions. He continued to be symptom-free without radiographic recurrence at 10 months postoperatively [22].

Conclusions

Although NTM infections are infrequent, they need to be considered in the differential of a patient who is immune deficient, particularly if acid-fast bacilli are found in a lesion in the CNS that does not yield *M. tuberculosis* on either culture or routine molecular methods [22].

References

1. Schluger, N.W. (2017). Moving non tuberculous mycobacteria infections into the 21st century. *Am. J. Respir. Crit. Care Med.* 196: 1507–1509.
2. Runyon, E.H. (1959). Anonymous mycobacteria in pulmonary disease. *Med. Clin. N. Am.* 43: 273–290.
3. Hawkins, C.C., Gold, J.W., Whimbey, E. et al. (1986). *Mycobacterium avium* complex infections in patients with the acquired immunodeficiency syndrome. *Ann. Intern. Med.* 105: 184–188.
4. Jacob, C.N., Henein, S.S., Heurich, A.E., and Kamholz, S. (1993). Non-tuberculous mycobacterial infection of the central nervous system in patients with AIDS. *South. Med. J.* 86: 638–640.
5. Gyure, K.A., Prayson, R.A., Estes, M.L., and Hall, G.S. (1995). Symptomatic *Mycobacterium avium* complex infection of the central nervous system. A case report and review of the literature. *Arch. Pathol. Lab. Med.* 119: 836–839.
6. Dickerman, R.D., Stevens, Q.E., Rak, R. et al. (2003). Isolated intracranial infection with *Mycobacterium avium* complex. *J. Neurosurg. Sci.* 2: 101–105; discussion 105.
7. Murray, R., Mallal, S., Heath, C., and French, M. (2001). Cerebral *Mycobacterium avium* infection in an HIV-infected patient following immune reconstitution and cessation of therapy for disseminated

Mycobacterium avium complex infection. *Eur. J. Clin. Microbiol. Infect. Dis.* 20: 199–201.
8. Kishida, S. and Ajisawa, A. (2008). Probable cerebral *Mycobacterium avium* complex-related immune reconstitution inflammatory syndrome in an HIV-infected patient. *Intern. Med.* 47: 1349–1354.
9. Gentry, R.H., Farrar, W.E., Mahvi, T.A. et al. (1977). Simultaneous infection of the central nervous system with *Cryptococcus neoformans* and *Mycobacterium intracellulare*. *South. Med. J.* 70: 865–868.
10. Zakowski, P., Fligiel, S., Berlin, G.W., and Johnson, L. Jr. (1982). Disseminated *Mycobacterium avium-intracellulare* infection in homosexual men dying of acquired immunodeficiency. *J. Am. Med. Assoc.* 248: 2980–2982.
11. Gray, F. and Sharer, L. (1993). Combined pathology. In: *Atlas of the Neuropathology of HIV Infection* (ed. F. Gray), 162–172. Oxford: Oxford University Press.
12. Pappolla, M.A. and Mehta, V.T. (1984). PAS reaction stains phagocytosed mycobacteria in paraffin sections. *Arch. Pathol. Lab. Med.* 108: 372–373.
13. Uldry, P.A., Bogousslavsky, J., Regli, F. et al. (1992). Chronic *Mycobacterium avium* complex infection in the central nervous system in a nonimmunosuppressed woman. *Eur. Neurol.* 32: 285–288.
14. Chowdhary, M., Narsinghani, U., and Kumar, R.A. (2015). Intracranial abscess due to *Mycobacterium avium* complex in an immunocompetent host: a case report. *BMC Infect. Dis.* 15: 281.
15. Morrison, A., Gyure, K.A., Stone, J. et al. (1999). Mycobacterial spindle cell pseudotumor of the brain: a case report and review of the literature. *Am. J. Surg. Pathol.* 23: 1294–1299.
16. Lim, M.-S., Bermingham, N., O'Broin, C. et al. (2016). Isolated cerebellar spindle cell pseudotumor caused by *Mycobacterium avium-intracellulare* complex in a patient without AIDS. *World Neurosurg.* 90: 703.e1–703.e3.
17. Chand, M., Lamagni, T., Kranzer, K. et al. (2017). Insidious risk of severe *Mycobacterium chimaera* infection in cardiac surgery patients. *Clin. Infect. Dis.* 64: 335–342.
18. Lindeboom, J.A., Bruijnesteijn van Coppenraet, L.E.S., van Soolingen, D. et al. (2011). Clinical manifestations, diagnosis, and treatment of *Mycobacterium haemophilum* infections. *Clin. Microbiol. Rev.* 24: 701–717.
19. Hernandez-Divers, S.J. and Shearer, D. (2002). Pulmonary mycobacteriosis caused by *Mycobacterium haemophilum* and *M marinum* in a royal python. *J. Am. Vet. Med. Assoc.* 220: 1661–1663.
20. Tufariello, J.M., Kerantzas, C.A., Vilchèze, C. et al. (2015). The complete genome sequence of the emerging pathogen *Mycobacterium haemophilum* explains its unique culture requirements. *MBio* 6: e01313–e0131315.
21. Merkler, A.E., Parlitsis, G., Patel, S. et al. (2014). Infection of the optic apparatus and hypothalamus by *Mycobacterium haemophilum*. *Neurology* 83: 659–660.
22. Barr, L.K., Sharer, L.R., Kunwar, E.K. et al. (2015). Intraventricular granulomatous mass associated with *Mycobacterium haemophilum*: a rare central nervous system manifestation in a patient with human immunodeficiency virus infection. *J. Clin. Neurosci.* 22: 1057–1060.
23. Buppajarntham, A., Apisarnthanarak, A., Rutjanawech, S. et al. (2015). Central nervous system infection due to *Mycobacterium haemophilum* in a patient with acquired immune deficiency syndrome. *Int. J. STD AIDS* 26: 288–290.
24. Kleinschmidt-DeMasters, B., Hawkins, K., and Franco-Paredes, C. (2018). Non-tubercular mycobacterial spinal cord abscesses in an HIV+ male due to *M. haemophilum*. (abstract). *J. Neuropathol. Exp. Neurol.* 77: 532.
25. Phowthongkum, P., Puengchitprapai, A., Udomsantisook, N. et al. (2008). Spindle cell pseudotumor of the brain associated with *Mycobacterium haemophilum* and *Mycobacterium simiae* mixed infection in a patient with AIDS: the first case report. *Int. J. Infect. Dis.* 12: 421–424.
26. Gordon, S.M. and Blumberg, H.M. (1992). *Mycobacterium kansasii* brain abscess in a patient with AIDS. *Clin. Infect. Dis.* 14: 789–790.
27. Bergen, G.A., Yangco, B., and Adelman, H.M. (1993). Central nervous system infection with *Mycobacterium kansasii*. *Ann. Intern. Med.* 118: 396.
28. Haworth, C.S., Banks, J., Capstick, T. et al. (2017). British thoracic society guidelines for the management of non-tuberculous mycobacterial pulmonary disease (NTM-PD). *Thorax* 72 (Suppl 2): ii1–ii64.

38 Spirochetal Infections of the CNS

Françoise Gray[1,2] and Catherine (Katy) Keohane[3]

[1] Retired from Department of Pathology, Lariboisière Hospital, APHP, Paris, France
[2] University Paris Diderot (Paris 7), Paris, France
[3] Department of Pathology and School of Medicine, University College Cork, Brookfield Health Science Complex, Cork, Ireland

Abbreviations

ACA	acrodermatitis chronica atrophicans
BBB	blood-brain barrier
CDC	Centers for Disease Control and Prevention
CNS	central nervous system
CS	congenital syphilis
CSF	cerebrospinal fluid
ELISA	enzyme-linked immunosorbent assay
EM	erythema migrans
ENMG	electroneuroyoraphy
FTA-ABS	fluorescent treponemal antibody-absorption
GPI	general paralysis (or paresis) of the insane
HIV	human immunodeficiency virus
LB	Lyme borreliosis
LD	Lyme disease
LNB	Lyme neuroborreliosis
MRI	magnetic resonance imaging
MSM	men who have sex with men
NS	neurosyphilis
PCR	polymerase chain reaction
US	United States
VDRL	venereal disease research laboratory test

Three genera of spirochetes cause infections in humans: *Treponema, Borrelia,* and *Leptospira.* All may involve the CNS.

Neurosyphilis

Definition of the disorder, major synonyms, and historical perspective

The name syphilis came from a Latin epic poem, *Syphilis, sive morbus gallicus,* written by Girolamo Fracastoro (1483–1553), a physician, astronomer, and poet of Verona in his work *De contagione et contagiosis morbis* in 1530 [1]. Syphilis is also known as luetic disease and historically was called "the great pox." It is a chronic bacterial infection caused by *Treponema pallidum,* usually transmitted by sexual contact with an infected partner or by maternal transmission to the fetus in congenital syphilis. Untreated syphilis can progress through four stages: primary (chancre, regional lymphadenopathy), secondary (disseminated skin eruptions, generalized lymphadenopathy), latent (fewer secondary-stage manifestations, absence of symptoms), and tertiary (gummas, cardiovascular syphilis, and late neurological symptoms). The CNS can be involved at any stage. Although the

---

Infections of the Central Nervous System: Pathology and Genetics, First Edition. Edited by Fabrice Chrétien, Kum Thong Wong, Leroy R. Sharer, Catherine (Katy) Keohane and Françoise Gray.
© 2020 John Wiley & Sons Ltd. Published 2020 by John Wiley & Sons Ltd.

leptomeninges are commonly invaded during secondary syphilis, symptomatic neurosyphilis (NS) occurs predominantly in the tertiary stage.

Syphilis has affected the lives of millions of people in all social strata for thousands of years. Following record high rates of infection in the World War II era, successful therapy with penicillin in 1943 dramatically reduced the incidence of primary and secondary syphilis in the second half of the twentieth century; NS also became rare [2]. With the advent of human immunodeficiency virus (HIV) infection in the early 1980s, there has been a resurgence of syphilis, most commonly in men who have sex with men (MSM) [3]. The number of newly diagnosed cases of congenital syphilis has also increased [4]. Currently, it is not clear how many individuals infected with syphilis subsequently develop the late manifestations, particularly NS.

Microbiology and genetics

Treponema pallidum subsp. *pallidum* belongs to a family of spiral-shaped bacteria, the Spirochaetaceae (spirochetes). It is differentiated from other pathogenic treponemes causing nonvenereal diseases – *T. pallidum* subsp. *endemicum* (bejel), *T. pallidum* subsp. *pertenue* (yaws), and *Treponema carateum* (pinta) – by their different clinical manifestations and by genetic differences [5, 6].

T. pallidum varies from 6 to 15 μm in length and is 0.2 μm in diameter. Its spiral-shaped body is surrounded by a cytoplasmic membrane, enclosed by a loosely associated outer membrane. A thin peptidoglycan layer between the membranes provides structural stability. Flagella located in the periplasmic space are anchored at each end of the organism, enabling its characteristic corkscrew motility [7].

Genome sequencing of the Nichols strain in 1998 [8], and later sequencing of additional strains, has shown a very high (>99.8%) sequence homology among the *T. pallidum* subspecies [9]. *T. pallidum* is a prime example of a pathogen that has undergone genome reduction to increase efficiency, having one of the smallest characterized prokaryote genomes. It depends completely on its host for most essential metabolic processes and so is remarkably fragile outside of a mammalian host and has not been continuously cultivated in vitro.

Nonetheless, *T. pallidum* is highly infectious and survives for decades in the untreated host [10]. Its molecular typing shows wide geographic variation in subtypes. Specific subtypes may be associated with macrolide resistance and NS, but this needs to be confirmed by wider studies [11].

Epidemiology

Humans are the only known natural host of *T. pallidum*. Syphilis is a sexually transmitted infection (STI) acquired by direct contact with active primary or secondary lesions. Congenital infection occurs when the fetus is infected via the placenta or during birth.

Syphilis affects virtually every rung of society, but it has a proclivity for the most vulnerable groups. It is endemic in low-income countries and occurs at lower rates in middle-income and high-income countries. The Centers for Disease Control and Prevention (CDC), reported the national rate of primary and secondary syphilis cases in the United States was 2.1 cases per 100 000 in 2000 and 2001; this represented the lowest rates since 1941. As of 2014, the incidence increased to 6.3 cases per 100 000 population [3], mainly among MSM [12], sex-industry workers, and drug users. Similar increases in MSM have occurred in Western Europe [9]. Most primary and secondary syphilis cases (84%) reported in 2004 to the CDC were in men [13]; over the past decade, increases in women with the infection have also occurred, affecting all age groups and ethnicities (i.e. Asian, black, Hispanic, and white). Reported congenital syphilis decreased from 10.5 to 8.4 cases per 100 000 live births between 2008 and 2012, but increased to 11.6 cases per 100 000 live births in 2014, the highest since 2001 [4].

Outbreaks among MSM are associated with unsafe sexual behavior, possibly reflecting improved antiretroviral treatment for HIV [14]. Other factors that drive the re-emergence and spread of syphilis include migration and travel, and economic and social changes that limit access to health care.

Although clinical NS remains rare, its epidemiology has largely paralleled that of syphilis in general [15]. The incidence of NS was 0.47 per 100 000 adults in a recent study from the Netherlands, and

75% of cases were men, mostly young, urban men. The incidence of NS was highest in men ages 35–65 years, and in women ages 75 years and older; the most common clinical manifestation was tabes dorsalis. In this study, 15% of the patients were HIV-seropositive [16]. Precise recent information is not available on the incidence and prevalence of the late complications of NS. Older studies showed that meningovascular syphilis decreased from 15 to 10% of patients with NS from the preantibiotic to the antibiotic era, respectively. Parenchymal syphilis was rare, even in the preantibiotic era (general paresis of the insane [GPI] occurred in 5%, tabes in 9% of patients with syphilis), and further declined in the antibiotic era [17].

Clinical features

CNS involvement is a sequel of undetected or inadequately treated primary syphilis. Asymptomatic NS may develop early in infection and is characterized by a positive venereal disease research laboratory test (VDRL) in cerebrospinal fluid (CSF) and a slight leukocyte pleocytosis. Symptoms can develop later. Early symptoms of NS may occur concurrently with primary or secondary syphilis or follow resolution of secondary syphilis. Late, symptomatic NS occurs predominantly at the tertiary stage.

Early neurosyphilis

Acute early meningitis presents typically with fever, headache, nausea, vomiting, and stiff neck. Early NS may also present with eye manifestations, such as iritis or uveitis. Less often, there are nonspecific or misleading clinical manifestations, including acute hydrocephalus, cranial nerve palsies (commonly II, III, VI, and VII), seizures or rarely, memory loss and mental confusion. Syphilis is classically described as "the great imitator." Occasionally, mesiotemporal changes on magnetic resonance imaging (MRI) mimicking herpes simplex encephalitis, paraneoplastic encephalitis, or early onset Alzheimer disease, have been reported [18]. Spinal cord disease, myelitis, or meningomyelitis is rarely seen.

Late neurological complications of syphilis

Late NS, affecting the cerebral vasculature, or brain or spinal cord parenchyma, presents 2–30 years after primary infection.

Patients with meningovascular syphilis present with stroke, usually within five years following infection. Prior to this, individuals may experience vertigo, insomnia, and personality changes; these symptoms are followed by diffuse or focal arterial involvement.

Late parenchymatous syphilis includes GPI and tabes dorsalis. GPI occurs 10–20 years after initial infection and is manifested by progressive personality disorder, affective and psychotic symptoms leading to cognitive decline and dementia. MRI typically shows severe frontotemporal atrophy with hippocampal involvement. Tabes dorsalis develops 15–25 years after initial infection. The features are "lightning pains" in the legs, paraesthesiae, loss of proprioception, ataxia, bowel and bladder incontinence, and Argyll Robertson pupil.

Classifying NS into meningovascular and parenchymatous forms is convenient, but both forms occasionally coexist, so individual patients have clinical signs of both syndromes. Nowadays, presentations such as GPI and tabes dorsalis are more often read about in textbooks than encountered in clinical practice, and milder forms with few symptoms make diagnosis difficult.

Late-stage syphilitic eye disease can present as optic neuritis or optic atrophy, both manifesting as progressive visual loss. Syphilitic otitis presents with sudden onset of sensorineural hearing loss and is regarded as NS involving cranial nerve VIII.

Diagnosis

CSF examination is mandatory for diagnosis. The CSF shows aseptic meningitis irrespective of the stage or type of NS. Lymphocytic pleocytosis may be mild with <50 leukocytes but can have 400 leukocytes per microliter. CSF protein is moderately elevated (usually <75 mg/dl) [19]. The CSF VDRL remains the diagnostic gold standard but is not invariably positive [15]; false positives occur when CSF is contaminated by peripheral blood. Treponemal tests such as the fluorescent treponemal antibody-absorption (FTA-ABS) have been used on CSF; they are more sensitive than CSF-VDRL, particularly in asymptomatic NS, but are less specific [20].

CSF is normal in up to 4% of all patients with symptomatic NS, particularly in the advanced stages. It has been reported that CSF abnormalities decline with the duration of disease, but abnormalities may persist even after appropriate treatment.

Pathology

Our knowledge largely comes from studies on patients from the 1940s [19], and because NS is rarer now, there are few case reports [21].

Meningovascular neurosyphilis

This is a combination of chronic meningitis, multifocal arteritis, and gummatous, necrotic lesions.

Chronic meningitis may be diffuse or localized to the base of the brain. Macroscopically the inflamed meninges contain a cloudy exudate and may be fibrosed. Microscopically, lymphocytes and a few plasma cells intermingle within fibrous tissue to form perivascular infiltrates around small blood vessels in the thickened meninges. Although plasma cells are not specific, their presence should always raise the possibility of syphilis. Occasionally the pia is damaged or destroyed, allowing bundles of fibrillary astrocytes to project from the cortex into the subarachnoid space. Inflammation extends into cranial and spinal nerves, and periarteritis may cause optic atrophy or cranial nerve palsies. Hydrocephalus is a frequent complication of meningeal fibrosis.

Syphilitic meningitis may be virtually confined to the spinal cord, in which case it is referred to as spinal arachnoiditis. Vascular involvement can produce a transverse myelitis. The infection may be confined to the cervical region, where the pia-arachnoid and both dural layers are thickened, adherent to, and encircle the cord, described as pachymeningitis cervicalis hypertrophica.

Meningovascular NS affects arteries of all sizes anywhere in the CNS. Heubner arteritis is the most common form of syphilitic arteritis and involves large and medium-size arteries. The features are concentric fibrous intimal thickening, associated with intimal proliferation (endarteritis obliterans) and corresponding thinning of the media. The elastic lamina remains intact (Figure 38.1). Lymphocytes and plasma cells infiltrate the thickened adventitia, penetrate the media, and "cuff" the vasa vasorum. Nissl-Alzheimer arteritis typically affects small vessels, which show endothelial

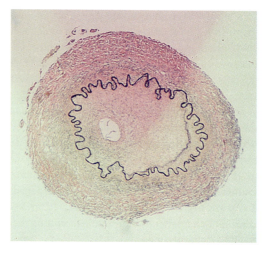

Figure 38.1 Heubner arteritis: A large artery shows concentric fibrous thickening of the intima associated with intimal proliferation (endarteritis obliterans) and thinning of the media. Note the elastic lamina is intact. Mononuclear cells infiltrate the thickened adventitia and penetrate the media. Weigert-Hart stain for elastic.

and adventitial thickening. Both types of arteritis produce lumenal stenosis and vascular occlusion resulting in ischemic lesions, mostly in the middle cerebral artery territory. Vertebrobasilar artery involvement with brainstem infarction is also common [21]. In the spinal cord the anterior spinal artery is most commonly involved [19].

Cerebral gumma is now rare in Europe and North America. Lesions in the meninges can involve the cerebral convexity but may be found in the midbrain, hypothalamus, and spinal cord. They are usually attached to both dura mater and brain and many become embedded in the brain parenchyma. They are round, red-tan-gray, focally firm rubbery lesions with central necrosis (Figure 38.2). Microscopically, the central gummatous necrosis shows ghost-like outlines of dead cells, surrounded by a granulomatous reaction including epithelioid cells, fibroblasts, and scattered multinucleated giant cells (Figure 38.3a). Spirochetes are rarely demonstrable (Figure 38.3b) because the gumma represents a hyperimmune form of tissue necrosis.

Parenchymatous neurosyphilis

This takes two forms: paretic dementia (the same as GPI) and tabes dorsalis. Both forms may coexist as "tabo-paresis."

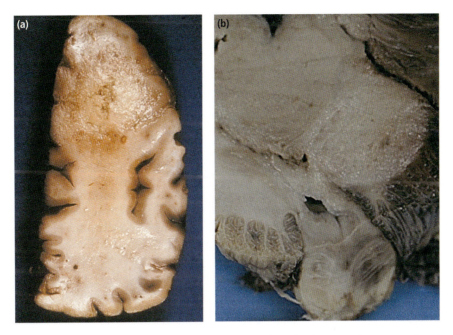

Figure 38.2 Cerebral gummas in patient with acquired immunodeficiency syndrome (AIDS) macroscopic appearance: Round, red, tan-gray, rubbery lesions with a central area of softening in the right occipital lobe (a) and the cerebellum (b). Source: Courtesy of the late Dr. Marius Valsamis.

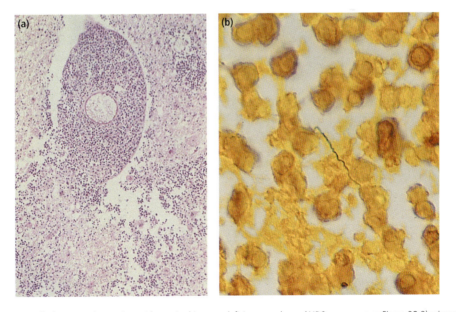

Figure 38.3 Cerebral gummas in a patient with acquired immunodeficiency syndrome (AIDS; same case as Figure 38.2) microscopic appearance: (a) Gummatous necrosis with ghost-like outlines of dead cells and granulomatous reaction with scattered multinucleated giant cells. Note mononuclear perivascular infiltration; hematoxylin and eosin (H&E). (b) Spirochete within a necrotic area (Modified Steiner stain.)

Formerly, in patients dying after several years of GPI, macroscopically the brain was shrunken, firm, and covered by a thick opaque pia-arachnoid, most marked frontally, decreasing posteriorly. The ventricles were enlarged, and the ependyma showed diffuse granular ependymitis. Nowadays, GPI is rare. In the healed stages, the brain is usually grossly normal except for ependymal granulations.

Microscopically, historic descriptions emphasized meningeal thickening and striking atrophy of the cerebral cortex, which showed loss of the normal laminar pattern, neuronal loss, and proliferation of reactive astrocytes and rod-shaped microglia. The lesions were distributed in scattered foci of different ages giving a "bush-fire" or wind-swept appearance. Perivascular cuffing by lymphocytes and plasma cells was found in the cortex and leptomeninges (Figure 38.4). Specific silver impregnation classically demonstrated the spirochete *T. pallidum* in many brains (Figure 38.5). Now, in patients with prolonged treatment, organisms can be difficult to find.

Tabes dorsalis consists of degeneration of the posterior columns (Figure 38.6) and spinal nerve roots with involvement of the dorsal roots and ganglia. It is apparently the result of inflammatory meningovascular lesions localized to the subarachnoid portion of the dorsal nerve roots. Spinal cord involvement is secondary to radiculo-ganglionic lesions and is characterized by wallerian degeneration of the dorsal columns. Macroscopically, the spinal posterior roots and posterior columns are shrunken. The lumbo-sacral nerve roots are most frequently affected, but cervical nerve roots may also be damaged. Microscopically, there is axonal and myelin loss in the posterior columns and prominent astrogliosis. The leptomeninges are thickened and show variable chronic inflammation, but inflammation is not seen in the cord parenchyma, and *T. pallidum* is absent (unlike GPI).

Syphilis and HIV infection

NS is not uncommon in patients with AIDS [22]. Syphilis and HIV share common risk factors and patients with HIV are at increased risk of NS. If coinfected with HIV, the clinical spectrum of syphilis can change; patients can progress rapidly to symptomatic NS, have an accelerated disease course, and treatment failure is also more frequent [23, 24]. Syphilitic ocular involvement seems particularly frequent [22]. In patients with HIV, NS is frequently asymptomatic; the most common manifestations are syphilitic meningitis and meningovascular syphilis. General paresis, syphilitic meningomyelitis, syphilitic polyradiculopathy, and cerebral gummas [25] have been reported in occasional cases.

Neuropathological reports are rare. Morgello and Laufer [26] reported a case with meningovascular syphilis including gummatous arteritis,

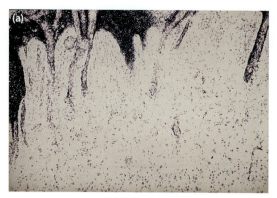
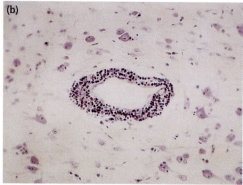

Figure 38.4 General paresis of the insane: (a) Severe mononuclear infiltration of the leptomeninges extending to the superficial cortex along the perivascular spaces. Note severe neuronal loss with disorganization of the normal laminar pattern and proliferation of rod-cell microglia (Nissl stain). (b) At higher magnification there is perivascular cuffing by lymphocytes and plasma cells. Note neuronal loss with mis-orientation of the remaining neurons and proliferation of reactive astrocytes and rod-shaped microglia (Nissl stain).

Congenital syphilis

Congenital NS is almost as rare as GPI at necropsy in Western countries but contributes to the high fetal mortality rates in developing countries. The risk of transplacental transmission is highest when the pregnant woman has primary- or secondary-stage syphilis. Fetal infection can occur at any time, including at birth, but symptomatic damage requires a fetal immature immune system; thus, most clinical effects occur between the fourth and seventh months of pregnancy. Penicillin therapy in early pregnancy prevents fetal infection, and maternal treatment late in pregnancy can cure the infected fetus. The later in gestation that therapy is started, the greater the chance the infant will develop stigmata of congenital syphilis.

Treponemes are inoculated directly into the circulation, so there is an immediate secondary stage with multiorgan damage, and compared with the vascular changes in other organs, brain involvement is often surprisingly mild [27].

Congenital stigmata of infection include interstitial keratitis, chorioretinitis, and perception deafness. The child who is congenitally infected is at risk of developing all the acquired NS syndromes. Basal meningitis can lead to infantile hydrocephalus, and juvenile GPI may occur from ages 6 to 21 years. Juvenile congenital tabes dorsalis is uncommon.

Animal models and pathogenesis
Animal models

Several mammals can be infected with *T. pallidum*, but only a few develop clinical disease. Rabbits have a naturally occurring venereal disease caused by the closely related *Treponema paraluiscuniculi* and are also susceptible to *T. pallidum* subspecies. As in human infection, *T. pallidum* infection of rabbits produces primary and secondary lesions, infection persists asymptomatically for the remainder of the animal's life, and the organism can invade the CNS and cross the placenta [28]; thus, they are the model of choice for studying pathogenesis and immunity.

Pathogenesis

T. pallidum invades the CNS early in infection and seeds into the meninges during the primary or, more commonly, the secondary stage of disease. In 30–50% of patients with primary or secondary

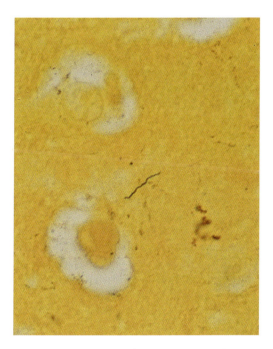

Figure 38.5 General paresis of the insane: Intracortical spirochete demonstrated by specific silver impregnation (Modified Steiner stain).

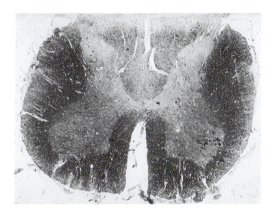

Figure 38.6 Tabes dorsalis: Horizontal section of the lumbar cord showing degeneration of the posterior columns (Loyez stain).

causing multiple cerebral infarcts and fulminant necrotizing encephalitis with massive treponemal invasion. The encephalitis was regarded as a hyperinfectious, anergic stage of the disease called "quaternary syphilis," occurring after an immune tertiary stage and demonstrating that HIV infection may alter the natural history of syphilis.

syphilis the CSF is abnormal, but only 1–5% exhibit signs or symptoms in the secondary stage. Most individuals clear the infection spontaneously, those who do not (<1%) are at risk of progressing to NS.

Two crucial properties enable *T. pallidum* establish and maintain a successful infection (i) a high-invasive capability [10] and (ii) a capacity to evade the immune response and persist for prolonged periods.

Invasive capability of T. pallidum
Within hours of infection in experimental animals, the highly motile *T. pallidum* disseminates widely via the bloodstream and lymphatics. In vitro studies have shown *T. pallidum* can penetrate intact membranes and endothelial cell monolayers. Invasion of tissues only occurs following its attachment to cells (e.g. endothelial cells that comprise capillary walls). Several proteins are active in this attachment to host cells, via extracellular matrix bridges [29].

Factors contributing to treponemal persistence
Primary and secondary syphilitic lesions are infiltrated by T lymphocytes, followed by macrophages. The vast majority of treponemes are cleared, with lesion resolution, shortly after macrophage infiltration. A subpopulation of treponemes are resistant to opsonophagocytosis by macrophages [30].

Theoretical explanations of the remarkable ability of treponemes to persist include their location in an "immunoprotective niche" such as the CNS, the eye, or inside cells other than professional phagocytes. Another likely contributory factor is the paucity of proteins on the treponemal surface, thereby limiting antigenic targets and enabling *T. pallidum* to evade functional immune responses [10]. A further factor is the antigenic diversity and variation among the *T. pallidum* repeat (Tpr) protein family, a subset of which are thought to be located on the treponemal surface. Antigenic variation of TprK abrogates specific antibody binding and may allow *T. pallidum* to evade host immunity and establish chronic infection [31].

Treatment, future perspective, and conclusions

Diagnosis and treatment of individuals infected and their contacts is key to syphilis control programs, as is sex education and promotion of condom use to prevent infection.

The treatment plan for syphilis, as detailed by the CDC, varies with the stage of infection [32]. Primary, secondary, and early-latent syphilis can be treated with a single intramuscular dose of 2.4 million units of penicillin G benzathine. Longer treatment with 2.4 million units of intramuscular penicillin G benzathine weekly for three weeks is recommended for late-latent syphilis, tertiary syphilis, or if infection duration is unknown. NS requires three to four million units of intravenous aqueous crystalline penicillin G every 4 hours for 10–14 days.

Follow-up of patients treated for NS depends on initial CSF findings. If pleocytosis is present, the CSF should be reexamined every six months until the leukocyte count is normal. Retreatment should be considered if the CSF leukocyte count does not reduce after six months or completely normalize after two years [33].

CSF also can be reexamined for serial decreases in VDRL antibodies or protein levels, although the management of persistent abnormalities is not well established. CSF parameters are expected to normalize within two years. Most treatment failures occur in patients who are immunocompromised.

Syphilis has many features of a disease that could be eradicated. It only affects humans, and there is no animal or environmental reservoir. There is ongoing development of easy, cheap, reliable diagnostic tests. Treatment with effective antibiotic therapy is inexpensive and the two- to six-week incubation period provides an opportunity to prevent spread by prophylactic treatment of sexual contacts. Considering the continuing global disease burden of syphilis, its correlation with increased transmission of HIV, and the significant morbidity and mortality of infectious syphilis and chronic syphilis, other therapies such as the development of a vaccine may be considered [34].

Borreliosis

Neuroborreliosis

Definition of the disorder, major synonyms, and historical perspective

Lyme borreliosis (LB) is a tick-borne multisystem infection caused by the spirochete *Borrelia burgdorferi* sensu lato (Bbsl). Infection usually begins with an expanding skin lesion, erythema migrans

(EM; stage 1), which if untreated, can be followed by early disseminated infection, often with neurological signs (stage 2), and by late infection, especially arthritis in North America or acrodermatitis chronica atrophicans (ACA) in Europe (stage 3).

Lyme arthritis was described in 1976 in clusters of children in Lyme, Connecticut, in the United States [35]. Later, Lyme arthritis was recognized as part of a complicated multisystem illness, which included EM, Bannwarth syndrome, and ACA and had already been described in Europe [36]. These syndromes were grouped together following the isolation of the spirochete B. burgdorferi from Ixodes scapularis [37] and its identification in patients with these clinical manifestations of infection [35]. The disease is now referred to as Lyme borreliosis. Involvement of the nervous system, Lyme neuroborreliosis (LNB), occurs in approximately 15% of all patients with LB [38].

Microbiology
Bbsl is a Gram-negative spirochete bacterium that comprises 20 different genospecies [39].

Like all spirochetes, members of the Bbsl complex are bound by an inner cytoplasmic membrane and an outer membrane. Characteristic periplasmic flagella are responsible for the bacteria's flat-wave morphology. Bbsl has a limited metabolic capacity and is highly dependent on its tick vector and vertebrate host for many essential factors.

All genospecies of the Bbsl complex have small, highly segmented genomes. The 1.5 million-base genome of B. burgdorferi strain B31 consists of a linear chromosome of 910 kilobases, 9 linear plasmids, and 12 circular plasmids of various sizes [40]. The linear chromosome is highly conserved among Bbsl genospecies, whereas the plasmids show a high degree of variation. Differences in plasmids among Bbsl are thought to contribute to the clinical variability in LB in different geographical regions.

Three genospecies are mainly responsible for human LB: B. burgdorferi sensu stricto (Bbss), Borrelia afzelii, and Borrelia garinii. These are transmitted by different tick species and cause LB in different geographical regions: Bbss is the main cause of LB in the United States, whereas B. afzelii and B. garini (and less often Bbss) cause LB in Europe and Asia. The different genospecies seem to have distinct clinical manifestations; B. garinii is more closely associated with NB than other species. Intraspecies genetic variation has also been noted for several Bbsl genospecies that correlate with the risk of blood-borne spread and clinical outcome [35].

Epidemiology
Lyme disease (LD) is the most common vector-borne illness in the Northern Hemisphere. Its prevalence is estimated at between 20 and 100 cases per 100 000 people in the United States and about 100 to 130 cases per 100 000 in Europe [35]. The usual vectors are small, hard-bodied ticks of the genus Ixodes; I. scapularis predominates in North America and I. ricinus in Europe. Small mammals, particularly rodents, are the principal reservoirs for the spirochete. The tick feeds only once at each of the three stages of its life cycle (i.e. larva, nymph, and adult). Human infections follow a tick bite and occur mostly in spring and summer during the tick's active nymph stage. The risk of transmission tends to be higher if the tick has been attached to the skin for more than 24 hours.

LD effects residents and visitors in endemic areas and occupations such as forest workers, hunters, rangers, gamekeepers, farmers, and military field personnel. Rates of infection are highest in children ages 5–15 years and adults older than 50 years of age. The incidence varies according to the genospecies of Bbsl and is also determined by the geographic distribution of vector tick species, ecologic factors that influence tick infection rates, and human behavior that facilitates tick bites [35, 39].

Clinical features
The clinical features of LB vary in each stage of the illness.

The characteristic clinical sign of early localized disease (stage 1) is a rash EM at the site of the tick bite. It occurs one to three weeks after the bite (typically 7–10 days) and disappears within weeks. It is recognized in approximately 90% of patients with confirmed infection and occurs mainly on the arms and legs. In the United States, EM is often accompanied by malaise, fatigue, headache, arthralgia, myalgia, fever, and regional lymphadenopathy. In Europe, EM expands more slowly and is not usually accompanied by other symptoms.

Borrelial lymphocytoma is a rare skin manifestation of early LB in Europe, typically located on the earlobe in children or on the nipple in adults [35].

The most common sign of early disseminated LB (stage 2) is multiple EM. Other common manifestations are mainly neurological. In the United States, LNB mainly manifests as lymphocytic meningitis with episodic headaches, mild neck stiffness, cranial neuropathy (particularly facial palsy), or motor or sensory radiculoneuritis. Cerebellar ataxia, encephalomyelitis, or mild late encephalopathy with subtle cognitive disturbance are rare. In Europe, B. garinii infection causes Bannwarth syndrome or tick-borne meningopolyneuritis, with painful radiculoneuritis associated with lymphocytic meningitis, often without headache, and may be followed by cranial neuropathy or pareses of the extremities. A severe chronic encephalomyelitis, characterized by spastic paraparesis, cranial neuropathy, or cognitive impairment has been described in rare instances. Strokelike signs and symptoms in patients with LB have been reported occasionally in both the United States and Europe. Peripheral nervous system (PNS) involvement including acute, sensory-motor painful radiculopathy, plexopathy, multiplex neuropathy, or polyneuropathy may occur in both American and European forms. Electroneuromyography (ENMG) usually suggests an axonal neuropathy, and CSF study reveals pleocytosis and elevated protein. Myocarditis occurs in approximately 10% of patients. Eye involvement (e.g. iritis, uveitis, and optic neuritis) may occur. Systemic symptoms including myalgia, arthralgia, headache, and fatigue occur frequently.

Late LD (stage 3) is quite rare and most often presents as arthritis. PNS involvement (axonal) is more or less latent, often associated with ACA. The CSF is normal.

At every stage, the diagnosis is suspected on clinical signs and confirmed by specific serology. Culture of Borrelia spp. from patient specimens gives a definitive diagnosis but is almost restricted to research studies because the organism grows slowly; it is present in very small numbers in CSF, blood, and tissues; and the necessary expertise and equipment are not routinely available in most laboratories.

In both the United States and Europe, serological testing usually by enzyme-linked immunosorbent assays (ELISAs) is the only practical and readily available method to support a diagnosis of LB. Specificity and sensitivity are important issues because some antigens detected by Lyme serological tests share immunological determinants with other bacteria. Nonetheless, in highly endemic areas, a positive test result has a high positive predictive value. Currently, two-step testing is recommended, whereby positive or borderline ELISA results are confirmed with Western blots.

CSF examination reveals abnormalities in virtually every case. A mild lymphocytic pleocytosis (usually <500 cells/mm^3) or an increased protein concentration should be present. In European LNB, both serum and CSF B. burgdorferi antibodies are measured to calculate the antibody index to determine intrathecal antibody production. The antibody index is not commonly used in the United States [35].

Pathology

Very few neuropathological reports have been published [41–43]. Macroscopically, brain atrophy or edema with leptomeningeal fibrosis was described in individual cases. Microscopically, there is chronic meningitis with lymphocytic infiltrates, some plasma cells, perivascular or vasculitic inflammation, diffuse astrocytosis, microglial activation, and multifocal areas of demyelination involving the periventricular white matter. Iritis leading to choroidal necrosis with polymorphonuclear infiltration has also been reported.

In stage 2, the PNS changes involve nerve roots, spinal ganglia, and distal nerve segments. Nerve biopsy shows acute axonal involvement. There is a strong inflammatory mononuclear reaction around blood vessels in the endoneurium, perineurium, and epineurium (Figure 38.7), mainly of B-type lymphocytes [44]. There are a few reports of axonal noninflammatory neuropathies associated with ACA in stage 3.

Pathogenesis and animal models

The nonhuman primate model of LNB accurately mimics aspects of the human illness. [45]. These studies were the first to demonstrate spirochetal

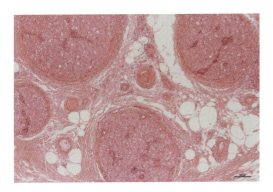

Figure 38.7 Lyme disease: Paraffin embedded section of sural nerve showing numerous perivascular cuffs of mononuclear cells around the vessels in the endoneurium, perineurium, and epineurium. Note the absence of vascular necrosis (hematoxylin and eosin [H&E]). (Source: Courtesy of Professor Jean Michel Vallat).

invasion of the subarachnoid space supporting the view that LNB pathogenesis is associated with direct spirochetal invasion. In humans, organisms were observed in a brain biopsy [46] and polymerase chain reaction (PCR) detection of *B. burgdorferi*. DNA was found in tissue samples from areas with inflammatory changes [42].

Current knowledge of LNB pathogenesis, from invasion to CNS inflammation is still incomplete. *B. burgdorferi* enters the host through a tick bite on the skin and may disseminate from there to secondary organs, including the CNS. To achieve this, *B. burgdorferi* first has to evade the host immune system [47], then reach the CNS and cross the blood-brain barrier (BBB). The process of dissemination may be different in Europe and the United States. Meningopolyradiculitis in Bannwarth syndrome might result from spread along nerves, whereas the more diffuse meningitis observed in the United States suggests hematogenous spread. Some authors suggest that *B. burgdorferi* spirochetes breach the BBB by penetrating between endothelial cells, and others favor transcellular passage. Once in the CSF, the spirochetes elicit an inflammatory response resulting in focal or diffuse neural dysfunction, but the pathophysiology is far from clear. Several mechanisms may apply: direct cytotoxicity, neurotoxic mediators, or triggered autoimmune reactions perhaps because of molecular mimicry [47].

Treatment
Antibiotics are beneficial for all clinical manifestations of LD. In stage 2, parenteral therapy with ceftriaxone or doxycycline or penicillin G should be used for three weeks. Patients with early disease usually have excellent outcomes. Recovery is slower and may be incomplete in patients with late disease.

Relapsing fever
Definition
Relapsing fever is caused by spirochetes of various *Borrelia* species and is characterized by recurrent fever, chills, and malaise.

Microbiology
These spirochetes are large with irregular spirals and readily stain with aniline dyes. Although *Borrelia* are technically Gram negative, they are most readily identified by Giemsa or Wright staining.

Epidemiology
The causative organism and associated vector vary in different geographic areas. *Borrelia recurrentis*, transmitted by the human body louse, causes epidemic relapsing fever and is most frequently reported in northern and eastern Africa. Other species causing relapsing fever in Africa include *Borrelia duttonii*, *Borrelia hispanica*, and *Borrelia crocidurae*. Humans are the only known host and reservoir for *B. recurrentis*, but small rodents and other mammals can be a reservoir for tick-borne *Borrelia* species. *Borrelia hermsii*, tick-borne relapsing fever, is reported in Colorado in the United States. Other responsible species in the United States include *Borrelia turicatae* and *Borrelia parkeri*. All are transmitted by bites from soft-bodied, night-feeding Ornithodoros ticks. In the northeastern United States, Japan, and Russia, *Borrelia miyamotoi* is a relapsing fever, similar to LD, transmitted by the Ixodes tick [48].

Physiopathology
The clinical manifestations are caused by an endotoxin-like substance produced by the spirochete. In the bloodstream, Borreliae are present during the febrile phase, disappear before the fever resolves, and

reappear during the next febrile episode. The initial febrile episode resolves because of the development of antibodies directed against the organism's surface proteins. During the afebrile phases, the organisms sequester in internal organs and re-emerge with a modified antigenic structure. The cycles of antigen variation, followed by specific antibody production, account for the relapsing course of the disease [48].

Clinical features
Clinically, the incubation period is typically 4–18 days following exposure to *Borrelia*. The symptoms of relapsing fevers are abrupt onset of fever and chills, often accompanied by malaise, arthralgia, and myalgia. Hemorrhagic and non-hemorrhagic rashes, nausea, vomiting, jaundice, and neurologic abnormalities may also occur. The first episode typically lasts a week and then resolves, and patients experience recurrent similar but shorter, less severe episodes, occurring every 5–10 days, which may persist for several cycles before resolution. In epidemic, or louse-borne, relapsing fever, there are typically only one or two episodes of fever. In endemic, tick-borne relapsing fever, three to seven episodes may occur before resolution of symptoms.

Neurological complications, including meningitis, encephalomyelitis, and cranial or peripheral neuropathies, occur in about 30% of louse-borne and 10% of tick-borne cases, particularly in infections by *B. turicatae* and *B. duttonii*. The CSF may be normal but, with neurological involvement, tends to show an increased opening pressure, mononuclear pleocytosis, and increased protein concentration with a proportional increase in immunoglobulin G (IgG) concentration. Spirochetes have been detected in CSF in nearly 12% of cases.

Laboratory evaluation may demonstrate leukopenia or leukocytosis and thrombocytopenia. Diagnosis is confirmed by detection of *Borrelia* in Giemsa-stained blood films, serologic analysis, or via PCR detection of the organism. These organisms are not identifiable on routine laboratory cultures. Diagnostic yield is highest with the earlier febrile episodes and decreases with each recurrence. Early in the illness, the number of spirochetes visible in blood can reach $100\,000/mm^3$. Between episodes and in later recurrences, spirochetes may not be visible at all. Serology is also used to diagnose tick-borne relapsing fever, particularly when the diagnosis is suspected late in the illness. In that situation, repeat testing with a rise in IgG suggests recent infection. Because these serologic tests cross-react with other spirochetes such as those causing leptospirosis and syphilis, they must be interpreted in the setting of clinical symptoms.

There are few postmortem studies, but brain edema [49] and subarachnoid hemorrhage have been described at autopsy in louse-borne relapsing fever [50].

Treatment
Relapsing fever is treated with doxycycline for 7 to 10 days. Fatalities are rare in tick-borne relapsing fever. With antibiotic treatment, the mortality of epidemic relapsing fever reduces from 10–40% to 2–4%. Mortality is mainly attributed to myocarditis. Patients must be observed for several hours after initiation of antibiotic therapy because a Jarisch-Herxheimer reaction is common; it is rarely fatal and is managed with supportive care. Some *Borrelia* infections may be self-limiting and resolve without treatment.

Leptospirosis

Definition and microbiology
Leptospirosis is a zoonosis caused by spirochetes belonging to the genus *Leptospira*. The pathogenic form, *Leptospira interrogans,* consists of 23 serogroups such as *icterohaemorrhagiae, canicola,* and *Pomona,* which are in turn comprised of nearly 200 serovars [51]. Rodents are reservoirs and are the most common source of human infection.

Epidemiology
Leptospirosis occurs throughout the world, especially in the tropics. Its epidemiology has changed in Western countries; it was an occupational disease for workers in sewers or abattoirs who were at risk of contact with rats and rat urine, but it is now increasingly seen in those pursuing recreational water sports [52]. Leptospirosis has a broader health impact as a disease of impoverished subsistence farmers, cash croppers, and field workers

from tropical regions. A recent study estimates that more than one million severe cases of leptospirosis occur annually, including 60 000 deaths [53].

Physiopathology

In humans *Leptospirae* enter the bloodstream through mucous membranes or skin abrasions. They replicate in the reticuloendothelial system, particularly in the liver. A leptospiraemia can follow and the organisms reach the brain and kidneys [51]. Involvement of the nervous system occurs in around 10–15% of the cases [54].

Clinical features

Clinically, leptospirosis is typically a biphasic illness. An early leptospiraemic phase occurs after an incubation period of 2–26 days; there is abrupt onset of high fever with headaches, malaise, chills, conjunctival injection, nausea, and vomiting; clinical meningitis; and occasionally cranial or peripheral nerve involvement may occur. Leptospira can be cultured from blood and CSF.

It is followed after four to seven days of illness, by a brief afebrile period lasting one to three days with clearing of symptoms. Then the immune phase begins, and patients again become ill. Most of the serious neurological complications occur during this phase. Meningitis is the most common manifestation and may be associated with encephalitis or myelitis in up to 7% of cases. A severe form of combined central and peripheral involvement (meningo-myelo-encephalo-polyneuritis) has been described [55]. Other presentations are polyradiculoneuropathy including Guillain-Barré-like syndrome, iridocyclitis, and optic neuritis.

Severe icteric leptospirosis (Weil disease) is characterized by liver and renal dysfunction, decreased level of consciousness, and widespread vasculitis with hemorrhage, including subarachnoid hemorrhage and intracerebral bleeding [56]. Untreated patients may shed leptospira from urine for weeks to months. Death occurs in 15–40% of cases; the prognosis is primarily dependent on the age and general condition of the patient.

Pathology

In fatal cases (mainly Weil syndrome), postmortem examination usually reveals petechiae and larger hemorrhages, focal hepatocellular necrosis, focal hemorrhagic myocarditis, and swelling and vacuolization of skeletal muscle cells. The brain is congested and swollen and may show meningeal and cortical petechial hemorrhages; intracerebral hemorrhage has also been observed [56]. Histological examination may show meningeal thickening, with a mononuclear cell infiltrate and perivascular lymphocytic infiltrate in the brain and spinal cord. Chromatolysis of cerebral cortical neurons and gliosis of the gray matter, along with patchy demyelination in the pons, may be present.

Animal models

Multiple animal models have been used. Guinea pigs and hamsters are good models, having a disease course resembling that in humans. Most studies are conducted using golden Syrian hamsters, reproducing human leptospirosis with manifestations of jaundice, hemorrhage, and interstitial nephritis. A recent model of self-healing leptospirosis in mice infected with a strain of *L. interrogans* serovar autumnalis showed characteristic manifestations including jaundice, subcutaneous and pulmonary bleeding but no kidney lesions [57].

Treatment

Treatment consists of antibiotics, crystalline penicillin being the drug of choice, which reduces the course of illness if given early. The role of steroids is controversial. The prognosis after primary neuroleptospirosis is generally good, but altered sensorium and seizures herald a worse prognosis.

References

1. Pearce, J.M.S. (2003). The origins of syphilis. In: *Fragments of Neurological History*, 558–563. London: Imperial College Press.
2. Nakashima, A.K., Rolfs, R.T., Flock, M.L. et al. (1996). Epidemiology of syphilis in the United States, 1941–1993. *Sex. Transm. Dis.* 23: 16–23.
3. Centers for Disease Control and Prevention (CDC) (2015). *2014 Sexually transmitted diseases surveillance: Syphilis*.https://www.cdc.gov/std/stats/archive/surv-2014-print.PDF (accessed 22 June 2019).
4. Bowen, V., Su, J., Torrone, E. et al. (2015). Increase in incidence of congenital syphilis - United States,

2012-2014. *MMWR Morb. Mortal. Wkly Rep.* 64: 1241–1245.
5. Šmajs, D., Norris, S.J., and Weinstoc, G.M. (2012). Genetic diversity in *Treponema pallidum*: implications for pathogenesis, evolution and molecular diagnostics of syphilis and yaws. *Infect. Genet. Evol.* 12: 191–202.
6. Centurion-Lara, A.C., Castro, R., Castillo, J.M. et al. (1998). The flanking region sequences of the 15-kDa lipoprotein gene differentiate pathogenic treponemes. *J. Infect. Dis.* 177: 1036–1040.
7. Charon, N.W. and Goldstein, S.F. (2002). Genetics of motility and chemotaxis of a fascinating group of bacteria: the spirochetes. *Annu. Rev. Genet.* 36: 47–73.
8. Fraser, C.M., Norris, S.J., Weinstock, G.M. et al. (1998). Complete genome sequence of Treponema pallidum, the syphilis spirochete. *Science* 281: 375–388.
9. Cejkoá, D., Zobaniká, M., Chen, L. et al. (2012). Whole genome sequences of three *Treponema pallidum* ssp. *pertenue* strains: yaws and syphilis treponemes differ in less than 0. 2% of the genome sequence. *PLoS Negl. Trop. Dis.* 6: e1471.
10. LaFond, R.E. and Lukehart, S.A. (2006). Biological basis for syphilis. *Clin. Microbiol. Rev.* 19: 29–49.
11. Peng, R.R., Wang, A.L., Li, J. et al. (2011). Molecular typing of Treponema pallidum: a systematic review and meta-analysis. *PLoS Negl. Trop. Dis.* 5: e1273.
12. Centers for Disease Control and Prevention (CDC) (2004). Trends in primary and secondary syphilis and HIV infections in men who have sex with men—San Francisco and Los Angeles, California, 1998-2002. *Morb. Mortal. Wkly Rep.* 53: 575–578.
13. Centers for Disease Control and Prevention (CDC) (2006). Primary and secondary syphilis—United States, 2003–2004. *Morb. Mortal. Wkly Rep.* 55: 269–273.
14. Chen, S.Y., Gibson, S., Katz, M.H. et al. (2002). Continuing increases in sexual risk behavior and sexually transmitted diseases among men who have sex with men: San Francisco, Calif., 1999-2001, USA. *Am. J. Public Health* 92: 1387–1388.
15. Berger, J.R. and Dean, D. (2014). Neurosyphilis. *Handb. Clin. Neurol.* 121: 1461–1472.
16. Daey Ouwens, I.M., Koedijk, F.D., Fiolet, A.T. et al. (2014). Neurosyphilis in the mixed urban-rural community of the Netherlands. *Acta Neuropsychiatr.* 26: 186–192.
17. Cahahine, L.M., Khoriaty, R.N., Tomford, W.J., and Hussain, M.S. (2011). The changing face of neurosyphilis. *Int. J. Stroke* 6: 136–143.
18. Saunderson, R.B. and Chan, R.C. (2012). Mesiotemporal changes on magnetic resonance imaging in neurosyphilis. *Intern. Med. J.* 42: 1057–1063.
19. Deckert, M. (2015). Spirochetal infections. In: *Greenfield's Neuropathology*, 9e (eds. S. Love, H. Budka, J.W. Ironside and A. Perry), 1215. Boca Raton: CRC Press.
20. Harding, A.S. and Ghanem, K.G. (2012). The performance of cerebrospinal fluid treponemal specific antibody tests in neurosyphilis: a systematic review. *Sex. Transm. Dis.* 39: 291–297.
21. Mao, C., Gao, J., Jin, L. et al. (2018). Postmortem histopathologic analysis of neurosyphilis: a report of 3 cases with clinicopathologic correlations. *J. Neuropathol. Exp. Neurol.* 77: 296–301.
22. Katz, D.A. and Berger, J.R. (1989). Neurosyphilis in acquired immunodeficiency syndrome. *Arch. Neurol.* 46: 895–898.
23. Johns, D.R., Tierney, M., and Felsenstein, D. (1987). Alteration in the natural history of neurosyphilis by concurrent infection with the human immunodeficiency virus. *N. Engl. J. Med.* 316: 1569–1572.
24. Musher, D.M., Hamill, R.J., and Baughn, R.E. (1990). Effect of human immunodeficiency virus (HIV) infection on the course of syphilis and on the response to treatment. *Ann. Intern. Med.* 113: 872–881.
25. Horowitz, H.W., Valsamis, M.P., Wicher, V. et al. (1994). Brief report: cerebral syphilitic gumma confirmed by the polymerase chain reaction in a man with human immunodeficiency virus infection. *N. Engl. J. Med.* 331: 1488–1491.
26. Morgello, S. and Laufer, H. (1989). Quaternary neurosyphilis in a Haitian man with human immunodeficiency virus infection. *Hum. Pathol.* 20: 808–811.
27. Guarner, J., Greer, P.W., Bartlett, J. et al. (1999). Congenital syphilis in a newborn: an immunopathologic study. *Mod. Pathol.* 12: 82–87.
28. Tantalo, L.C., Lukehart, S.A., and Marra, C.M. (2005). Treponema pallidum strain-specific differences in neuroinvasion and clinical phenotype in a rabbit model. *J. Infect. Dis.* 191: 75–80.
29. Houston, S., Hof, R., Honeyman, L. et al. (2012). Activation and proteolytic activity of the *Treponema pallidum* metalloprotease, pallilysin. *PLoS Pathog.* 8: e1002822.
30. Lukehart, S.A., Shaffer, J.M., and Baker-Zander, S.A. (1992). A subpopulation of *Treponema pallidum* is resistant to phagocytosis: possible mechanism of persistence. *J. Infect. Dis.* 166: 1449–1453.
31. LaFond, R.E., Molini, B.J., Van Voorhis, W.C., and Lukeh art, S.A. (2006). Antigenic variation of TprK V regions abrogates specific antibody binding in syphilis. *Infect. Immun.* 74: 6244–6251.

32. Workowski, K.A., Berman, S.M., and Centers for Disease Control and Prevention (2010). Sexually transmitted diseases treatment guidelines[published correction appears in *MMWR Recomm Rep.* 2011;60:18]. *MMWR Recomm. Rep.* 59 (RR-12): 1–110.
33. Centers for Disease Control and Prevention (2002). Sexually transmitted diseases treatment guidelines. *MMWR Recomm. Rep.* 51: 1–78.
34. Cameron, C.E. and Lukehart, S.A. (2014). Current status of syphilis vaccine development: need, challenges, prospects. *Vaccine* 32: 1602–1609.
35. Steere, A.C., Strle, F., Wormser, G.P. et al. (2016). Lyme borreliosis. *Nat. Rev. Dis. Primers* 2: 16090.
36. Garin, C. and Bujadoux, C. (1922). Paralysie par les tiques. *J. Med. Lyon* 71: 765–767.
37. Burgdorfer, W., Barbour, A.G., Hayes, S.F. et al. (1982). Lyme disease - a tick-borne spirochetosis? *Science* 216: 1317–1319.
38. Halperin, J.J. (2012). Lyme disease: a multisystem infection that affects the nervous system. *Continuum* 18: 1338–1350.
39. Mead, P.S. (2015). Epidemiology of Lyme disease. *Infect. Dis. Clin. N. Am.* 29: 187–210.
40. Fraser, C.M., Casjens, S., Huang, W.M. et al. (1997). Genomic sequence of a Lyme disease spirochaete, Borrelia burgdorferi. *Nature* 390: 580–586.
41. Miklossy, J., Kuntzer, T., Bogousslavsky, J. et al. (1990). Meningovascular form of neuroborreliosis: similarities between neuropathological findings in a case of Lyme disease and those occurring in tertiary neurosyphilis. *Acta Neuropathol.* 80: 568–572.
42. Oksi, J., Kalimo, H., Marttila, R.J. et al. (1996). Inflammatory brain changes in Lyme borreliosis. A report on three patients and review of literature. *Brain* 119: 2143–2154.
43. Bertrand, E., Szpak, G.M., Piłkowska, E. et al. (1996). Central nervous system infection caused by Borrelia burgdorferi. Clinico-pathological correlation of three post-mortem cases. *Folia Neuropathol.* 37: 43–51.
44. Vallat, J.M., Hugon, J., Lubeau, M. et al. (1987). Tick-bite meningo-radiculoneuritis. *Neurology* 37: 749–753.
45. Pachner, A.R., Delaney, E., O'Neil, T., and Major, E. (1995). Inoculation of nonhuman primates with the N40 strain of Borrelia burgdorferi leads to a model of Lyme neuroborreliosis faithful to the human disease. *Neurology* 45: 165–172.
46. Pachner, A.R., Duray, P., and Steere, A.C. (1989). Central nervous system manifestations of Lyme disease. *Arch. Neurol.* 46: 790–795.
47. Rupprecht, T.A., Koedel, U., Fingerle, V., and Pfister, H.W. (2008). The Pathogenesis of Lyme Neuroborreliosis: From Infection to Inflammation. *Mol. Med.* 14: 205–212.
48. Snowden, J. and Bhimji, S.S. (2017). *Relapsing Fever*. Treasure Island (FL): StatPearls Publishing.
49. Judge, D.M., Samuel, I., Periné, P.L., and Vukotic, D. (1974). Louse-borne relapsing fever in man. *Arch. Pathol.* 97: 136–140.
50. Salih, S.Y., Mustafa, D., Abdel Wahab, S.M. et al. (1977). louse-borne relapsing fever: I.A clinical and laboratory study of 363 cases in the Sudan. *Trans. R. Soc. Trop. Med. Hyg.* 71: 43–48.
51. Speelman, P. (1998). Leptospirosis. In: *Harrison's Principles of Internal Medicine*, 14e (eds. A.S. Fauci, E. Braunwald, K.J. Isselbacher, et al.), 1036–1038. New York: McGraw-Hill.
52. Palaniappan, R.U., Ramanujam, S., and Chang, Y.F. (2007). Leptospirosis: pathogenesis, immunity, and diagnosis. *Curr. Opin. Infect. Dis.* 20: 284–292.
53. Costa, F., Hagan, J.E., Calcagno, J. et al. (2015). Global morbidity and mortality of leptospirosis: a systematic review. *PLoS Negl. Trop. Dis.* 9: e0003898.
54. Mathew, T., Satishchandra, P., Mahadevan, A. et al. (2006). Neuroleptospirosis revisited: experience from a tertiary care neurological centre from south India. *Indian J. Med. Res.* 124: 155–162.
55. Lepur, D., Himbele, J., Klinar, I. et al. (2007). Antiganglioside antibodies-mediated leptospiral meningomyeloencephalopolyneuritis. *Scand. J. Infect. Dis.* 39: 472–475.
56. Forwell, M.A., Redding, P.J., Brodie, M.J., and Gentleman, D.D. (1984). Leptospirosis complicated by fatal intracerebral haemorrhage. *Br. Med. J.* 289: 1583.
57. Xia, B., Sun, L., Fan, X. et al. (2017). A new model of self-resolving leptospirosis in mice infected with a strain of Leptospira interrogans serovar Autumnalis harboring LPS signaling only through TLR4. *Emerg. Microbes Infect.* 6: e36.

39 Neurobrucellosis

Marine Le Dudal[1,2], Fabrice Chrétien[1,3,4,]*, and Grégory Jouvion[1,]*

[1] Experimental Neuropathology Unit, Pasteur Institute, Paris, France
[2] Embryology, Histology and Pathology Unit, The National Veterinary School of Alfort, University Paris-Est, Maison-Alfort, France
[3] Paris University, Paris, France
[4] Department of Neuropathology, Sainte Anne Hospital, Paris, France

Abbreviations

CSF   cerebrospinal fluid
Ig   immunoglobulin
WHO   World Health Organization

Introduction, definition, major synonyms, and historical perspective

Brucellosis is the most frequent zoonosis worldwide and is usually an occupational disease mostly affecting veterinarians, animal breeders and shepherds, laboratory technicians, and workers in the dairy industry or abattoirs. It is endemic in sub-Saharan Africa, the Middle East, and South America [1, 2]. The World Health Organization (WHO) estimates that 500 000 new cases are diagnosed each year worldwide [3]. Around 5–10% of patients display neurological signs. Clinical signs of neurobrucellosis are numerous and non-specific; the diagnosis is difficult and usually made by exclusion. With early treatment, the prognosis is quite good, but relapses are frequent, especially during the first year.

Brucella species are a category B priority pathogen according to the US National Institute of Health, which means they spread easily, result in moderate morbidity and low mortality, and require specific measures for accurate diagnosis and disease surveillance, similar to hepatitis A or Zika virus [4].

Brucellosis was also known as undulant fever, Mediterranean fever, and Malta fever.

Its discovery in humans was attributed to Sir David Bruce in 1886, when a cocco-bacillus was isolated from the spleen of a fatal case of "Malta Fever" [5]. Subsequently, the organism was isolated from goats, cows, and swine.

Microbiological characteristics of the agent

Brucella spp. is a facultative intracellular, nonsporulating, Gram-negative bacteria. More than 10 species exist, and some are still under discovery, but 4 are considered zoonotic. In order of virulence these are: *Brucella melitensis* (biovars 1–3, acquired from

*Fabrice Chrétien and Grégory Jouvion share senior co-authorship.

Infections of the Central Nervous System: Pathology and Genetics, First Edition. Edited by Fabrice Chrétien, Kum Thong Wong, Leroy R. Sharer, Catherine (Katy) Keohane and Françoise Gray.
© 2020 John Wiley & Sons Ltd. Published 2020 by John Wiley & Sons Ltd.

small ruminants), *Brucella suis* (biovars 3–5, acquired from swine), *Brucella abortus* (biovars 1–6, 9, acquired from cattle), and *Brucella canis* (acquired from dogs) [1]. *B. suis* was the first agent categorized by the US Army as a potential biological weapon. It has been estimated by the Centers for Disease Control and Prevention (CDC) that release of an aerosolized form of *Brucella* in a suburb of a major city would cause 82 500 cases and 413 fatalities under optimal conditions (i.e. thermal stability, relative humidity, wind direction and speed, and passage of the aerosol cloud over the target area within two hours) [6]. Laboratory-acquired brucellosis is a perfect example of airborne spread of the disease [7].

Epidemiology

The bacteria are transmitted to humans through consumption of unpasteurized dairy products or by close contact, usually with infected domestic animals. Some cases of infection from wild animals have been reported, raising concerns of a reservoir in the wild [2, 8]. Bacterial load in muscle tissues is low, but consumption of undercooked animal liver or spleen has been implicated in human infections [2]. A few cases have been reported of human-to-human transmission by sexual contact or vertical transmission [9]. The incubation period usually ranges from two to four weeks. Brucellosis is not regarded as an opportunistic infection [2].

Clinical signs

General signs include (but are not limited to) undulating fever (Malta fever), malaise, fatigue, headache, gastrointestinal disturbance, weight loss, and aching joints [8]. Malodorous perspiration is almost pathognomonic. The following systems are involved in order of decreasing frequency: osteoarticular (spondylodiscitis especially lumbosacral and osteomyelitis), neurological, reproductive, gastrointestinal. The most common cause of mortality is endocarditis, sometimes complicated by respiratory failure. Relapses are frequent, especially in the first year, and tend to be less severe than the primary infection [2]. Childhood brucellosis generally takes a more benign course with less complications and responds to treatment [10].

Neurobrucellosis occurs in 5–10% of brucellosis cases [2], but up to one-third of patients with *Brucella* develop neurological complications, probably secondary to immune dysfunction. Neurological signs are numerous and non-specific: behavioral changes, psychosis, dementia, insomnia, blurred vision, hearing loss, confusion, muscle weakness, paresthesia, ataxia, facial paralysis, and others [11]. Transient cerebral ischemic attacks are also reported, probably because of vascular and perivascular inflammation or vascular spasms caused by *Brucella* [12].

Diagnosis of neurobrucellosis

The diagnosis of brucellosis is primarily made by exclusion. Several factors need to be taken into account: epidemiologic data (possible exposure to the agent, living in endemic areas), serum agglutination titer >1:160, cerebrospinal fluid (CSF) agglutination titer >1:80, lymphocytosis and increased proteins in CSF, no signs of an alternative neurological disease, and symptomatic improvement or reduction of lesion size on imaging with appropriate treatment [13, 14]. The prognosis is usually good if treatment starts early enough.

Histopathology and pathogenesis

The pathophysiology of CNS infection by *Brucella* spp. involves allergic reactions, inappropriate immune response, or apoptosis [15]. Two histological patterns have been described: (i) chronic granulomatous infection with multinucleated giant cells and numerous lymphocytes around vessels or (ii) abscesses, which can be large enough to simulate a brain tumor, surrounded by an astroglial scar. The brain, meninges, spinal cord, and cranial or peripheral nerves (especially the vestibulocochlear cranial nerve) may all be involved. Lymphocytic perivascular cuffs may be prominent. Other lesions include vasculitis, thrombosis, infarcts, and foci of demyelination of possible autoimmune origin [16].

Brucella bacteria invade the mucosa via nonprofessional phagocytes [17] that migrate to the regional lymph nodes and then enter the general circulation. The main bacterial target is the reticuloendothelial system (i.e. liver, bone marrow, lymph nodes, and spleen) where the bacteria multiply. They can also localize in other tissues such as nervous system, joints, heart, and kidney [2]. *B. melitensis* tends to elicit small granulomas but strong toxemia, *B. suis* is often associated with chronic abscess formation in joints and spleen, and *B. abortus* can infect and multiply within brain endothelial cells and activate glial cells via interleukin (IL)-1β [18].

These bacteria do not have classic virulence factors such as endotoxins or exotoxins but possess the two-component system BvrS/BvrR, which codes for a kinase sensor and controls the expression of molecular determinants required for cell invasion [19]. After phagocytosis, 15–30% of bacteria survive [20], in gradually evolving compartments, which rapidly acidify, providing protection from antibiotics [2]. Bacterial replication takes place in endoplasmic reticulum without affecting host-cell integrity. Bacteria are released with the help of hemolysins, inducing cell necrosis [21].

Genetic factors

No specific studies have addressed genetic predisposition to neurobrucellosis. However, it appears that patients homozygous for the interferon gamma (INF-γ) +874A allele may be relatively more susceptible to brucellosis (and interestingly also to tuberculosis) [22]. INF-γ has a key role in the defense against *Brucella* because it is clearly involved in macrophage activation, production of reactive oxygen and reactive nitrogen intermediates, apoptosis, immune cell differentiation, and production of cytokines, immunoglobulin (Ig) G to IgG2a conversion, and increase of antigen-presenting molecule expression [23].

Treatment

Brucellosis is hard to cure and relapse is common. There are no real guidelines for neurobrucellosis. Doxycycline in combination with rifampin, trimethoprim and sulfamethoxazole, ciprofloxacin, or ceftriaxone are suitable because of their good CSF diffusion, tolerability, and high gastrointestinal absorption [24, 25], whereas streptomycin and tetracyclines do not seem to penetrate CSF effectively. Currently, no human vaccine is available [2].

Conclusions

Neurobrucellosis is still a diagnosis of exclusion, taking multiple criteria into account. Histopathologic lesions are not specific, and neurobrucellosis should be considered in the differential diagnosis of neurological infection in endemic areas. Adequate treatment has a good rate of success even though relapses are frequent.

References

1. Boschiroli, M.-L., Foulongne, V., and O'Callaghan, D. (2001). Brucellosis: a worldwide zoonosis. *Curr. Opin. Microbiol.* 4: 58–64.
2. Pappas, G., Akritidis, N., Bosilkovski, M., and Tsianos, E. (2005). Brucellosis. *N. Engl. J. Med.* 352: 2325–2336.
3. Oueslati, I., Berriche, A., Ammari, L. et al. (2016). Epidemiological and clinical characteristics of neurobrucellosis case patients in Tunisia. *Med. Mal. Infect.* 46: 123–130.
4. National Institute of Allergy and Infectious Diseases (2018). *NIAID emerging infectious diseases/pathogens.* https://www.niaid.nih.gov/research/emerging-infectious-diseases-pathogens (accessed 16 July 2019).
5. Bruce, D. (1887). Note on the discovery of a microorganism in Malta fever. *Practitioner* 39: 161–170.
6. Kaufmann, A.F., Meltzer, M.I., and Schmid, G.P. (1997). The economic impact of a bioterrorist attack: are prevention and postattack intervention programs justifiable? *Emerg Infect Dis* 3: 83–94.
7. Ergönül, Ö., Çelikbaş, A., Tezeren, D. et al. (2004). Analysis of risk factors for laboratory-acquired brucella infections. *J. Hosp. Infect.* 56: 223–227.
8. Lee, K.M., Chiu, K.B., Sansing, H.A. et al. (2013). Aerosol-induced brucellosis increases TLR-2 expression and increased complexity in the microanatomy of astroglia in rhesus macaques. *Front. Cell. Infect. Microbiol.* 3: 86.
9. Ceylan, A., Köstü, M., Tuncer, O. et al. (2012). Neonatal brucellosis and breast Milk. *Indian J. Pediatr.* 79: 389–391.

10. Shaalan, M.A., Memish, Z.A., Mahmoud, S.A. et al. (2002). Brucellosis in children: clinical observations in 115 cases. *Int. J. Infect. Dis.* 6: 182–186.
11. Guven, T., Ugurlu, K., Ergonul, O. et al. (2013). Neurobrucellosis: clinical and diagnostic features. *Clin. Infect. Dis.* 56: 1407–1412.
12. Ay, S., Tur, B.S., and Kutlay, Ş. (2010). Cerebral infarct due to meningovascular neurobrucellosis: a case report. *Int. J. Infect. Dis.* 14: e202–e204.
13. Memish, Z., Mah, M.W., Mahmoud, S.A. et al. (2000). Brucella bacteraemia: clinical and laboratory observations in 160 patients. *J Infect* 40: 59–63.
14. al Deeb, S.M., Yaqub, B.A., Sharif, H.S., and Phadke, J.G. (1989). Neurobrucellosis: clinical characteristics, diagnosis, and outcome. *Neurology* 39: 498–501.
15. Zhang, J., Chen, Z., Xie, L. et al. (2017). Treatment of a subdural empyema complicated by intracerebral abscess due to Brucella infection. *Braz. J. Med. Biol. Res.* 50: e5712.
16. Erdem, H., Senbayrak, S., Meriç, K. et al. (2016). Cranial imaging findings in neurobrucellosis: results of Istanbul-3 study. *Infection* 44: 623–631.
17. Gross, A., Terraza, A., Ouahrani-Bettache, S. et al. (2000). In vitro Brucella suis infection prevents the programmed cell death of human Monocytic cells. *Infect. Immun.* 68: 342–351.
18. Miraglia, M.C., Franco, M.M.C., Rodriguez, A.M. et al. (2016). Glial cell–elicited activation of brain microvasculature in response to Brucella abortus infection requires ASC Inflammasome–dependent IL-1β production. *J. Immunol.* 196: 3794–3805.
19. Guzmán-Verri, C., Manterola, L., Sola-Landa, A. et al. (2002). The two-component system BvrR/BvrS essential for Brucella abortus virulence regulates the expression of outer membrane proteins with counterparts in members of the Rhizobiaceae. *Proc. Natl. Acad. Sci. U. S. A.* 99: 12375–12380.
20. Arenas, G.N., Staskevich, A.S., Aballay, A., and Mayorga, L.S. (2000). Intracellular trafficking of Brucella abortus in J774 macrophages. *Infect. Immun.* 68: 4255–4263.
21. Gorvel, J.P. and Moreno, E. (2002). Brucella intracellular life: from invasion to intracellular replication. *Vet. Microbiol.* 90: 281–297.
22. Bravo, J.M., de Dios Colmenero, J., Alonso, A., and Caballero, A. (2003). Polymorphisms of the interferon gamma and interleukin 10 genes in human brucellosis. *Eur. J. Immunogenet.* 30: 433–435.
23. Zhan, Y. and Cheers, C. (1993). Endogenous gamma interferon mediates resistance to Brucella abortus infection. *Infect. Immun.* 61: 4899–4901.
24. Erdem, H., Ulu-Kilic, A., Kilic, S. et al. (2012). Efficacy and tolerability of antibiotic combinations in Neurobrucellosis: results of the Istanbul study. *Antimicrob. Agents Chemother.* 56: 1523–1528.
25. Akdeniz, H., Irmak, H., Anlar, Ö., and Demiröz, A.P. (1998). Central nervous system brucellosis: presentation, diagnosis and treatment. *J. Infect.* 36: 297–301.

40 Legionellosis

Edward S. Johnson
Department of Laboratory Medicine and Pathology, University of Alberta, Edmonton, Alberta, Canada

Abbreviations

16S rRNA PCR	16S ribosomal RNA polymerase chain reaction
ADEM	acute disseminated encephalomyelitis
ALL	acute lymphoblastic leukemia
APS	antiphospholipid syndrome
BYCYEα	buffered charcoal yeast extract alpha ketoglutarate supplement agar
CLL	chronic lymphocytic leukemia
CSF	cerebrospinal fluid
CT	computed tomography
DFA	direct fluorescent antibody
Dot/Icm	defective for organelle trafficking/intracellular multiplication
EEG	electroencephalography
EIA	enzyme immunoassay
ER	endoplasmic reticulum
F	female
GBS	Guillain-Barré syndrome
ICT	immune chromatographic assay
L	left
LCV	*Legionella*-containing vacuole
LD	Legionnaires' disease
Lp	*Legionella pneumophilia*
LPS	lipopolysaccharide
M	male
mip	macrophage infectivity potentiator
MRI	magnetic resonance imaging
NAAT	nucleic acid amplification test
PM	postmortem
PMNs	polymorphonuclear leukocytes
R	right
SCID	severe combined immunodeficiency
SLE	systemic lupus erythematosus
TNFα	tumor necrosis factor alpha

Introduction, synonyms, and historical perspective

Legionella is a genus of small Gram-negative aerobic bacteria that comprises 58 species, of which 30 species are pathogenic for humans. The isolation and identification of *Legionella* as a new genus arose from investigations of an epidemic of a mysterious pneumonia among attendees at an American Legion convention in Philadelphia in 1976 during which 34 people, out of 221 patients, died [1].

The term "Legionellosis" encompasses all forms of human illness caused by *Legionella* [1]. By far the most common form is Legionnaires' disease (LD), a noncontagious acute pneumonia, which occurs sporadically or as epidemics. In 65–90% of cases, it is attributable to infection with *Legionella pneumophilia* serogroup 1 (*Lp*1). Extrapulmonary *Legionella* infection without pneumonia is uncommon, usually

Infections of the Central Nervous System: Pathology and Genetics, First Edition. Edited by Fabrice Chrétien, Kum Thong Wong, Leroy R. Sharer, Catherine (Katy) Keohane and Françoise Gray.
© 2020 John Wiley & Sons Ltd. Published 2020 by John Wiley & Sons Ltd.

caused by non-*Lp*1 species, and more likely in patients who are immunocompromised. "Pontiac fever" in contrast, is a noninfectious, self-limited, acute febrile illness resulting from exposure to *Legionella* species in contaminated aerosols. Symptoms are nonspecific, so the incidence is difficult to ascertain though the illness tends to occur in epidemics; its etiology remains speculative [1]. Legionellosis can involve the nervous system as a direct or indirect consequence of infection.

Microbiology

In its natural microbiological environment, *Legionella* bacteria ubiquitously exist within a variety of freshwater sources (e.g. lakes, streams, and ponds) as well as diverse artificial water reservoirs. In these settings, the microorganism thrives in biofilms at an optimum temperature between 25 to 40 °C in its replicative phase as an intracellular parasite of ameba and, less commonly, ciliated protozoa and slime molds [1, 2]. In adverse conditions, it can persist within the encysted form of ameba or in a low metabolic free-living phase, thwarting cultivation or inactivation by biocides, and imparting a tenacious survivability [1].

Because of its requirement for protein rather than carbohydrates as an energy source, *Legionella* can only be cultured in the laboratory with a special medium containing L-cysteine supplemented by soluble iron and 0.1% α-ketoglutarate. Buffered charcoal yeast extract alpha ketoglutarate supplement agar (BCYEα) at pH 6.7–6.9 fulfills these specifications, which when plated and incubated at 35 °C under high humidification and 2–5% carbon dioxide (CO_2), produces a characteristic colony growth that aids in identification along with Gram stain employing 0.1% basic fuchsin. For confirmatory species identification, however, a battery of diverse tests is required [1, 2].

Epidemiology

Epidemiologic information on *Legionella* infection is skewed toward LD because it is the predominant form of illness. Even this data is imprecise because of underdiagnosis and underreporting. Thus, the 13.5 cases/million reported in the United States in 2011 is most likely an underestimate [1]; published incidences in other countries vary widely [2]. The seasonal peak of infection tends to be summer-autumn. Sporadic LD is four times more common than epidemics; 74% are community acquired, 18% arise during travel, and 7% are nosocomial [2]. Mortality rates range from 10–15% [1].

Inhalation of liquid aerosols infested by *Legionella* is the most common mode of transmission; microaspiration and exposure of skin wounds to contaminated water are other routes [1, 2]. Box 40.1 lists the sources of aerosol production from artificial reservoirs, the underlying principle being stagnant or low flow of warm water facilitating biofilm growth. Other factors influencing infectivity include stability and efficient dissemination of aerosol, bacterial load, and species virulence. *Legionella longbeachae,* however, is an exception because it contaminates potting soil. Person-to-person spread is rare, if not exceptional [3].

Factors increasing the risk of Legionellosis, often interacting in combination, are listed in Table 40.1. Of these, the most salient is iatrogenic immunosuppression, which increases vulnerability to nosocomial infections, predisposes to more severe pneumonia with abscess formation, increases the likelihood of extrapulmonary manifestations, and places children at risk [1]. Anti-tumor necrosis factor

---

Box 40.1 Examples of aerosol sources from artificial water reservoirs involved in *Legionella* dissemination

- Air conditioning and other cooling towers[a,b]
- Ornamental fountains
- Whirlpool spas and hot tubs
- Water heaters[c] and humidifiers
- Domestic plumbing and drains
- Hospital hot water systems[d]
- Hospital respiratory devices and nebulizers
- Nasogastric tube irrigation

[a] Dissemination of aerosol 1–6 km.
[b] ≤80% colonized.
[c] 5–30% colonized.
[d] 12–70% colonized.
Sources: Edelstein and Roy [1]; Burillo, Pedro-Botet, and Bouza [2].

Table 40.1 Risk factors associated with *Legionella* infection.[a]

Factor	Comment
Age	Risk increases ≥50 years
Sex	2 M : 1 F
Cigarette smoking	2–7 times increase in risk
Chronic illness	Chronic lung and heart disease
	Chronic renal failure
	Diabetes mellitus
Anti-TNFα therapy	Adalimumab > infliximab > etanercept
	No increased risk with concurrent steroid therapy
Corticosteroid therapy	2–6 times increase in risk
Solid-organ transplantation	Associated increased risk with:
	• azathioprine
	• prednisone
	• Cyclosporine A
	• rejection episodes
Malignancy	Associated increased risk with:
	• lung cancer
	• hematological malignancies with concurrent chemotherapy
	• (hairy cell leukemia, ALL, CLL)

ALL, acute lymphoblastic leukemia; CLL, chronic lymphocytic leukemia; F, female; M, male; TNF α, tumor necrosis factor alpha.
[a] Legionnaires' disease and extrapulmonary disease.
Sources: Edelstein and Roy [1]; Htwe and Khardoi [4].

alpha (TNF-α) therapy in rheumatoid arthritis, psoriasis, Crohn disease, and other illnesses functions as an antagonist to inflammation-induced macrophage resistance and clearance of *Legionella*, leading to unchecked infestation [4]. Corticosteroid therapy, as a single agent or in association with other immunosuppressive drugs in organ transplantation, increases the risk; recipients of kidney, heart, and bone marrow transplants are particularly susceptible. In addition to a greater predisposition to infection, these patients and those with lung cancer and hematological malignancy have a higher mortality (≈40%) and increased possibility of coinfection with another *Legionella* species or opportunistic microorganism, and need longer duration of treatment [1, 4].

Clinical features and diagnosis

Since the earliest reports, an association between an assortment of neurological conditions and LD was recognized [5]. As reviewed by Halperin [6], the proportion of affected patients ranges from 14% to approximately 50%, and the disorders are grouped into two categories:
• Encephalopathy with varied alterations in consciousness, with or without seizures;
• Less-frequent often transient syndromes with focal neurological signs, commonly cerebellar ataxia, or more rarely, transverse myelitis.

Investigations including electroencephalography (EEG), cerebrospinal fluid (CSF) analysis, and radiologic imaging have been normal or disclosed nonspecific findings. Correlating with these clinical observations, postmortem studies have shown no features of *Legionella* brain infection; the neuropathology findings were associated with underlying comorbidities [7, 8]. There is little to connect the neurological features to an abnormal immune response, notwithstanding documentation of cases of acute disseminated encephalomyelitis (ADEM) and Guillain-Barré syndrome (GBS). A longstanding presumed etiology has been an idiosyncratic reaction to an unknown endotoxin released by the bacteria. However, in his analysis, Halperin [6] proposes that these neurological manifestations are similar to those that occur in other severe infections with pneumonia and sepsis, and due to similar causes.

Documented instances of direct extrapulmonary brain infection (Table 40.2, Figure 40.1), are uncommon, but suggest a clinical profile with the following features [9–13]:
- predilection for male sex;
- altered immune status;
- presence of brain abscess, diagnosed by imaging studies or postmortem examination;
- unlikelihood of LD as a precondition;
- species other than *Lp* as an etiology.

Brain abscess is also a consideration in the case report by Perpoint et al. [12] with the emergence, after a month, on magnetic resonance imaging (MRI) of a white matter nodule of T2 signal hyperintensity that resolved with macrolide therapy. Although not consistently reported, CSF analysis shows mild to moderate pleocytosis with corresponding increase in protein but normal glucose levels. In all the reported cases, the environmental source for infection is unknown or not stated; only one patient had LD [9].

The tests available for the laboratory diagnosis of Legionellosis (Table 40.3) offer high specificity, but there are notable differences in the range of sensitivity and applicability. Culture on BCYEα medium remains the reference standard [1, 2, 14]. It provides diagnostic confirmation for other tests and is crucial in the isolation of cultivable non-*Lp* species. Because BCYEα cultures are not undertaken routinely, it is necessary to communicate the clinical suspicion of Legionellosis. The range in sensitivity is wide and dependent on the type and quality of sample submitted and severity of clinical illness [2]. Nucleic acid amplification tests (NAAT, e.g. 16S ribosomal RNA polymerase chain reaction [16S rRNA PCR] and macrophage infectivity potentiator [mip gene] sequencing) are emerging as important adjuncts to bacterial culture and have comparable or increased sensitivity [2, 14]. A variety of sample types can be tested, but species identification is dependent on selection of gene sequences analyzed. Because *Lp*1 exceeds all other species as the cause of LD and Pontiac fever, other tests focus primarily on its detection. Urine antigen testing is restricted to detection of *Lp*1 infection, which in conjunction with sensitivity entails an inherent risk of false negativity [1, 2, 14]. Serology lacks effectiveness as a diagnostic tool: there is a long delay in seroconversion; 25% of patients, including those who are immunocompromised, do not seroconvert; testing for antibodies other than *Lp*1 is undependable [1, 2]. The direct fluorescent antibody (DFA) test was once popular, but its use is limited because of methodological problems and restricted specificity to the battery of antibodies employed [1, 2]. For reasons discussed above, the optimum standard to detect *Legionella* is to use two or more diagnostic tests [1].

Pathology

The principal histopathologic features of *Legionella* infection [15] are:
- fibrinopurulent exudates consisting of polymorphonuclear leukocytes (PMNLs) and macrophages in varying proportions;
- leukocytoclastic fields of nuclear debris;
- focal coagulative necrosis;
- abscess formation.

Legionella bacilli are best demonstrated by silver impregnation techniques (Dieterle, Steiner, or Warthin-Starry) and are present in extracellular exudates, preferentially in macrophages (Figure 40.1). Furthermore, Ziehl-Neelsen or Fite stains can demonstrate *Legionella micdadei*. DFA methodology has been adapted for immunohistochemical and in situ hybridization techniques. By electron microscopy (EM) [16], the microorganisms are commonly found in macrophage phagosomes, a single phagosome containing as many as 30 to 40 bacteria. The bacilli range from 2 to 5 μm in length and 0.3–0.9 μm in width and display features typical of Gram-negative bacteria: envelopment by two trilaminar unit membranes with an intervening lucent space, and central "pinching" nonseptate division.

The lung is the most common organ involved; the infection is represented by consolidating bronchopneumonia that can coalesce into a lobar pattern [15]. Complications include abscess formation, empyema, and seeding to other organs (i.e. lymph

Table 40.2 Reported laboratory confirmed cases of legionella infection of the central nervous system.

Report	Age (years)	Sex	Concurrent Illnesses	Neurologic Features	Lesion	Diagnostic Methodology	Species Identified
Cutz et al. [9]	0.4	M	SCID	Not stated	Midbrain abscess (PM)	Culture (lung) DFA (lung, brain) Dieterle stain	L. pneumophila
Andersen and Sogaard [10]	33	M	None	Confusion R Hemiparesis Aphasia	Left Temporoparietal abscess (CT)	Serology	L. jordanis
Fukuta et al. [11]	57	F	SLE,[a] APS Perivalvular prosthetic valve abscess	Confusion Left Hemiparesis	R Frontal abscess (MRI)	16S rRNA PCR (valve) Warthin-Starry stain (abscess aspirate)	L. micdadei
Perpoint et al. [12]	44	M	None	Confusion Neck stiffness	Meningoencephalitis (CSF) White matter mass (MRI)	16S rRNA PCR (CSF) Serology	L. bozemani
Charles et al. [13]	59	M	Waldenstrom macroglobulinemia[b]	Confusion Left Hemiparesis Aphasia	R Frontal abscess (MRI, PM)	16S rRNA PCR (abscess aspirate) Culture (abscess) Warthin-Starry stain (abscess cavity)	L. micdadei

APS, Antiphospholipid syndrome; CSF, cerebrospinal fluid; CT, computed tomography; DFA, direct fluorescent assay; F, female; L, Legionella; M, male; MRI, magnetic resonance imaging; PM, postmortem; R, right; SCID, severe combined immunodeficiency; SLE, systemic lupus erythematosus.

[a] Treated with prednisone and azathioprine.
[b] Received prior six-month course of chemotherapy with rituximab (anti-CD 20 agent) and fludarabine (DNA synthesis inhibitor).

Infections of the Central Nervous System

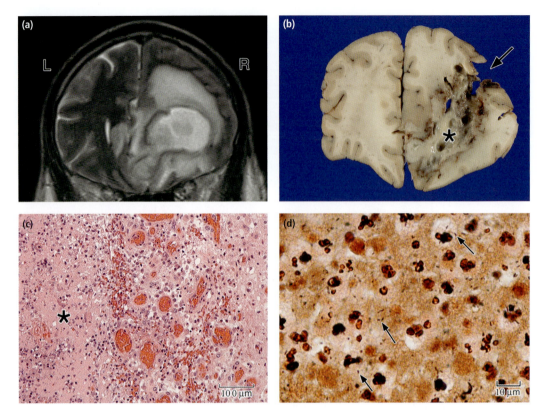

Figure 40.1 *Legionella micdadei* brain abscess. (a) Preoperative magnetic resonance imaging (MRI) scan, T2 coronal window, showing a large abscess in the right frontal lobe surrounded by vasogenic edema. (L, left; R, right). (b) Corresponding coronal section of frontal lobes at autopsy demonstrating tracking of the abscess (asterisk) from the corticectomy site (arrow) deep into the white matter to undermine the orbital cortex. The abscess wall is highlighted by a rim of hyperemia. (c) Microscopic section of abscess wall showing the fibrinopurulent exudate (asterisk) bordered by a zone of engorged proliferating blood vessels between, which are interspersed macrophages and acute inflammatory cells. Hematoxylin and eosin (H&E). (d) Warthin-Starry stain reveals numerous rod-shaped bacteria (arrows) among acute inflammatory cells and less often within cells (top right arrow) within the fibrinopurulent exudate. Source: Figure reproduced courtesy of the authors from [13] by permission of *Journal of Clinical Microbiology*, American Society for Microbiology.

nodes, spleen, liver, bone marrow, heart, kidney, skin, and joints), presumably by blood or lymphatics as a manifestation of bacteremia [1, 7, 9, 15].

Extrapulmonary infection in the absence of LD is less frequent and similarly involves prosthetic heart valves, joints, subcutaneous tissues, and skin [1]. Brain involvement is rare and can present as an abscess [10, 11, 13]. With the increased application of NAAT to the investigation of "sterile" brain abscesses, diagnosis of *Legionella* brain infection may become more common.

Pathogenesis and animal models

Studies on pathogenesis have predominantly focused on infectivity of mammalian macrophages by *Lp* in mice and guinea pig models. Whether the mechanism for *Lp* parallels that in other species remains uncertain, but in general *Legionella*, as an intracellular parasite, has adroitly adapted its strategies for protozoal infection to macrophages [1]. As outlined in Box 40.2, by subterfuge through

Table 40.3 Laboratory tests for diagnosis of legionellosis.

Laboratory Test	Comments	Specificity[a]	Sensitivity[b]
Bacterial Culture	Requires BCYEα agar, special conditions Variety of sample types Yield varies: • Sample type • Severity of illness Needed for identification of non-*Lp* species Confirms diagnosis by other tests	100%	20–95%
Nucleic Acid Amplification Tests • 16S rRNA PCR • mip gene sequence	Variety of sample types Utility depends on range of gene targets used Diagnostic sensitivity ≥30% of culture	90–95%	70–95%
Urine Antigen Test	Restricted to urine Detects soluble cell wall LPS antigen (EIA or ICT assay) Positive weeks to months Limited to *Lp1* Risk of false-negative result	>99%	60–95%
Serology	Need acute and convalescent sera (4, 8, and 12 weeks) Requires 4× increase in titer ≥1:128 No seroconversion – 25% patients Most applicable for diagnosis of *Lp1*	95–99%	20–70%
Direct Fluorescent Antibody Test	Limited applicability and sample type Specificity restricted to antibody panel used Low sensitivity Requires specialized laboratory procedures Risk of false-positive result	99%	20–50%

BCYEα, buffered charcoal yeast extract alpha-ketoglutarate supplemented agar; EIA, enzyme immunoassay; ICT, immune chromatographic; *Lp1*, *Legionella pneumophila* serogroup 1; LPS, Lipopolysaccharide; mip, macrophage infectivity potentiatior; non-*Lp*, non-*Legionella pneumophila*; PCR, polymerase chain reaction.
[a,b] From Edelstein and Roy [1]; refers to diagnosis of *Legionella pneumophilia*.
Sources: Edelstein and Roy [1]; Burillo, Pedro-Botet, and Bouza [2]; Dunne, Picot, and Belkum [14].

secreting eukaryotic-like effector proteins, phagocytized bacilli are able to elude lysosomal degradation and subvert host cell metabolic pathways to allow replication in a modified phagosome, the *Legionella*-containing vacuole (LCV). At completion, the bacterium triggers a pathogen-induced apoptosis of the macrophage causing lysis and bacilli are shed for further infection cycles and amplification of bacterial load. PMNs can phagocytize bacilli but do not permit replication.

In the mammalian host, macrophage infection initiates an innate immune response and provokes an inflammatory reaction with release of chemokines and cytokines, notably TNFα, interleukins, and interferon gamma (IFN-γ). Toll-like receptors (TLRs) on macrophages and other cells appear to modulate the immune response. Stimulation of T cells, in particular natural killer (NK) cells, promotes production of IFN-γ, a crucial factor in activating macrophages to transform from permissive hosts into killers of *Legionella*. One of the important factors in this reversal is the reduction of intracellular iron, a metal necessary for *Lp* replication [1]. Humoral immunity is not as vital for clearing the infection.

> **Box 40.2 Infection cycle of *Legionella* in mammalian macrophages**
>
> 1. Entry of *Legionella* into Macrophages
>   - Bacilli adhesion to macrophage cell surface
>   - Phagocytosis:
>   - conventional
>   - coiling
>   - Facilitating factors:
>   - bacterial surface proteins (e.g. outer membrane protein, mip protein, heat shock protein Hsp60)
>   - pili and flagella
>   - Dot/Icm type IV secretion system
> 2. Engulfment in Phagosome
>   - Blockage of:
>   - phagosome acidification
>   - fusion with endosomes and lysosomes[a]
>   - Redirection of macrophage ER vesicular trafficking to phagosome[a]
>   - Formation of LCV
> 3. Replication of Bacilli in LCV
>   - Subversion of macrophage metabolic pathways to LCV[a]
>   - Multiplication of bacilli in LCV
>   - Nutrient (amino acid) depletion in macrophage cytoplasm
>   - Conversion of bacilli to flagellated form
> 4. Pathogen- Induced Apoptosis of Macrophage[a]
> 5. Cell Lysis and Release of *Legionella* Bacilli
> 6. Repetition of Cycle of Infection and Amplification of Bacterial Load
>
> [a] Mediated by Dot/Icm type IV secretion system.
>
> Dot/Icm, defective for organelle trafficking/intracellular multiplication; ER, endoplasmic reticulum; LCV, *Legionella* containing vacuole; mip, macrophage infectivity potentiator.
>
> Source: Edelstein and Roy [1].

Treatment

Successful treatment of *Legionella* infection is contingent on an agent that is concentrated and bioactive within the LCV, narrowing selection to one of three families of antibiotics: macrolides, quinolones, and tetracyclines [1]. Azithromycin and levofloxacin are the most effective in killing the intracellular bacilli, whereas clarithromycin, erythromycin, and tetracyclines inhibit bacterial replication. Drug dosage and treatment duration depend on the severity of infection, patient immune status, and the presence of extrapulmonary disease. Another factor is coinfection by other microorganisms. Although treatment may rapidly be effective, convalescence is prolonged.

Acknowledgments

The author wishes to thank Mr. Tom Turner for assembling the original photomontage that appeared in the Journal of Clinical Microbiology 2013, 51(2): 701. DOI: 10.1128/JCM.02160-12, and the Journal of Clinical Microbiology for granting use of this image.

References

1. Edelstein, P.H. and Roy, C.R. (2015). Legionnaire's Disease and Pontiac Fever. In: *Mandell, Douglas, and Bennett's Principles and Practice of Infectious Diseases*,

1. 8e (eds. J.E. Bennet, R. Dolin, M.J. Blaser, et al.), 2633–2644. Philadelphia, PA: Elsevier/Saunders.
2. Burillo, A., Pedro-Botet, M.L., and Bouza, E. (2017). Microbiology and epidemiology of Legionnaire's disease. *Infect Dis Clin N Am* 31: 7–27.
3. Correia, A.M., Goncalves, J., Gomes, J.P. et al. (2016). Probable person-to-person transmission of Legionnaires' disease. *N Eng J Med* 374: 497–498.
4. Htwe, T.H. and Khardori, N.M. (2017). Legionnaire's disease and immunosuppressive drugs. *Infect Dis Clin N Am* 31: 29–42.
5. Johnson, J.D., Raff, M.J., and Van Arsdall, J.A. (1984). Neurologic manifestations of Legionnaires' disease. *Medicine* 63: 303–310.
6. Halperin, J.J. (2017). Nervous system abnormalities and Legionnaire's disease. *Infect Dis Clin N Am* 31: 55–68.
7. Weisenberg, D.D., Helms, C.M., and Renner, E.D. (1981). Sporadic Legionnaires' disease. A pathologic study of 23 fatal cases. *Arch Pathol Lab Med* 105: 130–137.
8. Pendlebury, W.W., Perl, D.P., Winn, W.C., and McQuillen, J.B. (1983). Neuropathologic evaluation of 140 confirmed cases of *Legionella* pneumonia. *Neurology* 33: 1340–1344.
9. Cutz, E., Thorner, P.S., Rao, C.P. et al. (1982). Disseminated *Legionella pneumophilia* infection in an infant with severe combined immunodeficiency. *J Pediatr* 100: 760–762.
10. Andersen, B.B. and Sogaard, I. (1987). Legionnaires' disease and brain abscess. *Neurology* 37: 333–334.
11. Fukuta, Y., Yildiz-Aktas, I.Z., Pasculle, A.W., and Veldkamp, P.J. (2012). Legionella micdadei prosthetic valve endocarditis complicated by brain abscess: Case report and review of the literature. *Scand J Infect Dis* 44: 414–418.
12. Perpoint, T., Jamilloux, Y., Descloux, E. et al. (2013). PCR-confirmed *Legionella* non-*pneumophilia* meningoencephalitis. *Med Mal Infect* 43: 32–34.
13. Charles, M., Johnson, E., Macyk-Davey, A. et al. (2013). *Legionella micdadei* brain abscess. *J Clin Microbiol* 51: 701–704.
14. Dunne, W.M., Picot, N., and van Belkum, A. (2017). Laboratory tests for Legionnaire's disease. *Infect Dis Clin N Am* 31: 167–178.
15. Winn, W.C. and Kissane, J.M. (1996). Chapter 33: Bacterial Diseases, Legionella species. In: *Anderson's Pathology, 10e*. St. Louis, MO (eds. I. Damjanov and J. Linder), 801–803. Mosby.
16. Chandler, F.W., Blackmon, J.A., Hicklin, M.D. et al. (1979). Ultrastructure of the agent of Legionnaires' disease in the human lung. *Am J Clin Pathol* 71: 43–50.

41 Neurosarcoidosis

Michael A. Farrell and Alan Beausang
Department of Neuropathology, Beaumont Hospital, Dublin, Ireland

Abbreviations

ACE	angiotensin-converting enzyme
CK	creatine kinase
CSF	cerebrospinal fluid
CT	computed tomography
EBUS-TBNA	endobronchial ultrasound guided transbronchial needle aspiration
FDG-PET	fluorodeoxyglucose positron emission tomography
HP	hypothalamic pituitary
HRCT	high resolution computed tomography
MRI	magnetic resonance imaging
ON	optic neuritis
PON	progressive optic neuropathy
SCS	spinal cord sarcoidosis
SS	systemic sarcoidosis
WASOG	World Association of Sarcoidosis and Other Granulomatous diseases

Definition, major synonyms, and historical perspective

Sarcoidosis is a systemic, noninfectious granulomatous disease of unknown etiology that primarily affects the lung and lymphoid tissues but frequently involves multiple organs in which characteristic granulomas develop. Each tissue or organ has its own unique symptom complex and organ-specific management difficulties. Typically involving those aged between 20 and 50 years, sarcoidosis is a complex disorder with strong genetic and prominent environmental influences that impact its prevalence and natural history. For those with neurologic involvement, sarcoidosis generates considerable morbidity and may be life-threatening [1, 2] Any area of the central and peripheral nervous systems, and frequently several areas in combination, may be involved at any time during the evolution of systemic sarcoidosis (SS). Although not regarded as an infection, the condition is discussed here because the differential diagnosis involves many granulomatous infections. It seems most likely that sarcoidosis represents an immunological granulomatous response to a variety of antigens.

Sarcoidosis is also known as Schaumann Syndrome and Besnier-Boeck-Schaumann disease. Involvement of the parotid gland and facial nerve palsy is known as Heerfordt syndrome, or Heerfordt- Waldenström syndrome when uveitis and fever are also present, (uveoparotid fever).

Infections of the Central Nervous System: Pathology and Genetics, First Edition. Edited by Fabrice Chrétien, Kum Thong Wong, Leroy R. Sharer, Catherine (Katy) Keohane and Françoise Gray.
© 2020 John Wiley & Sons Ltd. Published 2020 by John Wiley & Sons Ltd.

Erythema nodosum and hilar lympadenopathy is known as Löfgren syndrome.

The first description of skin sarcoidosis is attributed to an English physician, J. Hutchinson in 1869 [3]. The Danish ophthalmologist Heerfordt described uveitis and parotitis in 1909 and recognized cranial neuropathies and cerebrospinal fluid (CSF) abnormalities as part of sarcoidosis [4]. The first international conference on sarcoidosis was held in London in 1958. For further history see [5].

Microbiological characteristics

Although a relationship with *Mycobacterium tuberculosis* has frequently been suspected as playing some role, an infectious agent has not been conclusively identified as causing sarcoidosis.

Epidemiology

Sarcoidosis occurs worldwide, predominantly in adults who are young and middle-aged and affects women more than men [6]. The highest incidence is in northern Europe (5–40 cases per 100 000 people. Black Americans have three times the incidence of whites. It is unclear if or how, the various inhaled environmental exposures known to contribute to the pathogenesis of pulmonary sarcoidosis, influence the development of sarcoidosis in nonrespiratory organs, especially the nervous system. Genetic factors are important, given the high morbidity and mortality in black women, notwithstanding this group's increased history of occupational exposure and higher disease prevalence of sarcoidosis. The Th-1 immune response to different environmental antigens varies and operates under strong genetic regulation [7].

Diagnosis of neurosarcoidosis

In patients in whom a confident diagnosis of sarcoidosis has already been established, the challenge when faced with emerging neurologic symptoms is to determine if these are the result of (i) sarcoidosis occurring in the brain, meninges, peripheral nerve, or muscle (ii) a complication of therapy, or (iii) an entirely unrelated disease. It is essential to be certain about the original diagnosis of sarcoidosis. Similarly, when granulomas are found on brain, nerve, or muscle biopsy, making a confident diagnosis of neurosarcoidosis in the absence of a prior diagnosis of SS is hugely challenging.

Establishing a diagnosis of SS depends on interpretation of the combined clinical, radiologic, and pathologic findings by an experienced physician who will determine the extent of investigation. Endobronchial ultrasound guided transbronchial needle aspiration (EBUS-TBNA) may not be necessary in patients in whom a chest high-resolution computed tomography (HRCT) has been performed. Fluorodeoxyglucose positron emission tomography (FDG-PET) may enhance the diagnostic specificity of radiologic findings and show evidence of systemic subclinical, nonrespiratory involvement. Despite such improvements, when new unanticipated, nonrespiratory findings develop in patients with established sarcoidosis, the original diagnosis should be reviewed.

Putting this into practice is facilitated by use of the World Association of Sarcoidosis and Other Granulomatous diseases (WASOG) assessment instrument. At its core, this insists that noncaseating granulomas be found in an organ other than the one under investigation and that other explanations for the clinical presentation be excluded before its attribution to sarcoidosis [8]. Other organ involvement may be graded as highly probable (likelihood at least 90%), probable, (likelihood 50–89%), or possible (less than 50%, i.e. nonspecific). The instrument is not designed to hunt down subclinical granulomas in organs and for the nervous system is best used to decide on the need for biopsy.

Highly probable neurosarcoidosis is defined as the emergence of a clinical syndrome consistent with granulomatous inflammation of the meninges, brain, ventricular CSF system, cranial nerves, pituitary gland, spinal cord, cerebral vasculature, or nerve roots combined with abnormal magnetic resonance imaging (MRI) characteristic of neurosarcoidosis with abnormal enhancement following gadolinium administration or an inflammatory CSF profile. Given these rather vague criteria, the original diagnosis of sarcoidosis must be watertight and other explanations for neurologic findings should be excluded. Infections and other complications of sarcoidosis therapy could satisfy the criteria for "highly probable" and mimic neurosarcoidosis, sometimes with fatal consequences.

Neurosarcoidosis may be considered at least probable in the presence of an isolated facial palsy for which an MRI does not show any possible cause. Similarly, a normal MRI and absence of an inflammatory CSF in the presence of one or more of the various clinical neurological syndromes described may be adequate to consider neurosarcoidosis at least probable, but again, physician experience and judgment is critical.

A negative MRI in the presence of seizures or cognitive impairment may be considered as no more than evidence of possible neurosarcoidosis in a patient with well-documented SS. International experts formulating the criteria for neurosarcoidosis have not agreed to incorporate an isolated inflammatory CSF, low CSF glucose, or any form of peripheral or cranial neuropathy other than facial into any of the three categories.

Positive imaging or a palpable muscle mass is considered evidence of at least probable sarcoid myopathy and myalgias as possible evidence of muscle involvement.

Clinicopathological presentation of neurosarcoidosis

Clinically apparent nervous system involvement is said to occur in 5% of patients with sarcoidosis but may be found in up to 25% of patients at postmortem. Evidence for specific genetic and environmental risk factors for neurosarcoidosis is not robust. Nervous system involvement may be the first manifestation of sarcoidosis; almost half such patients show no evidence of SS at presentation and of these, 50% will never show signs of SS. Involvement of more than one area of the nervous system is frequent. In the absence of SS, several clinical neurological scenarios may necessitate biopsy. If granulomas are a feature on nervous system biopsy, considerable diagnostic challenges arise for the pathologist, and an adequately-sized biopsy is needed to perform a complete repertoire of investigations. Detailed are the common clinical presentations of neurosarcoidosis together with a differential diagnosis for granulomatous disease in each area.

Cranial neuropathy

Any cranial nerve or more than one cranial nerve may be involved in neurosarcoidosis. Facial nerve involvement is no longer considered to occur through direct extension of parotid granulomas into the facial nerve (Heerfordt syndrome). As with any mononeuritis, the cause is usually found locally in the form of granulomatous infiltration of the epineurium or perineurium with or without vascular involvement (Figure 41.1). More usually, cranial nerves are involved by meningeal granulomatous inflammation, which may be reflected in a CSF pleocytosis and in MRI-visible meningeal thickening with or without enhancement. Opportunities to confirm the precise mechanism of cranial nerve injury through biopsy or even autopsy are rare but arise when the granulomatous process is nodular, simulating tumor.

Rarely, optic nerve involvement may develop concurrently with the onset, or later in the course of SS, and may be bilateral. About one-third of patients with optic nerve involvement have coexistent intraocular inflammation, which may be indistinguishable from optic neuritis (ON) with a painful

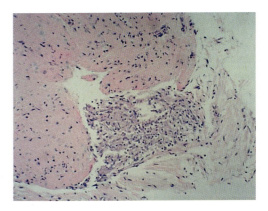

Figure 41.1 Ill-defined granuloma located at the interface between lateral pons and cranial nerve V.

reduction in visual acuity [9]. MRI demonstration of an enlarged optic nerve or of its sheath, with or without signal change, may extend to the chiasm, orbital apex, or anterior and middle cranial fossae. Alternatively, there may be a slowly progressive optic neuropathy (PON) with meningeal enhancement extending to the orbital apex. Unlike ON, PON does not readily respond to immunosuppressive therapy. Treatment relapse is common in the ON group. Rarely ON may be found in the absence of either a confirmatory diagnosis of multiple sclerosis or of SS in ethnic groups such as those of Caribbean origin, known to be at risk for neurosarcoidosis.

An isolated granulomatous orbital mass may be the only manifestation of sarcoidosis and present with proptosis and diplopia [10]. Occasionally only the extraocular muscles may be involved [11]. Bilateral third nerve involvement has also been reported [12]. Involvement of the trochlear nerve may occur at the dorsal midbrain regions where the differential diagnosis of a granulomatous mass includes granulomatous response to germinoma [13]. An abducens nerve palsy may be the result of nodular granulomas in Dorello's canal but is more likely to occur through cavernous sinus involvement. Sarcoidosis of the basal meninges may be isolated nodular, *en-plaque*, or multinodular. Unless there is compelling evidence of SS, there should be little hesitation in obtaining a biopsy, even if the suspect lesion involves the cavernous sinus because radiology cannot safely diagnose or exclude meningeal carcinoma, lymphoma, or meningioma. Trigeminal ganglion involvement may mimic schwannoma [14].

Deafness is rare in sarcoidosis and the precise pathologic mechanism(s) remain(s) poorly documented. Sarcoid vasculitis of the vestibulocochlear nerve, perivascular lymphocytic and granulomatous perineural inflammation at the nerve's junction with the brain, and vasculitis-mediated destruction of the organ of Corti may all be blamed [15]. Vagal nerve involvement may lead to recurrent laryngeal nerve palsy [16].

Meningeal involvement

In sarcoidosis, direct meningeal involvement (Figure 41.2) by granulomas or vasculitis may or may not be associated with underlying superficial parenchymal brain involvement (Figure 41.3). The onset of meningeal symptoms is gradual with persisting headache. Neck stiffness may not be prominent. Even if the patient has known established SS, when confronted with radiologic evidence of patchy or diffuse meningeal thickening or signal change and CSF findings of lymphocytosis, elevated protein, sterile cultures, negative cytology, and possibly a low glucose, the initial suspicion should be of infection especially tuberculosis or of meningeal carcinomatosis or lymphomatosis. Additionally, treatment-related infection must be considered. Every effort must be made to exclude cryptococcosis, and failure to do so may have fatal consequences [17].

Where evidence for SS is not robust and where culture and polymerase chain reaction (PCR) have

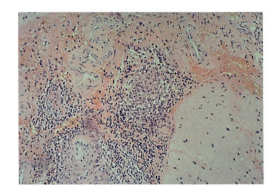

Figure 41.2 Non-necrotizing meningeal granuloma showing epithelioid cells and dense lymphocytic inflammation.

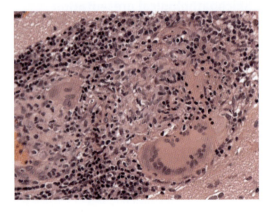

Figure 41.3 Cerebral intraparenchymal granulomas with prominent multinucleate giant cells in a patient with systemic sarcoidosis (SS).

failed to identify a causative organism (i.e. tuberculosis, syphilis, Lyme disease, fungal infection), there should be little hesitation in obtaining a meningeal biopsy of sufficient size to facilitate both histology and the full gamut of microbiological investigations. Once meningeal granulomatous inflammation is identified and infection has been excluded, causes other than sarcoidosis such as immunoglobulin-G-4 (IgG-4)–related disease, Wegener granulomatosis, rheumatoid arthritis, and idiopathic hypertrophic pachymeningitis should be considered.

Cerebral parenchymal involvement

Meningeal involvement may extend for a variable distance into brain parenchyma and simulate single or multiple mass lesions necessitating biopsy, particularly if CSF examination is precluded by the presence of any mass lesion. Dural (Figure 41.4) rather than meningeal granulomas are not usually associated with parenchymal brain disease. Neurosurgeons should be advised that dural biopsy is likely to be less informative than a combined meningeal–parenchymal 10-mm cube that includes arachnoid, gray, and white matter.

Sarcoid granulomas follow perivascular spaces (Figure 41.5) and penetrate the brain parenchyma. Typically involving small to medium-sized arteries, both granulomatous arteritis and fibrinoid necrosis may be found. Venous involvement may result in a destructive phlebitis. Brain hemorrhages may be small and incidental or large and occasionally fatal

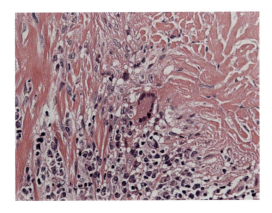

Figure 41.4 Dural granulomatous inflammation in sarcoidosis. Multinucleate giant cell in center with mononuclear and plasma cells separating dense collagen fibers.

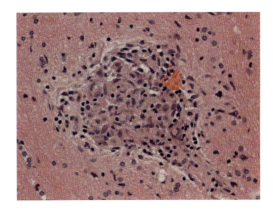

Figure 41.5 Cortical perivascular non-necrotizing granuloma.

[18]. Problems are generated by finding granulomatous angiitis on brain biopsy [19]. A granulomatous response to amyloid is readily diagnosed by immunohistochemical detection of βA4-peptides within giant cells. Varicella-zoster may be excluded by immunohistochemical detection of its antigens. Underlying Hodgkin's lymphoma should be suspected in cases of granulomatous angiitis of the nervous system, in which circumstance hilar adenopathy could mistakenly have been attributed to sarcoidosis rather than lymphoma.

Clinical cerebral involvement in sarcoidosis is a little like cerebral lupus, often lacking a definitive pathologic correlate. Seizures with behavioral and cognitive problems may be present in patients with SS in the absence of MRI abnormalities. In rare detailed autopsy studies, vascular involvement may be microscopic and cause sarcoid-related encephalopathy. Conversely, brain imaging findings are frequent and varied, but their underlying pathology is often not known. Periventricular white matter lesions may be attributed to microvascular involvement including small venules or mimic multiple sclerosis plaques.

In every case, the possibility must be considered that parenchymal changes are therapy-related, for instance, due to progressive multifocal leukoencephalopathy.

Neuroendocrine sarcoidosis

Hypothalamic pituitary (HP) dysfunction may be the first manifestation of SS [20]. Virtually all such patients have clinical and biochemical evidence of anterior pituitary dysfunction, and up to 50% have concurrent posterior pituitary dysfunction. Deficiency of any pituitary hormone or elevated prolactin may be accompanied by biochemical and clinical evidence of diabetes insipidus. Anti-tumor necrosis factor (TNF)-α therapy may lead to a return of anterior and posterior pituitary function. In most instances, even with radiologic improvement, pituitary endocrine insufficiency persists. Up to a quarter of patients with HP involvement have coexistent optic pathway involvement. Clinically evident hypothalamic involvement in the form of appetite, temperature, and sleep alterations rarely occurs. Biopsy of a pituitary mass lesion which yields unsuspected granulomatous inflammation necessitates a search for SS, and granulomatous infection especially tuberculosis [21], Wegener granulomatosis, Erdheim–Chester disease, and so-called idiopathic giant cell granulomatous hypophysitis. Cogan syndrome and Crohn disease may also involve the pituitary gland. A pathologic diagnosis of lymphocytic hypophysitis should not be entertained until multiple levels have been examined for granulomas and until lymphoma has been excluded by clonality studies. Granulomatous infiltration of the pituitary may be simulated by rupture of a Rathke cleft cyst [22].

Spinal cord and CSF involvement

Spinal cord sarcoidosis (SCS) may be the initial presentation of SS, may occur at any spinal level including the cauda equina, and may involve one or more covering spinal layers or spinal compartments including the central canal [23]. Sarcoid involvement of vertebra may lead to vertebral collapse and cord compression. Demonstration of the Trident sign [24] on spinal imaging in the context of a subacute myelitis is said to be suspicious of SCS. In the absence of previously diagnosed SS, distinguishing new-onset primary SCS from any of the immune-related myelopathies especially the neuromyelitis optica spectrum disorders is extraordinarily difficult and requires an in-depth search for occult malignancy and occult sarcoidosis and access to a comprehensive panel of auto-antibodies.

If these prove negative, the difficult decision to biopsy spinal cord, prior to commencement of immune-suppressive treatments, must be balanced by the likelihood of causing further spinal cord-related morbidity.

CSF examination is invariably abnormal with any combinations of elevated protein, high white cell count, and low glucose but these findings are non-specific. A combination of low CSF glucose and elevated CSF angiotensin-converting enzyme levels (c-ACE) levels is highly specific for SCS, although not very sensitive. In general, the overall sensitivity and specificity of c-ACE is relatively low and not clinically useful for the diagnosis of neurosarcoidosis [25].

Sarcoid neuropathy and myopathy

Peripheral nerve and muscle involvement in sarcoidosis may be involved in up to 20% of patients with neurosarcoidosis and is described in Peripheral Nerve Disorders Pathology and Genetics [26, 27].

Genetics

There is an 80-fold increased risk of developing sarcoidosis in co-twins of affected monozygotic brothers or sisters compared with a 7-fold increased risk in dizygotic twins, when compared with the general population [28]. However, mapping the pathways through which genetic and epigenetic influences operate will likely require large numbers of homogeneous clinical sarcoidosis cohorts, given the complex interplay of environmental, racial, and immunological forces [29] at work in the development of pulmonary sarcoidosis. It is not certain that these factors have similar relevance for extrapulmonary sarcoidosis. Understanding the relationships between the highly variable clinical phenotype and genotype is limited. Even though high-throughput genetic research has generated vast amounts of data on sarcoidosis, the significance of several newly-identified candidate genes remains to be determined [30].

Animal models

In myeloid cells, on being freed from the inhibitory effects of tuberous sclerosis 2 gene [*Tsc2*], checkpoint kinase mTORC1 may cause spontaneous formation of granulomas in a variety of mouse organs [31]. Furthermore, TSC2-deficient bone marrow when transferred to control mice is capable of inducing granulomas. Additionally, in response to stimulation by colony-stimulating factor 1, TSC2-deficient bone marrow-derived macrophages showed enhanced proliferation when compared with controls. Mediated by cyclin-dependent kinase 4, this enhanced macrophage proliferation is reversed through inhibition of mTORC1 by everolimus. In patients with sarcoidosis, investigators found enhanced activity of genes lying downstream of mTORC1 signaling, which resulted in increased phosphorylation of ribosomal S6 in up to one third of sarcoidosis granulomas. Although these insights into granuloma formation are fascinating, the environments and immune systems of mice and man differ substantially. In mice mTORC1 activation through loss of TSC1 (rather than TSC2 inhibition) results in a nongranulomatous disorder, and progressive sarcoidosis in humans is associated with loss of *TSC1* expression.

Pathogenesis: the sarcoid granuloma

Typically, irrespective of the tissue involved, the sarcoid granuloma is composed of a central zone of epithelioid histiocytes or differentiated macrophages and multinucleate giant cells surrounded by CD4+ T helper lymphocytes. "Epithelioid" refers to the resemblance of the interdigitated macrophage cell membranes to similar features in epithelial cells. Granuloma macrophages have become reprogrammed to express cell adhesion molecules such as E-cadherin, a step in the formation of multinucleate giant cells in granulomas [32].

Necrosis may be present and ranges from minimal to extensive. Involvement of blood vessels by granulomas may contribute to development of necrosis. A thorough search including several tissue levels and elastic stains to show blood vessels may reveal granulomatous angiitis. Involvement of veins more than arteries is the norm. Exclusion of infectious agents mandates that standard staining for acid-fast bacilli and fungi be performed, and tissue culture and PCR-based methods may also be required. Preoperative dialogue is mandatory to guarantee the biopsy size is adequate for maximum diagnostic yield.

What is responsible for formation and maintenance of granulomas in sarcoidosis is at the heart of all sarcoidosis research, and so far, it is unclear if granuloma dynamics are common to all organs. Superficially, sarcoid granulomas may appear to be relatively quiescent, but each granuloma constantly undergoes replenishment of its histiocytes from circulating activated monocytes, which show greater expression of surface Fc gamma (Fcγ) receptors than control subjects.

Though the nature of any persisting immunostimulatory material within a sarcoid granuloma remains to be determined, there is emerging evidence that in certain circumstances, granulomas may form spontaneously in the absence of any immunostimulatory material (see Animal Models).

Treatment, future perspectives, and conclusions

Because sarcoidosis can be a self-limiting disease, the decision to treat patients must be balanced against the potential harmful side effects of corticosteroid or immunosuppressive therapy including intravenous cyclophosphamide, methotrexate, mycophenolate, and azathioprine. In neurosarcoidosis, significant improvements in patient outcomes have been achieved recently by using infliximab, although recurrence rates on its cessation are more than 50%. Increasing application of high-throughput whole-genome sequencing of cohorts of patients with neurosarcoidosis will hopefully help predict responsiveness to treatment with the new monoclonal antibodies. Additionally, the development of national registries of patients with organ-specific sarcoidosis that use the Grades of Recommendation, Assessment, Development and Evaluation Working Group (GRADE Working Group) system for grading the quality of evidence will go a long way to improving understanding of the natural history and treatment responses of neurosarcoidosis [33].

References

1. Hoitsma, E., Drent, M., and Sharma, O.P. (2013). A pragmatic approach to diagnosing and treating neurosarcoidosis in the 21st century. *Curr Opin Pulm Med* 16: 472–479.
2. Fritz, D., Voortman, M., van de Beek, D. et al. (2017). Many faces of neurosarcoidosis: from chronic meningitis to myelopathy. *Curr Opin Pulm Med* 23: 439–446.
3. Hutchinson, J. (1877). Anomalous diseases of skin and fingers: case of livid papillary psoriasis. In: *Illustrations of Clinical Surgery* (ed. J. Hutchinson), 42–43. London: J. and A. Churchill.
4. Heerfordt, C.F. (1909). On febris uveo-parotidea subchronica localized in the parotid gland and uvea of the eye, frequently complicated by paralysis of the cerebrospinal nerves. *Graefes Arch Ophthal* 70: 254–258.
5. Iannuzzi, M.C., Rybicki, B.A., and Teirstein, A.S. (2007). Sarcoidosis. *N Engl J Med* 357: 2153–2165.
6. Pietinalho, A., Hiraga, Y., Hosoda, Y. et al. (1995). The frequency of sarcoidosis in Finland and Hokkaido, Japan: a comparative epidemiological study. *Sarcoidosis* 12: 61–67.
7. Broos, C.E., Hendriks, R.W., and Kool, M. (2016). T-cell immunology in sarcoidosis: disruption of a delicate balance between helper and regulatory T-cells. *Curr Opin Pulm Med* 22: 476–483.
8. Judson, M.A., Costabel, U., Drent, M. et al. (2014). The WASOG sarcoidosis organ assessment instrument: an update of a previous clinical tool. *Sarcoidosis Vasc Diffuse Lung Dis* 31: 19–27.
9. Kidd, D.P., Burton, B.J., Graham, E.M. et al. (2016). Optic neuropathy associated with systemic sarcoidosis. *Neurol Neuroimmunol Neuroinflamm* 2 (3): e270.
10. Sah, B.P., Sharma, B., and Iannuzzi, M.C. (2016). Isolated extraocular orbital mass: a rare presentation of sarcoidosis. *Sarcoidosis Vasc Diffuse Lung Dis* 33: 302–304.
11. Hayashi, Y., Ishii, Y., Nagasawa, J. et al. (2016). Subacute sarcoid myositis with ocular muscle involvement; a case report and review of the literature. *Sarcoidosis Vasc Diffuse Lung Dis* 33: 297–301.
12. Velazquez, A., Okun, M.S., and Bhatti, M.T. (2001). Bilateral third nerve palsy as the presenting sign of systemic sarcoidosis. *Can J Ophthalmol* 36: 416–419.
13. Klainguti, G., Spahn, B., and Borruat, F.X. (2004). Selective and sequential therapy of oculomotor and palpebral sequelae resulting from biopsy of dorsal midbrain sarcoidosis. *Klin Monbl Augenheilkd* 221: 404–407.
14. Lyra, T.G., Lee, H.W., Vellutini Ede, A. et al. (2015). Gasserian ganglion neurosarcoidosis mimicking trigeminal schwannoma. *Arq Neuropsiquiatr* 73: 173–174.
15. Cama, E., Santarelli, R., Muzzi, E. et al. (2011). Sudden hearing loss in sarcoidosis: otoneurological study and neuroradiological correlates. *Acta Otorhinolaryngol Ital* 31: 235–238.
16. Yamasue, M., Nureki, S., Ushijima, R. et al. (2016). Sarcoidosis presenting as bilateral vocal cord paralysis due to bilateral vagal nerve involvement. *Intern Med* 55: 1229–1233.
17. Lane, H., Browne, L., Delanty, N. et al. (2005). 40-year-old man with headaches and dyspnea. *Brain Pathol* 15: 89–90, 95.
18. O'Dwyer, J.P1., Al-Moyeed, B.A., Farrell, M.A. et al. (2013). Neurosarcoidosis-related intracranial haemorrhage: three new cases and a systematic review of the literature. *Eur J Neurol* 20: 71–78.
19. Mandal, J. and Chung, S.A. (2017). Primary Angiitis of the central nervous system. *Rheum Dis Clin North Am* 43: 503–518.
20. Langrand, C., Bihan, H., Raverot, G. et al. (2012). Hypothalamo-pituitary sarcoidosis: a multicenter study of 24 patients. *QJM* 105: 981–995.
21. Zia-Ul-Hussnain, H.M., Farrell, M., Looby, S. et al. (2017). Pituitary tuberculoma: a rare cause of sellar mass. *Ir J Med Sci* 187: 461–464.
22. Janeczko, C., McHugh, J., Rawluk, D. et al. (2009). Hypophysitis secondary to ruptured Rathke's cyst mimicking neurosarcoidosis. *J Clin Neurosci* 16: 599–60023.
23. Durel, C.A., Marignier, R., Maucort-Boulch, D. et al. (2016). Clinical features and prognostic factors of spinal cord sarcoidosis: a multicenter observational study of 20 BIOPSY-PROVEN patients. *J Neurol* 263: 981–990.
24. Zalewski, N.L., Krecke, K.N., Weinshenker, B.G. et al. (2016). Central canal enhancement and the trident sign in spinal cord sarcoidosis. *Neurology* 87: 743–744.
25. Bridel, C., Courvoisier, D.S., Vuilleumier, N. et al. (2015). Cerebrospinal fluid angiotensin-onverting enzyme for diagnosis of neurosarcoidosis. *J Neuroimmunol* 285: 1–3.
26. Vital, A. (2014). Sarcoid neuropathy. In: *Peripheral Nerve Disorders Pathology and Genetics* (eds. J.M.

Vallat and J. Weiss), 210–213. Oxford: Wiley Blackwell.
27. Vital, A. (2014). Combined muscle and nerve Biopsy. In: *Peripheral Nerve Disorders Pathology and Genetics* (eds. J.M. Vallat and J. Weiss), 12–14. Oxford: Wiley Blackwell.
28. Sverrild, A., Backer, V., Kyvik, K.O. et al. (2008). Heredity in sarcoidosis: a registry-based twin study. *Thorax* 63: 894–896.
29. Chen, E.S. (2016). Innate immunity in sarcoidosis pathobiology. *Curr Opin Pulm Med* 22: 469–475.
30. K1, H., A1, M., Kunej, T. et al. (2018). Sarcoidosis related novel candidate genes identified by multi-omics integrative analyses. *OMICS* 22: 322–331.
31. Linke, M., Pham, H.T., Katholnig, K. et al. (2017). Chronic signalling via the metabolic checkpoint kinase mTORC1 induces macrophage granuloma formation and marks sarcoidosis progression. *Nat Immunol* 18: 293–302.
32. Rosen, Y. (2015). Four decades of necrotizing sarcoid granulomatosis: what do we know now? *Arch Pathol Lab Med* 139: 252–262.
33. James, W.E. and Baughman, R. (2018). Treatment of sarcoidosis: grading the evidence. *Expert Rev Clin Pharmacol.* 11: 677–687.

42 Hypertrophic Pachymeningitis

Françoise Gray[1,2] and Leroy R. Sharer[3]

[1] Retired from Department of Pathology, Lariboisière Hospital, APHP, Paris, France
[2] University Paris Diderot (Paris 7), Paris, France
[3] Division of Neuropathology, Department of Pathology, Immunology, and Laboratory Medicine, Rutgers New Jersey Medical School and University Hospital, Newark, NJ, USA

Abbreviations

ANCA	anti-neutrophil cytoplasmic antibody
CNS	central nervous system
CSF	cerebrospinal fluid
CT	computed tomography
CTL	cytotoxic T lymphocytes
HCP	hypertrophic cranial pachymeningitis
HP	hypertrophic pachymeningitis
HPF	high power field
HSP	hypertrophic spinal pachymeningitis
HTLV-1	human T-cell leukemia/lymphoma virus 1
Ig	immunoglobulin
IgG4-RD	IgG4-related disease
IgG4-RHP	IgG4-related hypertrophic pachymeningitis
IHP	idiopathic hypertrophic pachymeningitis
MRI	magnetic resonance imaging
SLAMF7	signaling lymphocytic activation molecule F7

Definition of the disorder, major synonyms, and historical perspective

Hypertrophic pachymeningitis (HP), also known as chronic pachymeningitis or hypertrophic chronic pachymeningitis, is an uncommon disorder that causes a localized or diffuse inflammatory fibrosis and thickening of the dura mater [1]. The condition most commonly involves the cranial dura, referred to as hypertrophic cranial pachymeningitis (HCP) but may also occur in the spinal dura, referred to as hypertrophic spinal pachymeningitis (HSP) [2]. Both may occur together in rare cases.

Although the majority of HP cases have no identifiable cause and are referred to as idiopathic hypertrophic pachymeningitis (IHP) [1], various causes of HP have been identified, including infections (such as tuberculosis [3], syphilis [4], neurocysticercosis [5] or human T cell leukemia/lymphoma virus-1 [HTLV-1] [6]), metabolic disease, intrathecal injections, autoimmune diseases

---

Infections of the Central Nervous System: Pathology and Genetics, First Edition. Edited by Fabrice Chrétien, Kum Thong Wong, Leroy R. Sharer, Catherine (Katy) Keohane and Françoise Gray.
© 2020 John Wiley & Sons Ltd. Published 2020 by John Wiley & Sons Ltd.

(e.g. rheumatoid arthritis or sarcoidosis), vasculitic disorders (granulomatosis with polyangiitis [7], giant cell arteritis, Churg Strauss Syndrome, and Behçet disease), and malignancy, mostly lymphoma (for review see [8, 9]). The first case of probable IHP was described in 1869 by Charcot and Joffroy [10].

Pachymeningitis is a diagnosis of exclusion and often remains elusive despite thorough investigations. However, many IHP cases share a common histology, namely a lymphoplasmacytic infiltrate with fibrosis, and are sometimes referred to as "inflammatory pseudotumors." They resemble and, in some instances may be associated with, similar inflammatory lesions elsewhere, including the orbit and thyroid gland [1, 9].

Immunoglobulin G4 (IgG4)-related disease (IgG4-RD) is a recently described condition that encompasses a spectrum of fibro-inflammatory disorders characterized by IgG4-positive plasma cell infiltration that can affect almost every organ [11]. The disease was first described in the pancreas and then, in salivary and lacrimal glands, thyroid, kidney, bile ducts, lungs, and retroperitoneum. CNS involvement is relatively rare and mostly seen as hypophysitis. Both IgG4-RD and IHP share similar demographic characteristics, histopathology, and natural history, so IHP is now thought to belong to the IgG4-RD spectrum [9].

Epidemiology

The prevalence of HP has been evaluated in a Japanese national survey and reported as 0.949 cases per 100 000, with pachymeningitis due to IgG4-RD being observed in 8.8%, second only to antineutrophil cytoplasmic antibody (ANCA)-related pachymeningitis [12]. Although IHP is a relatively uncommon disease, reviews suggest that men are affected more than women and that patients typically present in the sixth or seventh decades of life [1]. The few large epidemiological studies of IgG4-RD from the United States, China, and Japan (for review see [13]) confirm that, in contrast to other autoimmune diseases, there is a male predominance of IgG4-RD with a peak onset of disease at 61–70 years. In all studies, neurological disease was relatively rare, although cases of pituitary, meningeal, and peripheral nervous system involvement were reported. In two smaller European studies, from Spain [14] and Italy [15], pachymeningitis was the only reported neurological manifestation – 2/55 (4%) and 3/41 (7%), respectively.

Clinical features

Clinical presentation

Whatever its etiology, symptoms of HP typically reflect either focal or widespread meningeal involvement (e.g. hemispheric or basal dura), leading to mechanical compression of structures (e.g. cranial palsies or vascular compromise) or to more diffuse symptoms (e.g. headache, seizures, and cognitive decline) [15]. Chronic headache and multiple cranial neuropathies are the most commonly reported symptoms. Symptoms resulting from mechanical compression are dependent on anatomical location. Involvement of the cavernous sinus or superior orbital fissure may cause paresis of cranial nerves II–VI and a combination of retro-orbital pain, altered vision, and extraocular muscle palsies, such as the Tolosa–Hunt syndrome. Involvement of the middle fossa, falx/tentorium, cerebellar tentorium, and posterior fossa typically causes paresis of cranial nerves VI–XII or cerebellar ataxia. Vertebral canal lesions are more common at the cervical and thoracic levels and may present with radiculopathies, limb paresis, or sphincter disturbances.

In a review of 33 cases of biopsy-proven IgG4-related HP (IgG4-RHP) [16], the presenting features were: headache (67%), cranial nerve palsies (33%), visual disturbance (21%, typically diplopia or decreased visual acuity), motor weakness (15%), limb numbness (12%), sensorineural hearing loss (9%), seizures (6%), and cognitive decline (3%). About 48% had systemic involvement, mostly bone (12%), salivary glands (9%), lungs (9%), kidney (6%), orbital pseudotumor (6%), and retroperitoneal fibrosis (6%). Isolated IgG4-RHP was present in 30% of the patients, although, notably, systemic involvement could not be excluded in 27% because of lack of available information.

Radiology

On computed tomography (CT) scans and magnetic resonance imaging (MRI) studies, HP appears either as a linear dural thickening or a focal mass and may be localized or diffuse [16]. The focal or pauci-focal distribution of changes within the meninges seems to be more frequent in pachymeningitis due to IgG4-RD, although this observation is based on a limited number of patients [9].

On T2-weighted MRI, fibrotic hypertrophic meninges are thickened and relatively hypointense, with foci of hyperintensity being suggestive of inflammation that can be confirmed using gadolinium-enhanced T1-weighted MRI [16]. Conversely, CT scans are more useful to assess concomitant bone involvement. On CT studies, dural lesions typically appear thickened, hyperdense, and enhanced with contrast [16]. In general, MRI is superior to CT to evaluate the optic chiasm, nerve roots, brainstem, and skull base. Gadolinium-enhanced T1-weighted MRI studies may also give superior spatial resolution to facilitate the identification of active inflammation along the dural edges.

Laboratory investigations

Serology is important to rule out infectious or neoplastic causes of HP and to identify vasculitic or autoimmune-associated systemic disorders.

An elevated serum IgG4 concentration is characteristic of IgG4-RD and when present supports the diagnosis [13]. However, on its own, it is neither necessary nor sufficient for a diagnosis of IgG4-RD. Serum IgG4 concentrations tend to be higher in patients with multi-organ involvement. High serum levels of IgG4 have been reported in healthy individuals and in patients with various diseases that can mimic IgG4-RD. About half of patients with biopsy-proven IgG4-RD may have normal serum IgG4 concentrations at the time of diagnosis [13].

More recently, Wallace et al. showed that circulating plasmablasts are elevated in active IgG4-RD (even in patients with normal serum IgG4 concentrations) and that plasmablast counts are a potentially useful biomarker for diagnosing IgG4-RD and assessing its response to treatment [17].

Cerebrospinal fluid (CSF) analysis is useful to exclude other pathologies, such as CNS infections or malignant disease. It usually reveals normal glucose levels, normal or slightly elevated protein levels, and a variable degree of pleocytosis (lymphocytic, monocytic).

A higher elevation of CSF IgG4 levels has also been reported in patients with IgG4-RHP when compared with patients with infectious, neoplastic, and inflammatory meningitis [18]. This may be of particular relevance in those with IHP, who can have increased intrathecal IgG4 synthesis despite normal serum levels of IgG4.

Pathology

Macroscopy

There are few autopsy cases of HP [19, 20]. There is marked dural thickening, which may be solitary or multiple, diffuse or nodular, and can involve both the cranial and spinal dura. HCP mainly affects the base of the skull and the posterior fossa, whereas HSP preferentially involves the cervical and thoracic levels. The lesion may adhere or not to the cerebral or spinal parenchyma, but the underlying parenchyma is generally not affected. Involvement of the leptomeninges or brain parenchyma has been reported infrequently in association with pachymeningitis or systemic IgG4-RD [21].

Surgical specimens show a solid yellow and white-colored focal thickening of the dura mater [8, 22].

Histopathology

Microscopic examination is required to establish the diagnosis of HP. Concentric layers of dense fibrous tissue underlie dural hypertrophy and are mixed with inflammatory cells (Figure 42.1a–c) consisting of lymphocytes, plasma cells (Figure 42.1b, c), and occasionally foreign body giant cells (Figure 42.2). The lymphoplasmacytic infiltrate may be very dense with a pseudofollicular arrangement (Figure 42.3). Russell bodies (Figure 42.4) are occasionally present.

In IgG4-RD, the histopathologic features are crucial to the diagnosis and dura mater biopsy remains the gold standard for diagnosing

Infections of the Central Nervous System

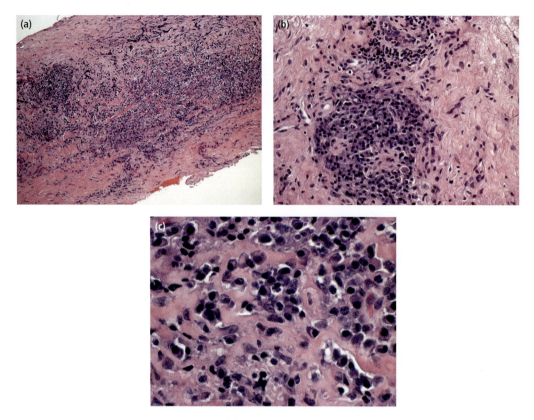

Figure 42.1 Hypertrophic pachymeningitis: characteristic fibrosis mixed with inflammatory cells. (a) Low magnification in a case of hypertrophic spinal pachymeningitis. (b) Note the perivascular lymphoplasmacytic infiltration. (c) Abundant plasma cells in the inflammatory infiltrate.

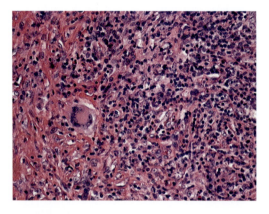

Figure 42.2 Hypertrophic pachymeningitis: A multinucleated giant cell is present at the border of the inflammatory infiltrate.

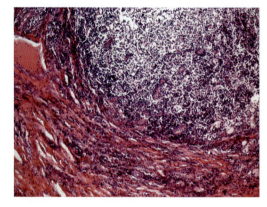

Figure 42.3 Dense inflammatory infiltrate with a pseudofollicular arrangement surrounded by concentric fibrosis.

Hypertrophic Pachymeningitis Chapter 42

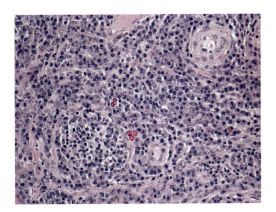

Figure 42.4 Very dense plasmacytic infiltrate with several Russell bodies. Note prominent endothelial cells in vessels almost enclosed by inflammation.

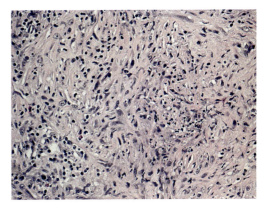

Figure 42.6 Churg Strauss Syndrome-related hypertrophic pachymeningitis. Interwoven fibrosis and mixed inflammation with numerous plasma cells and occasional eosinophils.

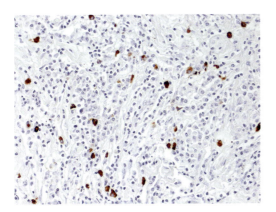

Figure 42.5 IgG4-RHP. Immunostain for immunoglobulin G4 (IgG4) showing many positive cells within the inflammatory infiltrate. (Source: Courtesy of Dr. Anthony Yachnis, University of Florida, USA.)

IgG4-related HP (IgG4-RHP). The major histopathologic features include a dense lymphoplasmacytic infiltrate, storiform fibrosis, and in many tissues, obliterative phlebitis. A mild to moderate infiltrate of eosinophils and nonobliterative phlebitis have also been associated with IgG4-RD [23]. There are no single immunohistochemical features that are pathognomonic for this disease. However, a cutoff value of 10 IgG4 + plasma cells per high-powered field, and an IgG4+/IgG+ plasma cell ratio >40%, are recognized as sufficient for the diagnosis of IgG4-RD of the meninges (Figure 42.5) [9].

Histopathology also helps exclude other causes of pachymeningitis: microorganisms cannot be demonstrated within the lesions by special stains, cultures of the inflammatory tissue are negative, and there is no evidence of malignancy. It may also identify other systemic diseases associated with HP. The presence of multinucleated giant cells or granulomas, although occasionally present in IgG4-RD, are more suggestive of granulomatous diseases such as rheumatoid arthritis and sarcoidosis. Necrotizing vasculitis is not a feature of IgG4-RD and may be found in systemic vasculitis such as granulomatosis with polyangiitis [7], Churg Strauss syndrome (Figure 42.6) [24], or systemic lupus erythematosus [25].

Pathogenesis

Although IgG4-RD has been recognized only recently, a plausible explanation of the pathogenesis has been put forward.

There is growing acceptance that IgG4 itself is unlikely to be pathogenic in IgG4-RD [26].

Instead, recent evidence suggests that CD4+ T-cells play a central role in IgG4-RD pathogenesis [27]. They are dispersed throughout IgG4-RD lesions and are the most abundant cell within affected tissues [23]. Mattoo et al. demonstrated that CD4$^+$ cytotoxic T lymphocytes (CTL) which also expressed signaling lymphocytic activation molecule F7 (SLAMF7) were clonally expanded in patients with IgG4-RD, and these cells expressed granzyme B, perforin, interleukin (IL)-1β, tumor growth factor (TGF)-β, and interferon gamma (IFN-γ), which may be important mediators of tissue damage [27].

Plasmablasts (CD19$^+$CD20$^-$CD27$^+$CD38$^+$) are found in high concentrations in IgG4-RD, regardless of the serum IgG4 concentration, and their number may correlate more closely with disease activity than IgG4 levels [17]. The circulating oligoclonal plasmablasts demonstrate intense somatic hypermutation, a hallmark of interaction with T cells within the germinal centers of lymph nodes [28, 29]. Furthermore, the presence of oligoclonal IgG4 bands in the CSF of subjects with IgG4-RHP supports the concept of an antigen-driven immune response [18] and the presence of oligoclonally restricted IgG4-positive plasma cells within inflammatory meningeal niches strongly suggests a specific response against a still unknown, possibly meningeal, antigen. Both B cells and plasmablasts may play a variety of roles in IgG4-RD, the most important of which may be presentation of antigen to T cells. How and why specific B cells are recruited to become clonally expanded IgG4-producing plasmablasts and plasma cells remains unknown, but T follicular helper cells appear to drive the class switch toward IgG4, perhaps through the secretion of IL-4 [29].

In summary, CD4$^+$ CTL may orchestrate IgG4-RD but be sustained themselves by continuous antigen presentation by B cells or by B-cell-dependent growth factors, self-perpetuating an immune response against a still unknown specific antigen [28]. Further characterization of the pathogenesis may offer an opportunity for a more rational and targeted therapeutic approach in the future.

Treatment

High-dose steroids are a first-line treatment, although toxicity can be dose-limiting. Methotrexate may be beneficial in steroid-refractory cases. Apart from pharmacological therapy, some patients have needed urgent surgical decompression in the face of ongoing neurological symptoms.

Treatment should also be targeted if the underlying systemic process is identified. For IgG4-RD, the standard first-line treatment is corticosteroids. Although often effective in reducing disease activity or inducing remission, they rarely have a durable effect. Alternative immunosuppressive agents such as azathioprine, cyclophosphamide, and methotrexate have been tested in patients who were refractory to steroids or developed steroid dependence, and these agents showed long-term success in a few patients.

Targeted treatments against the B-cell lineage, particularly Rituximab, appear promising [30], and therapy focused on the CD4+ SLAMF7+ CTL may also be feasible.

References

1. Kupersmith, M.J., Martin, V., Heller, G. et al. (2004). Idiopathic hypertrophic pachymeningitis. *Neurology* 62: 686–694.
2. Qin, L.X., Wang, C.Y., Hu, Z.P. et al. (2015). Idiopathic hypertrophic spinal pachymeningitis: a case report and review of literature. *Eur. Spine J.* 24 (Suppl. 4): S636–S643.
3. Guidetti, B. and La Torre, E. (1967). Hypertrophic spinal pachymeningitis. *J. Neurosurg.* 26: 496–503.
4. Vale, T.C., Moraes, T.E.C., Lara, A. et al. (2012). Hypertrophic cervical spinal cord pachymeningitis due to Treponema pallidum infection. *Neurol. Sci.* 33: 359–362.
5. Vale, T.C., Duani, H., Macedo, D.L., and Christo, P.P. (2013). Cranial hypertrophic pachymeningitis secondary to neurocysticercosis. *Neurol. Sci.* 34: 401–403.
6. Kawano, Y. and Kira, J. (1995). Chronic hypertrophic cranial pachymeningitis associated with HTLV-I infection. *J. Neurol. Neurosurg. Psychiatry* 59: 435–437.
7. Kato, E., Tahara, K., Hayashi, H. et al. (2018). Granulomatosis with polyangiitis complicated by hypertrophic pachymeningitis presenting with simultaneous multiple intracerebral hemorrhages. *Intern. Med.* 57: 1167–1172.
8. Bureta, C.A., Abematsu, M., Tominaga, H. et al. (2018). Hypertrophic spinal pachymeningitis associated with human T-cell lymphotrophic virus-1 infection and Sjogren's syndrome: a case report and brief literature review. *Int. J. Surg. Case Rep.* 45: 22–28.
9. Wallace, Z.S., Carruthers, M., Khosroshahi, A. et al. (2013). IgG4-related disease and hypertrophic pachymeningitis. *Medicine (Baltimore)* 92: 206–216.

10. Charcot, J.M. and Joffroy, A. (1869). Deux cas d'atrophie musculaire progressive avec lesions de la substance grise et des faisceaux anterolateraux de la moelle epiniere. *Arch. Physiol. Norm. Pathol.*: 354–367.
11. Stone, J.H., Zen, Y., and Deshpande, V. (2012). IgG4-related disease. *N. Engl. J. Med.* 366: 539–551.
12. Yonekawa, T., Murai, H., Utsuki, S. et al. (2014). A nationwide survey of hypertrophic pachymeningitis in Japan. *J. Neurol. Neurosurg. Psychiatry* 85: 732–739.
13. Baptista, B., Casian, A., Gunawardena, H. et al. (2017). Neurological manifestations of IgG4-related disease. *Curr. Treat. Options Neurol.* 19: 14.
14. Fernandez-Codina, A., Martinez-Valle, F., Pinilla, B. et al. (2015). IgG4-related disease: results from a multicenter Spanish registry. *Medicine (Baltimore)* 94: e1275.
15. Campochiaro, C., Ramirez, G.A., Bozzolo, E.P. et al. (2016). IgG4-related disease in Italy: clinical features and outcomes of a large cohort of patients. *Scand. J. Rheumatol.* 45: 135–145.
16. Lu, L.X., Della-Torre, E., Stone, J.H., and Clark, S.W. (2014). IgG4-related hypertrophic pachymeningitis: clinical features, diagnostic criteria, and treatment. *JAMA Neurol.* 71: 785–793.
17. Wallace, Z.S., Mattoo, H., Carruthers, M. et al. (2015). Plasmablasts as a biomarker for IgG4-related disease, independent of serum IgG4 concentrations. *Ann. Rheum. Dis.* 74: 190–195.
18. Della-Torre, E., Passerini, G., Furlan, R. et al. (2013). Cerebrospinal fluid analysis in IgG4-related hypertrophic pachymeningitis. *J. Rheumatol.* 40: 1927–1929.
19. Kaga, H., Komatsuda, A., Saito, M. et al. (2018). Anti-neutrophil cytoplasmic antibody-associated vasculitis complicated by periaortitis and cranial hypertrophic pachymeningitis: a report of an autopsy case. *Intern. Med.* 57: 107–113.
20. Masson, C., Hénin, D., Hauw, J.J. et al. (1993). Cranial pachymeningitis of unknown origin: a study of seven cases. *Neurology* 43: 1329–1334.
21. Regev, K., Nussbaum, T., Cagnano, E. et al. (2014). Central nervous system manifestation of IgG4-related diseases. *JAMA Neurol.* 71: 767–770.
22. Takeuchi, S., Osada, H., Seno, S., and Nawashiro, H. (2014). IgG4-related intracranial hypertrophic pachymeningitis: a case report and review of the literature. *J. Korean Neurosurg. Soc.* 55: 300–302.
23. Deshpande, V., Zen, Y., Chan, J.K. et al. (2012). Consensus statement on the pathology of IgG4-related disease. *Mod. Pathol.* 25: 1181–1192.
24. Lio, M., Fukuda, S., Maguchi, S. et al. (2001). Churg-Strauss syndrome with pachymeningitis refractory to steroid therapy-a case report. *Auris Nasus Larynx* (28 Suppl): S121–S125.
25. Han, F., Zhong, D.R., Hao, H.L. et al. (2016). Cranial and lumbosacral hypertrophic pachymeningitis associated with systemic lupus erythematosus: a case report. *Medicine (Baltimore)* 95: e4737.
26. Stone, J.H., Zen, Y., and Deshpande, V. (2012). IgG4 related disease. *N. Engl. J. Med.* 366: 539–551.
27. Mattoo, H., Mahajan, V.S., Maehara, T. et al. (2016). Clonal expansion of CD4 cytotoxic T lymphocytes in patients with IgG-related disease. *J. Allergy Clin. Immunol.* 138: 825–838.
28. Stone, J.H. (2016). IgG4-related disease: pathophysiologic insights drive emerging treatment approaches. *Clin. Exp. Rheumatol.* 34 (Suppl 98): 66–68.
29. Mattoo, H., Mahajan, V.S., Della-Torre, E. et al. (2014). De novo oligoclonal expansions of circulating plasmablasts in active and relapsing IgG4-related disease. *J. Allergy Clin. Immunol.* 134: 679–687.
30. Jang, Y., Lee, S.T., Jung, K.H. et al. (2017). Rituximab treatment for idiopathic hypertrophic pachymeningitis. *J. Clin. Neurol.* 13: 155–161.

43 Toxin-Induced Neurological Diseases

Pierre L. Goossens[1,2], Cédric Thépenier[1], and Michel R. Popoff[3]

[1] Experimental Neuropathology Unit, Pasteur Institute, Paris, France
[2] Yersinia, Pasteur Institute, Paris, France
[3] Bacterial Toxins Unit, Pasteur Institute, Paris, France

Abbreviations

BBB	blood-brain barrier
BoNT	botulinum neurotoxin
CNS	central nervous system
CSF	cerebrospinal fluid
DAMP	damage-associated molecular pattern
ER	endoplasmic reticulum
ETX	epsilon toxin
FPR	formyl peptide receptors
GABA	gamma amino butyric acid
HC	high chain
HUS	hemolytic uremic syndrome
LC	light chain
LCGT	large clostridial glucosylating toxins
LPS	lipopolysaccharide
LTA	lipoteichoic acid
MAL	myelin and lymphocyte protein
PAMP	pathogen-associated molecular pattern
PNS	peripheral nervous system
STEC	shiga toxin-producing *Escherichia coli*
SNAP25	synaptosome-associated protein 25
SNARE	N-ethylmaleimide-sensitive-factor attachment protein receptor
Stx	shiga-toxin
TeNT	tetanus neuro-toxin
VAMP	vesicle-associated membrane protein

Introductory remarks

Toxins are diffusible molecules that act at a distance from their site of production. In this respect:

1. Toxin-induced neurological diseases resulting from bacteria are usually not linked to actual infection of the central nervous system (CNS). The involved bacteria enter, colonize, and multiply remotely from the CNS and use specific means to allow their toxins ultimately reach or interact with the CNS.

Bacterial toxins may act either directly or indirectly on the CNS (Figure 43.1).
- Directly via neural pathways (such as for the *Clostridium tetani* tetanus neurotoxin, [TeNT]) or via the bloodstream (such as *Clostridium perfringens* Epsilon toxin) – i.e. reaching the CNS through the blood-brain barrier (BBB).
- Indirectly, thus strictly speaking not reaching the CNS but modulating host systems that interact with the CNS. Two main systems are involved: the peripheral nervous system (PNS) that relays information from the periphery (with the paradigm being botulinum neurotoxin [BoNT]) and the blood compartment that bathes the brain (i.e. signal transmission through the highly adapted BBB interface).

Infections of the Central Nervous System: Pathology and Genetics, First Edition. Edited by Fabrice Chrétien, Kum Thong Wong, Leroy R. Sharer, Catherine (Katy) Keohane and Françoise Gray.
© 2020 John Wiley & Sons Ltd. Published 2020 by John Wiley & Sons Ltd.

Infections of the Central Nervous System

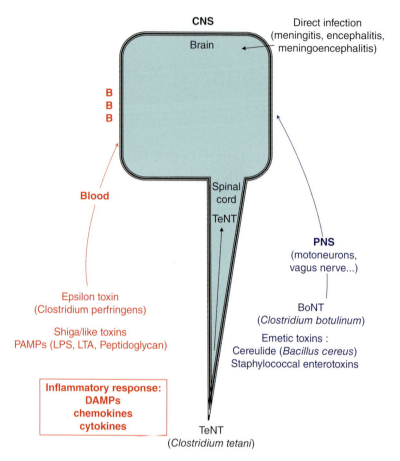

Figure 43.1 Tetanus neurotoxin (TeNT) reaches the CNS directly, in contrast to botulinum neurotoxin (BoNT) that reaches it indirectly through the peripheral nervous system (PNS). Emetic toxins interact with the CNS via stimulation of the vagus nerve. Alternatively, toxins can reach the CNS via the blood compartment (*Clostridium perfringens* Epsilon toxin, *Shigella dysenteriae* shiga toxins, or *Escherichia coli* Shiga-like toxins). In a broader sense, bacterial products (pathogen-associated molecular pattern [PAMPs]) and infected host molecules (damage-associated molecular pattern [DAMPs], cytokines, and chemokines) circulating in the blood could exert toxic effects on the CNS. BBB, blood brain barrier; LPS, lipopolysaccharide; LTA, lipoteichoic acid.

2. As detailed in other chapters of this book, bacteria can also reach the meninges and the CNS and locally multiply. The bacteria then deliver their toxins directly into the cerebrospinal fluid (CSF) and CNS parenchyma.

Toxins with direct toxic activity against the CNS

The main pathological effects of toxins that directly affect the CNS are observed on neurons, so these cells have been the most extensively investigated. Because neurons extend very far from the brain, they are more likely to be affected than microglial cells, astrocytes, and oligodendrocytes, where toxins have to reach them locally. Toxins may directly reach the CNS either via a neural or hematogenous route or locally through direct infection of the CNS.

The most frequent toxins and their corresponding bacterial producer and culprit are presented.

Toxins affecting the CNS via a neural route

TeNT produced by *C. tetani* is the classic example of a toxin using this route.

Definition, historical perspectives, and synonyms

Tetanus is a neurological disease characterized by spastic paralysis. The word is derived from the Greek *tétanos* meaning "muscular stretch" or "spasm." It has been known since antiquity and was described by Hippocrates of Kos in the fourth century BCE as a horrible disease. A detailed clinical description was given by Sir Charles Bell in a soldier wounded at Corunna during the British-French war (1809). Carle and Rattone as well as Nicolaier (1884) demonstrated that the disease was caused by a bacterium, which Kitasato (1889) later isolated and named *C. tetani*. Subsequently, Faber, Tizzoni, and Cattani (1889–1890) and Bruschettini (1892) discovered that the symptoms were due to the result of a protein (TeNT), which travels to the CNS [1]. Tetanus is also known as "lockjaw" or "trismus."

Microbiological characteristics of the agent

C. tetani is a Gram-positive, anaerobic bacillus that forms round terminal and enlarged spores with the appearance of drumsticks. It is a ubiquitous organism found in soil samples worldwide, particularly in warmer countries. *C. tetani* strains belong to a homogeneous bacterial species and produce only one type of TeNT during the end of the exponential growth phase and the beginning of the stationary phase. TeNT gene is localized on large size plasmids in *C. tetani* strains.

TeNT is synthesized as a single chain protein of about 150 kDa, which is proteolytically activated in the extracellular medium into a light chain (LC, ~50 kDa) and heavy chain (HC, ~100 kDa), which remain linked by a disulfide bridge. TeNT structure is similar to that of BoNT with three main domains: LC containing the catalytic active site, the HC N-terminal with two long helices being the translocation domain, and the HC C-terminal subdivided into two subdomains (HC_N and HC_C), involved in recognizing specific receptors on target neurons [2].

Epidemiology and importance

Tetanus is a major infectious disease resulting from wounds contaminated with *C. tetani*. All people regardless of age and sex are susceptible. Currently, the main forms are neonatal and maternal tetanus, notably in the tropical countries of Africa and Asia. Deaths from neonatal tetanus decreased from 780 000 in 1988 to 34 000 in 2015, thanks to vaccination [3]. Tetanus is a rare disease in France (36 cases reported from 2008 to 2011).

Clinical features and diagnosis

Tetanus symptoms are characterized by spastic paralysis. In local tetanus, persistent muscle spasms occur in close proximity to the infected site. Generalized tetanus is the most commonly recognized form, manifested by trismus (lockjaw), *risus sardonicus,* opisthotonic posturing, limb rigidity, general convulsions, and respiratory distress.

The diagnosis is mainly based on the characteristic clinical symptoms. Biological investigations involve detection of *C. tetani* in the contaminated wound. However, the initial wound is often no longer visible at the onset of the symptoms.

Pathology

C. tetani spores germinate in the contaminated wound under anaerobic conditions in the presence of necrotic tissue (deep wound with weak surface opening). The umbilical stump is a common portal of entry. TeNT is produced locally during bacterial growth and disseminates to proximal neuron endings, mainly motor neurons. TeNT binds to specific neuronal receptors – polysialogangliosides, nidogen, and possibly other specific membrane proteins – enters neural endocytic vesicles, and undergoes retrograde transport to the spinal cord and brain. TeNT is released and gains access to glycinergic and γ-aminobutyric acid (GABA)-ergic inhibitory interneurons. Upon entry via endocytosis into acidified vesicles, the L-chain is translocated into the cytosol and proteolytically cleaves vesicle-associated membrane protein (VAMP), one of the three soluble N-ethylmaleimide-sensitive-factor attachment protein receptors (SNARE) involved in neuroexocytosis. This prevents the release of glycine and GABA and the control of motor reflex responses [1].

Histopathological changes are not seen in the CNS in tetanus cases.

Treatment and Prevention

Tetanus treatment is mainly symptomatic. In patients who are not vaccinated, anti-TeNT immunoglobulins are indicated to prevent tetanus if wounds are suspected to be contaminated with *C. tetani*. Vaccination with tetanus toxoid (or anatoxin) is the most effective preventive measure.

Toxins affecting the CNS via the hematogenous route: *C. perfringens* epsilon toxin

Definition and historical perspectives

C. perfringens is responsible for various diseases in man and animals including gangrene, puerperal septicemia, and intestinal disorders such as diarrhea, enteritis, necrotic enteritis, food poisoning, and enterotoxemia. The bacterium was discovered by Achalme (1891) from a human case of arthritis, and since the beginning of the twentieth century epsilon toxin (ETX)-producing *C. perfringens* was recognized as an important pathogen in animals. Recently, chronic infection with ETX-producing *C. perfringens* has been suspected to be implicated in multiple sclerosis [4].

Microbial characteristics of the agent

C. perfringens is a ubiquitous Gram-positive, anaerobic, spore-forming bacterium, which is widespread in the environment. It produces numerous toxins and is divided into five types based on the alpha, beta, epsilon, and iota toxins. ETX is produced by *C. perfringens* types B and D.

ETX is a pore-forming toxin of 33 kDa, activated by trypsin and other proteases. Its structure is related to that of aerolysin. ETX is one of the most lethal toxins (lethal dose in mouse 70 ng/kg by intraperitoneal route). In sensitive cells, ETX induces a rapid loss of intracellular potassium (K^+) and adenosine triphosphate (ATP) and subsequent cell death by necrosis.

Epidemiology, importance

C. perfringens type D is the causative agent of enterotoxemia in animals, mainly sheep, in whom it is a fatal, economically important global disease. In some countries *C. perfringens* type B is responsible for lamb dysentery; other animals are more rarely affected.

The epidemiology and importance of ETX-producing *C. perfringens* infections that might be involved in multiple sclerosis in human are not known.

Clinical features and diagnosis

In the hyperacute form, animal enterotoxemia is characterized by sudden death without premonitory symptoms. Neurological symptoms (i.e. violent convulsions, opisthotonos, nystagmus, ataxia, and lateral recumbency) are prominent in the acute form, which is rapidly fatal in minutes to hours.

Enterotoxemia in animals is mainly diagnosed on epidemiological and clinical grounds and observation of the lesions and confirmed by finding ETX-producing *C. perfringens* in biological samples (i.e. intestinal contents, kidney, spleen, and liver).

Pathology

ETX targets cells expressing the specific receptor myelin and lymphocyte protein (MAL). In enterotoxemia, ETX is produced in the intestinal contents due to *C. perfringens* overgrowth. ETX increases intestinal permeability and passes into the blood circulation and then targets different organs, mainly brain and kidneys. ETX crosses the BBB and accumulates in the brain, causing perivascular edema mainly in the white matter, and swelling of perivascular astrocytes. In the chronic form, foci of necrosis and hemorrhage are observed in the brain [5].

ETX binds to oligodendrocytes and glutamatergic neurons such as granule cells and induces glutamate release, which is the most abundant excitatory neurotransmitter. In addition, ETX induces demyelination of CNS axons, which could be a virulence factor involved in human multiple sclerosis [6, 7].

Treatment and prevention

No specific treatment is available. Prevention in animals is provided by vaccination with detoxified ETX.

Toxins with indirect toxic activity against the CNS

BoNT produced by *Clostridium botulinum*, is the best example of a toxin that acts indirectly on the CNS, through stimulation of the PNS.

Botulinum neurotoxins and *C. botulinum*

Definition and historical perspectives

Botulism (from the Latin name *botula*, meaning "sausage") is a neurological disease in man and animals, characterized by flaccid paralysis and inhibition of secretions. The first detailed clinical descriptions were in the late eighteenth century in southern Germany by Kerner and were associated with the consumption of sausages. *C. botulinum* was first isolated by van Ermengen (1895) and was found to produce a potent neurotoxin. Later, other neurotoxigenic bacteria and different BoNT types were reported [8].

Microbial characteristics of the agent

C. botulinum is a Gram-positive, anaerobic, spore-forming bacterium from the environment (i.e. soil, dust, sediment), which forms a heterogeneous species divided into four genetically and physiologically different groups. In addition, atypical strains from other *Clostridium* species (*Clostridium baratii*, *Clostridium butyricum*) and nonclostridial species (*Weisella oryzae*, *Enterococcus faecium*, and *Chryseobacterium piperi*) synthetize a BoNT.

BoNTs are divided into 10 types (A to J) based on neutralization with specific antibodies, and more than 40 subtypes according to variant protein sequences. All BoNTs are paralytic neurotoxins, type A being the most potent. BoNT types A, B, E, and less frequently F are responsible for human botulism, whereas BoNT types C and D are mainly involved in animal botulism.

BoNTs retain a similar structure to that of TeNT, including a LC containing the catalytic site linked by a disulfide bridge to a HC.

It is noteworthy that BoNTs are highly poisonous substances, but they are widely used as therapeutic agents.

Epidemiology and importance

Botulism occurs worldwide. It is a rare but severe disease, often fatal without treatment. The incidence varies between countries because of different diets and food-preservation methods.

Foodborne botulism is caused by ingestion of preformed BoNT in food. Homemade preserved foods and commercial minimally heated and chilled foods are the most frequent sources.

Infant botulism or botulism by intestinal colonization results from growth of *C. botulinum* in the intestinal contents and in situ production of toxin. Contamination of infants age <1 year is most often from the environment (ingestion of dusts containing *C. botulinum* spores).

Clinical features and diagnosis

Botulism is a flaccid descending paralysis with diplopia, blurred vision, dysphagia, dysphonia, dry mouth, paresis and paralysis of limbs, constipation, and respiratory distress in the severe forms. Sensation and consciousness are not affected.

The diagnosis is based on the characteristic symptoms and detection of BoNT in the patient's serum and food, as well as isolating *C. botulinum* in stool and food samples.

Pathology

BoNTs are stable in the digestive tract because they associate with nontoxic proteins from *Clostridium* to form *botulinum* complexes. BoNTs can cross the intestinal barrier by transcytosis without alteration of intestinal epithelial cells and then gain access to motorneuron endings where they recognize specific receptors (sialogangliosides, synaptic vesicle proteins: SV2 or synaptotagmin). They enter peripheral motorneurons by endocytosis and release the L chain into the cytosol. BoNT L chain cleaves soluble SNARE proteins (VAMP, synaptosome-associated protein 25 [SNAP25], or syntaxin according to BoNT type) and blocks the release of acetylcholine at the neuromuscular junction, inducing a flaccid paralysis [9].

BoNTs (mainly BoNT type A) can be transported retrogradely along motorneurons to reach the CNS. Central effects have been documented in some patients with botulism or people who have received BoNT injection [10].

Although in animal experiments sprouting of nerve endings occurred and new neuromuscular junctions were formed following botulinum toxin intramuscular injection [11, 12], no specific histopathological changes have been observed in human botulism.

Treatment and prevention

Treatment of botulism is mainly symptomatic. Anti-BoNT sera are effective if administrated shortly (24 hours) after the onset of symptoms. Vaccination is effective and is only used for persons at risk.

Emetic toxins

These toxins act through stimulation of the vagus nerve, leading to activation of the vomiting centers in the CNS: two of the most frequently encountered molecules are cereulide from *Bacillus cereus* and the staphylocccal enterotoxins (SEs) from *Staphyloccus aureus*. Both bacteria are important food-poisoning pathogens [5].

Staphylococcal food poisoning includes nausea, vomiting, abdominal cramps, and diarrhea. *S. aureus* synthesizes a set of enterotoxins which cross intestinal epithelial or goblet cells by transcytosis. They then target mast cells, inducing 5-HT/serotonin release, which interacts with vagus nerve extensions. This results in stimulation of the CNS vomiting center in the medulla oblongata [13, 14]. Some *B. cereus* strains also produce cereulide, an emetic toxin, along with several enterotoxins. They are responsible for food poisoning emetic syndrome characterized by vomiting and nausea. Cereulide is a K+ ionophore similar to valinomycin: it stimulates the vagus nerve through 5-HT/serotonin receptor and then the CNS vomiting center. However, the molecular mechanism of action of cereulide is not yet known [5].

Alternative toxins

Some toxins induce neuronal changes, though these effects do not represent their main pathogenic mechanisms.

Shiga toxin and shiga-like toxins

Shigella dysenteriae serotype 1 and Shiga toxin-producing *Escherichia coli* (STEC) are responsible for hemorrhagic colitis [5, 15]. Systemic complications such as hemolytic uremic syndrome (HUS) and neurological disorders occur when Shiga toxin (Stx) gains access to the blood circulation, probably circulating through low-affinity interactions with neutrophils or monocytes.

CNS complications are frequent in infants with HUS (20–50%) and accompany severe adult STEC infections. CNS symptoms associated with HUS include hyperexcitability with increased muscle reflexes, anxiety, memory deficit, ataxia, cranial nerve palsy, epileptic seizures, hallucinations, and changes in consciousness ranging from lethargy to coma.

CNS lesions include anoxic and ischemic foci with focal edema and necrosis and microhemorrhages with little evidence of cell death. However, these lesions do not seem to be responsible for the neurologic damage.

Life-threatening complications in humans seem to be associated with strains producing the Stx2 subtype a (Stx2a). In a mouse model, Stx2a is found in susceptible tissues (kidneys and brain). Stx recognizes the globotrioside Gb3 as a cell membrane receptor. Gb3 is expressed by neurons in numerous brain regions in mice. After entering the cell, Stx undergoes retrograde intracellular trafficking (i.e. from an early endosome to the trans-Golgi network, through the Golgi apparatus, to the endoplasmic reticulum [ER]). The enzymatic domain is delivered into the cytosol leading to inhibition of protein synthesis in the host cell, and depending on cell type and toxin concentration, apoptosis, and ER-stress, autophagy, and inflammatory responses.

The passage of Stx2 through the BBB is still unclear. Stx2-treated mice show microglial activation corresponding to early neural injury but no histopathological changes in the brain [16]. This neuroinflammatory response is most probably due to activation of a systemic inflammatory cascade leading to BBB weakening [17]. Astrocytes are reported as negative for Gb3 but show cell lesions, also suggesting indirect effects of the toxins.

The diagnosis is based on bacteriological identification from stools.

Clostridium difficile and *clostridium sordellii* large clostridial toxins

These toxins are responsible for enteritis as well as gangrene and toxic shock syndrome, respectively. They inactivate Rho/Ras-GTPases through UDP-glucosylation. In addition to their activity on epithelial cells, large clostridial glucosylating toxins (LCGTs) can target neurons leading to impairment of neuroexocytosis subsequent to Rac inactivation. However, neuronal morphological changes are not common in *C. difficile* and *C. sordellii* infections [5].

Concluding remarks: a broader definition of toxin

During a bacterial infection, the CNS senses homeostasis perturbations in a highly coordinated way – either through neural transmission from the periphery via the nociceptive pathways or the vagus nerve or via the bloodstream through the highly adapted BBB cellular interface.

Bacteria release pathogen-derived molecules (pathogen-associated molecular pattern [PAMPs], such as lipopolysaccharide [LPS], lipoteichoic acid [LTA], peptidoglycan and induce cytotoxic effects leading to the release of damaged tissue-derived molecules (damage-associated molecular pattern [DAMPs] or alarmins, such as ATP, high motility group box 1, S100A8/9, mitochondrial DNA). Furthermore, these signals are sensed and translated by classical and nonprofessional immune cells into eukaryotic signaling messengers of inflammation including cytokines and chemokines, gas (nitric oxide species and reactive oxygen species), and lipid mediators (prostaglandins, leukotrienes, and thromboxanes) [18].

Both peripheral neurons and BBB express receptors for PAMPs (such as toll-like receptors, formyl peptide receptors [FPRs]), DAMPs, or soluble effectors of the stimulated immune system (chemokines, cytokines) [19, 20]. Interestingly, some of these receptors, in an economical and elegant way, are able to recognize both PAMPs and DAMPs (e.g. FPR also binds mitochondrial formylated peptides [21]), whereas some receptors usually associated with pain or heat perception, such as TRPA1, also react to bacterial products such as LPS [22–24]. Ultimately, if the BBB functional integrity as a barrier is impaired, the PAMPS, DAMPS, and soluble mediators of inflammation can gain direct access to and modulate cells in the CNS [25–27].

As all pathways are stimulated concomitantly, attributing more importance to one over the other would be difficult and might be pathophysiologically irrelevant (i.e. the effects of bona fide toxins, of PAMPs, of DAMPs, or of the mediators of the inflammatory response); these effects being local or systemic, direct or indirect. Furthermore, depending on the nature and intensity of these signals, BBB and CNS parenchymal cells will amplify, modulate, or counter these signals through complex interactions that we are only beginning to unravel. A comprehensive review is given in [25]. The classic example of these events is sepsis in which all these diffusible signal molecules are released and lead to CNS alterations [28].

Taking into account the global toxic effects that bacteria can produce by stimulating various CNS cells, directly or indirectly, the definition of "toxin" can be modified from its strictly defined meaning (exhibiting a specific activity targeting a specific pathway in the CNS) to a wider viewpoint (i.e. signaling via PAMPs, DAMPs, chemokines, and cytokines). In this respect, bacterial and endogenous molecules could be considered toxins if produced in pathologic conditions (e.g. increased quantity, additive effects with other molecules, abnormal localization).

Finally, over a much longer time scale, recent studies suggest that altered gut microbiota may detrimentally participate in the initiation and progression of several chronic CNS pathologies (e.g. Alzheimer disease or Parkinson disease; reviewed by [29]). Although still lacking direct evidence, these hypotheses rely on the same pathways previously described for acute neuroinflammation during non-CNS infections and often on the same PAMPs. In a more physiological context, the extent and complexity of bacterial-host interactions (symbiosis/dysbiosis microbiota/host) are only beginning to be explored [22].

References

1. Rossetto, O., Scorzeto, M., Megighian, A. et al. (2013). Tetanus neurotoxin. *Toxicon* 66: 59–63.
2. Masuyer, G., Conrad, J., and Stenmark, P. (2017). The structure of the tetanus toxin reveals pH-mediated domain dynamics. *EMBO Rep.* 18: 1306–1317.
3. WHO (2017). Tetanus vaccines: WHO position paper – February 2017. *Wkly Epidemiol. Rec.* 92: 53–76.
4. Rumah, K.R., Vartanian, T.K., and Fischetti, V.A. (2017). Oral multiple sclerosis drugs inhibit the in vitro growth of epsilon toxin producing gut bacterium, *Clostridium perfringens. Front. Cell. Infect. Microbiol.* 7: 11.

5. Popoff, M.R. and Poulain, B. (2010). Bacterial toxins and the nervous system: neurotoxins and multipotential toxins interacting with neuronal cells. *Toxins* 2: 683–737.
6. Wagley, S., Bokori-Brown, M., Morcrette, H. et al. (2018). Evidence of *Clostridium perfringens* epsilon toxin associated with multiple sclerosis. *Mult. Scler.*: 1–8.
7. Wioland, L., Dupont, J.L., Doussau, F. et al. (2015). Epsilon toxin from *Clostridium perfringens* acts on oligodendrocytes without forming pores, and causes demyelination. *Cell. Microbiol.* 17: 369–388.
8. Peck, M.W., Smith, T.J., Anniballi, F. et al. (2017). Historical perspectives and guidelines for botulinum neurotoxin subtype nomenclature. *Toxins (Basel)* 9: 38.
9. Rossetto, O., Pirazzini, M., and Montecucco, C. (2014). Botulinum neurotoxins: genetic, structural and mechanistic insights. *Nat. Rev. Microbiol.* 12: 535–549.
10. Mazzocchio, R. and Caleo, M. (2015). More than at the neuromuscular synapse: actions of botulinum neurotoxin A in the central nervous system. *Neuroscientist* 21: 44–61.
11. Duchen, L.W. and Stritch, S.J. (1968). The effects of botulinum toxin on the pattern of innervation of skeletal muscle in mouse. *Q. J. Exp. Physiol. Cogn. Med. Sci.* 53: 84–89.
12. Duchen, L.W. (1971). An electron microscopic study of the changes induced by botulinum toxin in the motor end-plates of slow and fast skeletal muscle fibres of the mouse. *J. Neurol. Sci.* 14: 47–60.
13. Fisher, E.L., Otto, M., and Cheung, G.Y.C. (2018). Basis of virulence in enterotoxin-mediated staphylococcal food poisoning. *Front. Microbiol.* 9: 436.
14. Hu, D.L., Zhu, G., Mori, F. et al. (2007). Staphylococcal enterotoxin induces emesis through increasing serotonin release in intestine and it is downregulated by cannabinoid receptor 1. *Cell. Microbiol.* 9: 2267–2277.
15. Obata, F., Tohyama, K., Bonev, A.D. et al. (2008). Shiga toxin 2 affects the central nervous system through receptor globotriaosylceramide localized to neurons. *J. Infect. Dis.* 198: 1398–1406.
16. Pradhan, S., Pellino, C., MacMaster, K. et al. (2016). Shiga toxin mediated neurologic changes in murine model of disease. *Front. Cell. Infect. Microbiol.* 6: 114.
17. Lee, M.S., Koo, S., Jeong, D.G. et al. (2016). Shiga toxins as multi-functional proteins: induction of host cellular stress responses, role in pathogenesis and therapeutic applications. *Toxins (Basel)* 8: pii: E77.
18. Olofsson, P.S., Metz, C., and Pavlov, V.A. (2017). The Neuroimmune communicatome in inflammation. In: *Inflammation: From Molecular and Cellular Mechanisms to the Clinic*, vol. 4 (eds. J.-M. Cavaillon and M. Singer), 1485–1516. Weinheim, Germany: Wiley VCH.
19. Chavan, S.S., Pavlov, V.A., and Tracey, K.J. (2017). Mechanisms and therapeutic relevance of neuro-immune communication. *Immunity* 46: 927–942.
20. Dantzer, R. (2018). Neuroimmune interactions: from the brain to the immune system and vice versa. *Physiol. Rev.* 98: 477–504.
21. Chiu, I.M., Heesters, B.A., Ghasemlou, N. et al. (2013). Bacteria activate sensory neurons that modulate pain and inflammation. *Nature* 501: 52–57.
22. Cohen, L.J., Esterhazy, D., Kim, S.H. et al. (2017). Commensal bacteria make GPCR ligands that mimic human signalling molecules. *Nature* 549: 48–53.
23. Lim, J.Y., Choi, S.I., Choi, G. et al. (2016). Atypical sensors for direct and rapid neuronal detection of bacterial pathogens. *Mol. Brain* 9: 26.
24. Meseguer, V., Alpizar, Y.A., Luis, E. et al. (2014). TRPA1 channels mediate acute neurogenic inflammation and pain produced by bacterial endotoxins. *Nat. Commun.* 5: 3125.
25. Erickson, M.A. and Banks, W.A. (2018). Neuroimmune axes of the blood-brain barriers and blood-brain interfaces: bases for physiological regulation, disease states, and pharmacological interventions. *Pharmacol. Rev.* 70: 278–314.
26. Vargas-Caraveo, A., Sayd, A., Maus, S.R. et al. (2017). Lipopolysaccharide enters the rat brain by a lipoprotein-mediated transport mechanism in physiological conditions. *Sci. Rep.* 7: 13113.
27. Zhan, X., Stamova, B., Jin, L.W. et al. (2016). Gram-negative bacterial molecules associate with Alzheimer disease pathology. *Neurology* 87: 2324–2332.
28. Sankowski, R., Mader, S., and Valdes-Ferrer, S.I. (2015). Systemic inflammation and the brain: novel roles of genetic, molecular, and environmental cues as drivers of neurodegeneration. *Front. Cell. Neurosci.* 9: 28.
29. Calvani, R., Picca, A., Lo Monaco, M.R. et al. (2018). Of microbes and minds: a narrative review on the second brain aging. *Front. Med. (Lausanne)* 5: 53.

44 Fungal Infections of the CNS

Michael Blatzer[1], Fanny Lanternier[2,3,4], Jean-Paul Latgé[5], Anne Beauvais[5], Stéphane Bretagne[2,6,7], Fabrice Chrétien[3,8,9,*], and Grégory Jouvion[9,*]

[1] Aspergillus and Experimental Neuropathology Units, Pasteur Institute, Paris, France
[2] Molecular Mycology Unit, French National Reference Centre for Invasive Mycoses and Antifungal Treatments, Pasteur Institute, Paris, France
[3] Paris University, Paris, France
[4] Department of Infectious Diseases and Tropical Medicine, Necker-Sick Children University Hospital and Imagine Institute, APHP, Paris, France
[5] Aspergillus Unit, Pasteur Institute, Paris, France
[6] Saint Louis Hospital, APHP, Paris, France
[7] University Paris Diderot, Sorbonne Paris Cité, Paris, France
[8] Department of Neuropathology, Sainte Anne Hospital, Paris, France
[9] Experimental Neuropathology Unit, Pasteur Institute, Paris, France

Abbreviations

CARD9	caspase recruitment domain adaptor 9
CSF	cerebrospinal fluid
CNS	central nervous system
DAMP	damage-associated molecular patterns
FDA	Food and Drug Administration
H&E	hematoxylin and eosin
HIV/AIDS	human immunodeficiency virus/acquired immunodeficiency syndrome
PAMP	pathogen-associated molecular patterns
PAS	periodic acid-Schiff
PCR	polymerase chain reaction
PRR	pattern recognition receptors
PIDs	primary immunodeficiencies

Introduction and historical perspective

Fungi are among the oldest recognized causes of infection in humans. Hippocrates seemingly wrote on "aphthae" in 500 BCE, which modern mycologists identify as thrush. In the modern era, fungi were of considerable scientific interest. The first reports of human fungal diseases were by David Gruby (1842–1844) [1].

In 2000, 396 fungal species were associated with infections in mammals; more than 20 species were associated with systemic or disseminated human infection [2]. Invasive fungal infections are a major cause of morbidity and mortality in the setting of iatrogenic immunosuppression or HIV infection. Fungal infections of the CNS are uncommon, often devastating and difficult to diagnose and treat, and are mainly confined to patients who are

*Fabrice Chrétien and Grégory Jouvion share senior co-authorship.

Infections of the Central Nervous System: Pathology and Genetics, First Edition. Edited by Fabrice Chrétien, Kum Thong Wong, Leroy R. Sharer, Catherine (Katy) Keohane and Françoise Gray.
© 2020 John Wiley & Sons Ltd. Published 2020 by John Wiley & Sons Ltd.

immunocompromised. Despite advances in imaging and microbiological techniques, the diagnosis remains challenging. Although developing molecular techniques may facilitate identification in the future, a significant percentage of patients still require invasive interventions for diagnosis and treatment. Polymerase chain reaction (PCR)-based detection of invasive fungal infections and sequencing of fungal DNA enable both identification of the infecting fungus and detection of drug resistance (e.g. azole resistance for *Aspergillus fumigatus*). Several commercial and noncommercial PCR assays are already available but their diagnostic benefit still has to be determined.

In the majority of cases, the fungus spreads to the CNS from another primary site of infection, most often the respiratory tract, because all individuals inhale airborne fungal spores daily. Once pulmonary infection is established, blood-borne spread of fungus to the CNS can occur [3]. Other routes into the CNS are as a result of contaminated medical devices, surgery, trauma, or following intravenous drug use.

Innate immune cells protect against invading fungal elements; they recognize fungal cell wall polysaccharide components as pathogen-associated molecular patterns (PAMP) and damage-associated molecular patterns (DAMP) via pattern recognition receptors (PRR). Fungal PAMP include α- and ß-glucans, mannans, or chitin. These polysaccharides are recognized by the major PRR, the toll-like receptors (TLRs), C-type lectin receptors, DC-SIGN, mincle, and the mannose receptors. PRR activate multiple intracellular pathways on binding specific PAMP and induce (i) the inflammasome, resulting in cytokine and chemokine release, (ii) phagocytosis of conidia and yeasts, and (iii) oxidative defense mechanisms, resulting in fungal killing. Additionally, cytokine release induces T helper (Th)-1 and Th-17 immune responses needed for phagocyte activation and Th-17 differentiation [4].

Risk factors for invasive fungal infections are immunosuppression resulting from human immunodeficiency virus (HIV) and acquired immunodeficiency syndrome (AIDS), certain lymphoreticular malignancies, diabetes mellitus, autoimmune disease, and conditions of iron overload. Immunosuppressant, antibiotic, and high-dose corticosteroid therapies, iron chelators, and intravenous drug use can also contribute to infection and pathogenesis [5]. Antibiotics also play a role in yeast infections. Direct inoculation into the CNS as a result of contaminated medical devices, surgery, or intravenous drug use can also occur in individuals who are immunocompetent [6].

Mortality rates for invasive fungal infections frequently exceed 50% [3]. Despite antifungal therapy, the mean time from diagnosis to death is alarmingly short; six weeks for some patients with cancer [7]. Dissemination to the CNS is the most serious and life-threatening complication of invasive fungal infections with mortality rates increasing to 90% [8].

Diagnosis is challenging and typically requires biopsies for histopathology and tissue culture [5]. Histopathology is the most effective method for fungal identification and should include (i) precise description of the fungus morphology using classical (hematoxylin and eosin [H&E] and periodic acid-Schiff [PAS]) and specific (Gomori Grocott, Fontana-Masson, Alcian Blue, mucicarmine) stains and immunohistochemistry with specific primary antibodies and (ii) host tissue response (i.e. type of necrosis, type of inflammation, vascular lesions, hemorrhages). For best results, biopsy findings should be supplemented by cerebrospinal fluid (CSF) analysis, culture and PCR, and serological tests for fungal biomarkers and neuroimaging.

General aspects of fungal pathogens: definitions and classification

Fungal pathogens can be subdivided into obligate pathogens that infect healthy individuals and opportunistic pathogens that invade susceptible and immunosuppressed hosts. The major primary fungal pathogens that cause CNS infections are *Coccidioides* spp., *Histoplasma* spp., *Blastomyces* spp., and *Sporothrix*. These pathogens are able to establish infections in individuals who are immunocompetent and immunosuppressed. Opportunistic pathogens like *Cryptococcus* spp., *Candida* spp., and *Aspergillus* spp. or Mucorales (formerly Zygomycetes) cause CNS infections in individuals who are immunocompromised. They occur only very rarely in individuals who are immunocompetent with high doses of infection. The epidemiology of fungal CNS infections is evolving because of the emergence of novel pathogens, antifungal drug resistance, and changes in the use of immune-suppressive agents.

According to their morphology, fungal pathogens can be grouped into three major forms: molds, yeasts, and dimorphic fungi. This categorization does not relate to the taxonomic groups, but it may be helpful in guiding diagnosis because each category shares similar clinical features.

Molds are ubiquitous saprophytes and occur naturally in the environment on decaying organic matter and soil to which humans are constantly exposed. Based on the appearance of their multicellular filaments and hyphae, they can be classified into three major categories: (i) pigmented (dematiaceous) or colorless (hyaline). Hyaline hyphae can either be (ii) septate or (iii) pauciseptate.

Yeasts are unicellular eukaryotic microorganisms that reproduce by asymmetric fission. They account for approximately 1% of fungal species. During their life cycles, yeasts such as the basidiomycetous yeast *Cryptococcus neoformans* may exhibit different morphotypes, both pseudohyphae and hyphae. However, these forms occur in the natural environment (the soil) and not in human hosts. In contrast, *Candida* spp. can form pseudohyphae in humans.

The third group consists of the dimorphic fungi. These organisms grow as molds (hyphae, filaments) at room temperature and in the environment but as yeast forms at body temperature. Conversion between the two morphotypes at 25–30 °C and 35–37 °C, respectively, is a classical identification method in culture. Interestingly, these fungi are endemic in certain geographical regions. The major fungi in this group, including *Blastomyces dermatiditis, Coccidioides immitis,* and *Coccidioides posadasii, Paracoccidioides brasiliensis,* and *Paracoccidioides lutzii, Histoplasma capsulatum, Sporothrix schenkii, Talaromyces marneffei* (formerly known as *Penicillium marneffei*), and *Emmonsia* spp. belong to the taxonomic phylum of Ascomycota.

Mold infections

Septate hyaline molds

Molds enter the human body mainly via inhalation of conidia and infection is commonly established in the lung. Angioinvasion accounts for hematogenous spread from the lung to other organs. CNS mold infections have a poor prognosis in patients who are immunocompromised and are mainly caused by a variety of opportunistic hyaline molds, namely *Aspergillus* spp. and Mucorales, which are ubiquitous saprophytic fungi usually found in the soil and decomposing organic matter. *A. fumigatus* is the most common organism identified.

Aspergillosis

Aspergillus spp., as hyaline septate molds, are the major cause of morbidity and mortality in individuals who are immunocompromised [7]. Invasive aspergillosis usually affects patients taking immunosuppressive medications and those with solid-organ transplants, hematological malignancies, or neutropenia. Patients who are critically ill with severe liver cirrhosis or chronic obstructive pulmonary disease are also at risk. Within the genus *Aspergillus,* only a few of the more than 300 described species can cause human infection, including *A. fumigatus, Aspergillus flavus, Aspergillus terreus, Aspergillus niger,* and *Aspergillus oryzae,* which occur in different geographical areas and clinical settings.

A. fumigatus is the most frequent cause of disseminated aspergillosis involving the CNS, individual cases are also reported for other species. Small spores (2–5 μm) enter the respiratory tract easily and spread (i) by the bloodstream, (ii) along lymphatics, and (iii) via airways. Infection of the CNS results in single or multiple abscesses and granulomas with central necrosis and sometimes central cavitation, petechiae, and hemorrhages (Figure 44.1).

The diagnosis of *Aspergillus* infections is challenging as radiologic findings are often nonspecific and CSF cultures are frequently negative, even in cases of *Aspergillus* meningitis [9, 10]. Definitive diagnosis requires evidence of tissue invasion by hyaline, thin (thickness <12 μm), septate, acute

Infections of the Central Nervous System

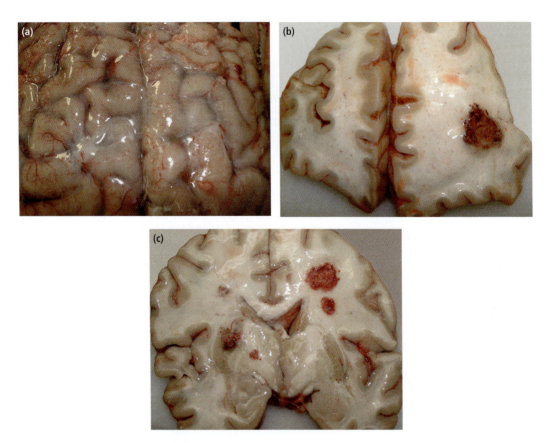

Figure 44.1 Macroscopic appearance of CNS aspergillosis (patient with immunosuppression with organ transplant). (a) Cloudy slightly green meningeal exudate. (b and c) Multiple bilateral hemorrhagic partly necrotic lesions in the deep white matter, and in the left putamen and internal capsule. Source: Courtesy Pr. Katy Keohane.

angle branching hyphae, strongly outlined by Gomori Grocott stain (Figure 44.2). Vascular lesions (e.g. blood vessel wall destruction, thrombi, hemorrhages, and edema) are frequently observed as well as infarction and invasion of blood vessel walls by the fungus (invasive form of the disease). Even though different *Aspergillus* species are morphologically specific, the distinction between them on histology is difficult and complementary diagnostic methods should be used. The differential diagnosis includes infections by other hyaline, septate, acute angle branching hyphae (e.g. *Scedosporium* spp. and *Fusarium* spp.) [11, 12].

Microbiological tests may be falsely negative despite fungal elements being seen in pathological specimens. The nature and volume of the sampled material and low fungal burden (e.g. in CSF) limit current microbiological definitive diagnosis. Centrifuged diagnostic material concentrates fungal elements and enhances the likelihood of directly observing fungi by microscopy using fluorescent optical brighteners (Calcofluor white binding to ß-1,3 ß-1,4 polysaccharides as in chitin or cellulose). Molecular detection of fungal DNA is more sensitive and more suited to CSF samples but lacks standardization and has contradictory sensitivity and specificity depending on the PCR assay. Detection of the *Aspergillus* cell wall component galactomannan in the CSF holds promise, but it is not validated by the EORTC/MSG as a microbiologic criterion for invasive aspergillosis [13]. The Platelia GM assay is only approved by the Food and Drug Administration (FDA) for use in serum and bronchoalveolar lavage samples [14, 15]. Of note,

Fungal Infections of the CNS **Chapter 44**

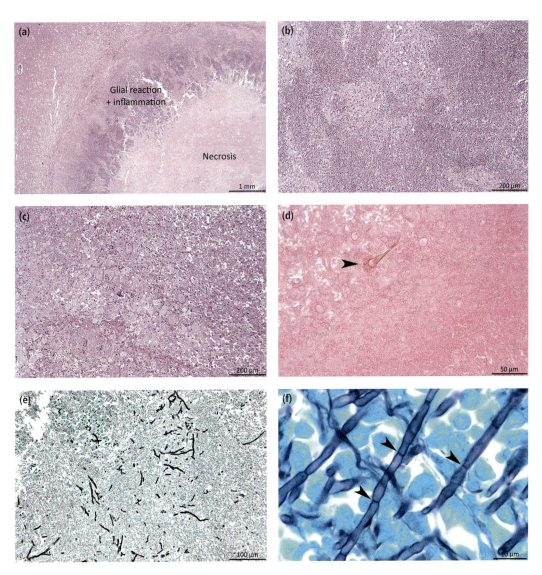

Figure 44.2 Morphological patterns of cerebral aspergillosis. (a–c) Focal well-delineated lesion with a concentric organization (a) central necrosis and peripheral glial reaction and inflammation. In the center (b), necrosis containing cell debris and fragmented neutrophils (suppuration: abscess). At the periphery (c), activated phagocytic microglial cells displaying foamy cytoplasm (Gitter cells) with activated astrocytes and neutrophils. (d) Compact accumulation of hyphae (fungus ball), *sella turcica*, with a pigmented head (Conidiophore; black arrowhead). (e) On low magnification, hyphae are thin (<12 μm), homogeneous, branched at an acute angle, and strongly positive with Gomori Grocott stain. (f) On high magnification, septa are easily detected (black arrowheads). a–d, hematoxylin and eosin (H&E) stain; e–f, Gomori Grocott stain.

the *Aspergillus* galactomannan antigen test can display cross reactivity with *Fusarium, Penicillium, Acremonium,* or *Histoplasma* species. Combining galactomannan and fungal DNA detection results in higher diagnostic accuracy [16].

Infection by *scedosporium* species

The *Scedosporium* species complex comprises other hyaline, septate, ubiquitous fungi that can cause CNS infections in people who are immunocompromised and immunocompetent. Members of this species complex are commonly found in temperate climates and are less frequent in tropical climates. *Scedosporium apiospermum* and *Lomentospora prolificans* (formerly *Scedosporium prolificans*) are the most frequent members that infect humans. They are poorly sensitive to antifungal drugs. *L. prolificans* is resistant to Amphotericin B, triazoles, and echinocandins [17]; therefore, for appropriate treatment, it is important to identify the organism.

These fungi have gained attention because of their relatively high frequency of airway colonization in patients with cystic fibrosis and increased infections in individuals who are immunocompromised. Spores are the causative agent. Similar to other molds, these fungi can disseminate in immunosuppressed hosts. In individuals who are immunocompetent, *Scedosporium* species can cause CNS infections in the context of near-drowning.

There are no distinguishing histopathologic features from other hyaline molds, so microbiologic and molecular biologic tests are required for precise identification. The serological test for 1,3-ß-D-glucan antigen detects *Scedosporium* spp., albeit the diagnostic accuracy has yet to be determined. PCR amplification and sequencing of the internal transcribed spacer regions of the ribosomal DNA allow rapid species identification, but these methods are not standardized or widely available.

Pauciseptate hyaline molds

Diabetes mellitus, hematological malignancies, and trauma are classical risk factors for mucormycosis. Mucorales are hyaline pauciseptate molds, the genera *Rhizopus*, *Lichtheimia* (formerly *Absidia*), and *Mucor* are the most frequent, followed by *Cunninghamella*, *Rhizomucor*, and *Apophysomyces* [18, 19]. Mucorales are ubiquitous fungi found in soil, air, and water. Their hyphae are non- or pauciseptate, wide-shaped ribbon-like structures, larger than *Aspergillus* hyphae. Of 101 cases of mucormycosis, 13 involved CNS; 10 were contiguous with a sinus and 3 had disseminated infection without sinus involvement [20]. When a sinus was involved, mucormycosis extended to the brain in 10 of 25 patients. The most significant risk factor for rhino-cerebral mucormycosis is diabetes mellitus [18, 21].

Histopathology is very useful for rapid diagnosis of mucormycosis. Hyphae are wide (5–20 μm), hyaline, with right-angle branching, and a "folded ribbon-like morphology" (Figure 44.3). They may appear empty in H&E-stained sections; Gomori Grocott staining is often only faintly positive, so PAS is the preferred stain. Vascular lesions are prominent and include tissue infarcts, hemorrhages, thrombi, and invasion of blood vessel walls and lumen by fungi. Rare lymphocytes can be detected in patients who are immunosuppressed even when neutrophilic inflammation is also present [22], in contrast to the marked granulomatous and suppurative inflammation that can be seen in

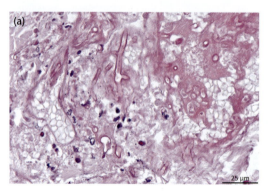
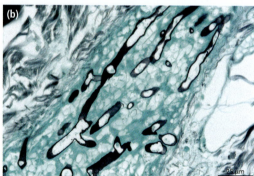

Figure 44.3 Mucormycosis. (a) Infarction, hemorrhage, edema, fibrin, and rare fragmented inflammatory cells (neutrophils) are visible. (b) High magnification of hyphae in a vascular space. Hyphae have a "ribbon-like" morphology, and there is almost no septum. Right-angle branching is seen. The center of hyphae seems empty. a, hematoxylin and eosin (H&E) stain; b, Gomori Grocott stain.

immunocompetent hosts. The histological differential diagnosis includes other hyaline hyphae such as *Aspergillus* spp., *Fusarium* spp., *Scedosporium* spp., and even *Candida* spp., which can form pseudohyphae.

There are no specific serological assays for the detection of Mucorales. Diagnosis is often made by isolation of the fungus. Mucorales do not contain (1, 3)-ß-D-glucan in the cell wall. Another complicating factor is that microbiological cultures often yield no growth, despite fungal elements being seen in histological samples [23]. The large pauciseptate hyphae may be unviable because of fragmentation during sample processing, and standard microbiologic growth media are not optimal for recovery of Mucorales from necrotic tissues [24]. Also, free DNA from damaged hyphae may be degraded more easily in patient samples. PCR-based methods to detect Mucorales are limited; however for mucormycosis, there have been recent improvements for detecting circulating DNA in human samples [25]. Cerebral mucormycosis is the most aggressive CNS mold infection, and early diagnosis and primary antifungal therapy with amphotericin B formulations influence successful treatment.

Dematiaceous molds

This group of molds is characterized by melanin-like pigments within the cell wall of hyphae, coloring the mycelia a pale brown to black. Dematiaceous molds may cause invasive infections (phaeohyphomycosis), including in the CNS [26]. Phaeohyphomycoses classically involve skin in patients who are immunocompromised. In contrast, some phaeohyphomycetes such as *Cladophialophora bantiana*, *Rhinocladiella mackenzii* and *Exophiala* spp. are associated with CNS infections in patients without known immunodeficiency. However, caspase recruitment domain adaptor 9 (CARD9) deficiency was identified in one of the patients [27].

Macroscopically, lesions are pigmented, brown-black to yellowish-brown; single or multiple (especially in immunosuppression) brain abscesses or pyogranulomas can also be seen. Histology is very useful for diagnosis. The lesions are necrotic with possible vasculitis and infiltrates of macrophages and neutrophils. Intralesional pigmented thin 2- to 6-µm wide hyphae with a heterogeneous morphology (i.e. irregular swelling, irregular branching, prominent septa, and constrictions) can be found (Figure 44.4). As the degree of pigmentation varies, some dematiaceous fungi with little melanin may appear hyaline. Fontana-Masson stain for melanin can help highlight hyphae in tissues. It is impossible to distinguish the different dematiaceous fungal species by histology, so for precise identification, cultures combined with sequence-based PCR assays may help.

Most fungi causing phaeohyphomycosis grow very slowly compared to *Aspergillus* spp. or Mucorales, and incubation times for their identification can take up to three weeks.

C. bantiana, Exophiala dermatitidis, Rhinocladiella mackenziei, and *Ochroconis gallopava* are the most commonly isolated species [26, 27]. The neurotropic fungi *R. mackenziei* and *C. bantiana* occur more frequently in geographically restricted areas such as the Middle East and India, respectively. In 2012 *Exerophilum rostratum*, an uncommon dematiaceous mold was the cause of a fatal fungal meningitis outbreak due to three contaminated preservative-free methylprednisolone lots from one compounding pharmacy. This outbreak caused 751 CNS infections and 64 deaths across the United States. *E. rostratum* can be diagnosed with the (1, 3)-ß-D-glucan antigen test and PCR assays. The Fontana-Masson stain for melanin may be useful to confirm diagnosis in tissue.

There are no standardized therapies, but the European Society of Clinical Microbiology and Infectious Diseases (ESCMID) and European Confederation of Medical Mycology (ECMM) guidelines advise voriconazole or posaconazole treatment as first choice where excision is not possible [28]. Combination treatment with a triazole plus an echinocandin plus flucytosine can be a first-line treatment and prolonged survival time is reported in murine infection models for disseminated *C. bantiana* infections [29]. A recent in vitro study indicates synergistic effects of amphotericin with flucytosine [30].

Yeasts

Cryptococcosis

Cryptococcus spp. as encapsulated yeasts are the leading cause of fungal meningitis. Cryptococcosis was considered rare before the

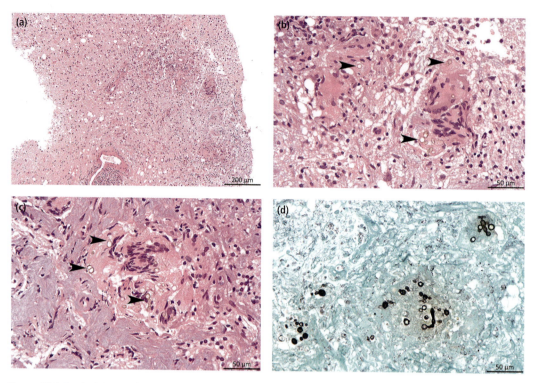

Figure 44.4 Cerebral phaeohyphomycosis. (a–c) Multifocal, randomly distributed inflammatory lesions characterized by (b–c) small granulomas with tissue necrosis and intralesional pigmented hyphae (black arrowheads). (d) These hyphae display a heterogeneous morphology, with irregular swelling and branching, and multifocal constrictions. a–c, hematoxylin and eosin (H&E) stain. d, Gomori Grocott stain.

AIDS pandemic; nowadays, nearly 223 000 new cases are reported each year with 181 100 deaths among people with HIV. Cryptococcal meningitis causes 15% of all AIDS-related deaths in the world, with an estimated mortality of approximately 20% [31].

Two species cause disease in humans, *C. neoformans* and *C. gattii*. Based on molecular and genetic factors, it is proposed to divide the pathogenic species complex into seven species. *C. neoformans* is the most frequently found pathogen with *C. neoformans* var. *grubii* accounting for 95% of infections. *C. neoformans* can cause disease in people who are immunocompetent and immunosuppressed, with a high prevalence in individuals with HIV. CNS infection with *C. gattii* is less frequent [32, 33].

In the environment, *Cryptococcus* is found in association with excreta of certain birds, particularly pigeons. Primary infection occurs in childhood via inhalation of basidiospores or dessicated yeasts [34] and is controlled by the immune system. Infection becomes latent and the yeast dormant [35]. If immunosuppression occurs, yeast cells reactivate, probably in the lung, and disseminate as yeast cells or within phagocytes through the bloodstream to different organs, including the CNS [36]. Three virulence factors have been described for *Cryptococcus*: formation of a polysaccharide capsule, melanin pigment production, and thermotolerance. The thick polysaccharide capsule composed of glucuronoxylomannan is unique to *Cryptococcus* species and affects host immunity. More importantly, this polysaccharide is used for capsular antigen testing in serological diagnosis [37]. On direct microscopy, the capsule also can be visualized as a halo against a black background on specimens stained with India ink [38].

Fungal Infections of the CNS **Chapter 44**

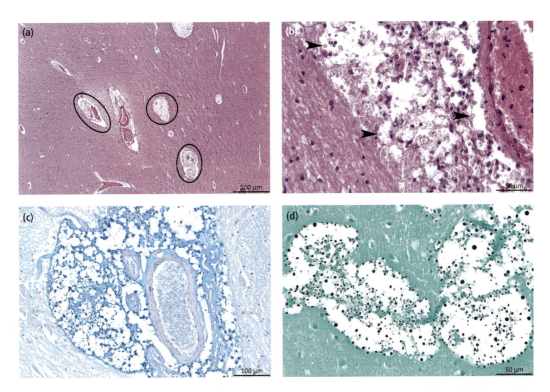

Figure 44.5 Cerebral cryptococcosis. (a, b). Multifocal lesions, centered on Virchow-Robin perivascular spaces (black circles), characterized by round refringent yeasts (black arrowheads) with abundant unstained amorphous material (capsule) at their periphery (hematoxylin and eosin [H&E]). (b) There are rare inflammatory cells but no gliosis. (c) The capsular material is stained by Alcian blue. (d) Gomori Grocott stain reveals very heterogeneous yeast size with narrow-based budding. a–b, H&E stain; c, Alcian blue stain; d, Gomori Grocott stain.

In the CNS, the most frequently observed lesion is meningitis at the base of the cerebral and cerebellar hemispheres. Microscopically, *Cryptococcus* is a spherical to ovoid encapsulated yeast, displaying a narrow-based budding, and measuring 5–20 μm. The capsule can increase the overall diameter to a maximum of 30 μm. With H&E staining, *Cryptococcus* appears as a refringent yeast with a peripheral clear space. The yeast wall stains with PAS and Gomori Grocott; while the capsule is Alcian blue and mucicarmine positive (Figure 44.5). Two different host reactions can be observed: (i) in immunodeficiency, there is minimal inflammation and gliosis with a high number of extracellular yeasts, and (ii) in immunocompetence, there is granulomatous inflammation with multinucleated giant cells containing yeasts. The differential diagnosis should include *Candida* spp. and *Histoplasma* spp. when the capsule is poorly developed [11].

Cryptococcal vaccine and specific monoclonal antibodies were developed more than two decades ago; however, their applicability has not yet been determined in clinical trials [32]. Cryptococcus is the only fungal pathogen included in the FDA-approved fully automated molecular diagnostic panel for meningitis and encephalitis [39].

Candidiasis

Candida albicans is the most common fungal pathogen causing invasive infections in humans. CNS mycoses resulting from this commensal yeast are rare, but in neonates are significantly increased with 466 per 100 000 cases of invasive candidiasis. Of these, 16% are meningitis and 4% other forms of CNS infection. *C. albicans* and other species (*C. glabrata, C. krusei, C. parapsilosis,* and *C. tropicalis*) can also cause disseminated lesions in association with predisposing factors [40]: diabetes mellitus, leukemia, lymphoma, intravenous drug

Infections of the Central Nervous System

use, AIDS, and inherited and acquired immunodeficiencies [41].

As *Candida* spp. invade blood vessels, cerebral lesions are characterized by hemorrhagic infarcts, abscesses, and granulomas. Microscopically, small yeasts measuring 3–5 µm (*C. glabrata* can be smaller, from 2 to 3 µm), associated with pseudohyphae (except for *C. glabrata*), stain positively with PAS and Gomori Grocott stains (Figure 44.6).

Dimorphic fungi

Dimorphic fungi, which are considered as true pathogens, exist in geographically defined regions. Although able to infect individuals who are immunocompetent, they are a real threat for immunosuppressed populations. Coccioidioidmycosis (also known as "Valley fever"), Histoplasmosis, and *T. marneffei* infection have been recognized as AIDS-defining illness.

Coccioidioidmycosis

Infections with *C. immitis* and its sibling *C. posadasii* occur predominantly in the Southwestern United States and in parts of Central and South America [42]. Disseminated coccidioidomycosis is rare; it occurs in less than 5% of symptomatic patients, 25–35% of disseminated infections involve the

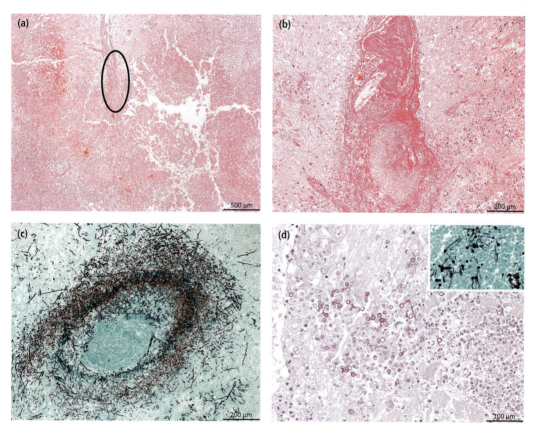

Figure 44.6 Cerebral candidiasis. (a) Extensive necrosis, centered on an artery (black circle). (b) Higher magnification of the artery, with destruction of its wall. The thrombosed lumen is filled with fibrin and cell debris, and there is peripheral infarction of the cerebral parenchyma. (c) Severe tissue invasion by the fungus, with complete invasion of the artery. (d and inset) At the periphery of the lesion, the fungus morphology is more easily seen: yeasts associated with pseudohyphae and filaments. a–b, hematoxylin and eosin (H&E) stain; c and inset, Gomori Grocott stain; d, periodic acid-Schiff (PAS).

CNS. Predisposing factors include compromised cellular immunity (HIV), immunosuppressive therapy for rheumatologic disorders, and antirejection therapy after organ transplant.

Histologically, chronic granulomatous meningitis is the most common finding; in the tissue, round spherules of varying diameter up to 100 μm, containing multiple endospores, can be observed even in H&E stains. The inflammatory reaction consists of abscesses and granulomas (Figure 44.7) [43, 44]. Interestingly, primary immunodeficiencies (PIDs) with defects in the interleukin-12/interferon gamma (IL-12/INF-γ) pathway and Th-17–mediated response are associated with susceptibility to certain endemic dimorphic fungal pathogens [45].

Histoplasmosis

H. capsulatum causes infections within certain areas of the United States (around 40 million people infected) [46], as well as South America, Southeast Asia, and Africa. Almost all described cases were infections by *H. capsulatum* var. *capsulatum*. Patients who are immunosuppressed, especially those with HIV, are particularly at risk and 3–5% develop disseminated histoplasmosis. Of these, 10–20% develop CNS infection, with lesions in the meninges, spinal cord, or brain. The mortality rate is 20–40% [47].

Histological lesions include necrosis and macrophages and granulomas; small oval yeasts (2–4 μm), surrounded by a clear space corresponding to the yeast wall, with narrow-based budding, are visible with H&E, PAS, or Gomori Grocott stains. Yeasts may be either extracellular or in the cytoplasm of macrophages (Figure 44.8). The differential diagnosis includes several other pathogens: *Blastomyces dermatitidis* (displaying broad-based budding), *Cryptococcus* spp. with a thin capsule, endospores of *Coccidioides* spp., and several Protozoa such as *Leishmania* spp. and *Toxoplasma* spp. (there is no clear space around these pathogens and a kinetoplast is present in *Leishmania* spp.) [11]. The clinical context is very important for a precise identification of the pathogen.

Blastomycosis

Blastomycosis, caused by *B. dermatitidis*, generally presents as pulmonary infection in both children and adults. Infection of the CNS is rare (1–3% in most studies) and is usually associated with another primary site of infection. Isolated CNS forms are rare. Macroscopic lesions can present as meningitis and single or multiple abscesses [48]. *B. dermatitidis* can be detected in H&E sections or after PAS or Gomori Grocott staining. Yeasts are round, 8–15 μm in diameter, with a refractive wall, and display broad-based budding (Figure 44.9).

Paracoccidioidomycosis

Paracoccidioides spp. are endemic to Latin America and the most common cause of deep mycoses. The estimated frequency of CNS involvement is 2.5% [49]. The definitive diagnosis

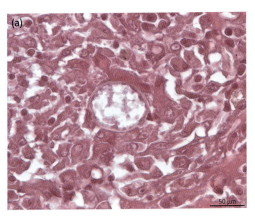
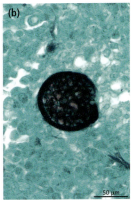
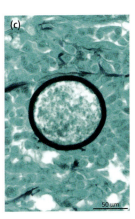

Figure 44.7 Coccidioidomycosis. (a–c) Spherule delineated by a thick, refringent wall, either empty (a and c), or containing endospores (b). a, hematoxylin and eosin (H&E) stain; b–c, Gomori Grocott stain.

Infections of the Central Nervous System

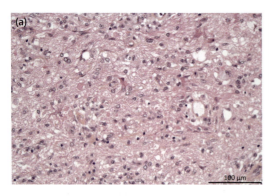 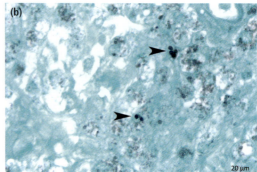

Figure 44.8 Cerebral histoplasmosis. (a) Gliosis with activation of microglial cells and rare multinucleated giant cells. (b) High magnification: small oval yeasts grouped in the cytoplasm of microglial cells or macrophages and multinucleated giant cells (black arrowheads). a, hematoxylin and eosin (H&E) stain; b, Gomori Grocott stain.

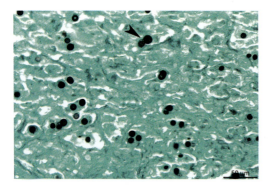 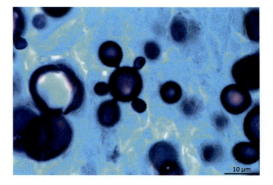

Figure 44.9 Blastomycosis. High magnification, Gomori Grocott stain: round yeasts, measuring 8–15 μm in diameter, showing broad-based budding (black arrowhead).

Figure 44.10 Paracoccidioidomycosis. Multiple narrow-based buds, resembling a "pilot wheel." Gomori Grocott stain.

of paracoccidioidomycosis depends on microscopic examination and positive culture, which may take up to four weeks. On histology, multiple narrow-based buds, resembling a "pilot wheel," should be identified (Figure 44.10). Combined histology, direct examination, and molecular-based methods enable early diagnosis. Because of increased global travel, these infections are also encountered outside endemic regions so the travel history of suspected patients is important [50].

All these aforementioned pathogens are acquired by inhalation of conidia. Within the body, the dimorphic fungi grow as yeast forms and systemic dissemination may occur in patients who are immunocompromised [45].

Genetic predispositions to fungal CNS infections

PIDs are rare inborn deficiencies of immunity and may interfere with pathogen recognition via PRR and downstream signaling events. C-type lectin receptors and downstream elements are central to the recognition of fungal pathogens and for induction of the innate and adaptive immune responses. CARD9 is involved in the signaling downstream of C-type lectin receptors, such as Dectin-1, Dectin-2, and Mincle and is a central player in antifungal innate immune response by inducing production of proinflammatory cytokines after recognition of fungal cell wall components [51]. Patients with autosomal recessive CARD9 mutations are predisposed to recurrent mucocutaneous and invasive fungal infections with *Candida* spp., *Aspergillus*, dermatophytes, and phaeohyphomycetes. Invasive dermatophytosis and phaeohyphomycosis CNS infections are the major clinical phenotypes in CARD9 deficient patients. More importantly CARD9 plays a major role in neutrophil trafficking in the CNS highlighting a central role in brain *Candida* immunity [51]. CNS infection with *A. fumigatus* has also been observed in persons with CARD9 deficiency. Chronic granulomatous disease, a defect in the NADPH oxidase complex, required for the oxidative burst against fungal pathogens in neutrophils, typically is associated with dissociated mold infections like *A. fumigatus*.

Other new PIDs are described every year (e.g. inborn errors of IFN-γ or Il-17 immunity), resulting in children and young adults being susceptible to diverse superficial and invasive fungal infections. Identifying these disorders hopefully will pave the way for better patient care and new treatments [52–54].

Animal models

Fungal pathogens can cause extinction in amphibians due to chytridiomycosis *(Batrachochytrium dendrobatidis)* or historic declines in mammalian populations (e.g. white nose syndrome in bats due to the ascomycete *Geomyces destructans*). There are several animal models to investigate fungal pathogenesis, host immune responses, and novel antifungal compounds (reviewed in [55]).

Mice are the best animal models to study clinical syndromes associated with pathogenic fungi; inbred laboratory strains and gene-deficient and transgenic variants enable examination of host genetic predispositions. Other vertebrate models (e.g. rats, guinea pigs, rabbits, hamsters, or zebrafish) have advantages of size or specific genetic strains. Transparent zebrafish larvae allow noninvasive imaging and the availability of modified antisense oligonucleotides (i.e. Morpholinos) to lower protein levels in zebra fish are also advantages.

Nonvertebrate animal models using fruit flies *(Drosophila melanogaster)*, wax moths *(Galleria mellonella)*, and nematodes like *Caenorhabditis elegans* as mini hosts have been adapted for high throughput screening of drug compound libraries, fungal mutant strains, or infection studies at ambient temperatures.

Human pathogenic fungi exhibit two main common features. As opportunistic pathogens, most fungi infect susceptible individuals; vertebrates also require immunosuppression to become susceptible. Second, the majority of pathogenic fungi are airborne pathogens, invade respiratory sites first, and disseminate under certain conditions to extrapulmonary locations. *Candida* spp. are the major exception as they are commensals in the human gut, and they cause infection by crossing gastrointestinal or mucosal barriers to reach the bloodstream.

The appropriate choice of animal model depends on the fungal strain, the host and immune suppression, inoculum dose, route of administration, and experimental read out. Different fungal strains can cause various immune responses as shown for clinical *A. fumigatus* isolates in murine pulmonary infection models [56] and different subsets of *C. albicans* strains [57]. *C. albicans* strains also show differences in pathogenicity depending on infection sites [58].

Biochemical pathways may be different between animals and humans. Murine chronic granulomatous disease (CDG) with a defect in the NADPH oxidase activity is associated with increased susceptibility to aspergillosis, similar to humans. However, murine CDG also causes defects in tryptophan metabolism (i.e. the formation of anti-inflammatory kynurenines) that increase inflammatory responses, but this does not occur in human patients with CDG [59].

Different immunosuppressive drugs (i.e. corticosteroids or myelotoxic chemotherapy), impact pathogenesis and disease progression. The route of administration also strongly influences disease development in animal models. The inoculum should be administered via the physiologically relevant route, and numerous protocols exist to model systemic (intravenous, intraperitoneal), pulmonary (intranasal, intratracheal, or inhalational), mucosal (oropharyngeal, vaginal), gastric (by gavage), superficial (skin abrasion or local application),

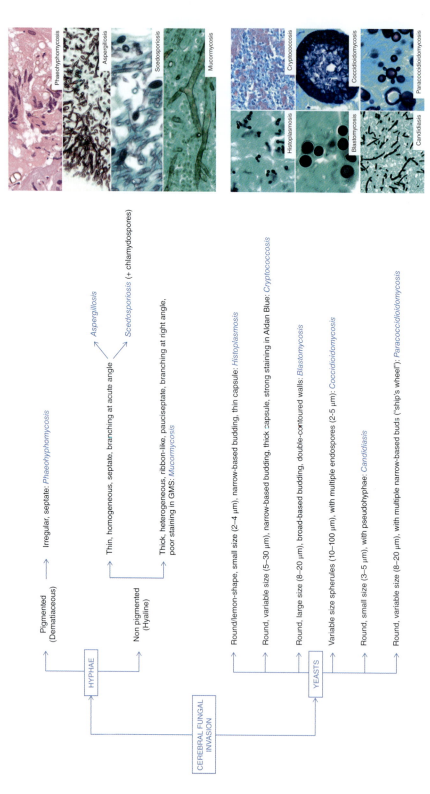

Figure 44.11 Histological diagnosis of fungal infections.

Table 44.1 Overview of the most common fungal pathogens causing CNS infection including risk factors, therapy strategies, and serological tests.

Pathogen	Risk factors	Therapy	Comments	Serological tests
Aspergillus spp.	neutropenia, glucocorticoids, immunosuppression, primary immunodeficiencies, CARD9 deficiency	Voriconazole, liposomal AmB second-line: AmB lipid complex, Casopfungin	Azole resistance might be a concern; A. terreus displays AmB resistance	Galactomannan antigen, LFA assay
Scedosporium apiospermum	neutropenia, glucocorticoids	Voriconazole, second line: Posaconazole	—	β-D-glucan all fungi except Mucorales and Cryptococcus
Lomentospora prolificans		—	Resistant to all major antifungals, surgical resection	—
Mucorales	neutropenia, glucocorticoids, diabetes mellitus	Liposomal AmB, AmB lipid complex	Sinus infections more common than lung infections	—
Dematiaceous molds	neutropenia, glucocorticoids	Voriconazole, Liposomal AmB	No antifungal effective against Cladophialophora bantaiana	β-D-glucan all fungi except Mucorales and Cryptococcus
Cryptococcus spp.	immunosuppression, HIV infection	Combined therapy AmB flucytosine Liposomal AmB or AmB deoxycholate + flucytosine or flucytosine	Flucytosine easily penetrates the CNS	Glucuronoxylo-mannan antigen, LFA Mannan AG test
CNS candidiasis	immunosuppression, CARD9 deficiency			
Dimorphic fungi	immunosuppression, HIV infection	Voriconazole or combined therapies with AmB or Echinocandin + flucytosine	Restricted geographic distribution	AG and AB detection for Histoplasma and Blastomyces, AB detection against Coccidioides

CARD9, capase recruitment domain–containing protein 9; CNS, central nervous system; HIV, human immunodeficiency virus; LFA, lateral flow assay.

dermal (subcutaneous), or CNS (intracranial, intracisternal, or intrathecal) mycoses.

Direct inoculation of fungal cells into the CNS via CSF can be readily reproduced and are particularly useful for pharmacologic studies.

In animal models, classical experimental parameters include fungal organ burden, histopathology, and survival. Released fungal antigens (e.g. galactomannan for *A. fumigatus*) can be monitored by serology and provide a quantitative result of fungal tissue burden in murine experiments. Host cytokines and inflammatory mediators can also be monitored, whereas fungal intermediates like iron chelating siderophores hold promise as biomarkers to improve diagnosis and monitor infection [60].

Conclusions

Diagnosis and therapy of CNS fungal infections have developed significantly in recent years. Morphological and histopathological features enable rapid and efficient diagnosis (Figure 44.11 and Table 44.1 for summary), especially when combined with molecular biology. Nevertheless, these infections are still difficult to treat and have a poor prognosis. Greater awareness of the numerous pathogens, diagnostic strategies, genetic predispositions, and appropriate drug treatments may result in earlier diagnosis and initiation of appropriate therapy to improve outcomes.

References

1. Homei, A. and Worboys, M. (eds.) (2013). Introduction. In: *Fungal Disease in Britain and the United States 1850–2000*, 225. Basingstoke (UK): Palgrave Macmillan Ed.
2. Li, D.M. and de Hoog, G.S. (2009). Cerebral phaeohyphomycosis – a cure at what lengths? *Lancet Infect. Dis.* 9: 376–383.
3. Brown, G.D., Denning, D.W., Gow, N.A.R. et al. (2012). Hidden killers: human fungal infections. *Sci. Transl. Med.* 4: 165rv13.
4. Romani, L. (2011). Immunity to fungal infections. *Nat. Rev. Immunol.* 11: 275–288.
5. De Pauw, B., Walsh, T.J., Donnelly, J.P. et al. (2008). Revised definitions of invasive fungal disease from the European Organization for Research and Treatment of cancer/invasive fungal infections cooperative group and the National Institute of Allergy and Infectious Diseases mycoses study group (EORTC/MSG) consensus group. *Clin. Infect. Dis.* 46: 1813–1821.
6. Perfect, J.R. (2012). Iatrogenic fungal meningitis: tragedy repeated. *Ann. Intern. Med.* 157: 825–826.
7. Economides, M.P., Ballester, L.Y., Kumar, V.A. et al. (2017). Invasive mold infections of the central nervous system in patients with hematologic cancer or stem cell transplantation (2000-2016): uncommon, with improved survival but still deadly often. *J. Inf. Secur.* 75: 572–580.
8. Walsh, T.J., Anaissie, E.J., Denning, D.W. et al. (2008). Treatment of aspergillosis: clinical practice guidelines of the Infectious Diseases Society of America. *Clin. Infect. Dis.* 46: 327–360.
9. Kourkoumpetis, T.K., Desalermos, A., Muhammed, M., and Mylonakis, E. (2012). Central nervous system aspergillosis: a series of 14 cases from a general hospital and review of 123 cases from the literature. *Medicine (Baltimore)* 91: 328–336.
10. Antinori, S., Corbellino, M., Meroni, L. et al. (2013). Aspergillus meningitis: a rare clinical manifestation of central nervous system aspergillosis. Case report and review of 92 cases. *J. Inf. Secur.* 66: 218–238.
11. Guarner, J. and Brandt, M.E. (2011). Histopathologic diagnosis of fungal infections in the 21st century. *Clin. Microbiol. Rev.* 24: 247–280.
12. Lee, S., Yun, N.R., Kim, K.-H. et al. (2010). Discrepancy between histology and culture in filamentous fungal infections. *Med. Mycol.* 48: 886–888.
13. Moling, O., Lass-Flörl, C., Verweij, P.E. et al. (2002). Case reports. Chronic and acute aspergillus meningitis. *Mycoses* 45: 504–511.
14. Tarrand, J.J., Lichterfeld, M., Warraich, I. et al. (2003). Diagnosis of invasive septate mold infections. A correlation of microbiological culture and histologic or cytologic examination. *Am. J. Clin. Pathol.* 119: 854–858.
15. Chong, G.M., Maertens, J.A., Lagrou, K. et al. (2016). Diagnostic performance of galactomannan antigen testing in cerebrospinal fluid. *J. Clin. Microbiol.* 54: 428–431.
16. Loeffler, J., Hafner, J., Mengoli, C. et al. (2017). Prospective biomarker screening for diagnosis of invasive aspergillosis in high-risk pediatric patients. *J. Clin. Microbiol.* 55: 101–109.
17. Denning, D.W. and Hope, W.W. (2010). Therapy for fungal diseases: opportunities and priorities. *Trends Microbiol.* 18: 195–204.
18. Roden, M.M., Zaoutis, T.E., Buchanan, W.L. et al. (2005). Epidemiology and outcome of zygomycosis: a

review of 929 reported cases. *Clin. Infect. Dis.* 41: 634–653.
19. Pana, Z.D., Seidel, D., Skiada, A. et al. (2016). Collaborators of http://Zygomyco.net and/or FungiScope™ registries*: invasive mucormycosis in children: an epidemiologic study in European and non-European countries based on two registries. *BMC Infect. Dis.* 16: 667.
20. Lanternier, F., Sun, H.Y., Ribaud, P. et al. (2012). Mucormycosis in organ and stem cell transplant recipients. *Clin. Infect. Dis.* 54 (11): 1629–1636.
21. Verma, A., Brozman, B., and Petito, C.K. (2006). Isolated cerebral mucormycosis: report of a case and review of the literature. *J. Neurol. Sci.* 240: 65–69.
22. Malik, A.N., Bi, W.L., McCray, B. et al. (2014). Isolated cerebral mucormycosis of the basal ganglia. *Clin. Neurol. Neurosurg.* 124: 102–105.
23. Lass-Flörl, C. (2009). Zygomycosis: conventional laboratory diagnosis. *Clin. Microbiol. Infect.* 15 (Suppl 5): 60–65.
24. Spellberg, B., Edwards, J., and Ibrahim, A. (2005). Novel perspectives on mucormycosis: pathophysiology, presentation, and management. *Clin. Microbiol. Rev.* 18: 556–569.
25. Millon, L., Herbrecht, R., Grenouillet, F. et al. (2016). Early diagnosis and monitoring of mucormycosis by detection of circulating DNA in serum: retrospective analysis of 44 cases collected through the French surveillance network of invasive fungal infections (RESSIF). *Clin. Microbiol. Infect.* 22: 810.e1–810.e8.
26. Revankar, S.G., Sutton, D.A., and Rinaldi, M.G. (2004). Primary central nervous system phaeohyphomycosis: a review of 101 cases. *Clin. Infect. Dis.* 38: 206–216.
27. Lanternier, F., Barbati, E., Meinzer, U. et al. (2015). Inherited CARD9 deficiency in 2 unrelated patients with invasive Exophiala infection. *J. Infect. Dis.* 211 (8): 1241–1250.
28. Chowdhary, A., Meis, J.F., Guarro, J. et al. (2014). ESCMID and ECMM joint clinical guidelines for the diagnosis and management of systemic phaeohyphomycosis: diseases caused by black fungi. *Clin. Microbiol. Infect.* 20 (Suppl 3): 47–75.
29. Mariné, M., Pastor, F.J., and Guarro, J. (2009). Combined antifungal therapy in a murine model of disseminated infection by Cladophialophora bantiana. *Med. Mycol.* 47: 45–49.
30. Deng, S., Pan, W., Liao, W. et al. (2016). Combination of amphotericin B and Flucytosine against neurotropic species of Melanized fungi causing primary cerebral Phaeohyphomycosis. *Antimicrob. Agents Chemother.* 60: 2346–2351.
31. Rajasingham, R., Smith, R.M., Park, B.J. et al. (2017). Global burden of disease of HIV-associated cryptococcal meningitis: an updated analysis. *Lancet Infect. Dis.* 17: 873–881.
32. Maziarz, E.K. and Perfect, J.R. (2016). Cryptococcosis. *Infect. Dis. Clin. N. Am.* 30: 179–206.
33. Krockenberger, M.B., Malik, R., Ngamskulrungroj, P. et al. (2010). Pathogenesis of pulmonary Cryptococcus gattii infection: a rat model. *Mycopathologia* 170: 315–330.
34. Kronstad, J.W., Attarian, R., Cadieux, B. et al. (2011). Expanding fungal pathogenesis: Cryptococcus breaks out of the opportunistic box. *Nat. Rev. Microbiol.* 9: 193–203.
35. Alanio, A., Vernel-Pauillac, F., Sturny-Leclère, A., and Dromer, F. (2015). Cryptococcus neoformans host adaptation: toward biological evidence of dormancy. *MBio* 6 pii e02580-14.
36. Chrétien, F., Lortholary, O., Kansau, I. et al. (2002). Pathogenesis of cerebral Cryptococcus neoformans infection after fungemia. *J. Infect. Dis.* 186: 522–530.
37. Jarvis, J.N., Percival, A., Bauman, S. et al. (2011). Evaluation of a novel point-of-care cryptococcal antigen test on serum, plasma, and urine from patients with HIV-associated cryptococcal meningitis. *Clin. Infect. Dis.* 53: 1019–1023.
38. Sato, Y., Osabe, S., Kuno, H. et al. (1999). Rapid diagnosis of cryptococcal meningitis by microscopic examination of centrifuged cerebrospinal fluid sediment. *J. Neurol. Sci.* 164: 72–75.
39. Hanson, K.E. (2016). The first fully automated molecular diagnostic panel for meningitis and encephalitis: how well does it perform, and when should it be used? *J. Clin. Microbiol.* 54: 2222–2224.
40. Figueiredo, S.M., Campolina, S., Rosa, C.A. et al. (2014). Cerebral macroabscess caused by Candida albicans in an immunocompetent patient: a diagnostic challenge. *Med. Mycol. Case Rep.* 3: 17–19.
41. Lanternier, F., Mahdaviani, S.A., Barbati, E. et al. (2015). Inherited CARD9 deficiency in otherwise healthy children and adults with Candida species-induced meningoencephalitis, colitis, or both. *J. Allergy Clin. Immunol.* 135: 1558–1568.
42. Stockamp, N.W. and Thompson, G.R. (2016). Coccidioidomycosis. *Infect. Dis. Clin. N. Am.* 30: 229–246.
43. Brown, J., Benedict, K., Park, B.J., and Thompson, G.R. (2013). Coccidioidomycosis: epidemiology. *Clin Epidemiol* 5: 185–197.
44. Motley, B.D., Grabowski, M., and Prayson, R.A. (2015). Coccidioides parenchymal cerebral abscess in the setting of lymphoma. *J. Clin. Neurosci.* 22: 40–41.

45. Lee, P.P. and Lau, Y.-L. (2017). Cellular and molecular defects underlying invasive fungal infections- revelations from endemic mycoses. *Front. Immunol.* 8: 735.
46. Kauffman, C.A. (2007). Histoplasmosis: a clinical and laboratory update. *Clin. Microbiol. Rev.* 20: 115–132.
47. Hariri, O.R., Minasian, T., Quadri, S.A. et al. (2015). Histoplasmosis with deep CNS involvement: case presentation with discussion and literature review. *J. Neurol. Surg. Rep.* 76: e167–e172.
48. Madigan, T., Fatemi, Y., Theel, E.S. et al. (2017). Central nervous system Blastomycosis in children: a case report and review of the literature. *Pediatr. Infect. Dis. J.* 36: 679–684.
49. de Almeida, S.M., Roza, T.H., Salvador, G.L.O. et al. (2017). Neurological and multiple organ involvement due to *Paracoccidioides brasiliensis* and HIV co-infection diagnosed at autopsy. *J. Neurovirol.* 23: 913–918.
50. Van Damme, P.A., Bierenbroodspot, F., Telgtt, D.S.C. et al. (2006). A case of imported paracoccidioidomycosis: an awkward infection in the Netherlands. *Med. Mycol.* 44: 13–18.
51. Pilmis, B., Puel, A., Lortholary, O., and Lanternier, F. (2016). New clinical phenotypes of fungal infections in special hosts. *Clin. Microbiol. Infect.* 22: 681–687.
52. Li, J., Vinh, D.C., Casanova, J.-L., and Puel, A. (2017). Inborn errors of immunity underlying fungal diseases in otherwise healthy individuals. *Curr. Opin. Microbiol.* 40: 46–57.
53. Maskarinec, S.A., Johnson, M.D., and Perfect, J.R. (2016). Genetic susceptibility to fungal infections: what is in the genes? *Curr. Clin. Microbiol. Rep.* 3: 81–91.
54. Lanternier, F., Cypowyj, S., Picard, C. et al. (2013). Primary immunodeficiencies underlying fungal infections. *Curr. Opin. Pediatr.* 25: 736–747.
55. Hohl, T.M. (2014). Overview of vertebrate animal models of fungal infection. *J. Immunol. Methods* 410: 100–112.
56. Rizzetto, L., Giovannini, G., Bromley, M. et al. (2013). Strain dependent variation of immune responses to a. fumigatus: definition of pathogenic species. *PLoS One* 8: e56651.
57. Marakalala, M.J., Vautier, S., Potrykus, J. et al. (2013). Differential adaptation of Candida albicans in vivo modulates immune recognition by dectin-1. *PLoS Pathog.* 9: e1003315.
58. Rahman, D., Mistry, M., Thavaraj, S. et al. (2012). Murine model of concurrent oral and vaginal Candida albicans colonisation. *Methods Mol. Biol. (Clifton NJ)* 845: 527–535.
59. Romani, L., Fallarino, F., De Luca, A. et al. (2008). Defective tryptophan catabolism underlies inflammation in mouse chronic granulomatous disease. *Nature* 451: 211–215.
60. Petrik, M., Haas, H., Laverman, P. et al. (2014). Decristoforo C: 68Ga-triacetylfusarinine C and 68Ga-ferrioxamine E for aspergillus infection imaging: uptake specificity in various microorganisms. *Mol. Imaging Biol. MIB Off. Publ. Acad. Mol. Imaging* 16: 102–108.

45 Cerebral Malaria

Patrícia Reis, Vanessa Estato, and Hugo Caire de Castro Faria Neto

Laboratory of Immunopharmacology, Oswaldo Cruz Institute, FIOCRUZ, Rio de Janeiro, Brazil

Abbreviations

BBB	blood-brain barrier
BDNF	brain-derived neurotrophic factor
CI	cognitive impairment
CM	cerebral malaria
CNS	central nervous system
DAMPs	damage-associated molecular patterns
ECM	experimental cerebral malaria
GFP	green fluorescent protein
GPI	glycosylphosphatidylinositols
ICAM-1	intercellular adhesion molecule 1
IFN-γ	interferon-gamma
LT	lymphotoxin
NK	natural killer
NO	nitric oxide
NOS	nitric oxide synthase
PAMP	pathogen associated molecular pattern
PbA	*Plasmodium berghei Anka*
PfEMP1	*P. falciparum* erythrocyte membrane protein 1
PRBCs	parasitized red blood cells
PRR	pattern recognition receptors
RBC(s)	red blood cell(s)
TGF	transforming growth factor
TH1	T helper 1
TNF	tumor necrosis factor

Introduction, synonyms, and historical perspective

Malaria, meaning "bad air," is caused by infection with protozoans of the genus *Plasmodium* and transmitted by female *Anopheles* mosquitoes to vertebrate hosts, including monkeys and humans. Five known species of *Plasmodium* infect humans (*Plasmodium falciparum, Plasmodium vivax, Plasmodium malariae, Plasmodium ovale,* and *Plasmodium knowlesi*). Most of them cause a benign or asymptomatic disease reflecting well-adapted parasite–host interactions and effective immune defense mechanisms, but complicated disease may arise from virtually any *Plasmodium* infection. *P. falciparum* is the one species most frequently associated with severe forms of malaria. In nonimmune hosts, *Plasmodium* infections (mainly *P. falciparum*) can become serious and life threatening, clinically presenting as malaria syndromes with metabolic acidosis, severe malarial anemia, or cerebral malaria (CM). These diverse presentations may indicate different underlying pathogenic mechanisms; however, they seem to share three major features: (i) sequestration of parasitized red blood cells (PRBCs) in target organs; (ii) increased concentrations of parasite products; and (iii) recruitment of inflammatory cells with production

---

Infections of the Central Nervous System: Pathology and Genetics, First Edition. Edited by Fabrice Chrétien, Kum Thong Wong, Leroy R. Sharer, Catherine (Katy) Keohane and Françoise Gray.
© 2020 John Wiley & Sons Ltd. Published 2020 by John Wiley & Sons Ltd.

of inflammatory mediators. The etiology of CM and other complicated malaria presentations is debated, but these three hallmarks impart a worse prognosis and appear to be fundamental pathophysiological processes.

Malaria has many synonyms, the best known are "ague" and "jungle fever."

In 2700 BCE, malaria symptoms were described in the *Nei Ching* ancient Chinese writings. By the fourth century BCE malaria was widely recognized in Greece. Hippocrates described the main symptoms. A relationship to swamps was noted by Roman writers, and in the Sanskrit text of Sushruta's compendium (seventh or sixth centuries BCE), symptoms were attributed to the bites of certain insects. In the seventeenth century *Peruvian bark*, a source of quinine was used to cure malaria. In 1880, Charles Laveran, a French surgeon described malaria parasites in the blood of a malaria patient and suspected mosquitoes were responsible for their transmission. The British officer Ronald Ross, working in the Indian medical service, showed that parasites could be transmitted from malaria patients to mosquitoes in 1897, and he studied the parasite life cycle. Although the Qinghao plant *Artemesia annua* was described in China during the second century BCE, it was not until 1971 its active ingredient, artemisinin, was identified by Chinese scientists. Artemisinins and quinine are used today as effective antimalarial drugs. For detailed malaria history see [1].

Life cycle

The parasite has two life cycles, sexual reproduction in an *Anopheles* mosquito vector and asexual reproduction and multiplication in the intermediate (human) host [2]. An infected biting mosquito injects sporozoites into the human bloodstream, from where they are taken up into hepatocytes. Hepatocytes rupture following multiplication of parasites, releasing thousands of merozoites after 7–10 days. Merozoites invade red blood cells (RBCs) and undergo their intra-erythrocyte development: ring forms, later trophozoites, and then schizonts. The parasite ingests and catabolizes host hemoglobin and releases its brown refractile pigmented breakdown product as haemozoin.

RBCs with schizonts hemolyze, releasing 24–32 newly infective merozoites, which reinvade noninfected RBCs. Some merozoites mature into male and female gametocytes, which can be taken up by a biting mosquito to initiate the sexual phase of the life cycle in the mosquito's gut and salivary gland.

The cycle of RBC invasion, parasite multiplication, and release occurs every 48 hours for *P. falciparum;* the release phase coincides with the spikes of fever characteristic of malaria.

Epidemiology and genetics

Malaria is one of the most important infectious diseases in the world. It affects around 207 million people, usually in low-income countries, and causes more than 600 000 deaths annually, mainly in children [3]. *P. falciparum* is endemic in sub-Saharan Africa but is present in other tropical areas worldwide. CM caused by *P. falciparum* is the deadliest of the severe malaria forms, with an estimated mortality rate of 18.6% [4]. Approximately 1% of all *P. falciparum* infections develop into CM, 90% of which occur in children in sub-Saharan Africa [3]. CM accounts for approximately 34% of severe pediatric malaria cases [5] and for 50% of adult malaria deaths in Southeast Asia [6].

The risk factors for CM are age, immunological status, overall health of the host, host genotype, and parasite diversity. Specific population risk groups are young children in stable transmission areas, women who are pregnant and nonimmune and semi-immune in areas of high transmission, people with human immunodeficiency virus (HIV) and acquired immunodeficiency syndrome (AIDS), and international travelers from nonendemic areas [7]

Some human genetic variations and phenotypes protect against malaria; these mainly involve host RBCs and immunological factors. They include: (i) RBC and hemoglobin (Hb) defects such as thalassemia, sickle cell trait, HbC, and HbE; (ii) enzyme defects such as glucose-6-phosphtae dehydrogenase (G6PD) deficiency and pyruvate kinase (PK) deficiency; (iii) membrane defects such as ovalocytosis; (iv) the Duffy blood group; (v) immunogenetic variants such as human leukocyte antigen (HLA) alleles; and (vi) immunological components such as complement receptor 1, nitric oxide synthase 2 (NOS2), tumor necrosis factor alpha (TNF-α), and the chromosome 5q31–q33 region (the cytokine region). These genetic variants are highly detected in malaria-endemic areas as a result of natural selection. The mechanism of protection is not yet clear. The reduction or failure of parasite invasion and multiplication in RBCs, induction of clearance by the immune system, and increased oxidative stress are all likely to contribute to malaria protection (see pathogenesis) [8].

Human genetic factors influence the outcome of malaria severity. Predisposition to CM could be explained by genetic polymorphisms of the genes involved in malaria pathobiology (most involve immunological responses and cell receptors). However, variation in the genetic background of each ethnic population contributes to differences in disease predisposition and severity [8].

Parasite virulence is also believed to contribute to the severity of malaria and risk of CM. Multiple studies have tried to identify virulent strains of *P. falciparum* using genetic polymorphisms as markers [9]. Although there are differences in virulence among *P. falciparum* strains, the virulent strains have not yet been sufficiently characterized to identify suitable virulence markers.

Clinical presentation

CM is defined clinically as impaired consciousness (coma) in the absence of hypoglycemia, drugs, meningitis, or other cause of coma in a patient with *P. falciparum* infection. CM presents as a diffuse symmetrical encephalopathy with fever and few or no focal neurological signs. Coma is defined by a Glasgow Coma Score <11 in adults or a Blantyre Coma score <3 in children. In children coma develops rapidly once fever sets in but is more gradual in adults, with confusion, drowsiness, and high fever [10–12]. Characteristically, adults develop encephalitis and multiorgan failure, features not seen in children. Convulsions are present in 80% of children and up to 50% have status epilepticus, but only 15% of adults develop convulsions [11, 13].

Fundoscopy reveals changes in vessel color, macular and extramacular whitening, and white-centered retinal hemorrhages [14]. In survivors, coma recovers in around 24 hours for children and 48 hours for adults [5]. Up to 12% of children and 1% of adults develop neurologic sequelae with hemiplegia, aphasia, and ataxia, but these deficits are self-limiting and disappear after 6–12 months [15]. Long-term cognitive impairment (CI) and epilepsy are reported in children, increasing the societal impact of malaria in developing countries [16–18].

In endemic areas, or in travelers recently returned from such areas, a CM diagnosis must be considered in any comatose patient with a fever history. Febrile convulsions must be distinguished from CM in children when coma persists for more than 1 hour after anticonvulsant therapy. Diagnosis is usually made by microscopy of stained blood smears (Figure 45.1). The rapid diagnostic test may be used if direct microscopy is not possible. Fundoscopy improves the specificity of CM diagnosis and may be prognostic in patients with severe malaria [12].

Pathology

The original description of the pathology of CM by Marchiafava and Bignami [19] more than 100 years ago, is still relevant.

Macroscopically the brain is swollen with dusky leptomeninges, and on section it appears pale or slate-gray. Diffuse petechial hemorrhages of various types are seen in the cerebral white matter (Figure 45.2), brainstem, and cerebellar white matter, particularly in children.

Microscopically the most common feature is sequestration of parasitized RBCs within cerebral microvessels, which also contain dark malarial pigment (Figure 45.3a and b). Vascular thrombosis or rupture may be associated with ring hemorrhages (Figure 45.3c). Focal areas of white matter necrosis with axonal and myelin damage, accompanied by a macrophage and microglial reaction, are called Dürck granulomas (Figure 45.3d) [20]. In chronic cases, hemozoin pigment deposition may be marked (Figure 45.3e).

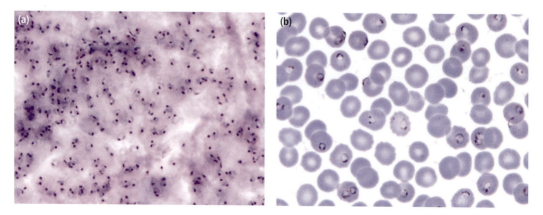

Figure 45.1 Stained blood smear showing erythrocytes containing parasites (Giemsa). (a) Most erythrocytes are parasitized. (b) Higher magnification shows erythrocytes parasitized by ring forms of trophozoites (Giemsa). Both images courtesy of Pr. Pierre Buffet, Faculté de Médecine Université Paris Descartes and Institut National de la Transfusion Sanguine.

Pathogenesis and animal models

The pathophysiology of CM is complex and has been debated for many decades [21–23], but none of the proposed hypotheses seem to fully explain all the findings in malaria patients and experimental models.

The hypotheses

One hypothesis is that PRBCs cause mechanical obstruction of microvessels. This feature was first described in 1894 [19] and has since been confirmed by numerous studies [23, 24]. Sequestration of PBRC and microvascular congestion are observed in all autopsies from patients who died with CM. However, it occurs in almost all cases infected by *P. falciparum*, even without cerebral complications [20, 25, 26]. Sequestration correlates with coma and early death in adults, but this correlation is not clear in children [27]. Cytoadherence and sequestration of PRBCs are observed in other organs such as lungs and gut, without associated pathology.

Cytoadherence of PRBCs correlates with expression of *P. falciparum* erythrocyte membrane protein 1 (PfEMP1). Parasites within RBCs transport PfEMP1 to the erythrocyte membrane, where it is expressed on RBC knobs creating points for endothelial attachment [28]. Counter-receptors on endothelial cells are CD 36 and intercellular adhesion molecule 1 (ICAM-1; mainly in the brain); endothelial protein C receptor has recently been identified as a binding receptor for PfEMP1 [12]. Increased cytoadhesion leads to blockage of the microcirculation and tissue hypoxia [29]. Further flow obstruction is caused by platelet-mediated agglutination and rosette formation (due to decreased deformability of both PRBCs and nonparasitized RBCs) [29, 30].

Another theory suggests that brain lesions can be explained by excessive activation and microvascular adhesion of immune cells leading to uncontrolled release of proinflammatory cytokines [31, 32]. In both humans with CM, and mouse models of CM, host leukocytes and platelets are sequestered in brain microvessels in addition to PRBCs [25, 33]. Macrophages also have pivotal effector roles in brain injury and edema in CM. Activation of endothelial cells and T lymphocytes also seem to play a role in the cascade reaction leading to CM [34]. All these host cells are likely to be involved in CM pathogenesis, either via local effects on brain microvessels or through distant effects mediated by potentially deleterious mediators, such as proinflammatory cytokines.

In both situations, blood-brain barrier (BBB) disruption seems to be an important consequence that contributes to cerebral edema and dysfunction. Structural and functional disruption of the BBB during CM is characterized by altered expression of the cell junction proteins occludin, vinculin, and

Cerebral Malaria Chapter 45

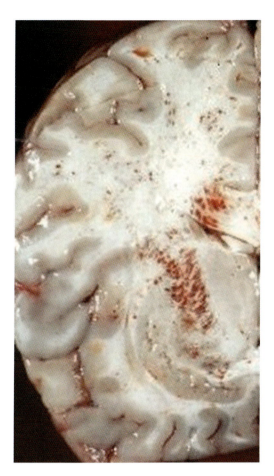

Figure 45.2 Cerebral malaria. Coronal section of the brain at the level of the thalamus showing diffuse white matter petechial hemorrhages. The brain is swollen with incipient uncal herniation.

ZO-1, as demonstrated in a study in Malawian children [35]. Breakdown of BBB and consequent cerebral edema is documented in both adults and children with CM, indicating endothelial activation and dysfunction [12, 36]. Several markers of endothelial activation are present in CM. *P. falciparum* infection upregulates ICAM-1, V-CAM, and E-selectin in brain microvasculature that colocalizes with PRBC sequestration. Some of these markers are shed into the plasma and soluble ICAM-1 seems to correlate with development of CM [22]. Endothelial microparticles are detected in the circulation of children with CM [24] and were higher in severe malaria cases, including CM, than in uncomplicated *P. falciparum* infections [37].

The main pathophysiologic events in CM are illustrated in Figure 45.4.

The contribution of animal models
Plasmodium berghei Anka (PbA) infection in CBA or CB57BL/6 mice is used widely as a murine model of human CM, despite different histopathological features. The murine model shows marked inflammation with little or no intracerebral sequestration of PRBC, whereas the reverse is seen in human CM (intense intracerebral sequestration, often with little inflammatory response) [38].

Microvascular and endothelial dysfunction
Low availability of nitric oxide (NO) may participate in the pathogenesis of human and experimental cerebral malaria (ECM). It is mainly related to the NO-scavenging effects of high concentrations of free oxyhemoglobin (HbO^{2+}) derived from hemolysis and to endothelial dysfunction. Mice with ECM show impaired responses of brain vessels to endothelial and neuronal NO synthase- (eNOS and nNOS) dependent vasodilators [39]. Recently, Bertinaria et al. showed that artemisinin-NO-donor hybrid compounds improved survival of mice with ECM when compared to artemisinin alone [40].

Impaired cerebral blood flow is associated with microvascular obstruction from sequestrated PRBCs adhering to the vascular endothelium, or binding to uninfected RBCs, resulting in formation of cell clusters called rosettes. In PbA-infected mice with ECM, we have shown a marked increase of rolling and adherent leukocytes colocalizing with adherent green fluorescent protein (GFP)-PRBCs in pial postcapillary vessel walls (Figure 45.5) [41].

Impairment of blood vessels goes beyond microvascular plugging in some ECM studies. Cabrales et al. demonstrated decreased RBC velocity in arterioles and venules [42]. We observed dramatically decreased cortical perfusion (Figure 45.6), attributed to vasoconstriction and reduced RBC velocity, leading to a collapse of cerebral microvessels.

Arteriolar dysfunction is also attributed to local inflammatory mediators triggering vasospasm in response to sequestered PRBCs [43]. This might correlate with the rapid onset of CM symptoms as a consequence of irregular capillary perfusion.

Infections of the Central Nervous System

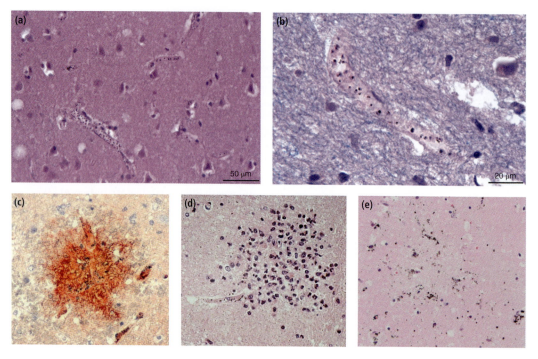

Figure 45.3 Microscopic changes in cerebral malaria. (a and b) Sequestration of parasitized red blood cells (PRBCs) within cerebral microvessels, which also contain dark malaria pigment. (c) A ruptured cerebral microvessel associated with a ring hemorrhage. (d) Dürck granuloma in the white matter, with numerous microglial cells and macrophages. (e) Deposition of hemozoin pigment in a chronic case of cerebral malaria.

The role of lymphocytes on CM

CM is often associated with a T helper 1 (TH1) immune response, implicating major roles for CD4$^+$ and CD8$^+$ T cells, natural killer (NK) cells, and the proinflammatory cytokines. CD8$^+$ T cells have been described as crucial for CM pathogenesis [44], and we have shown that anti-CD8$^+$ T cell antibody treatment reduces CM mortality and prevents cognitive decline [45].

Other studies showed that cross-presentation of malaria antigens on CNS endothelial cells recognized by CD8$^+$ cytotoxic lymphocytes led to endothelial damage [46] and parasite-specific CD8$^+$ T cells engaged endothelial cells in an antigen-dependent manner, which led to vascular breakdown, edema, loss of brainstem neurons, and subsequent death [47].

The role of platelets in CM

The characteristic thrombocytopenia in *P. falciparum* infection suggested a role for platelets in CM pathogenesis [48] and was supported by quantitative proteomic analysis of frontal lobe samples from patients with CM [49]. Infected mice treated with anti-CD11a/CD18 antibody (which selectively abrogates cerebral platelet sequestration), prevented a fatal outcome and correlated with CM prevention [50]. Animals rendered thrombocytopenic were protected against CM. Interestingly, platelet accumulation was significantly higher in the brains of patients who died of CM than in those who died of other causes [25]. In vitro, platelets are effectors of vascular endothelial damage after TNF stimulation and potentiate PRBC cytotoxicity to endothelial cells [51].

Cytokine response

Distinct patterns of cytokine responses have been shown in human CM studies. Transforming growth factor (TGF)-β, TNF-α, interleukin (IL)-10, IL-12, IL-1β, and interferon gamma (IFN-γ) are the most frequently reported as differentially elevated (comparing CM to non-CM). Elevated TNF levels

Cerebral Malaria **Chapter 45**

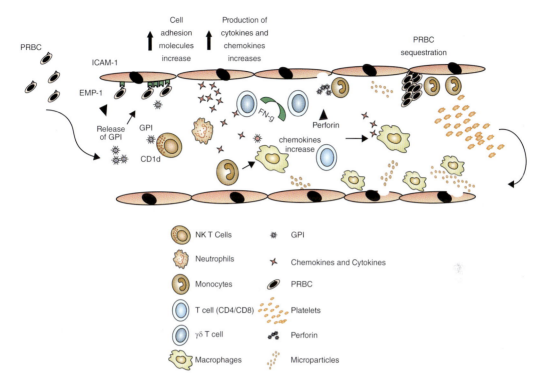

Figure 45.4 Pathophysiologic events likely to lead to severe malarial disease, particularly in the brain. Parasitized red blood cell (PRBC) expressing *Plasmodium falciparum* erythrocyte membrane protein 1 (PfEMP1) are sequestered in brain microvessels. Intravascular macrophages, lymphocytes, and platelets may also get trapped forming heterogeneous aggregates. Blood flow is affected and tissue hypoxia and oxidative stress set in. Activation of endothelial cells and leukocytes trigger production of inflammatory mediators and increase permeability of blood-brain barrier. Cerebral dysfunction is manifested as a diffuse encephalopathy with coma. EMP-1, erythrocyte membrane protein 1; GPI, glycosylphosphatidylinositols; ICAM-1: intercellular adhesion molecule 1; NK, natural killer; PRBC, parasitized red blood cell.

in cerebrospinal fluid were associated with long-term cognitive impairment after CM in children [52]. IL-12, IL-18, and TGF levels were elevated in all children with malaria; IL-12 levels were reliable in predicting disease progression [53, 54].

TNFα, lymphotoxin (LT)-alpha, and IFN-γ also have a central role in ECM pathogenesis [55–58].

However, individual cytokines are unlikely to account for the systemic or organ-specific manifestations of CM, and a common pattern of cytokine response predisposing to CM or CM severity has not yet been identified.

Neuroinflammation

Neuroinflammation can be triggered by systemic infectious diseases (Figure 45.7), leading to BBB disruption and efflux of proinflammatory cytokines, pathogen-associated molecular patterns (PAMPs) and damage-associated molecular patterns (DAMPs). These molecules activate glial cells, which assume inflammatory profiles, releasing cytokines and chemokines and reactive oxygen and nitrogen species exerting direct and indirect neuronal cytotoxicity [59, 60].

In ECM, we found intense inflammation in mouse brain coinciding with the onset of clinical signs at day 6 post infection. Inflammation was characterized by increased levels of TNF-α, IL-1β, monocyte chemotactic protein 1(MCP-1), and IL-12 [41], and microglial activation (Figure 45.8) and astrogliosis on histology. We also observed alterations in synaptic proteins and neuronal death. In ECM, increased brain glutamate levels lead to neuronal death by both excitotoxicity and ferroptosis. Ferroptosis, related to

Infections of the Central Nervous System

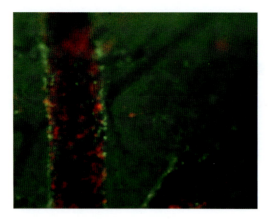

Figure 45.5 Postcapillary venule with adherent and rolling rhodamine-labeled leukocyte (red) co-localized with green fluorescent protein-red blood cells (GFP-RBCs, green) in the cerebral microcirculation of *Plasmodium berghei* ANKA (PbA, 10^{-6} PRBCs) infected C57BL/6 mice.

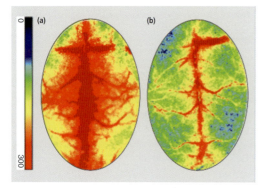

Figure 45.6 Image of cerebral microvascular blood flow assessed by laser speckle contrast imaging on exposed intact skull of C57BL/6 mice infected with *Plasmodium berghei* ANKA (PbA, 10^{-6} PRBCs) (a) or noninfected red blood cell (RBC) control mice (b).

excessive oxygen species production, lipid peroxidation, and excessive glutamate, leads to thiol reduction and may trigger neuronal death in CM and neurodegenerative disease [61].

Long-term sequelae of CM

Approximately 35% of those who survive CM have some form of impairment in neurological function or neurodevelopmental disorder. Usually neurological impairment is self-limiting and disappears after a year. However, long-term CI is underestimated and may be an additional societal burden of malaria in developing nations.

Neurological and CI was found in at least 21.4% of Ugandan children six months after CM [62] and was also found in Kenyan children 90 years following recovery from CM [63].

Most of the knowledge about mechanisms that cause CI results from ECM. Mice infected with PbA, develop long-term CI if rescued from lethal outcome by antimalarial drugs [45]. CI appears to be a consequence of neuroinflammation. Also, low levels of brain-derived neurotrophic factor (BDNF) have been detected in brain tissue after CM and inversely correlate to the degree of CI [64]. BDNF is key to long-term potentiation (LTP) and memory consolidation, so low BDNF levels could be linked to cognitive decline after CM.

In general, children are most affected by CM, and prone to developing CI, while experimental models usually use adult mice. Using infant mice, we observed CI of spatial and aversive memory that lasted until adulthood. These animals also had signs of depression and anxiety in behavioral tasks, suggesting that CM might be associated with late neuropsychiatric conditions.

The mechanisms by which malaria leads to neurocognitive impairment are not fully defined and consequently there is no specific treatment available.

In the experimental setting, antioxidant treatment can prevent cognitive decline [45]. Statins can prevent CI by controlling proinflammatory responses and reducing oxidative stress [41]. Minocycline is already used to treat some cases of malaria. It is an effective inhibitor of microglial activation, and unpublished data from our laboratory show it was effective in preventing cognitive decline.

Treatment

Treatment of CM is based on two main strategies: early initiation of antimalarial drugs and supportive care. Quinine was the traditional antimalarial drug used, but artesunate significantly reduces mortality in children and adults so the World

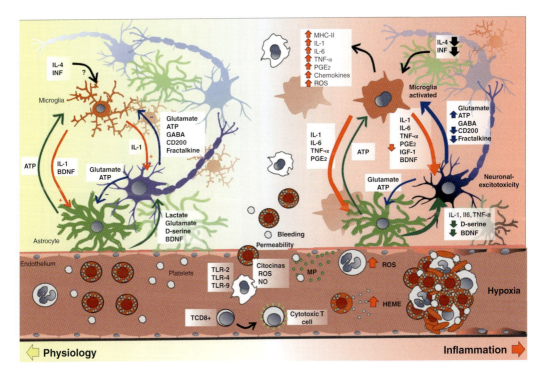

Figure 45.7 Under physiological conditions, low cytokine levels contribute to protein synthesis for cross-talk among neuron and glial cells. During cerebral malaria, adhesion of parasitized red blood cells (PRBCs) to endothelium due to Plasmodium falciparum erythrocyte membrane protein 1 (PfEMP1) triggers endothelial and immune cell activation. Cytokine and chemokine release and hijacking of red blood cells (RBCs), leukocytes, and platelets to endothelium leads to blood vessel occlusion and blood-brain barrier (BBB) breakdown. Astrocytes and microglial cells are activated, releasing cytokine and chemokine and reactive oxygen and nitrogen species. Microglial activation exacerbates cell damage, especially in neurons and endothelial cells. Astrocyte activation, despite releasing cytokines and contributing to BBB breakdown and cerebral edema, reduces glutamate intake, leading to its accumulation on synaptic clefts. Excessive glutamate triggers excitotoxicity and neuronal death. Tripartite cross talk is lost, contributing to development of neurological sequelae, particularly cognitive impairment). ATP, adenosine triphosphate; BDNF, brain-derived neurotrophic factor; GABA, gamma-aminobutyric acid; IGG-1, insulin growth factor-1; IL, interleukin; MHC, major histocompatibility complex; NO, nitric oxide; PGE$_2$, prostaglandin E2; ROS, reactive oxygen species; TLR, toll-like receptor; TNF-α, tumor necrosis factor alpha. Source: image kindly provided by MSC. Filipe Dutra.

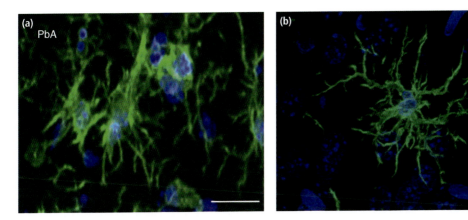

Figure 45.8 Immunostain of Iba-1 (green) in cortical brain tissue, showing activation of microglial cells in mice infected with *Plasmodium berghei Anka* (PbA) at day 6 post infection, when the first signs of cerebral malaria are observed. (a) Photomicrography shows changes in cell shape, with reduction of cellular process (amoeboid shape) in infected mice, (b) whereas uninfected cells have the normal appearance of resting microglia. Scale bar 20 μm.

Health Organization (WHO) recommends artesunate as the first-line treatment. Artemether and quinine are second choices [12].

In addition to artesunate therapy, supportive care is fundamentally important to reduce mortality. Patients who are comatose need endotracheal intubation, mechanical ventilation, urinary catheters, and nasogastric tubes. Monitoring glycemia and fever control with paracetamol is mandatory. Although convulsions are frequent in children with CM, prophylactic anticonvulsants are not recommended due to the risk of respiratory depression [12]. To date, therapies directed toward reducing malarial sequelae are unproven.

Conclusions

CM is the most severe form of malaria. It is caused by *P. falciparum* infection, mainly affects children and has a high mortality in children and adults. Cytoadherence of PRBCs, platelets, and leukocytes leading to microvascular obstruction, BBB dysfunction, neuroinflammation, and oxidative damage seem to be fundamentally important pathophysiologic events. CM is highly lethal but can cause long-term CI in survivors. Additional understanding of CM mechanisms and new adjunctive therapies are desperately needed to improve patient outcomes.

References

1. Centers for Disease Control and Prevention (CDC) (2018). *Malaria*. https://www.cdc.gov/malaria/about/history/index.html (accessed 9 November 2018).
2. Lucas, S. (2015). Parasitic infections. In: *Greenfield's Neuropathology*, 9e (eds. S. Love, H. Budka, J.W. Ironside and A. Perry), p1232–p1233. Boca Raton: CRC press.
3. World Health Organization (WHO) (2016). *2016 World Malaria Report*. Geneva, Switzerland: WHO.
4. Newton, C.R. and Krishna, S. (1998). Severe falciparum malaria in children: current understanding of pathophysiology and supportive treatment. *Pharmacol. Ther.* 79: 1–53.
5. Dondorp, A.M., Fanello, C.I., Hendriksen, I.C. et al. (2010). Artesunate versus quinine in the treatment of severe falciparum malaria in African children (AQUAMAT): an open-label, randomised trial. *Lancet* 376: 1647–1657.
6. Idro, R., Jenkins, N.E., and Newton, C.R. (2005). Pathogenesis, clinical features, and neurological outcome of cerebral malaria. *Lancet Neurol.* 4: 827–840.
7. World Health Organization (2013). *Management of severe malaria: a practical handbook*, 3e. Geneva, Switzerland: WHO.
8. Wah, S.T., Hananantachai, H., Kerdpin, U. et al. (2016). Molecular basis of human cerebral malaria development. *Trop. Med. Health* 44: 33.
9. Chaorattanakawee, S., Nuchnoi, P., Hananantachai, H. et al. (2018). Sequence variation in Plasmodium falciparum merozoite surface protein-2 is associated with virulence causing severe and cerebral malaria. *PLoS One* 13: e0190418.
10. Dondorp, A., Nosten, F., Stepniewska, K. et al. (2005). Artesunate versus quinine for treatment of severe falciparum malaria: a randomised trial. *Lancet* 366: 717–725.
11. Molyneux, M.E., Taylor, T.E., Wirima, J.J., and Borgstein, A. (1989). Clinical features and prognostic indicators in paediatric cerebral malaria: a study of 131 comatose Malawian children. *Q. J. Med.* 71: 441–459.
12. Plewes, K., Turner, G.D.H., and Dondorp, A.M. (2018). Pathophysiology, clinical presentation, and treatment of coma and acute kidney injury complicating falciparum malaria. *Curr. Opin. Infect. Dis.* 31: 69–77.
13. (2014). Severe malaria. *Tropical Med. Int. Health* 19 (Suppl 1): 7–131.
14. Lewallen, S., Taylor, T.E., Molyneux, M.E. et al. (1993). Ocular fundus findings in Malawian children with cerebral malaria. *Ophthalmology* 100: 857–861.
15. Nguyen, T.H., Day, N.P., Ly, V.C. et al. (1996). Post-malaria neurological syndrome. *Lancet* 348: 917–921.
16. Bangirana, P., Opoka, R.O., Boivin, M.J. et al. (2014). Severe malarial anemia is associated with long-term neurocognitive impairment. *Clin. Infect. Dis.* 59: 336–344.
17. Birbeck, G.L., Molyneux, M.E., Kaplan, P.W. et al. (2010). Blantyre malaria project epilepsy study (BMPES) of neurological outcomes in retinopathy-positive paediatric cerebral malaria survivors: a prospective cohort study. *Lancet Neurol.* 9: 1173–1181.
18. Brim, R., Mboma, S., Semrud-Clikeman, M. et al. (2017). Cognitive outcomes and psychiatric symptoms of retinopathy-positive cerebral malaria: cohort description and baseline results. *Am. J. Trop. Med. Hyg.* 97: 225–231.

19. Marchiafava, E. and Bignami, A. (1894). On summer-autumnal malaria fevers. In: *Malaria and the Parasites of Malarial Fever*, vol. 15 (ed. T.S. Society), 1–234. London: The Sydenham Society.
20. Dorovini-Zis, K., Schmidt, K., Huynh, H. et al. (2011). The neuropathology of fatal cerebral malaria in Malawian children. *Am. J. Pathol.* 178: 2146–2158.
21. Berendt, A.R., Ferguson, D.J., Gardner, J. et al. (1994). Molecular mechanisms of sequestration in malaria. *Parasitology* 108 (Suppl): S19–S28.
22. Storm, J. and Craig, A.G. (2014). Pathogenesis of cerebral malaria – inflammation and cytoadherence. *Front. Cell. Infect. Microbiol.* 4: 100.
23. White, N.J., Turner, G.D., Day, N.P., and Dondorp, A.M. (2013). Lethal malaria: Marchiafava and Bignami were right. *J. Infect. Dis.* 208: 192–198.
24. Coltel, N., Combes, V., Hunt, N.H., and Grau, G.E. (2004). Cerebral malaria – a neurovascular pathology with many riddles still to be solved. *Curr. Neurovasc. Res.* 1: 91–110.
25. Hunt, N.H. and Grau, G.E. (2003). Cytokines: accelerators and brakes in the pathogenesis of cerebral malaria. *Trends Immunol.* 24: 491–499.
26. Taylor, T.E., Fu, W.J., Carr, R.A. et al. (2004). Differentiating the pathologies of cerebral malaria by postmortem parasite counts. *Nat. Med.* 10: 143–145.
27. Ponsford, M.J., Medana, I.M., Prapansilp, P. et al. (2012). Sequestration and microvascular congestion are associated with coma in human cerebral malaria. *J. Infect. Dis.* 205: 663–671.
28. Magowan, C., Wollish, W., Anderson, L., and Leech, J. (1988). Cytoadherence by Plasmodium falciparum-infected erythrocytes is correlated with the expression of a family of variable proteins on infected erythrocytes. *J. Exp. Med.* 168: 1307–1320.
29. Silamut, K., Phu, N.H., Whitty, C. et al. (1999). A quantitative analysis of the microvascular sequestration of malaria parasites in the human brain. *Am. J. Pathol.* 155: 395–410.
30. Dondorp, A.M., Pongponratn, E., and White, N.J. (2004). Reduced microcirculatory flow in severe falciparum malaria: pathophysiology and electron-microscopic pathology. *Acta Trop.* 89: 309–317.
31. Grau, G.E. and de Kossodo, S. (1994). Cerebral malaria: mediators, mechanical obstruction or more? *Parasitol. Today* 10: 408–409.
32. Clark, I.A. and Rockett, K.A. (1994). The cytokine theory of human cerebral malaria. *Parasitol. Today* 10: 410–412.
33. Grau, G.E., Mackenzie, C.D., Carr, R.A. et al. (2003). Platelet accumulation in brain microvessels in fatal pediatric cerebral malaria. *J. Infect. Dis.* 187: 461–466.
34. Turner, G.D., Morrison, H., Jones, M. et al. (1994). An immunohistochemical study of the pathology of fatal malaria. Evidence for widespread endothelial activation and a potential role for intercellular adhesion molecule-1 in cerebral sequestration. *Am. J. Pathol.* 145: 1057–1069.
35. Brown, H., Rogerson, S., Taylor, T. et al. (2001). Blood-brain barrier function in cerebral malaria in Malawian children. *Am. J. Trop. Med. Hyg.* 64: 207–213.
36. Davis, T.M., Suputtamongkol, Y., Spencer, J.L. et al. (1992). Measures of capillary permeability in acute falciparum malaria: relation to severity of infection and treatment. *Clin. Infect. Dis.* 15: 256–266.
37. Sahu, U., Sahoo, P.K., Kar, S.K. et al. (2013). Association of TNF level with production of circulating cellular microparticles during clinical manifestation of human cerebral malaria. *Hum. Immunol.* 74: 713–721.
38. White, N.J., Turner, G.D., Medana, I.M. et al. (2010). The murine cerebral malaria phenomenon. *Trends Parasitol.* 26: 11–15.
39. Ong, P.K., Melchior, B., Martins, Y.C. et al. (2013). Nitric oxide synthase dysfunction contributes to impaired cerebroarteriolar reactivity in experimental cerebral malaria. *PLoS Pathog.* 9: e1003444.
40. Bertinaria, M., Orjuela-Sanchez, P., Marini, E. et al. (2015). NO-donor dihydroartemisinin derivatives as multitarget agents for the treatment of cerebral malaria. *J. Med. Chem.* 58: 7895–7899.
41. Reis, P.A., Estato, V., da Silva, T.I. et al. (2012). Statins decrease neuroinflammation and prevent cognitive impairment after cerebral malaria. *PLoS Pathog.* 8: e1003099.
42. Cabrales, P. and Carvalho, L.J. (2010). Intravital microscopy of the mouse brain microcirculation using a closed cranial window. *J. Vis. Exp.* (45): pii 2184.
43. Polder, T.W., Jerusalem, C.R., and Eling, W.M. (1991). Morphological characteristics of intracerebral arterioles in clinical (Plasmodium falciparum) and experimental (Plasmodium berghei) cerebral malaria. *J. Neurol. Sci.* 101: 35–46.
44. Howland, S.W., Claser, C., Poh, C.M. et al. (2015). Pathogenic CD8+ T cells in experimental cerebral malaria. *Semin. Immunopathol.* 37: 221–231.
45. Reis, P.A., Comim, C.M., Hermani, F. et al. (2010). Cognitive dysfunction is sustained after rescue therapy in experimental cerebral malaria, and is reduced by additive antioxidant therapy. *PLoS Pathog.* 6: e1000963.

46. Howland, S.W., Poh, C.M., Gun, S.Y. et al. (2013). Brain microvessel cross-presentation is a hallmark of experimental cerebral malaria. *EMBO Mol. Med.* 5: 984–999.
47. Swanson, P.A. 2nd, Hart, G.T., Russo, M.V. et al. (2016). CD8+ T cells induce fatal brainstem pathology during cerebral malaria via luminal antigen-specific engagement of brain vasculature. *PLoS Pathog.* 12: e1006022.
48. Gramaglia, I., Velez, J., Combes, V. et al. (2017). Platelets activate a pathogenic response to blood-stage Plasmodium infection but not a protective immune response. *Blood* 129: 1669–1679.
49. Kumar, M., Varun, C.N., Dey, G. et al. (2018). Identification of host-response in cerebral malaria patients using quantitative proteomic analysis. *Proteomics Clin. Appl.* 12: e1600187.
50. Lou, J., Lucas, R., and Grau, G.E. (2001). Pathogenesis of cerebral malaria: recent experimental data and possible applications for humans. *Clin. Microbiol. Rev.* 14: 810–820, table of contents.
51. Wassmer, S.C., Combes, V., Candal, F.J. et al. (2006). Platelets potentiate brain endothelial alterations induced by Plasmodium falciparum. *Infect. Immun.* 74: 645–653.
52. Shabani, E., Ouma, B.J., Idro, R. et al. (2017). Elevated cerebrospinal fluid tumour necrosis factor is associated with acute and long-term neurocognitive impairment in cerebral malaria. *Parasite Immunol.* 39 https://doi.org/10.1111/pim.12438.
53. Malaguarnera, L., Pignatelli, S., Simpore, J. et al. (2002). Plasma levels of interleukin-12 (IL-12), interleukin-18 (IL-18) and transforming growth factor beta (TGF-beta) in Plasmodium falciparum malaria. *Eur. Cytokine Netw.* 13: 425–430.
54. Musumeci, M., Malaguarnera, L., Simpore, J. et al. (2003). Modulation of immune response in Plasmodium falciparum malaria: role of IL-12, IL-18 and TGF-beta. *Cytokine* 21: 172–178.
55. Rudin, W., Eugster, H.P., Bordmann, G. et al. (1997). Resistance to cerebral malaria in tumor necrosis factor-alpha/beta-deficient mice is associated with a reduction of intercellular adhesion molecule-1 up-regulation and T helper type 1 response. *Am. J. Pathol.* 150: 257–266.
56. Engwerda, C.R., Mynott, T.L., Sawhney, S. et al. (2002). Locally up-regulated lymphotoxin alpha, not systemic tumor necrosis factor alpha, is the principle mediator of murine cerebral malaria. *J. Exp. Med.* 195: 1371–1377.
57. Garcia, I., Miyazaki, Y., Araki, K. et al. (1995). Transgenic mice expressing high levels of soluble TNF-R1 fusion protein are protected from lethal septic shock and cerebral malaria, and are highly sensitive to listeria monocytogenes and Leishmania major infections. *Eur. J. Immunol.* 25: 2401–2407.
58. Grau, G.E., Piguet, P.F., Vassalli, P., and Lambert, P.H. (1989). Tumor-necrosis factor and other cytokines in cerebral malaria: experimental and clinical data. *Immunol. Rev.* 112: 49–70.
59. Sankowski, R., Mader, S., and Valdes-Ferrer, S.I. (2015). Systemic inflammation and the brain: novel roles of genetic, molecular, and environmental cues as drivers of neurodegeneration. *Front. Cell. Neurosci.* 9: 28.
60. Kopitar-Jerala, N. (2015). Innate immune response in brain, NF-kappa B signaling and cystatins. *Front. Mol. Neurosci.* 8: 73.
61. Lewerenz, J., Ates, G., Methner, A. et al. (2018). Oxytosis/Ferroptosis-(re-) emerging roles for oxidative stress-dependent non-apoptotic cell death in diseases of the central nervous system. *Front. Neurosci.* 12: 214.
62. Boivin, M.J., Nakasujja, N., Sikorskii, A. et al. (2018). Neuropsychological benefits of computerized cognitive rehabilitation training in Ugandan children surviving severe malaria: a randomized controlled trial. *Brain Res. Bull.* pii S0361-9230(17)30718-9.
63. Carter, J.A., Mung'ala-Odera, V., Neville, B.G. et al. (2005). Persistent neurocognitive impairments associated with severe falciparum malaria in Kenyan children. *J. Neurol. Neurosurg. Psychiatry* 76: 476–481.
64. Comim, C.M., Reis, P.A., Frutuoso, V.S. et al. (2012). Effects of experimental cerebral malaria in memory, brain-derived neurotrophic factor and acetylcholinesterase acitivity in the hippocampus of survivor mice. *Neurosci. Lett.* 523: 104–107.

46 *Toxoplasma* Infection of the CNS

Stéphane Bretagne[1-3], Catherine (Katy) Keohane[4], and Homa Adle-Biassette[5,6]

[1] Saint Louis Hospital, APHP, Paris, France
[2] University Paris Diderot, Sorbonne Paris Cité, Paris, France
[3] Molecular Mycology Unit, French National Reference Centre for Invasive Mycoses and Antifungal treatments, Pasteur Institute, Paris, France
[4] Department of Pathology and School of Medicine, University College Cork, Brookfield Health Science Complex, Cork, Ireland
[5] Department of Pathology, Lariboisière Hospital, APHP, Paris, France
[6] Paris University, NeuroDiderot, INSERM F-75019, Paris, France

Abbreviations

AIDS	acquired immune deficiency syndrome
CNS	central nervous system
CTx	congenital toxoplasmosis
DSC	dynamic susceptibility contrast
DWI	diffusion-weighted magnetic resonance imaging
EVT	extravillous trophoblasts
HAART	highly active antiretroviral therapy
HSCT	hematopoietic stem cell transplants
HCT	hematopoietic cell transplantation
IRIS	immune reconstitution inflammatory syndrome
MRI	magnetic resonance imaging
MS	microsatellite analysis
PCR	polymerase chain reaction
PET	positron emission tomography
PML	progressive multifocal leukoencephalopathy
SPECT	single photon emission computed tomography

Introduction, definition of the disorder, and historical perspective

Toxoplasmosis is a common infection by the protozoon *Toxoplasma gondii*. The name derives from the Greek words *toxon* meaning "arc" or "bow," *plasm* meaning "shape," and *gundi* or *gondi*, the name of the rodent species in which it was first identified.

The parasite was first isolated in *Ctenodactylus gondi* rodents in 1908 by Nicolle and Manceaux [1] and recognized as causing human disease in 1939 in a congenitally-infected infant [2]. The Sabin-Feldman antibody dye test was developed in 1948 and subsequently *T. gondii* was discovered worldwide, in warm-blooded mammals, humans, and some birds. The life cycle identified cats as the definitive hosts in the 1970s.

Toxoplasmosis causes encephalitis or focal brain mass lesions in patients who are immunocompromised and congenital encephalitis in newborns infected transplacentally. Before the availability of highly active antiretroviral therapy (HAART), toxoplasmosis was a frequent complication in the acquired immune deficiency syndrome (AIDS) [3]. It still occurs regularly in recipients of hematopoietic allogeneic stem cell transplants (HSCT) and less often in recipients of solid-organ transplants [4]. Drug prophylaxis and rapid early diagnosis help limit the disease in these populations, but biopsy may still be required for diagnosis. Early treatment is important because there is usually a good response to appropriate medication.

Microbiological characteristics

T. gondii is an obligate intracellular protozoon, which is heteroxenous (requiring more than one host to complete its life cycle) and polyxenous (infecting more than one species). The sexual phase of its life cycle takes places only in domestic cats and their relatives, which are the definitive hosts. Oocysts excreted in cat feces sporulate and become infective; these contaminate water, soil, or plants. The oocysts are ingested by a wide variety of animals, who are the intermediate hosts, as are humans. In the intermediate hosts, oocysts undergo asexual replication and form tachyzoites (approximately 5 µm long and 2 µm wide), which replicate intracellularly within six to eight hours (in vitro) by internal budding (endodyogeny) and then exit the cell to infect neighboring cells. In infected animals, tachyzoites differentiate into bradyzoites and form tissue cysts 7–10 days post infection. Cysts are found predominantly in the CNS and muscle, where they may reside for the life of the host [5]. Sporulated oocysts in the environment, or bradyzoites in refrigerated meat, can survive for several weeks [6]. The life cycle cannot be completed in animals other than the cat. Cats ingest tissue containing bradyzoites, and sexual replication of the organisms leads to excretion of oocysts, completing the cycle. Because *T. gondii* can self-mate, the resultant offspring are clonal if cats are infected with one strain; however recombinant progeny can be produced if the cat is infected with more than one strain [7]. Bradyzoites are traditionally regarded as being "dormant" in tissue, but recent analysis showed they were more active than originally thought [8].

Epidemiology

Humans become infected by ingesting raw or undercooked meat containing bradyzoites or inadvertent ingestion of oocysts passed in cat feces through contact with litter boxes, soil, or plants [1, 9]. Humans develop a life-threatening infection in three circumstances: profound impaired cellular immunity, maternal-fetal transmission, and infection with atypical virulent strains [10].

In patients who are immunocompromised, reactivation of latent cysts is the main mechanism of infection. Because *T. gondii* tachyzoites can invade all nucleated cells, cysts can be found in virtually any site. However, brain, eye and muscle are the main affected organs.

In mothers who are immunocompetent, the organisms are transmitted to the fetus from maternal blood across the placenta; this occurs mostly when mothers develop a primary infection during pregnancy. Transmission to the fetus has also occurred in women infected before pregnancy or reinfected with a second serotype during pregnancy. Intrauterine transmission has been reported as long as 20 years after maternal infection [11]. Immunosuppression can reactivate infection, with increased risk of transmission to the fetus [12]. The incidence of congenital toxoplasmosis (CTx) increases with the stage of pregnancy. For untreated women, the transmission rate is approximately 25% in the first trimester, 54% in the second trimester, and 65% in the third trimester [13]. Fetal disease is more severe when infection occurs early in gestation [14]; the highest risk for severe CTx is between 10 and 24 weeks gestation.

The prevalence of toxoplasmosis is inferred from serology surveys in women who are pregnant and blood donors [15, 16]. Seroprevalence varies geographically, is strongly linked to culinary habits such as the consumption of undercooked meat [16], and increases with age. Estimated seroprevalence in women who are pregnant has fallen from 84% in the 1960s to 44% in 2003 in France [17] and other populations [18]. Deep-freezing of meat carcasses for long periods in current industrial practice may contribute to this reduction [17].

Incidence in patients who are immunocompromised

The geographic differences in seroprevalence in the general population explains the different rates reported in patients who are immunocompromised. In the United States, 789 toxoplasmosis deaths were identified during the period 2000–2010, (56% codiagnosed with human immunodeficiency virus [HIV], lymphoma, leukemia, and connective tissue disorders) [19]. Currently, toxoplasmosis deaths in patients with AIDS have declined, partly attributed to environmental and healthcare factors [20]. The incidence of *Toxoplasma* encephalitis was low in patients with AIDS with a sustained CD4 cell count >200 as a result of HAART [20].

The incidence of toxoplasmosis following HSCT varies between 0.4 and 8.7%, depending on the endemic region [21–24]. Post-transplant disease typically occurs within six months following the transplant but may be delayed.

Toxoplasmosis is also reported in recipients of solid-organ transplants. As muscles more often contain parasite cysts, patients undergoing a heart transplant are more at risk than those undergoing a liver or kidney transplant [4, 25].

Incidence of congenital toxoplasmosis

Transplacental transmission increases during gestation, whereas the severity of infection inversely correlates with gestational age [26]. The role of other factors influencing congenital transmission is poorly known, but there is greater virulence with atypical genotype strains [27].

In France, national surveillance (in 272 cases) found a prevalence of 5.5 per 10 000 live births [28], somewhat similar to Poland (4.3 per 10 000 live births), Switzerland (3.3 per 10 000 live births), and Brazil (3.3 per 10 000 live births)] but higher than that estimated in Denmark (1.6 per 10 000 live births) [29], and Massachusetts (1 per 10 000 live births) [6]. In the French series, the estimated incidence of symptomatic CTx was 0.34 cases per 10 000 live births. Among symptomatic children, 21 of 28 had moderate and 7 (3%) had severe disease, comparable to the rate of symptomatic CTx in England and Ireland [28].

Clinical features including appropriate investigations and important differential diagnosis

Human infection is usually asymptomatic. After ingestion, the parasite multiplies in blood. This phase is sometimes associated with fever, enlarged lymph nodes, or other nonspecific signs. Serological conversion occurs, but cysts are believed to stay alive for a long time despite permanent immune stimulation. However, the immune response prevents subsequent infections by repeat ingestion of the parasite, unless reinfection with another strain occurs (see below).

In patients who are immunocompromised

Most commonly, neurologic symptoms are subacute with headache, fever, changes in mental status, lethargy, confusion, loss of consciousness, convulsions, and focal neurologic deficits. Fever is inconsistent, and clinical manifestations may be masked by immunosuppressive therapy. Definitive diagnosis in patients who are immunocompromised formerly relied on identifying the parasite in tissues, mainly brain biopsies, or finding tachyzoites in respiratory specimens. These methods were poorly sensitive, and only positive late in the disease, hence the poor prognosis. Polymerase chain reaction (PCR) enables more rapid diagnosis and should be performed as soon as the disease is suspected [30].

Imaging studies in patients who are immunocompromised

Typically, cerebral toxoplasmosis manifests as multiple necrotizing, hemorrhagic foci of cerebritis or organizing abscesses, with a predilection for the basal ganglia, thalami, or periventricular regions [31]. Involvement of the corpus callosum can mimic neoplasm.

On computed tomography (CT) scans, the lesions are typically hypodense, with nodular or ring enhancement and on magnetic resonance imaging (MRI) [32] are iso- or hypodense and surrounded by edema. On T2-weighted images, hyperdense lesions probably correspond to necrotizing encephalitis and isodense lesions to organizing abscesses [33]. Hemorrhage is uncommon, and lesions may just be edematous without gadolinium enhancement. The "eccentric target sign" (a small eccentric cortical nodule alongside an enhancing ring) is considered pathognomonic but is not consistently found [34]. The "'concentric target sign" (alternating hypo- and hyperdense zones in deep parenchymal lesions) is regarded as more specific [35]. Steroid treatment reduces enhancement, edema, and mass effect. Even in a single focus, an iso- or hypodense signal on T1-weighted images, perilesional edema, and ring-enhancement suggest cerebral toxoplasmosis.

Magnetic resonance spectroscopy displays an increased lipid-lactate peak. Dynamic susceptibility contrast (DSC)-MRI scanning and single photon emission computed tomography (SPECT) may help distinguish toxoplasmosis from lymphoma [36]. On positron emission tomography (PET)/CT scan and thallium SPECT, the lesions are "cold"; there is minimal or no uptake.

Antibody detection for patients who are immunocompromised

Many commercial assays are available and provide similar results [6]. Immunoglobulin G (IgG) antibody levels indicate the patient's status, but low titers do not help diagnose current infection and can be negative in cerebral toxoplasmosis [37]. Immunoglobulin M (IgM) antibodies indicate active toxoplasmosis but are rarely relevant in patients who are immunocompromised.

Serology screening is important to identify the risk of reactivation of latent infection, prior to HSCT, renal and heart transplant [38–41], and in patients with HIV [42].

PCR diagnosis

Using PCR, *Toxoplasma* DNA was detected earlier in the disease than using microscopy [43, 44]. The European Group for Blood and Marrow Transplantation Infectious Diseases Working Party Guidelines classified (i) *T. gondii infection* in patients with positive PCR performed on blood samples, with or without fever, but no evidence of organ involvement, (ii) *probable toxoplasmosis* in those with positive PCR on a blood or another sample from the involved organ (usually CSF or bronchoalveolar lavage fluid) with clinical signs and symptoms and radiological evidence of active disease, and (iii) *definite toxoplasmosis* as histological evidence of active toxoplasmosis in a clinically and radiologically involved organ [45]. PCR screening is widely used to investigate unexplained fever in at-risk patients [4].

Differential diagnosis

Patients who are immunocompromised are susceptible to multiple opportunistic infections and malignancies; therefore, identifying a single cause for the patient's symptoms is often difficult. Imaging can help distinguish the major differential diagnoses of CNS toxoplasmosis including primary glial, lymphoid, and metastatic tumors. CNS lymphoma is characterized by patchy, uniform enhancement on MRI and, occasionally, low-density areas reflecting necrosis and bleeding.

In patients with AIDS, the differential diagnosis also includes: CNS tuberculoma or other mycobacterial infections, cryptococcosis, pyogenic abscesses, and neurocysticercosis [32]. Progressive multifocal leukoencephalopathy (PML) lesions typically involve white matter, are non- or faintly contrast enhancing, and produce no mass effect but may show ring lesion on diffusion-weighted magnetic resonance imaging (DWI) [46].

The most common focal CNS infections in HCT are *Toxoplasma* encephalitis (up to 74%) and aspergillosis (18%) [24]. Bacteria, apart from *Nocardia*, are rarely associated with brain abscesses in transplant recipients. Meningoencephalitis in transplant recipients is predominantly due to herpes viruses and less often to *Listeria monocytogenes*, *T. gondii*, and *Cryptococcus*.

Congenital toxoplasmosis

The classic features of CTx are hydrocephalus, choroidoretinitis, and intracranial calcification. Other manifestations include anemia, thrombocytopenia-induced petechiae, rash, hepatic disorder, and pneumonitis.

Severe cases are evident in the fetus and birth is often premature, with neonatal erythroblastosis and hydrops fetalis. The spectrum of disease includes mild cases recognized early (in infancy) or late (in childhood or adolescence). Infants asymptomatic at birth may develop late sequelae with mental retardation, psychomotor deficiency, seizures, microcephaly, hydrocephalus, deafness, and ocular manifestations. In early pregnancy, severe eye involvement leads to uveitis, chorioretinitis, microphthalmia, cataract, strabismus, optic neuritis, and retinal necrosis [47]. There is no conclusive evidence to indicate that toxoplasmosis causes congenital malformations.

Imaging studies for congenital toxoplasmosis
Brain ultrasound displays calcifications, echogenic nodular foci, abnormal germinal matrix echogenicity and thickening, and hydrocephalus; congenital cysts and ventriculitis may be observed. Systemic findings include a hyperechogenic mesentery and hepatosplenomegaly. In fetal toxoplasmosis, the prognosis of cerebral hyperechogenic lesions without ventriculomegaly may be favorable [48].

Laboratory findings
Maternal infection can be diagnosed by serology, with increasing IgG titers and presence of anti-toxoplasma IgM; IgM can persist for over a year. Low-avidity IgG testing can be useful to identify recent infection. Fetal IgM is not sensitive for infection in early gestation. Testing in a reference laboratory is recommended to distinguish recent from chronic infection [49]. PCR of amniotic fluid is both sensitive and specific for identifying fetal infection [50].

Differential diagnosis
CTx has to be differentiated from other congenital infections, such as cytomegalovirus (CMV), which can be clinically similar (see Chapter 7).

Pathology

Cerebral toxoplasmosis in patients who are immunocompromised
In patients who are immunocompromised, toxoplasmosis mainly affects just the CNS but can be associated with eye lesions and systemic disease [51]. The characteristic features are multifocal lesions in the cerebral hemispheres, particularly the basal ganglia [52] and the cortico-subcortical junctions (Figure 46.1a), but anywhere in the CNS can be involved including the cerebellum, brainstem, and spinal cord.

Depending on the stage of infection, treatment, and the degree of tissue reaction or immunosuppression, three patterns can be seen; all can occur within the same brain [52].

i. Necrotizing lesions and abscesses (Figure 46.1) are found mostly in recent infections or following brief treatment. These have central eosinophilic ill-defined foci of coagulative necrosis (Figure 46.1c), surrounded by a cellular infiltrate with polymorphs and some macrophages and microglial cells. There are numerous parasites either within pseudocysts (bradyzoites) (Figure 46.1e, f) or present as free forms (tachyzoites) (Figure 46.1d). Occlusive endarteritis obliterans is frequent, with concentric lamellar proliferation, thrombosis and necrosis of the arterial wall and hemorrhages. Ventriculitis with a fibrinous exudate and periventricular petechiae or periventricular necrotizing encephalitis (Figure 46.1b) [38] may also be seen.

ii. Organizing well-demarcated abscesses (Figure 46.2a) with central coagulative necrosis surrounded by a granulomatous reaction, including inflammatory cells (Figure 46.2b), vascular proliferation, lipid and hemosiderin-laden macrophages are found in more chronic lesions or in patients treated for one to two weeks.

iii. Chronic scars may be observed after successful treatment. These are circumscribed orange-yellow cystic lesions (Figure 46.3) forming gliotic scars, and containing lipid-laden macrophages and hemosiderin pigment.

These chronic "burnt out" forms of toxoplasmosis, devoid of inflammation and organisms, have been increasingly noted in patients receiving HAART and are presumed to relate to prolonged survival in clinically and biologically cured patients who die from other causes [53]. Despite apparently adequate treatment for toxoplasmosis and HIV infection, some patients with extensive multifocal toxoplasmosis progress clinically and radiologically and show progressive demyelination and deterioration of mental status. It may be that, when

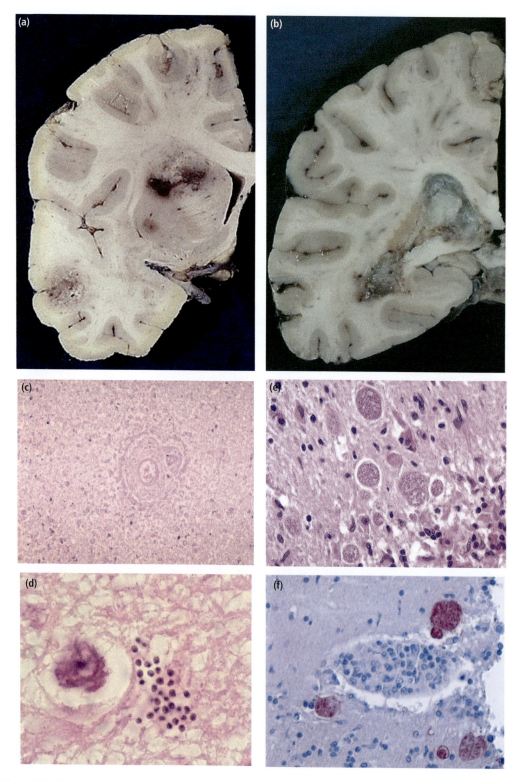

Figure 46.1 Necrotizing lesions in patients with acquired immunodeficiency syndrome (AIDS). (a) Coronal section of the left cerebral hemisphere at the level of the anterior commissure: Multifocal necrotic and hemorrhagic abscesses are present in the basal ganglia and temporal lobe at the cortico-subcortical junction. (b) Coronal section of the left cerebral hemispheres at the level of the splenium of corpus callosum: Ventriculitis with intraventricular fibrinous exudate. (c) Eosinophilic coagulative necrosis in the center of an abscess (hematoxylin and eosin [H&E]). (d) Free forms (tachyzoites) of toxoplasma in the parenchyma surrounding the necrosis (H&E). (e) Pseudocysts (bradyzoites) are numerous in the cerebellar parenchyma surrounding an abscess (H&E). (e) These are identified more clearly by immunohistochemistry. *(Courtesy of Pr. Francoise Gray).*

Toxoplasma Infection of the CNS **Chapter 46**

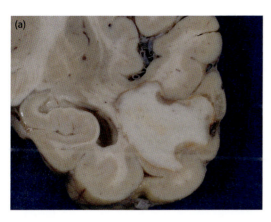
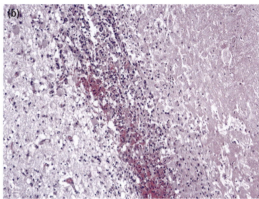

Figure 46.2 Organizing circumscribed abscess in a patient with acquired immunodeficiency syndrome (AIDS). (a) Coronal section of the right temporal lobe. A well-demarcated abscess with central necrosis and hemorrhagic capsule is present in the white matter at the cortico-subcortical junction. (b) The central coagulative necrosis is surrounded by a granulomatous reaction with inflammatory cells and vascular proliferation. Note reactive astrocytosis in the surrounding parenchyma (hematoxylin and eosin [H&E]). *(Courtesy of Pr. Francoise Gray).*

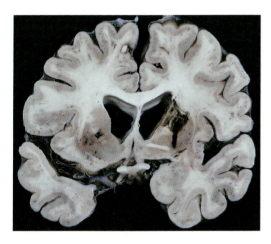
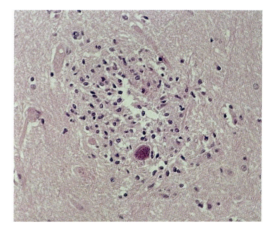

Figure 46.3 Chronic scar lesions in a patient with acquired immune deficiency syndrome (AIDS). Coronal section of the cerebral hemispheres at the level of the anterior commissure. Bilateral well-demarcated orange-yellow cystic lesions are present in the basal ganglia. Note a small organizing abscess at the cortico-subcortical junction in F1, on the left. *(Source: courtesy of Pr. Francoise Gray.)*

Figure 46.4 Diffuse, non-necrotic, nodular "encephalitic" toxoplasmosis. A microglial nodule contains an encysted bradyzoite (hematoxylin and eosin [H&E]). *(Source: Courtesy of Pr. Francoise Gray.)*

treatment is administered too late, irreversible cerebral destruction occurs, with secondary progressive Wallerian degeneration [54].

Disseminated cysts without a parenchymal reaction are not uncommon in AIDS and may be the only manifestation of cerebral toxoplasmosis.

Diffuse, non-necrotic, nodular "encephalitic" toxoplasmosis with disseminated micronodules containing tachyzoites or encysted bradyzoites (Figure 46.4) is also described and can be a treatable cause of diffuse encephalopathy in AIDS [55].

Other opportunistic infections (e.g. CMV, HIV encephalitis, cryptococcosis, and PML), tumors such as lymphoma, and cerebrovascular lesions may be present in addition to toxoplasmosis in patients with AIDS or who are immunosuppressed [51, 56].

Congenital toxoplasmosis

In fatal cases, external brain examination shows multiple well-outlined, soft, yellow lesions, randomly scattered on the surface, so-called "thumb-print" lesions (Figure 46.5a). Coronal brain sections show ventricular enlargement and friable, necrotic yellow tissue lining the ventricles, often destroying the basal ganglia (Figure 46.5b). Multiple necrotic and calcified lesions are dispersed throughout the brain, brainstem, spinal cord, and cerebellum [57].

Microscopically, there is a chronic meningoencephalitis with microglial nodules and extensive vascular involvement with fibrinoid necrosis of blood vessel walls and intravascular thrombosis (Figure 46.6). Necrotic areas (Figure 46.6a, b) are often surrounded by granulation tissue with abundant macrophages. There is extensive periventricular inflammation and a nodular ependymitis that often occludes the aqueduct of Sylvius. There is both fine mineralization outlining cells and blood vessels and coarse mineralization in zones of necrosis. Organisms are often abundant near areas of necrosis, microglial nodules, or perivascular inflammation but may also be seen in noninflamed tissue. Intense inflammation is present around tachyzoites, which are oval, 2- to 3-μm structures in tissue sections. There may be little or no inflammation around cysts and pseudocysts (Figure 46.6c). Tachyzoites can be difficult to identify on hematoxylin and eosin (H&E) stains (Figure 46.6d) but are clearly visible on immunohistochemistry, particularly when cysts are not identified (Figure 46.6e).

Genetics

Genetic diversity in *T. gondii* strains is important in human toxoplasmosis. Three major lineages were described, based on DNA polymorphisms at the SAG2 locus, encoding tachyzoite surface antigen p22 [58]. Restriction fragment length polymorphisms in PCR-amplified SAG2 products used to determine the genotypes in patient samples showed that Type II strains were found in 81%. Type I and III strains were much fewer [58]. Further studies using eight microsatellite markers on stocks of *T. gondii*, found that group III was a subgroup of Group II and could be distinguished by allele 117 of TgM-A [59]. This allele is also detectable in a subgroup of Group I, possibly the results of genetic transfer between the two main groups.

Four lineages account for the majority of strains responsible for human infections in Europe and North America (clonal types I, II, and III and type 12), whereas in South America strains have more genetic diversity and lack a clonal structure. Type I strain is highly virulent. "Atypical" highly virulent

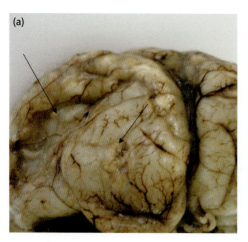 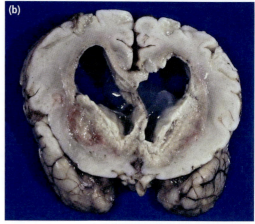

Figure 46.5 Congenital toxoplasmosis macroscopic appearance: Premature infant who died at age two months. (a) "Thumbprint" lesions (arrows) with depressed cortical surface and yellow necrotic areas on the surface of the brain. (b) Coronal slice of the frontal lobes showing extensive friable necrosis and calcification especially in the periventricular regions. The lateral ventricles are widely dilated.

Toxoplasma Infection of the CNS **Chapter 46**

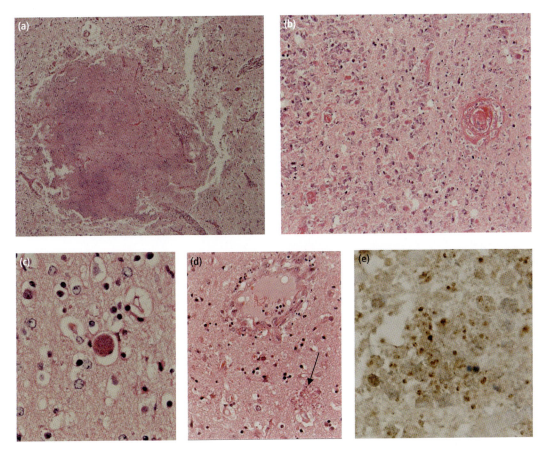

Figure 46.6 Congenital toxoplasmosis histology: (a) Circumscribed area of necrosis (hematoxylin and eosin [H&E]). (b) At higher magnification there is intense inflammation and necrosis mixed with tachyzoites, surrounding a blood vessel showing fibrinoid necrosis of the wall (H&E). (c) Toxoplasma pseudocyst in noninflamed tissue (H&E). (d) Tachyzoites (arrow) are present in the parenchyma surrounding the microabscess (H&E). (e) Tachyzoites and bradyzoites are clearly visible on immunohistochemistry.

strains can cause severe clinical sepsis in patients who are immunocompetent, mainly in South America. These strains have unusual allelic combinations and a new allele for the *TGM-A* locus. [10].

Animal models and pathogenesis

To study transmission, host response to different parasite strains and effects of treatment, most animal studies use BALB/c, C57BL/6 and severe combined immune deficiency (SCID) mice. Other rodents (Rat, calomys), zebrafish, guinea pig, golden hamsters, sheep, and pigs have also been used. A porcine model is said to be more comparable to human infection (including CTx) than the murine model [60].

Ingested organisms enter the intestines and either invade cells directly or are phagocytosed. Type 1 strains have more invasive capacity in the intestine than type II or type III strains. Tachyzoites replicate intracellularly, destroy those cells, invade adjacent cells, and eventually invade all tissues. Spread occurs via (i) the migration of free parasites in blood and tissues, (ii) by intracellular dissemination by hijacking migrating leukocytes, or (iii) by extracellular migration with the parasite attached to the outside of migrating leukocytes [61].

Both cell-mediated and humoral immunity are required to control the spread of tachyzoites.

Natural killer (NK) and T cells produce interferon gamma (IFN-γ), which controls the acute infection. The immune response also leads to the parasite forming cysts, which can persist in tissues (especially the brain, eye, and muscles), providing sites for later reactivation when immunosuppression occurs. It is rare to find such cysts as incidental findings in autopsies. Entry to the brain might be via endothelial cells, which can be infected in vitro. Cell adhesion molecules (ICAM-1 and VCAM) are upregulated in toxoplasmosis [61]. The extensive necrosis and vasculitis in cerebral toxoplasmosis probably involves direct cellular injury to brain parenchyma and vessels from contact with the parasite, as well as cytokine-induced necrosis. Virulence in *T. gondii* appears related to the parasite-encoded rhoptry effectors ROP5and ROP18, which antagonize the hosts interferon-induced immunity-regulated GTPases [7]. Another factor affecting virulence is the dense granule protein, GRA25, secreted outside the parasites, which, in experimental studies, promotes parasite expansion [62].

For CTx, extravillous trophoblasts (EVT) that attach the placenta to the uterus are more vulnerable to infection than syncytiotrophoblasts that are bathed in maternal blood. It is likely that following primary infection, parasitemia leads to intracellular uterine infection, then to EVT infection because tachyzoites move from cell to cell, with eventual infection of the fetus. Infected maternal leukocytes may also possibly cross the placenta and contribute to fetal infection, which could explain the apparent delay between primary maternal infection and fetal infection [13]. There appears to be a trend toward increased placental transmission by type 1 genotype [13].

Treatment, future perspective, and conclusions

The use of MRI, together with clinical and laboratory findings, reduces the need for cerebral biopsies [63]. Patients with "typical" imaging findings of toxoplasmosis are usually treated empirically. In general, biopsy is not required. Following treatment, follow-up imaging is necessary to demonstrate lesion response, especially as lymphoma has similar findings. Shrinkage of lesions may take from two to four weeks up to six months. All lesions need to be followed to resolution because multiple pathologies may coexist in patients who are immunocompromised.

The initial therapy of choice is a combination of pyrimethamine plus sulfadiazine, with folinic acid (leucovorin) to reduce the hematologic adverse effects. Adjunctive steroids can be administrated [64]. For patients unable to take or intolerant of sulfadiazine, clindamycin, pyrimethamine, and folinic acid are the second-line therapy. Immune reconstitution inflammatory syndrome associated with toxoplasmosis appears to be rare.

References

1. Dubey, J.P. (2008). The history of *Toxoplasma gondii* – the first 100 years. *J. Eukaryot. Microbiol.* 55: 467–475.
2. Wolf, A., Cowen, D., and Paige, B. (1939). Human toxoplasmosis: occurrence in infants as an encephalomyelitis verification by transmission to animals. *Science* 89: 226–227.
3. Porter, S.B. and Sande, M.A. (1992). Toxoplasmosis of the central nervous system in the acquired immunodeficiency syndrome. *N. Engl. J. Med.* 327: 1643–1648.
4. Robert-Gangneux, F., Meroni, V., Dupont, D. et al. (2018). Toxoplasmosis in transplant recipients, Europe, 2010-2014. *Emerg. Infect. Dis.* 24: 1497–1504.
5. Black, M.W., John, C., and Boothroyd, J.C. (2000). M. Lytic cycle of *Toxoplasma gondii. Mol. Biol. Rev.* 64: 607–623.
6. Robert-Gangneux, F. and Dardé, M.L. (2012). Epidemiology of and diagnostic strategies for toxoplasmosis. *Clin. Microbiol. Rev.* 25: 264–296.
7. Jensen, K.D., Camejo, A., Melo, M. et al. (2015). Toxoplasma gondii superinfection and virulence during secondary infection correlate with the exact *ROP5/ROP18* allelic combination. *MBio* 6 (2): e02280–e02214. https://doi.org/10.1128/mBio.02208-14.
8. Watts, E., Zhao, Y., Dhara, A. et al. (2015). Novel approaches reveal that toxoplasma gondii Bradyzoites within tissue cysts are dynamic and replicating entities in vivo. *MBio* 6 (5): e01155–e01115. https://doi.org/10.1128/mBio.01155-15.
9. Cook, A.J., Gilbert, R.E., Buffolano, W. et al. (2000). Sources of toxoplasma infection in pregnant women: European multicentre case-control study. European

research network on congenital toxoplasmosis. *BMJ* 321: 142–147.
10. Carme, B., Bissuel, F., Ajzenberg, D. et al. (2002). Severe acquired toxoplasmosis in immunocompetent adult patients in French Guiana. *J. Clin. Microbiol.* 40: 4037–4044.
11. Silveira, C., Ferreira, R., Muccioli, C. et al. (2003). Toxoplasmosis transmitted to a newborn from the mother infected 20 years earlier. *Am J. Ophthalmol.* 136: 370–371.
12. Mitchell, C., Erlich, S., Mastrucii, M. et al. (1990). Congenital toxoplasmosis occurring in infants perinatally infected with human immunodeficiency virus 1. *Pediatr. Infect. Dis. J.* 9: 512–518.
13. McAuley, J.B. (2014). Congenital toxoplasmosis. *J. Pediatr. Infect. Dis. Soc.* 3 (suppl1): S30–S35.
14. Foulon, W., Villena, I., Stray-Petersen, B. et al. (1999). Treatment of toxoplasmosis during pregnancy: a multicenter study of impact on fetal transmission and children's sequalae at age 1 year. *Am. J. Obstet. Gynecol.* 180: 410–415.
15. Foroutan-Rad, M., Majidiani, H., Dalvand, S. et al. (2016). Toxoplasmosis in blood donors: a systematic review and meta-analysis. *Transfus. Med. Rev.* 30: 116–122.
16. Pappas, G., Roussos, N., and Falagas, M.E. (2009). Toxoplasmosis snapshots: global status of toxoplasma gondii seroprevalence and implications for pregnancy and congenital toxoplasmosis. *Int. J. Parasitol.* 39: 1385–1394.
17. Nogareda, F., Strat, Y.L., Villena, I. et al. (2014). Incidence and prevalence of toxoplasma gondii infection in women in France, 1980–2020: model based estimation. *Epidemiol. Infect.* 142: 1661–1670.
18. Guigue, N., Léon, L., Hamane, S. et al. (2018). Continuous decline of *Toxoplasma gondii* seroprevalence in hospital: a 1997-2014 longitudinal study in Paris, France. *Front. Microbiol.* 9: 2369.
19. Cummings, P.L., Kuo, T., Javanbakht, M., and Sorvillo, F. (2014). Trends, productivity losses, and associated medical conditions among toxoplasmosis deaths in the United States, 2000-2010. *Am. J. Trop. Med. Hyg.* 91: 959–964.
20. Abgrall, S., Rabaud, C., and Costagliola, D. Clinical epidemiology Group of the French Hospital Database on HIV (2001) incidence and risk factors for toxoplasmic encephalitis in human immunodeficiency virus-infected patients before and during the highly active antiretroviral therapy era. *Clin. Infect. Dis.* 33: 1747–1755.
21. Martino, R., Maertens, J., and Bretagne, S. (2000). Toxoplasmosis after hematopoietic stem cell transplantation. *Clin. Infect. Dis.* 31: 1188–1195.
22. Meers, S., Lagrou, K., Theunissen, K. et al. (2010). Myeloablative conditioning predisposes patients for toxoplasma gondii reactivation after allogeneic stem cell transplantation. *Clin. Infect. Dis.* 50: 1127–1134.
23. Hakko, E., Ozkan, H.A., Karaman, K., and Gulbas, Z. (2013). Analysis of cerebral toxoplasmosis in a series of 170 allogeneic hematopoietic stem cell transplant patients. *Transpl. Infect. Dis.* 15: 575–580.
24. Maschke, M., Dietrich, U., and Prumbaum, M. (1999). Opportunistic CNS infection after bone marrow transplantation. *Bone Marrow Transplant.* 23: 1167–1176.
25. Fischer, S.A. and Lu, K. AST infectious diseases Community of Practice (2013) screening of donor and recipient in solid organ transplantation. *Am. J. Transplant.* 13 (Suppl 4): 9–21.
26. Desmonts, G. and Couvreur, J. (1974). Toxoplasmosis in pregnancy and its transmission to the fetus. *Bull. N. Y. Acad. Med.* 50: 146–159.
27. Ajioka, J.W. and Soldati, D. (eds.) (2007). *Toxoplasma: Molecular and Cellular Biology*. Norfolk, United Kingdom: Horizon Biosciences.
28. Villena, I., Ancelle, T., Delmas, C. et al. (2010). Congenital toxoplasmosis in France in 2007: first results from a national surveillance system. *Euro Surveill.* 15: 19600.
29. Röser, D., Nielsen, H.V., Petersen, E. et al. (2010). Congenital toxoplasmosis--a report on the Danish neonatal screening programme 1999-2007. *J. Inherit. Metab. Dis.* 33 (Suppl 2): S241–S247.
30. Costa, J.M., Pautas, C., Ernault, P. et al. (2000). Real-time PCR for diagnosis and follow-up of toxoplasma reactivation after allogeneic stem cell transplantation using fluorescence resonance energy transfer hybridization probes. *J. Clin. Microbiol.* 38 (2): 929–932.
31. Lummus, S. and Kleinschmidt-DeMasters, B.K. (2014). Predominantly periventricular necrotizing encephalitis due to toxoplasmosis: two unusual cases and review of literature. *Clin. Neuropathol.* 33: 29–37.
32. Smith, A.B., Smirniotopoulos, J.G., and Rushing, E.J. (2008). From the archives of the AFIP: central nervous system infections associated with human immunodeficiency virus infection: radiologic-pathologic correlation. *Radiographics* 28: 2033–2058.
33. Brightbill, T.C., Post, M.J., Hensley, G.T., and Ruiz, A. (1996). MR of toxoplasma encephalitis: signal characteristics on T2-weighted images and pathologic correlation. *J. Comput. Assist. Tomogr.* 20: 417–422.
34. Gupta, K., Vasishta, R.K., Bansal, A. et al. (2011). Cortical cysts with hydrocephalus and ventriculitis: an unusual presentation of congenital toxoplasmosis at autopsy. *J. Clin. Pathol.* 64: 272–274.

35. Mahadevan, A., Ramalingaiah, A.H., Parthasarathy, S.J. et al. (2013). Neuropathological correlate of the "concentric target sign" in MRI of HIV-associated cerebral toxoplasmosis. *Magn. Reson. Imaging* 38: 488–495.
36. Dibble, E.H., Boxerman, J.L., Baird, G.L. et al. (2017). Toxoplasmosis versus lymphoma: cerebral lesion characterization using DSC-MRI revisited. *Clin. Neurol. Neurosurg.* 152: 84–89.
37. Bretagne, S., Gray, F., and Costa, J.M. (1993). Central nervous system toxoplasmosis in AIDS. *N. Engl. J. Med.* 328: 1353–1354.
38. Gea-Banacloche, J., Masur, H., da Arns, Cunha, C. et al. (2009). Regionally limited or rare infections: prevention after hematopoietic cell transplantation. *Bone Marrow Transplant.* 44: 489–494.
39. Ullmann, A.J., Schmidt-Hieber, M., Bertz, H. et al. (2016). Infectious diseases in allogeneic haematopoietic stem cell transplantation: prevention and prophylaxis strategy guidelines 2016. *Ann. Hematol.* 95: 1435–1455.
40. Haute Autorité de Santé (2015). *Recommandation de Bonne Pratique. Transplantation rénale Accès à la liste d'attente nationale Méthode Recommandations pour la pratique Clinique*. https://www.has-sante.fr/portail/upload/docs/application/pdf/2015-12/rbp_recommandations_greffe_renale_vd_mel.pdf (accessed 29 August 2018).
41. Fischer, S.A. and Lu, K. AST infectious diseases Community of Practice (2013) screening of donor and recipient in solid organ transplantation. *Am. J. Transplant.* 13 (Suppl 4): 9–21.
42. Kaplan, J.E., Benson, C., Holmes, K.K. et al. (2009). Guidelines for prevention and treatment of opportunistic infections in HIV-infected adults and adolescents: recommendations from CDC, the National Institutes of Health, and the HIV medicine Association of the Infectious Diseases Society of America. *MMWR Recomm. Rep.* 58: 1–207.
43. Bretagne, S., Costa, J.M., Vidaud, M. et al. (1993). Detection of toxoplasma gondii by competitive DNA amplification of bronchoalveolar lavage samples. *J. Infect. Dis.* 168: 1585–1588.
44. Bretagne, S., Costa, J.M., Foulet, F. et al. (2000). Prospective study of toxoplasma reactivation by polymerase chain reaction in allogeneic stem-cell transplant recipients. *Transpl. Infect. Dis.* 2: 127–132.
45. Martino, R., Bretagne, S., Einsele, H. et al. (2005). Early detection of toxoplasma infection by molecular monitoring of toxoplasma gondii in peripheral blood samples after allogeneic stem cell transplantation. *Clin. Infect. Dis.* 40: 67–78.
46. Finelli, P.F. and Foxman, E.B. (2014). The etiology of ring lesions on diffusion-weighted imaging. *Neuroradiol. J.* 27: 280–287.
47. Remington, J., McLeod, R., Thulliez, P., and Desmonts, G. (2001). Toxoplasmosis. In: *Infectious Diseases of the Fetus and Newborn Infant*, 5e (eds. J. Remington and J. Klein), 205–346. Philadelphia: WB Saunders.
48. Dhombres, F., Friszer, S., Maurice et al. (2017). Prognosis of Fetal parenchymal cerebral lesions without Ventriculomegaly in congenital toxoplasmosis infection. *Fetal Diagn. Ther.* 41: 8–14.
49. Dhakal, R., Gajurel, K., Christelle Pomares, C. et al. (2015). Significance of a positive *Toxoplasma* immunoglobulin M test result in the United States. *J. Clin. Microbiol.* 53: 3601–3605.
50. Grover, C., Thulliez, P., Remington, J., and Boothroyd, J. (1990). Rapid prenatal diagnosis of congenital toxoplasma infection by using polymerase chain reaction and amniotic fluid. *J. Clin. Microbiol.* 28: 2297–2301.
51. Martinez, A.J., Sell, M., Mitrovics, T. et al. (1995). The neuropathology and epidemiology of AIDS. A Berlin experience. A review of 200 cases. *Pathol. Res. Pract.* 191: 427–443.
52. Scaravilli, F. and Gray, F. (1993). Opportunistic infections. In: *Atlas of the Neuropathology of HIV Infection* (ed. F. Gray), 103–117. Oxford, New York, Tokyo: Oxford University Press.
53. Strittmatter, C., Lang, W., Wiestler, O.D., and Kleihues, P. (1992). The changing pattern of human immunodeficiency virus-associated cerebral toxoplasmosis: a study of 46 postmortem cases. *Acta Neuropathol.* 83: 475–481.
54. Gray, F., Chretien, F., Vallat-Decouvelaere, A.V., and Scaravilli, F. (2003). The changing pattern of HIV neuropathology in the HAART era. *J. Neuropathol. Exp. Neurol.* 62: 429–440.
55. Gray, F., Gherardi, R., and Wingate, E. (1989). Diffuse "encephalitic" cerebral toxoplasmosis in AIDS. Report of four cases. *J. Neurol.* 236: 273–277.
56. Gray, F. and Sharer, L. (1993). Combined pathologies. In: *Atlas of the Neuropathology of HIV Infection* (ed. F. Gray), 162–171. Oxford, New York, Tokyo: Oxford University Press.
57. Keohane, C. and Adle-Biassette, H. (2018). Intrauterine infections. In: *Developmental Neuropathology*, 2e (eds. H. Adle-Biassette, B.N. Harding and J.A. Golden), 500–502. Hoboken, NJ: Wiley Blackwell.
58. Howe, D.K., Honoré, S., Derouin, F. et al. (1997). Determination of genotypes of toxoplasma gondii strains isolated from patients with toxoplasmosis. *J. Clin. Microbiol.* 35: 1411–1414.

59. Ajzenberg, D., Dumètre, A., and Dardé, M.L. (2005). Multiplex PCR for typing strains of *Toxoplasma gondii*. *J. Clin. Microbiol.* 43 (4): 1940–1943.
60. Nau, J., Eller, S.K., and Wenning, J. (2017). Experimental porcine *Toxoplasma gondii* infection as a representative model for human toxoplasmosis. *Mediators of Inflammation*. (Volume 2017) (Article ID 3260289) https://doi.org/10.1155/2017/3260289.
61. Randall, L.M. and Hunter, C.A. (2011). Parasite dissemination and the pathogenesis of toxoplasmosis. *Eur. J. Microbiol. Immunol.* 1: 3–9.
62. Shastri, A.J., Marino, N.D., Franco, M. et al. (2014). GRA25 is a novel virulence factor of toxoplasma gondii and influences the host immune response. *Infect. Immun.* 82 (6): 2595–2605.
63. Greenway, M.R.F., Sacco, K.A., and Burton, M.C. (2017). In deep: cerebral toxoplasmosis. *Am. J. Med.* 130: 802–804.
64. Sonneville, R., Schmidt, M., Messika, J. et al. (2012). Neurologic outcomes and adjunctive steroids in HIV patients with severe cerebral toxoplasmosis. *Neurology* 79: 1762–1766.

47 Other Protozoal Infections

Leila Chimelli[1,2] and Catherine (Katy) Keohane[3]
[1] Laboratory of Neuropathology and Molecular Genetics, State Brain Institute Paulo Niemeyer, Rio de Janeiro, Brazil
[2] Federal University of Rio de Janeiro (UFRJ), Rio de Janeiro, Brazil
[3] Department of Pathology and School of Medicine, University College Cork, Brookfield Health Science Complex, Cork, Ireland

Abbreviations

AIDS	acquired immunodeficiency syndrome
BBB	blood-brain barrier
CL	cutaneous leishmaniasis
CNS	central nervous system
CSF	Cerebrospinal fluid
GAE	granulomatous amoebic encephalitis
HIV	human immunodeficiency virus
MCL	mucocutaneous lesishmaniasis (MCL)
PAM	primary amoebic meningoencephalitis
PCR	polymerase chain reaction
VL	visceral leishmaniasis
WHO	World Health Organization

Introduction

Apart from *Plasmodium falciparum* causing cerebral malaria and *Toxoplasma gondii* causing toxoplasmosis, the main protozoa responsible for human infections are amoebae, trypanosomes, microsporidia, *Sarcocystis,* and *Leishmania.* Although not common, these infections are endemic to certain regions but can occur throughout the world because of increased travel and migration [1, 2]. In addition, immunosuppression predisposes to more severe manifestations and failure to respond to treatment [2]. The nervous system may be the only affected system (but often the most severe and lethal) or be involved as part of a generalized infection. The main clinical presentations are as meningoencephalitis or multiple pseudo-tumoral lesions. Although clinical, laboratory, and imaging investigations provide crucial information, and narrow the differential diagnosis, some cases need biopsy or autopsy to confirm the diagnosis. Tissue samples provide morphological proof of infection and also supply material for culture and molecular diagnosis [3, 4].

Amoebiasis

The first detailed description of amoebic dysentery and liver abscess was by Fedor Loasch, a Russian physician in 1875, although previous descriptions had been made [5]. *Naegleria fowleri* was discovered in 1899, but the human CNS disease was described in Australia in 1965 by Fowler and Carter [6].

The main amoebic infections of the CNS in humans are cerebral amoebic abscesses and amoebic encephalitis. *Entamoeba histolytica,* the best-known amoeba, causes cerebral amoebic abscesses, albeit rarely [7], and amoebic encephalitis is caused by mitochondria-bearing, free-living eukaryotic

---

Infections of the Central Nervous System: Pathology and Genetics, First Edition. Edited by Fabrice Chrétien, Kum Thong Wong, Leroy R. Sharer, Catherine (Katy) Keohane and Françoise Gray.
© 2020 John Wiley & Sons Ltd. Published 2020 by John Wiley & Sons Ltd.

amoebae. These two types of organism can both survive independently of the host but differ with regard to their epidemiology, clinical presentation, and morphological features. There are two types of amoebic encephalitis: primary amoebic meningoencephalitis (PAM) and granulomatous amoebic encephalitis (GAE). Both are rare and highly lethal CNS infections [8, 9]. PAM is caused by *N. fowleri* and GAE is caused by *Acanthamoeba* spp. and *Balamuthia mandrillaris*. Both *Acanthamoeba* spp. and *B. mandrillaris* also cause a disseminated disease involving the lungs, skin, kidneys, and uterus. Another free-living amoeba *Sappinia pedata*, previously described as *Sappinia diploidea*, caused a single case of amoebic meningoencephalitis [10].

Cerebral amoebic abscess

Cerebral amoebic abscess is a rare and late complication of intestinal, pulmonary, or hepatic amoebiasis that is usually fatal. The etiologic agent is *E. histolytica*, a common intestinal parasite, particularly in tropical and subtropical climates that exists in two forms: trophozoites, found in the colon, and cysts, excreted in the feces. Trophozoites invade the brain through hematogenous routes from a primary focus. Very occasionally, amoebic brain abscesses develop without an obvious extraneural infection.

Patients present with a combination of nonspecific features of encephalitis or meningoencephalitis and manifestations of a mass lesion. Common presentations include severe headache, vomiting, and altered mental status. The most common signs are meningeal signs, facial nerve (VII) palsy, motor paralysis, and seizure. Most patients have abnormal cerebrospinal fluid (CSF), although there is no special or characteristic abnormality. Diagnosis is by serology and polymerase chain reaction (PCR) of brain abscess aspirate or CSF, and treatment is with metronidazole [7].

Macroscopically, the cerebral lesion is usually single and located in the cortical gray matter, basal ganglia, or at the junction between cortex and white matter. Occasionally there are multiple abscesses. Early lesions appear as small foci of hemorrhagic softening, which become necrotic, with yellow–green centers, and later cavitate. The walls are irregular without evidence of encapsulation.

Microscopically, the abscesses are made up of inflamed necrotic tissue. The wall has an inner zone of necrosis and a broad outer zone with prominent congestion and vascular proliferation. It may be difficult to distinguish *E. histolytica* trophozoites from macrophages. Trophozoites are spherical or oval, 15–25 µm in diameter, have vacuolated cytoplasm with abundant glycogen and a single nucleus (Figure 47.1). Occasionally, pseudopodia can be seen. The round nuclei have a small central karyosome and peripheral chromatin. Reactive gliosis and an infiltrate of lymphocytes, plasma cells, macrophages, and some neutrophils are seen in the surrounding brain [7].

Primary amoebic meningoencephalitis

PAM, is a rare form of acute, fulminant necrotizing, and hemorrhagic meningoencephalitis caused by the free-living amoeba *N. fowleri*. This parasite is also known as the "brain-eating bug." It has been recognized in most parts of the world [11, 12]. Infections are usually associated with aquatic activities during the summer months. The organism gains entry to the brain via the nasal cavity through the olfactory epithelium. Transmission via the domestic water supply has also been reported. *N. fowleri* has been isolated from fresh water, soil, sewage, heating, ventilation and air conditioning units, dental units, gastrointestinal washings, and dust. There are no known predisposing medical conditions, and the infection usually affects

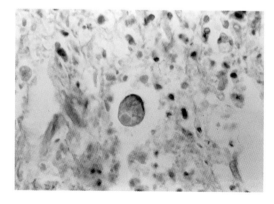

Figure 47.1 Amoebic abscess. *Entamoeba histolytica* (center) with single nucleus and large vacuolated periodic acid-Schiff (PAS)-positive cytoplasm.

previously healthy children and young adults who have recent exposure to warm freshwater, often from swimming [7, 11]. The incubation period of 1–14 days is followed by a rapidly progressive course, which is almost always fatal.

Symptoms include meningism with severe frontal headache, fever, and vomiting, followed rapidly by seizures, coma, and death. The main differential diagnosis is bacterial meningitis, which can be distinguished by clinical recognition of the syndrome and finding amoebae in CSF. These can easily be missed, and a high index of suspicion is needed. Fresh CSF should be examined under phase-contrast or dark-field illumination. The organisms can also be seen on Giemsa preparations as trophozoites of 15–25 μm in diameter. Microscopy to identify motile trophozoites on wet CSF preparations and PCR are recommended for early diagnosis and management. Cyst forms are generally not present in the CSF or on histopathological examination of the brain.

Macroscopically, there is often cerebral edema, swollen, and congested cerebral hemispheres and cerebellum, in addition to a hemorrhagic meningeal exudate over the cerebrum, brainstem, and cerebellum. The olfactory bulbs and tracts and the adjacent parts of the frontal and temporal lobes show areas of hemorrhagic necrosis.

Microscopically, a scanty mononuclear inflammatory infiltrate with focal hemorrhage is seen in the meninges, and there is usually extensive necrosis of brain parenchyma, the features of a fulminant acute meningoencephalitis. Variable numbers of amoebic trophozoites can be identified in the subarachnoid space and around vessels in the necrotic parenchyma. Their diameter (8–15 μm) is slightly less than that of *E. histolytica*. They resemble macrophages but are distinguished by their vesicular nucleus with its large central nucleolus. A scanty polymorphonuclear inflammatory cellular reaction and reactive astroglial response secondary to the extensive areas of hemorrhagic necrosis may be seen [9].

Granulomatous amoebic encephalitis

Several species of *Acanthamoeba* belonging to different genotypes cause a chronic insidious disease, GAE. They have a worldwide distribution and have been isolated from a range of sources in soil and water. GAE occurs principally in immunocompromised hosts including individuals infected with human immunodeficiency virus (HIV) who have acquired immunodeficiency syndrome (AIDS) [8, 9]. Other free-living amoebae, such as those belonging to the order Leptomyxida classified as *B. mandrillaris* [8, 13] and *S. pedata* (previously described as *S. Diploidea*) [8], can also cause GAE. Transmission of *B. mandrillaris* by organ transplantation has also been reported [14].

The route of entry into the brain is hematogenous, probably from a primary focus in the lower respiratory tract or skin. The infection is predominantly encountered in individuals who are chronically ill and debilitated or immunosuppressed. The main risk factors are HIV infection, lymphoma, malnutrition, cirrhosis, and diabetes.

The clinical presentation of meningitis and encephalitis is gradual, with headache, fever, stiff neck, focal neurologic abnormalities, seizures, and personality changes. Despite the subacute or chronic course, the disease is usually fatal, although there are rare reports of successful treatment with surgery and ketoconazole.

The CSF shows a pleocytosis with lymphocytes and polymorphs, often raised protein, and slightly decreased glucose. The neuroimaging appearances are variable because the lesions can mimic either space-occupying lesions or infarcts.

Macroscopically, the brain is swollen, may be covered by a leptomeningeal exudate, especially overlying the most affected cortical regions, and show confluent areas of multifocal hemorrhagic necrosis and encephalomalacia. All cortical lobes are affected. Other areas of the brain and cervical spinal cord may also be involved.

Histologically, there is a chronic, angiocentric inflammatory encephalitis, with foci of necrotic parenchyma surrounding trophozoites and cysts (Figure 47.2a) and a mixed inflammatory cell pattern, with mononuclear cells predominating (Figure 47.2b). Multinucleated giant cells may be encountered (Figure 47.2c), but only a few cases show typical granulomas. There is also a chronic inflammatory infiltrate in the meninges. Organisms are commonly seen in the perivascular space and can elicit severe angiitis, with fibrinoid necrosis of blood vessels and perivascular cuffing (Figure 47.2d).

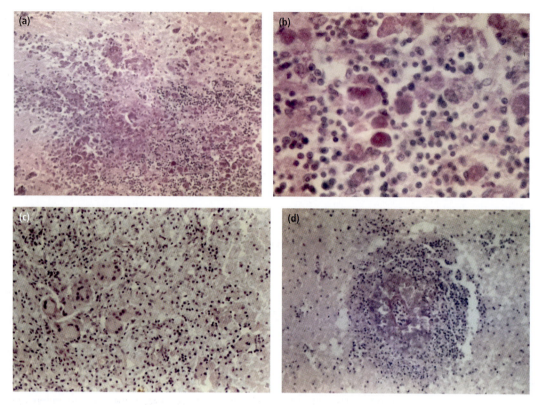

Figure 47.2 Granulomatous amoebic encephalitis. (a) Focus of necrotic parenchyma surrounding trophozoites and cysts with mononuclear inflammatory cell infiltrate. (b) Mixed inflammatory cell pattern, predominantly mononuclear cells, and numerous amoebae. (c) Multinucleated giant cells in the inflammatory infiltrate. (d) Parasites are present in the perivascular space, and there is angiitis with fibrinoid necrosis of a central blood vessel and perivascular cuffing by mononuclear inflammatory cells.

In contrast to PAM, the encysted parasite forms can be seen. Both *Acanthamoeba* and *Balamuthia* species have slightly larger trophozoites and cysts than *N. fowleri*. The amoebae are 15–40 µm in diameter and have a prominent vesicular nucleus with a dense central nucleolus. The cysts are surrounded by a double membrane. Although the organisms and the lesions are morphologically identical to those of *Acanthamoeba*, *B. mandrillaris* can be distinguished immunohistochemically. In the case reported to be caused by *S. diploidea*, the necrotizing hemorrhagic inflammatory mass contained free-living amoebae. Immunofluorescence microscopy showed that the organism was not an amoeba species previously known to cause encephalitis. Trophozoites had a highly distinctive double nucleus, and transmission electron microscopy confirmed they contained two nuclei closely apposed along a flattened surface [10].

Acanthamoeba keratitis

Acanthamoeba keratitis, caused by *Acanthamoeba* spp., has been associated with corneal trauma, infection through contaminated contact lenses and infected corneal transplants. The neuropathologist may encounter the disease in corneal biopsy specimens, where the parasite may be identified along with a polymorph inflammatory cell infiltrate, which can be minimal (Figure 47.3) [9].

Trypanosomiasis

Trypanosomes are unicellular hemoflagellate protozoan parasites of the family Trypanosomatidae. Depending on the geographic area where the disease is contracted, human infection presents in different forms. African trypanosomiasis causes

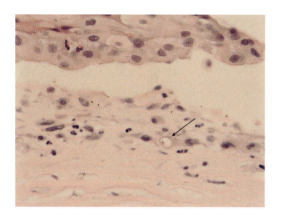

Figure 47.3 Acanthameba keratis. Corneal resection for chronic acanthameba keratitis. Parasite (arrowed) beneath the corneal epithelium with a scant polymorphonuclear inflammatory response. Hematoxylin and eosin (H&E).

"sleeping sickness" and is caused by two different species: *Trypanosoma brucei gambiense* (Gambian or West African trypanosomiasis) and *Trypanosoma brucei rhodesiense*, responsible for Rhodesian or East African trypanosomiasis. South American trypanosomiasis or Chagas disease is caused by the *Trypanosoma cruzi*. The diseases are clinically distinct, although both are characterized by acute phases involving direct parasitization of the CNS and chronic disease resulting from immunopathogenic reactions [15].

African trypanosomiasis

Definition of the disorder, major synonyms, and historical perspective

African trypanosomiasis ("sleeping sickness") is transmitted by the bite of the tsetse fly (genus *Glossina*). It was discovered in 1902, when the epidemic killed two-thirds of the population of 300 000 in Uganda. Although African trypanosomiasis is predominantly a zoonosis, millions of people are at risk of infection. In the early 1950s, it became controlled in West and Central Africa through population surveillance and in East Africa through vector control. Later, having gained independence, various countries failed to implement prophylactic measures, which led to the disease reappearing so that it is still a major concern in some regions [16, 17].

Microbiological characteristics and epidemiology

The parasite undergoes part of its life cycle in the gut and salivary gland of the fly. Exposure to the disease depends on the habitat of the vector. In West Africa it leads to endemic transmission, although epidemics can occur. Primary human exposure is rarer in the East African form, where vector contact is rarer, and the disease exists as a zoonosis in numerous species of wild and domestic animals. Blood-borne and congenital infections have been recorded but are rare forms of transmission.

Clinical features

Infection causes a localized skin reaction at the site of the bite (the "chancre"), which may be followed by a generalized rash. Spread occurs via the bloodstream, causing fever. The disease primarily affects the hematolymphoid system, the cardiovascular system, and the CNS. Direct infection of the CNS occurs within weeks of the initial infection, with focal blood-brain barrier (BBB) breakdown and parasite colonization of the choroid plexus. Trypanosomes can be detected in the CSF, although they are often rare and repeated examination or concentration of deposits may be required. They may also be detected in fluid from the primary chancre or peripheral blood smear (Figure 47.4a). They have rarely been reported in histological sections of the brain.

Neurological and psychiatric manifestations include irritability, meningism, mood and personality change, and headache. Involuntary episodes of daytime somnolence and reversal of normal sleep patterns develop—hence, the name of the disease. Depression, withdrawal and libido changes can occur. Motor and sensory symptoms are also common with a characteristic syndrome of excessive delayed pain response to trivial injury (Kerandel or Key sign). As symptoms worsen, the periods of somnolence increase, leading to coma and death. The electroencephalogram shows marked changes, with characteristic slow delta wave oscillations mimicking those of normal sleep.

Chronic CNS involvement and deterioration are rare in East African sleeping sickness, which tends to follow a more rapid course, although terminal

Infections of the Central Nervous System

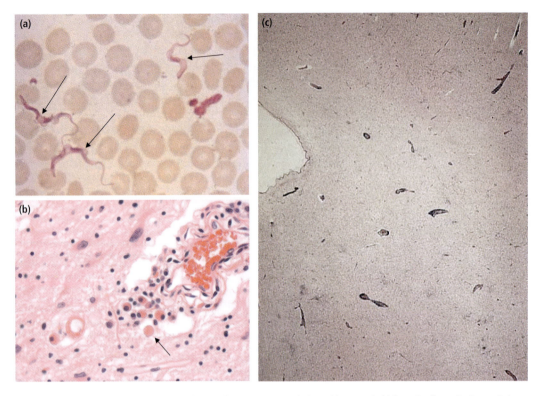

Figure 47.4 African trypanosomiasis. (a) Blood smear showing organisms (indicated by arrows). (b) "Mott" cell morular forms of plasma cells with prominent eosinophilic cytoplasmic surrounding a cerebral blood vessel, and a Russell body (arrowed) formed from immunoglobulin. (c) Brainstem. Perivascular lymphocytic inflammation, most noticeable in the periaqueductal region.

symptoms of tremor, drowsiness, and coma occur. In contrast, the West African form is characterized by chronic, progressive deterioration of CNS function lasting from months to years. Meningoencephalitis is characteristic of the later stages, and death usually results from intercurrent infection or malnutrition.

Pathology

The primary neuropathological changes of African trypanosomiasis are meningitis and encephalitis.

Macroscopically, the brain may be normal or the leptomeninges are cloudy and the brain swollen and congested. Patients who have been treated with melarsoprol may develop acute hemorrhagic leukoencephalopathy.

Microscopically, lymphocytes, macrophages, and plasma cells surround the cerebral blood vessels and infiltrate the subarachnoid space. They include numerous B cells and plasma cells, including the "Mott cell" morular forms of plasma cells with prominent eosinophilic cytoplasmic Russell bodies formed from immunoglobulins (Figure 47.4b). These "morular cells" are characteristic but not specific. Traveling via the subarachnoid and perivascular Virchow–Robin spaces, parasites enter the brain. This causes characteristic intense subarachnoid and perivascular inflammation, which tends to be most marked in the brainstem (Figure 47.4c) and cerebellum. Other features include reactive gliosis, clusters of mononuclear inflammatory cells or typical microglial nodules, especially in *T. b. rhodesiense* encephalitis, often associated with lymphophagocytosis. Trypanosomes are rarely demonstrable in histologic sections. Parasites may also invade sensory ganglia, the spinal cord (causing meningomyelitis), and colonize the choroid plexus, from where they can spill over into CSF. The dense perivascular cuffing and meningeal infiltrate are accompanied by a developing white matter reaction in the brain parenchyma, including widespread astrocyte activation and microglial nodules surrounding blood vessels.

Pathogenesis
It is postulated that parasites initially spread into the brain parenchyma in areas where the BBB is deficient, such as the choroid plexus, area postrema, median eminence, and periventricular nuclei, followed by release of cytokines such as interferon gamma (IFN-γ), which induce trypanosomal growth. Various immunopathogenic mechanisms have been proposed to explain the pathological effects of trypanosomes in the CNS, mainly as a result of studies in animal models [18].

It is also suggested that the reactive acute hemorrhagic lethal leukoencephalopathy, which occurs in 5–10% of patients treated in the late stage, is triggered by viable organisms remaining within the brain following inadequate drug therapy [15].

South American trypanosomiasis
Definition of the disorder major synonyms, and historical perspective
South American trypanosomiasis is transmitted via contamination of wounds and bites by the feces of the triatomine bug. Transmission can also occur by blood transfusion, through organ transplants, breastfeeding, transplacentally and accidentally in laboratories [15]. Carlos Chagas described the disease in Brazil in 1909 and, uniquely for a parasitic infection, reported not only a new human disease but also described the agent, its morphology, life cycle, the form of transmission, and the clinical symptoms in humans [16].

Microbiological characteristics and epidemiology
T. cruzi is an obligate intracellular parasite, which can take up the undulating, flagellate trypomastigote form, or the *Leishmania*-like amastigote form. These multiply inside a variety of cells, particularly macrophages, nerve, and muscle cells.

The disease is a significant health problem in many areas of the continent, affecting patients in South and Central America, in Mexico, and also in Java and India. It has become a concern in the United States as a result of human emigration from Latin America. Surveillance remains important in states with large populations of immigrants or frequent travelers from endemic regions. Surveillance can increase awareness in health providers and facilitate patient access to treatment to help prevent cardiac and gastrointestinal complications [19].

Clinical features
At the site of the bite a firm nodule develops, the parasite reaches the blood or lymphatic circulation and infects other tissues. Acute Chagas disease may be asymptomatic or cause a mild meningoencephalitis. About 10% of patients, mostly young children, develop acute myocarditis and encephalitis, which is fatal in approximately 10% of cases. *T. cruzi* organisms can be identified in the CSF. After recovery from the acute stage, patients enter an intermediate stage, where neurological symptoms are absent and circulating parasites disappear. However, scanty parasitized cells persist as a latent infection, remaining as inflammatory foci in cardiac and extracardiac tissues. During this phase, the host immune response is assumed to suppress both recrudescence of infection and the autoimmune reactions that characterize the chronic disease [15, 20].

The CNS may be involved in the acute infective stage. In the subsequent intermediate stage symptoms regress. In the later chronic stage autoimmune damage may be responsible for chronic CNS involvement, but this is controversial and overshadowed by the long-term consequences of autonomic neuropathy and destruction of muscle fibers in the heart (causing cardiomyopathy) and gut (causing megacolon) [20]. Patients who are immunosuppressed are liable to *T. cruzi* reactivation in the brain and new pathological presentations of the disease have been recorded, manifesting as abscess or meningoencephalitis [21–24], including cases with moderate [25] and unknown [26] immunosuppression.

Various neurological syndromes have been reported in chronic Chagas disease, including spastic paralysis, mental restriction, and cerebellar symptoms. Only 20–40% of patients with acute Chagas disease are believed to progress to the chronic form. This includes several types. First, a true chronic Chagasic encephalopathy is not only rare but also unconvincing in patients who are not immunocompromised. Neuronal loss and focal inflammatory changes may be the result of chronic hypoxia secondary to the cardiomyopathy accompanying chronic Chagas disease [20].

In reactivated Chagas disease with immunosuppression resulting from tumors, transplantation, drug treatment, or HIV infection, there is an acute necrotizing hemorrhagic encephalitis including a syndrome that presents as a space-occupying, tumor-like lesion [15, 20].

Pathology

In the acute phase, macroscopically the brain appears swollen and congested with scattered petechial hemorrhages. Microscopically, amastigote (*Leishmania*-like) forms of the parasites are present within glial cells or less frequently at the center of microglial nodules, composed of microglia and macrophages, which are scattered within the brain parenchyma. The parasites can be seen within microglia, macrophages, endothelial cells, and neurons. These lesions are also seen in the meninges and choroid plexus. Individual case reports have described a diffuse granulomatous process or an isolated hemorrhagic tumor-like mass consisting of multiple areas of necrosis with perifocal glial reaction and identifiable parasites.

In the chronic phase, macroscopically, the brain usually appears normal. On microscopy, a few microglial nodules and aggregates of lymphoid cells may be found but no parasites are.

Reactivated disease takes the form of multifocal necrotizing encephalitis with nodules of microglia, associated hemorrhage, and abundant amastigote forms of the parasite detected by conventional histology (Figure 47.5a, b, c) and confirmed immunohistochemically (Figure 47.5d) and by immunofluorescence and in situ hybridization, electron microscopy, and PCR methods, using formalin-fixed and paraffin-embedded tissues. Although parasites are found most often in astrocytes and macrophages [15, 27], neurons can also rarely be infected (personal experience).

Pathogenesis

There are several proposed mechanisms to explain the progression of Chagas disease, including parasite persistence, immune responses against the parasite, or host that persist in the heart, vascular compromise, involvement of autonomic nervous system and CNS, macrophage activation, mitochondrial dysfunction, and oxidative stress [20, 28].

Other causes of CNS pathology in chronic Chagas disease include ischemic or hemorrhagic vascular lesions related to the chronic cardiomyopathy that courses with congestive heart failure, dysrhythmias, and thrombo-embolic phenomena. Secondary hypoxic nerve cell changes, cerebral infarcts, and hemorrhages can all occur. Patients with Chagas disease are at increased risk for stroke, so identifying risk factors for thromboembolism in this disease may expedite therapy and improve outcomes [20, 29].

Congenital Chagas disease

Mild meningoencephalitis with epithelioid and giant cells may occur in congenital Chagas disease. In the chronic phase, the risk of maternal transmission to the fetus during pregnancy is very low, probably <1% [15, 30].

Peripheral nervous system involvement

The peripheral nervous system may also be affected in the acute phase of Chagas disease. The autonomic tissue of the heart, esophagus, and gut are especially susceptible, leading to chronic cardiopathy with cardiomegaly, dilatation, and enlargement of digestive viscera. Peripheral somatosensory neuropathies with involvement of dorsal root ganglia, anterior horn neurons, and peripheral sensory and motor nerve fibers are less frequent than autonomic neuropathies. Clinical, electrophysiological, and histological reports in human and experimental infections show both axonal and demyelinating neuropathies are probably the result of autoimmune mechanisms [15–20].

Microsporidiosis

Microsporidia are obligate intracellular spore-forming organisms. More than 20 genera of microsporidium are pathogenic in mammals, but *Encephalitozoon* species more commonly affect individuals who are immunosuppressed. *Trachipleistophora anthropophthera* may also cause encephalitis. In humans,

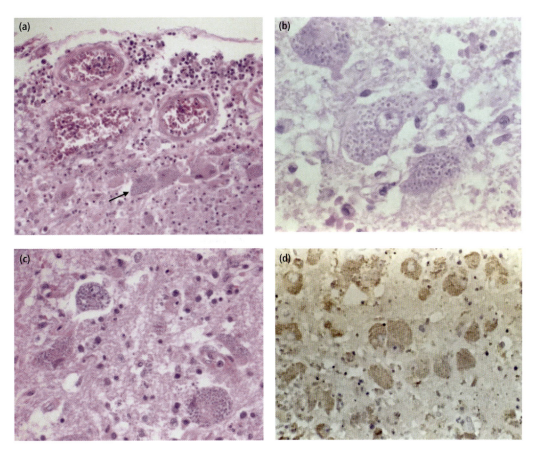

Figure 47.5 South American trypanosomiasis Chagas disease. (a) Multifocal necrotizing encephalitis with nodules of microglia, associated hemorrhage, and abundant amastigote forms of the parasite (arrowed). (b) Amazygotes within macrophages and astrocytes. (c) Amastigote within a neuron in a personal case of trypanosomiasis associated with AIDS. (d) Amastigotes staining positively with antibody to *Trypanosoma cruzi*.

microsporidium can be transmitted via contaminated water or air droplets and via the fecal-oral route. Sexual transmission of *Encephalitozoon* species may also occur. The parasites have an internal coiled tube through which infectious sporoplasm is extruded into the cytoplasm of the host cell by piercing and injecting [31].

The spectrum of disease varies from diarrhea and keratoconjunctivitis to disseminated infection involving multiple organs. Disseminated infection with CNS involvement is rare but can occur following kidney, pancreas, and bone marrow transplantation; there are rare reports in immunocompetent hosts. Clinically, CNS involvement presents with signs and symptoms of encephalitis and seizures.

Diagnosis often requires brain biopsy, but spores can occasionally be found in other sites. Albendazole and fumagillin have been successfully used in treating microsporidiosis at other sites, but their role in CNS infection is unclear [31, 32].

Macroscopically, mild meningeal opacity has been reported. There is a diffuse, nodular encephalitis, sometimes with necrotic foci. The multifocal lesions in gray or white matter can mimic cerebral toxoplasmosis.

Microscopically, there may be small foci of necrosis. The parasites can be detected in tissue biopsies (Figure 47.6). They are seen as clusters of hematoxyphilic nuclear dots within refractive clear cytoplasm, often gram and Ziehl-Neelsen

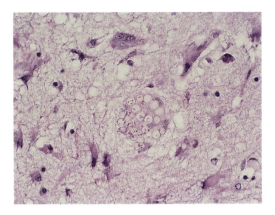

Figure 47.6 Microsporidiosis. Clusters of hematoxyphilic nuclear dots within refractive clear cytoplasm seen within a parasitized astrocyte.

positive. Astrocytes are parasitized (but not neurons), and there is localized microglial proliferation. Electron microscopy is more successful than light microscopy in identifying the organisms; molecular diagnosis with PCR of biopsy samples is highly sensitive but is not widely available. During CNS infection, spores are often present in peripheral blood [30, 31].

Sarcocystosis

Sarcocystis spp. are global intestinal infections of carnivores, taxonomically related to *T. gondii*. Humans becomes infected by accidentally ingesting sarcocyst-containing meat (beef or pork) or water or food contaminated by fecal oocysts. The parasite spreads to cardiac and skeletal muscle (including tongue). Most cases are incidental findings on muscle biopsy or autopsy material. There are a few reported outbreaks of myositis attributable to *Sarcocystis* infection [33–35].

To our knowledge, human CNS disease has not been reported. A severe meningoencephalitis with numerous schizonts and merozoites associated with extensive focal necrosis was described in a nine-months-old bull calf [36]. Individual *Sarcoystis* merozoites were seen in neurons, astrocytes, oligodendrocytes, leukocytes, vascular endothelial cells, and in the nuclei of mononuclear cells.

Leishmaniasis

Definition of the disorder, synonyms, and historical perspective

Leishmaniasis is a vector-borne infection resulting from parasites of the genus *Leishmania*. There are more than 23 *Leishmania* species. Around 70 animal species (including humans) are natural reservoir hosts. There are three clinical forms in humans: visceral leishmaniasis (VL), the most severe and potentially fatal form, is characterized by bouts of fever, enlarged liver and spleen, and anemia; cutaneous leishmaniasis (CL) is less severe but often disfiguring and manifests as skin ulcers that heal leaving scars; mucocutaneous leishmaniasis (MCL) causes destructive lesions of the mucosa of the nose, mouth, and throat, leading to severe deformities.

VL is also known as kala-azar (meaning black fever in Hindi) or Dumdum fever, and CL was known as white leprosy, Andean fever, valley fever, Aleppo boil, or Oriental sore.

There are descriptions in ancient texts from Assyria in the seventh century BCE, but they possibly derive from even older records 1500–2500 BCE [37]. The causative organism of VL, *Leishmania donovani*, originally thought to be a trypanosome, was named after the Scottish pathologist William Leishman and the Irish physician Charles Donovan, who both worked in India. In 1903 each independently and almost simultaneously identified the parasite from autopsy spleen [38, 39].

Epidemiology

VL caused by *L. donovani* is a relatively common infection in all continents except Australasia. It is mainly transmitted to humans by the bites of female sandflies and spreads via the bloodstream. VL is a major health problem and a neglected disease affecting the poorest populations, especially children, in many regions of the world. The World Health Organization (WHO) estimates that 50 000–90 000 new cases occur annually. and in 2015, more than 90% of new cases reported to WHO occurred in seven countries: Brazil, Ethiopia, India, Kenya, Somalia, South Sudan, and Sudan [40]. In Europe, since the advent of HIV, about half the cases are in adults.

Clinical presentation

CNS involvement is extremely rare in humans [2]. A case of pontine involvement in VL is reported in a 54-year-old man from Southwest Iran with a three-week history of headache, fever, chills, weakness, anorexia, and weight loss [41]. A child with VL refractory to treatment had meningitis with parasites in CSF [42].

Pathology

Fatal cases of VL have enormous hepatosplenomegaly and profound anemia. The organisms (amastigotes) are mainly seen in the liver and spleen as intracellular nonflagellate round or oval hematoxyphilic dots 2–4 μm in diameter usually in macrophages (Leishman-Donovan bodies). Despite detecting *Leishmania* parasites in the brain and CSF of human patients and dogs [43], epidemiological data and information about the mechanisms of CNS and peripheral nervous system alterations are poorly described. Both brain infection and inflammation were detected in a mouse model of VL. Live parasites were identified in an early phase; there were signs of BBB disruption, providing convincing evidence that *L. donovani* can indeed infect and inflame the brain [44].

Conclusion and future perspective

Because of globalization, mass movement of people because of political instability, breakdown of health provision, and increased immunosuppression, parasitic infections traditionally confined to certain regions can be found worldwide and are likely to persist. Control of their specific vectors and early effective supportive or specific drug therapy offer the best hopes for a successful outcome, but even so, some of these CNS infections are almost always lethal.

References

1. Chacko, G. (2010). Parasitic diseases of the central nervous system. *Semin. Diagn. Pathol.* 27: 167–185.
2. Walker, M., Kublin, J.G., and Zunt, J.R. (2006). Parasitic central nervous system infections in immunocompromised hosts: malaria, microsporidiosis, leishmaniasis, and African trypanosomiasis. *Clin. Infect. Dis.* 42: 115–125.
3. Chimelli, L. (2011). A morphological approach to the diagnosis of protozoal infections of the central nervous system. *Pathol. Res. Int.* 2011: 290853.
4. Jansen, M., Corcoran, D., Bermingham, N. et al. (2010). The role of biopsy in the diagnosis of infections of the central nervous system. *Ir. Med. J.* 103: 6–8.
5. Imperato, P.J. (1981). A historical overview of amoebiasis. *Bull. N. Y. Acad. Med.* 57 (3): 175–187.
6. Fowler, M. and Carter, R.F. (1965). Acute pyogenic meningitis probably due to Acanthamoeba sp.: a preliminary report. *Br. Med. J.* 2: 740–742.
7. Petri, W.A. and Haque, R. (2013). Entamoeba histolytica brain abscess. *Handb. Clin. Neurol.* 114: 147–152.
8. Martinez, A.J. and Visvesvara, G.S. (1997). Free-living, amphizoic and opportunistic amoebas. *Brain Pathol.* 7: 583–598.
9. Visvesvara, G.S. (2013). Infections with free-living amoebae. *Handb. Clin. Neurol.* 114: 153–156.
10. Gelman, B.B., Popov, V., Chaljub, B. et al. (2003). Neuropathological and ultrastructural features of amoebic encephalitis caused by Sappinia diploidea. *J. Neuropathol. Exp. Neurol.* 62: 990–998.
11. Kaushal, V., Chhina, D.K., Ram, S. et al. (2008). Primary amoebic meningoencephalitis due to Naegleria fowleri. *J. Assoc. Physicians India* 56: 459–462.
12. Ghanchi, N.K., Jamil, B., Khan, E. et al. (2017). Case series of Naegleria fowleri primary amoebic meningoencephalitis from Karachi, Pakistan. *Am. J. Trop. Med. Hyg.* 97: 1600–1602.
13. Chimelli, L., Hahn, M.D., Scaravilli, F. et al. (1992). Granulomatous amoebic encephalitis due to Leptomyxid amoebae: report of the Brazilian case. *Trans. R. Soc. Trop. Med. Hyg.* 86: 635.
14. Farnon, E.C., Kokko, K.E., Budge, P.J. et al. (2016). Transmission of Balamuthia mandrillaris by organ transplantation. *Clin. Infect. Dis.* 63: 878–888.
15. Chimelli, L. and Scaravilli, F. (1997). Trypanosomiasis. *Brain Pathol.* 7: 599–611.
16. Scaravilli, F. (1997). Historical perspective of tropical infections. *Brain Pathol.* 7: 561–567.
17. Cox, F.E. (2004). History of sleeping sickness (African trypanosomiasis). *Infect. Dis. Clin. N. Am.* 18: 231–245.
18. Kristensson, K., Nygård, M., Bertini, G., and Bentivoglio, M. (2010). African trypanosome infections of the nervous system: parasite entry and effects on sleep and synaptic functions. *Prog. Neurobiol.* 91: 152–171.

19. Bennett, C., Straily, A., Haselow, D. et al. (2018). Chagas disease surveillance activities – seven states, 2017. *MMWR Morb. Mortal. Wkly Rep.* 67: 738–741.
20. Pittella, J.E. (2009). Central nervous system involvement in chagas disease: a hundred-year-old history. *Trans. R. Soc. Trop. Med. Hyg.* 103: 973–978.
21. Diazgranados, C.A., Saavedra-Trujillo, C.H., Mantilla, M. et al. (2009). Chagasic encephalitis in HIV patients: common presentation of an evolving epidemiological and clinical association. *Lancet Infect. Dis.* 9: 324–330.
22. Cordova, E., Boschi, A., Ambrosioni, J. et al. (2008). Reactivation of Chagas disease with central nervous system involvement in HIV-infected patients in Argentina, 1992-2007. *Int. J. Infect. Dis.* 12: 587–592.
23. Lattes, R. and Lasala, M.B. (2014). Chagas disease in the immunosuppressed patient. *Clin. Microbiol. Infect.* 20: 300–309.
24. Rossi Spadafora, M.S., Céspedes, G., Romero, S. et al. (2014). Trypanosoma cruzi necrotizing meningoencephalitis in a Venezuelan HIV+-AIDS patient: pathological diagnosis confirmed by PCR using formalin-fixed- and paraffin-embedded-tissues. *Anal. Cell. Pathol. (Amst.)* 2014: 124795.
25. Buccheri, R., Kassab, M.J., Freitas, V.L. et al. (2015). Chagasic meningoencephalitis in an HIV infected patient with moderate immunosuppression: prolonged survival and challenges in the haart era. *Rev. Inst. Med. Trop. Sao Paulo* 57: 531–535.
26. Fernandes, H.J., Barbosa, L.O., Machado, T.S. et al. (2017). Meningoencephalitis caused by reactivation of chagas disease in patient without known immunosuppression. *Am. J. Trop. Med. Hyg.* 96: 292–294.
27. Gomez, C.A. and Banaei, N. (2018). Trypanosoma cruzi reactivation in the brain. *N. Engl. J. Med.* 378: 1824.
28. Lopez, M., Tanowitz, H.B., and Garg, N.J. (2018). Pathogenesis of chronic Chagas disease: macrophages, mitochondria, and oxidative stress. *Curr. Clin. Microbiol. Rep.* 5: 45–54.
29. Nunes, M.C., Kreuser, L.J., Ribeiro, A.L. et al. (2015). Prevalence and risk factors of embolic cerebrovascular events associated with chagas heart disease. *Glob. Heart* 10: 151–157.
30. Martins-Melo, F.R., Lima Mda, S., Ramos, A.N. Jr. et al. (2014). Prevalence of chagas disease in pregnant women and congenital transmission of Trypanosoma cruzi in Brazil: a systematic review and meta-analysis. *Tropical Med. Int. Health* 19: 943–957.
31. Weiss, L.M. (2005). Microsporidiosis. In: *Mandell, Douglas and Bennett's Principles and Practice of Infectious Diseases*, 6e (eds. G.L. Mandell, J.E. Bennett and R. Dolin), 3237–3254. Pennsylvania: Elsevier Churchill Livingstone.
32. Ashfaq, A. and White, A.C. Jr. (2013). Microsporidiasis. *Handb. Clin. Neurol.* 114: 183–191.
33. Gutierrez, Y. (2000). *Diagnostic Pathology of Parasitic Infections with Clinical Correlations*, 2e. Oxford: Oxford University Press.
34. Arness, M.K., Brown, J.D., Dubey, J.P. et al. (1999). An outbreak of acute eosinophilic myositis attributed to human Sarcoystis parasitism. *Am. J. Trop. Med. Hyg.* 61: 548–553.
35. Italiano, C.M., Wong, K.T., AbuBakar, S. et al. (2014). Sarcocystis nesbitti causes acute, relapsing febrile myositis with a high attack rate: description of a large outbreak of muscular Sarcocystosis in Pangkor Island, Malaysia, 2012. *PLoS Negl. Trop. Dis.* 8 (5): e2876.
36. Dubey, J.P., Calero-Bernal, R., Verma, S.K. et al. (2016). Pathology, immunohistochemistry, and ultrastructural findings associated with neurological sarcocystosis in cattle. *Vet. Parasitol.* 223: 147–152.
37. Steverding, D. (2017). The history of leishmaniasis. *Parasit Vectors* 10: 82. https://doi.org/10.1186/s13071-017-2028-5.
38. Leishman, W.B. (1903). On the possibility of the occurrence of trypanosomiasis in India. *Br. Med. J.* 1: 1252–1254.
39. Donovan, C. (1903). On the possibility of the occurrence of trypanosomiasis in India. *Br. Med. J.* 2: 79.
40. World Health Organization (WHO). *Leishmaniasis*. http://www.who.int/leishmaniasis/visceral_leishmaniasis/en (accessed 8 November 2018).
41. Sedaghattalab, M. and Azizi, A. (2018). Brain parenchyma (pons) involvement by visceral leishmaniasis: a case report. *Iran. J. Parasitol.* 13: 145–148.
42. Prasad, L.S.N. and Sen, S. (1996). Migration of leishmania donovani amastigotes in the cerebrospinal fluid. *Am. J. Trop. Med. Hyg.* 55: 652–654.
43. Maia, C.S., Monteiro, M.C., Gavioli, E.C. et al. (2015). Neurological disease in human and canine leishmaniasis – clinical features and immunopathogenesis. *Parasite Immunol.* 37: 385–393.
44. Melo, G.D., Goyard, S., Fiette, L. et al. (2017). Unveiling cerebral leishmaniasis: parasites and brain inflammation in leishmania donovani infected mice. *Sci. Rep.* 7: 8454.

48 Helminth Infections of the CNS

Marine Le Dudal[1,2], Stéphane Bretagne[3,4,5], David Hardy[1], Fabrice Chrétien[1,6,7,*], and Grégory Jouvion[1,*]

[1] Experimental Neuropathology Unit, Pasteur Institute, Paris, France
[2] Embryology, Histology and Pathology Unit, The National Veterinary School of Alfort, University Paris-Est, Maison-Alfort, France
[3] Saint Louis Hospital, APHP, Paris, France
[4] University Paris Diderot, Sorbonne Paris Cité, Paris, France
[5] Molecular Mycology Unit, French National Reference Centre for Invasive Mycoses and Antifungal treatments, Pasteur Institute, Paris, France
[6] Paris University, Paris, France
[7] Department of Neuropathology, Sainte Anne Hospital, Paris, France

Abbreviations

CE	cystic echinococcosis
CNS	central nervous system
CSF	cerebrospinal fluid
CT-scan	computed tomography
ELISA	enzyme-linked immunosorbent assay
H&E	hematoxylin and eosin
HIV/AIDS	human immunodeficiency virus/acquired immunodeficiency syndrome
MRI	magnetic resonance imaging
NCC	neurocysticercosis
NTD	neglected tropical diseases

Introduction and historical perspective

Helminths are important causes of disease in humans and all species of animals. The first descriptions of probable human parasitic infections were written 3000–400 BCE (Egyptian civilization), and calcified helminth eggs were incidentally detected in mummies dating from 1200 BCE [1]. In the eighteenth century, Linnaeus was the first to name and precisely describe six helminths: *Ascaris lumbricoides*, *Ascaris vermicularis* (*Enterobius vermicularis*), *Gordius medinensis* (*Dracunculus medinensis*), *Fasciola hepatica*, *Taenia solium*, and *Taenia lata* (*Diphyllobothrium latum*) [1]. At the beginning of the twentieth century, only 28 species were known in man; today, more than 340 parasitic helminths have been identified in humans, many of which have little or no impact on public health. A few parasites have an important impact with serious complications [1, 2] (see Table 48.1 [3]). After invasion, helminths may produce a wide variety of harmful effects by: (i) mechanical interference with different functions, (ii) tissue invasion and displacement, (iii) consuming blood or other host tissues, (iv) inducing or predisposing to neoplasia, (v) introducing bacteria or other infections, and (vi) secreting toxic products [4].

*Fabrice Chrétien and Grégory Jouvion share senior co-authorship.

Infections of the Central Nervous System: Pathology and Genetics, First Edition. Edited by Fabrice Chrétien, Kum Thong Wong, Leroy R. Sharer, Catherine (Katy) Keohane and Françoise Gray.
© 2020 John Wiley & Sons Ltd. Published 2020 by John Wiley & Sons Ltd.

Table 48.1 Helminths infecting human CNS.

Helminths	Distribution	Clinical signs	Imaging	Histopathology
Cestodes				
Taenia solium	Worldwide	Headache, epilepsy, hydrocephalus, vasculitis, spastic paraparesis	Parenchymal/extraparenchymal cysts	Larval form: *Cysticercus* Cyst wall: outer cuticular layer, middle cellular layer, and inner reticular layer. Scolex bearing a double row of hooklets and four suckers.
Echinococcus granulosus	Worldwide	Headache, epilepsy, visual disturbances, papilledema	Single or multiple intra-axial spherical or oval cysts with mass effect	Larval form: Hydatid cyst Delineated by an inner germinal layer (endocyst) and a thick concentrically laminated outer layer (ectocyst). From the germinal layer: Scolices bearing hooklets (can be absent: sterile cyst), brood capsules and daughter cysts.
Taenia multiceps	Worldwide	Signs of increased intracranial pressure: headache, vomiting, papilledema	Single or multiple cysts, sometimes in the ventricle with possible obstructive hydrocephalus	Larval form: *Coenurus* Cyst without laminar concentric structure containing up to 500 scolices
Spirometra mansoni	Tropics	Headache, seizures, hemiparesis, sensory disturbances, weakness, bleeding	Single, enhancing mass lesion, edema, tunnel sign, atrophy, calcification	Larval form; solid noncavitated body, no bladder wall and hooked scolices Migration tracts.
Trematodes				
Schistosoma spp.	Worldwide	Headache, language dysfunction, seizures, weakness, visual disturbance, ataxia, hemiparesis, paralysis	Edema, multiple, small, contrast-enhancing lesions, tumor-like lesions	Egg morphology. Terminal spine: *Schistosoma hematobium* Lateral spine: *Schistosoma mansoni* Spine absent/inconspicuous: *Schistosoma japonicum*.
Paragonimus westermani	Tropics	Seizures, headache, personality changes, visual disturbances, weakness, sensory deficits	Multiple conglomerate, calcified masses or nodules, ring-like lesions	Egg morphology. Unembryonated operculated oval shape, encapsulated by a double shell, absence of spine.
Nematodes				
Angiostrongylus cantonensis	Tropics	Headache, paraesthesia, weakness, sensory disturbance, meningitis, coma, convulsion, epilepsy	T2-hyperintense, enhancing lesions, hydrocephalus	Eosinophilic meningitis, necrosis, hemorrhages, granulomas, nonspecific vascular lesions, intralesional larvae

Gnathostoma spinigerum	Tropics	Headache, seizures, coma, bleeding, encephalitis, myelitis	Intracranial bleeding, enhancing white matter lesions, dilated myelin	Necrotic tracts, edema, hemorrhages, eosinophilic meningitis, intralesional larvae (more severe than *Angiostrongylus*)
Toxocara canis	Worldwide	Multi-organ involvement, meningoencephalitis, vasculitis, epilepsy, stroke, dementia	Vesicular, colloid-vesicular, granular-nodular, or nodular-calcified lesions	Eosinophilic meningitis, encephalitis, vasculitis, arachnoiditis, necrotic migration tracts, rare larvae in the lesions
Trichinella spiralis	Worldwide	Disorientation, focal deficits, somnolence, apathy, unequal pupils, facial nerve paralysis, memory and behavioral disturbance	Multifocal lesions in cortex/white matter, microinfarcts	Larvae rarely found, granulomas, eosinophilic meningoencephalitis, small hemorrhages and thrombi
Strongyloides stercoralis	Tropics	In general mild or asymptomatic Patients with immunosuppression: Hyperinfection syndrome	Multifocal lesions, microinfarcts	Microinfarcts, necrotic foci, abscesses, presence of larvae

Source: modified from [3].

The public health problems caused by helminths largely occur in low-income countries. Sporadic cases are described in nonendemic regions, targeting immigrants, international travelers, and patients who are immunosuppressed.

The CNS is a protected environment. Except for larvae of the Nematode *Angiostrongylus cantonensis* and larvae (cysticerci) of the tapeworm *T. solium,* which are definitely neurotropic, the CNS is most often accidentally infected during migration of helminth larvae or eggs. Invasion occurs by two routes: (i) the bloodstream (the main route for infection by *A. cantonensis, Toxocara* spp., *T. solium, Echinococcus* spp., and rarely *Schistosoma* spp.) and (ii) through soft tissues (i.e. along nerves, vessels and muscles [*Gnathostoma* spp., *Spirometra mansoni,* and *Paragonimus westermani*]) [5]. Clinical signs vary, depending on the number and localization of parasites and on host factors; they are non-specific, and so diagnosis can be difficult. Classical clinical features include headache, dizziness, root pain, epileptic seizures, increased intracranial pressure, sensory disturbance, meningeal syndrome, cerebellar ataxia, and core syndromes [6]. In general, diagnosis relies on imaging appearances on computed tomography (CT) and magnetic resonance imaging (MRI) scans and histology to identify the nature and location of the lesions (i.e. calcifications, cysts, vesicles, granulomas and abscesses) or direct visualization of the parasites (e.g. hooklets, eggs, or larvae). Immunodiagnosis, enzyme-linked immunosorbent assay (ELISA), and serology of cerebrospinal fluid (CSF) or serum may also be useful.

General description of helminths in tissue sections

Precise identification of helminths can be challenging because only fragments of the parasites are present in tissue sections. Host factors to assist in narrowing the possibilities include geographic origin and history of international travel, immune status (normal or nature and type of immunosuppression), anatomic location of the parasites, and tissue reaction (lesion profiles). Parasite factors are the morphologic features (Figure 48.1). Helminths are metazoan parasites. The major criteria used for identification are: (i) absence of a body cavity and digestive tract, body flattened dorsoventrally, presence of a scolex and calcareous corpuscles (Cestodes); (ii) absence of a body cavity but presence of digestive tract, body flattened dorsoventrally, and absence of calcareous corpuscles (Trematodes); and (iii) presence of a body cavity and a digestive tract, body not flattened, and smooth musculature (Nematodes) [7]. Organization of the muscle layer is an important parameter for Nematode identification and differentiates meromyarian platymyarian muscle cells (e.g. Oxyurids and Strongyles except Metastrongyles) from polymyarian coelomyarian muscle cells (e.g. Ascarids, Spirurids, Filarids) (Figure 48.2).

Infection by cestodes

Neurocysticercosis

Cysticercosis is infection by the larval stage (cysticerci) of the tapeworm *T. solium.* Larvae located in the CNS are the most common preventable cause of epilepsy in developing countries, with an estimated two million cases [8]. This high frequency led the World Health Organization (WHO) to add cysticercosis to the list of major neglected tropical diseases (NTD) in 2010.

Humans are the natural definitive hosts, harboring the sexual stage of *T. solium* and can develop taeniasis with little clinical consequences. Taeniasis occurs after ingestion of live cysticerci contained in pig meat. Pigs, the intermediate hosts, are infected through ingestion of eggs found in contaminated human feces. Humans ingest eggs through fecal-oral transmission or by autoinfection; these *T. solium* eggs can develop into larvae, which seed well-vascularized organs such as subcutaneous tissue, skeletal muscles, lungs, brain, eyes, liver, and heart, similar to what occurs in pigs. Proximity between pigs and humans allows the parasite life cycle to perpetuate.

The localization of larvae in brain leads to neurocysticercosis (NCC). Cysts evolve through

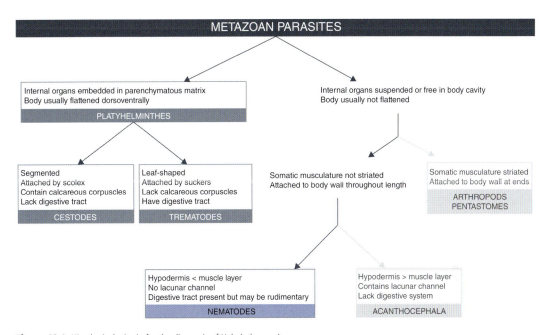

Figure 48.1 Histological criteria for the diagnosis of Helminth parasites.

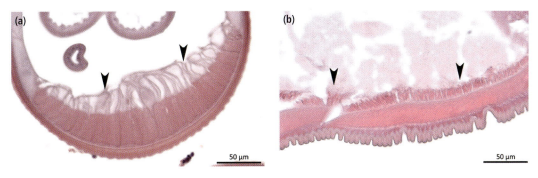

Figure 48.2 Organization of the muscle layer for Nematode identification. Organization of the muscle layer (black arrowheads) is important for Nematode identification. (a) Polymyarian (numerous muscle cells) and coelomyarian muscle cells (contractile portions extend up the side of the cell body) characteristic of Ascarids, Spirurids, and Filarids), (b) Meromyarian (= section has only few muscle cells) platymyarian muscle cells (= contractile elements are all pressed to the hypodermis with an empty cell body above them) characteristic of Oxyurids and Strongyles except Metastrongyles. Hematoxylin and eosin (H&E) stain.

different stages; only the first stages contain live larvae amenable to anti-helminthic drugs [9]. Seizures occur when an immune reaction is elicited to larvae, feeding the debate on the respective roles of anticysticercal drugs (i.e. praziquentel and albendazole) and corticosteroids. Despite treatment, seizures can recur, even when CT scan lesions resolve.

Two forms of NCC are described: parenchymal NCC involving brain tissue and extraparenchymal NCC involving intraventricular spaces (most often the fourth ventricle), subarachnoid space, meninges, and spinal cord [10]. Parenchymal NCC is the most common type, affecting cerebral hemispheres, basal ganglia, brainstem, and cerebellum. Lesions are generally at the gray and white matter junctions, similar to other blood-borne infections because of the smaller caliber of blood vessels in these sites [11]. Five appearances are described on imaging, correlating with the different parasite stages: non-cystic, vesicular (viable parasite), colloidal vesicular (degenerating parasite), granular nodular (scolex is completely degenerated), and calcified (parasite is completely calcified) [12].

Parenchymal NCC generally has a better prognosis than the extraparenchymal form. Seizures and headaches occur, but they tend to disappear with time [13]. Psychiatric syndromes are rare, accounting for only 5% of NCC cases [14].

Extraparenchymal NCC is more variable. The parasite load is generally higher and cysticerci are larger (less restriction of growth) and irregular [15]. Severe complications are described with massive inflammation leading to arachnoiditis, obstruction of CSF flow causing hydrocephalus, optic and cranial nerves palsies leading to visual impairment, and vasculitis [15, 16]. Spinal NCC is rare and may be associated with motor and sensory dysfunction [17, 18].

The macroscopic appearance varies, from the presence of a single to several hundred cysts, measuring up to 1 cm, located in the brain (Figure 48.3a), meninges, or ventricles. Cysts may or may not be pedunculated, projecting into the ventricles or protruding from the cortical surface. When the parasite is viable, the cyst is delineated by a translucent wall and contains clear fluid. In larger cysts, a single yellowish spot representing the embryo can be observed on the cyst surface [4, 19]. When the parasite degenerates the fluid becomes turbid, the cyst wall is thicker and whitish/gray, and microscopy reveals three layers: an outer cuticle layer, a middle cellular layer, and an inner reticular layer. The scolex has a double row of hooklets and four suckers (Figure 48.3b–e) [7].

The inflammatory response in humans varies depending on the stage of the parasite. When cysticercus is viable, it can modulate the immune environment to survive, by forcing dendritic cells to adopt a tolerogenic phenotype [20]. Inflammation around the parasite is minimal, with rare lymphocytes, plasma cells, and eosinophils [21]. This immune evasion can last up to 10 years. When the parasite degenerates, inflammation is more severe; in the early stages there is a predominant T helper (Th)-1 response, characterized by natural killer (NK) cell infiltration associated with macrophages and T cells [22]. In the late stages, when the scolex has degenerated and calcified, granulomas with foreign body multinucleated giant cells are observed, associated with infiltrates of neutrophils and eosinophils, surrounded by dense connective tissue, with marked astrocytic gliosis and microglial cell proliferation [23].

Age seems to affect the sensitivity to cysticercosis. Children have fewer parasites than adults but a higher frequency of degenerating parasites [24–26], suggesting that potential protective immune mechanisms exist in children and that age-related factors may influence host immune responses [24].

The racemose form of extraparenchymal NCC has clusters of larger nonviable cysts, which exert local mass effects. The cysts have interconnected "bladders" of different sizes, and external small protrusions often lacking scolices. There is marked inflammation associated with fibrosis, sometimes leading to hydrocephalus [27–29].

In nonendemic areas, diagnosis and management of NCC are challenging because of unfamiliarity with the disease [30]. Clinical signs are non-specific (Table 48.2 [15, 31]). Neuroimaging with CT scan and MRI detects the number and location of cysticerci and, with experience, identify the parasite's evolutionary stage. MRI is the superior method but is often unavailable in endemic regions [15, 32, 33]. Antibody tests in serum are less sensitive and less specific [34]) than in CSF (sampling is difficult and painful [35]). Both are limited as late calcified lesions are not detected. A search for cysticerci outside the CNS may enable easier tissue sampling than brain biopsy.

Cerebral echinococcosis

Echinococcus granulosus is the tapeworm causing cystic echinococcosis (CE). Canids are the definitive hosts, harboring the worms in their intestines; herbivores or omnivores are intermediate hosts,

Helminth Infections of the CNS **Chapter 48**

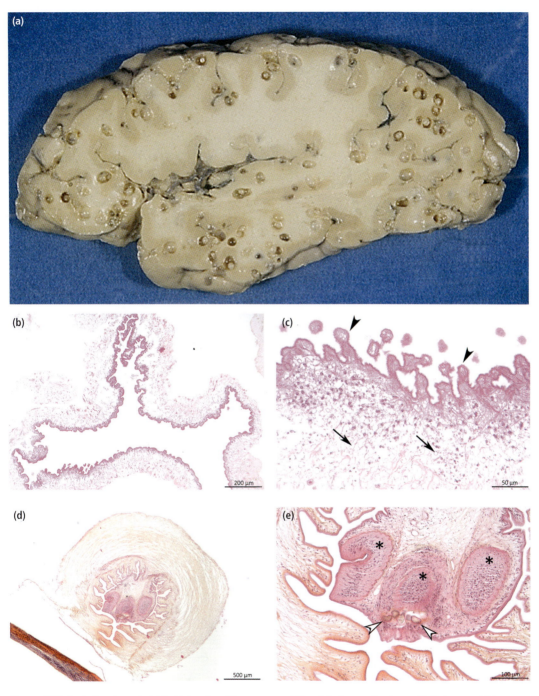

Figure 48.3 Cerebral cysticercosis. (a) Sagittal section of the cerebral hemisphere showing numerous small-sized cysts mainly located at the gray and white matter junction. (b) Cyst at a low magnification. (c) High magnification of a cyst wall with three distinct layers: an outer cuticular layer (black arrowheads), a middle cellular layer, and an inner reticular layer, containing a network of small canaliculi (black arrows). (d) Entire scolex. (e) High magnification of the scolex bearing a row of hooklets (white arrowheads) and suckers (black stars). Hematoxylin and eosin (H&E) stain.

Table 48.2 Diagnosis of NCC.

Absolute criteria (AbsC)	Major criteria (MajC)	Minor criteria (MinC)	Epidemiological criteria (EpiC)	Diagnosis
Histology: visualization of the parasite	**Neuroimaging:** lesions highly suggestive of NCC	**Neuroimaging:** lesions suggestive of NCC	Patient's country of origin endemic for NCC	**Definitive:** 1 AbsC OR
Neuroimaging: cysts + scolex	**Immunological assays:** detection of *T. solium* antibodies	**Clinical manifestations:** symptoms suggestive of NCC	Patient currently resides in NCC endemic area	2 MajC + 1 MinC/EpiC **Probable:** 1 MajC + 1 MinC
Fundoscopy: subretinal parasites	**Cystocidal drug therapy:** lesion resolution	**CSF ELISA:** positive detection of *T. solium* antibodies or antigens Evidence of cysticercosis outside the CNS	Patient frequently travels to endemic areas Patient household has had contact with *T. solium* infection	OR 1 MajC + 1MinC + 1 EpiC OR 3 MinC + 1 EpiC

CNS, central nervous system; CSF, cerebrospinal fluid; ELISA, enzyme-linked immunosorbent assay; NCC, neurocysticercosis.
Sources [15, 31].

harboring the cysts in different organs. Humans can become intermediate hosts by ingesting eggs dispersed by dogs on fur and in the environment [36]. Once ingested, eggs hatch in the intestine and enter the portal circulation. The liver is the most commonly affected organ, followed by the lungs. Once in the circulation, larvae may develop into hydatid cysts in other organs, including the brain [37]. Cysts containing multiple scolices develop slowly and are usually detected by imaging after five years of evolution. The cycle between dogs and cattle, particularly the dog-sheep association, explains the high prevalence of CE in sheep-breeding regions. This disease is worldwide because of travel and population movements, but it is endemic in the Mediterranean region, Middle East, and South America. Sporadic human cases are encountered in Australia, New Zealand, and the United States, particularly in people in close contact with sheep and cattle [38, 39].

Recent genetic studies revealed that *E. granulosus* is not a single species [40]. At least five cryptic species are described including the predominant *E. granulosus* (dog-sheep strain; 75% of CE) followed by *Echinococcus canadensis* (22% of CE). Cerebral CE cases with molecular identification are too rare to determine the causal agent. However, *E. canadensis* CE seems more prevalent in children [41]. Currently, species identification has no impact on diagnosis or treatment.

Around 1% of patients with *Echinococcus* develop a cerebral form. Depending on the location of the cyst(s), clinical symptoms include nausea, headache, vomiting, seizure, weakness, or visual disturbances; papilledema is usually present at the time of diagnosis [42]. Hydatid cysts may be found anywhere in the brain, but the middle cerebral artery territory (parietal lobe) is the most common site [43, 44]. Most cerebral cysts are acquired during childhood and grow silently at a rate of 1.5–10 cm per year [45] until their size is sufficient to increase intracranial pressure, compress the brain, and provoke symptoms. Consequently, 50–70% of cerebral echinococcosis cases are seen in children and young adults, potentially more frequently in males [42, 46]. Most patients present with a solitary cyst; multiple cysts (Figure 48.4a) are usually the result of cyst rupture after trauma or surgery and most cysts are not fertile. Ten percent of cases have hydatid cysts in other organs, particularly liver and lungs [42]. The recurrence rate is 30–40% for fertile cysts, and negligible for infertile cysts [47].

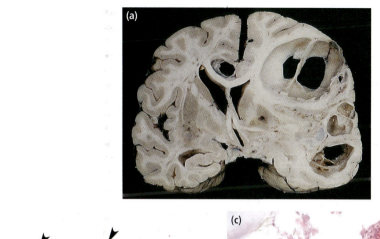

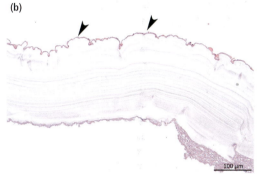
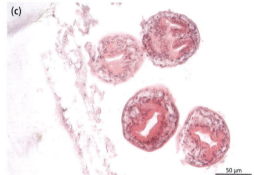

Figure 48.4 Cerebral echinococcosis. (a) Frontal section of the cerebral hemispheres at the level of the anterior commissure showing multiple cysts mainly involving the right side in the territory of the middle cerebral artery. A smaller cyst is present in the left cingulum. (b) Wall of a hydatid cyst, delineated by an inner translucent germinal layer (endocyst, black arrowheads) and a thick concentrically laminated outer layer (ectocyst). (c) From the germinal layer, scolices can be observed. Hematoxylin and eosin (H&E) stain.

Spinal involvement is rare, encountered in less than 1% of hydatid disease [36]; patients usually present with cauda equina or cord compression symptoms.

Diagnosis relies on serology and imaging. MRI is the most helpful in detecting cysts and outlining their relationship to adjacent structures [42]. In intracranial hydatid disease, the antibody response is usually absent or low, especially if the cyst is calcified [44] (calcification of hydatid cysts occur in <1% of cases [42]).

Histology is the most reliable method of diagnosis [42]; the differential diagnosis includes primarily cerebral cysticercosis [48], porencephalic or arachnoid cysts, cystic tumors, and pyogenic abscesses [42]. The hydatid cyst inner translucent germinal layer is called the endocyst (only in fertile cysts); the thick concentrically laminated outer layer is the ectocyst (Figure 48.4b). They are surrounded by the host fibrous capsule reaction, the pericyst, which contains blood vessels providing nutrients for the parasite via the ectocyst. From the germinal layer, scolices (embryonic forms; each scolex is ovoid, bears 32–40 hooklets), brood capsules (containing as many as 40 scolices), and daughter cysts are formed by endoproliferation (internal budding) [42, 44] (Figure 48.4c). Hydatid cysts may be sterile, lacking scolices.

Surgery is the treatment of choice to remove hydatid cysts, with pre- and postoperative medical treatment with albendazole to reduce recurrence and sterilize the cyst wall [38, 49]. Dowling's technique [38, 50] is mainly used for intact cyst excision, which can be difficult in large thin-walled cysts. Rupture during surgery is estimated to occur in 28% of cases [44], sometimes leading to anaphylactic shock.

Coenurosis

Human coenurosis is caused by infection with the coenurus (metacestode or larval stage) of several *Taenia*. Only *Taenia multiceps* coenurus infects the CNS, displaying a predilection for the CNS and eye [51]. Domestic and wild canids (i.e. dogs, foxes) are the definitive hosts. Diverse herbivores including sheep, rodents, rabbits, horses, and cattle are the intermediate hosts, with sheep being the most important. Coenurosis is mainly distributed in sheep-breeding areas of the Americas, parts of Europe, and Africa. In sheep, the disease is known as "gid" or "staggers," and the coenurus is located in the CNS, causing circling, ataxia, incoordination, paralysis, blindness, and coma [52]. Very few human cases have been described, mostly in Africa, but also in Europe, South America, United States, and Canada. Humans, especially children, become infected by ingesting eggs shed in the feces of a definitive host. After ingestion, eggs release oncospheres that penetrate the intestinal wall to enter the bloodstream and then reach target organs such as the eye, brain, and spinal cord [52].

There may be an interval of several years between egg ingestion and the first symptoms; symptoms and signs vary depending on the site of the cysts and include headache, vomiting, papilledema as a result of raised intracranial pressure, and other neurological deficits [52]. Cysts may be single or multiple, located in the ventricles (usually the fourth) attached to the wall or free-floating, or in the CSF pathways, often associated with obstructive hydrocephalus, chronic meningitis, and arachnoiditis.

The cyst size ranges from 2 mm to several cm. Differential diagnoses include NCC and CE. Features that help in their distinction are (i) the *coenurus* wall, which is thick, opaque, and milky white, without a laminar concentric structure [19], and (ii) cysts, which are filled with clear fluid containing up to 500 scolices [4] (Figure 48.5).

Diagnosis is based on imaging, most often CT scan or pathologic analysis following surgical removal. Serology has a limited value because of shared antigens between *T. multiceps* and *E. granulosus* [52]. The prognosis of coenurosis is always serious, and the primary treatment is surgery to remove the parasite and allow precise identification.

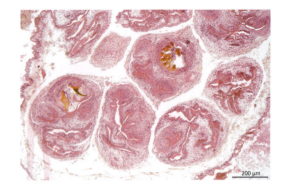

Figure 48.5 Cerebral coenurosis. High magnification of scolices with brownish hooklets. Hematoxylin and eosin (H&E) stain.

Sparganosis

Sparganosis is a zoonosis caused by infestation with a plerocercoid larvae (spargana) of the tapeworm belonging to the genus *Spirometra*, a member of the Diphyllobothriidae family [53]; three main species infest humans: *S. mansoni* (or *Spirometra erinaceieuropaei*), *Spirometra mansonoides*, and *Spirometra proliferum*.

The adult cestode (60–110 cm in length) lives in the small intestine of several mammalian carnivorous hosts, mainly dogs and cats. Eggs shed in their feces into freshwater are ingested by copepods (small crustaceans; first-intermediate hosts). Copepods are ingested by mice, frogs, and snakes (second-intermediate hosts) and develop into plerocercoid larvae. Humans rarely harbor adult *Spirometra* worms and act as a second-intermediate host. Human infestation follows: (i) ingestion of water contaminated by copepods, (ii) ingestion of raw second-intermediate hosts (frogs or snakes), (iii) application of a poultice of raw mammalian flesh onto human wounds and mucous membranes and (iv) ingestion of a plerocercoid larva through carriers [54]. In humans, the spargana can invade the brain, eyes, spinal cord, and many subcutaneous tissues.

Cerebral sparganosis is rare but has been reported worldwide, mainly in China, South Korea, Japan, and Thailand [55–58], less frequently in the Americas and Australia and very rarely in Europe [59]. Despite its rarity, the disease seems more frequent in children, young persons, and males [60]. The parasite can survive in the human body from 5 to 20 years [59].

In humans, clinical signs depend on the site of the lesions. The most commonly observed symptoms include seizures, hemiparesis, headache, sensory disturbances, confusion, weakness [57, 61], and cerebral hemorrhages [62].

Macroscopically, the parasite is white and flat, measuring approximately 1–50 cm long and 1–2 mm wide. Microscopically it has a dense eosinophilic integument with microvilli, contains bundles of smooth muscle and excretory ducts in a myxoid matrix, and is surrounded by dense inflammation with foreign body type granulomas [63] (Figure 48.6). An important particular diagnostic feature is that the live sparganum migrates with an undulating motion, forming a tunnel [64]. Migration of the parasite is also partly responsible for clinical signs changing between the initial attack and hospital admission [61].

Diagnosis is based on imaging, MRI being superior to CT. Demonstration of the tunnel sign on the postcontrast MRI, representing the moving track of the parasite, and granulomas are characteristic findings. Pathologic diagnosis can be made following surgical removal of the parasite. Serology is of limited value because of cross-reactivity with other Cestodes [59]. The differential diagnosis includes brain tumors and infestation by other tapeworm larvae. Histology can differentiate sparganosis by its solid noncavitated body, hooked scolices, and absence of a bladder wall (Figure 48.6) [7]. There is no specific medical treatment; the best available treatment is complete surgical removal of larvae because a retained scolex can lead to recurrence [53].

Infection by trematodes

Schistosomiasis

Schistosomiasis, caused by Trematodes of the genus *Schistosoma*, is socioeconomically the second-most devastating parasitic disease worldwide. Around 240 million people in 77 countries are affected, and 800 million are currently at risk for the disease [65]. Humans are the definitive hosts. They release eggs in feces or urine, which can be used for diagnosis; after hatching in freshwater, ciliated embryos (miracidia) infect the intermediate host, a species-specific aqueous snail in which they develop into cercariae. Cercariae released in water (infective stage), can swim, and are responsible for human infection; they penetrate human skin, reach the bloodstream, mature within the portal vasculature, and migrate to the target organs (i.e. gastrointestinal tract or bladder according to the species) [66].

Three main *Schistosoma* species infect the human CNS: *Schistosoma hematobium*, *Schistosoma mansoni*, and *Schistosoma japonicum*. Rare cases are described for other *Schistosoma* species, e.g. *Schistosoma mekongi* [67]; see appendix. *Schistosoma* are snail-species–specific and thus frequently geographically limited to tropical Africa, Near East and South America (*S. mansoni*), Africa and Middle East (*S. hematobium*), and Asia (*S. japonicum*) [68]. Cases are increasing in Europe, having been imported from endemic areas via immigration and travel.

CNS infection is rare and is due to ectopic dissemination of worms or eggs via the bloodstream, the leading hypothesis being via retrograde flow into Batson's vertebral epidural venous plexus [69]. *S. japonicum* typically infects the brain; *S. hematobium* and *S. mansoni* infect the spinal cord [68]. These differences can be explained partly by the egg morphology: *S. mansoni* and *S. hematobium*

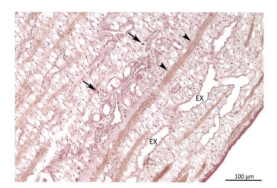

Figure 48.6 Sparganosis. High magnification of *Sparganum* plerocecoid larva, characterized by a pale myxoid matrix, and calcareous corpuscles (black arrows) with branches of the excretory system (EX) and numerous longitudinal smooth muscle fibers (black arrowheads), extending throughout the entire parasite. Scolex is absent in contrast to Cysticerci. Hematoxylin and eosin (H&E) stain.

are large (110–150 μm long and 40–60 μm wide), have protruding spines, and are retained in the lower spinal cord and rarely affect the brain. *S. japonicum* eggs are smaller and shed in much greater numbers; they reach the brain and cross the blood–brain barrier (BBB) more easily [70, 71]. Clinical signs appear soon after infection or may be delayed for months or years [72–74]; they include headache, language dysfunction, acute encephalopathy, epilepsy, visual disturbance, motor weakness, hemiparesis, or paralysis when lesions are in the spinal cord. In *S. hematobium*-endemic areas, spinal schistosomiasis is the leading cause of spinal cord injury [66, 75]. The host's inflammatory reaction certainly plays an important role in explaining the variability in clinical signs.

Lesions of cerebral schistosomiasis can be detected in cerebral hemispheres, cerebellum, or brainstem [66]. Cerebral and spinal schistosomiasis are characterized by necrosis and intense granulomatous inflammation, associated with the presence of eggs in the lesions. The position of the parasite spine on the eggshell is pathognomonic for each species: terminal for *S. hematobium*, lateral for *S. mansoni*, and absent or inconspicuous for *S. japonicum* (Figure 48.7). *S. mansoni* ova can interact with endothelial cells, provoking inflammation with necrotizing vasculitis and thrombosis [70].

For diagnosis, a history of travel to endemic areas and exposure to contaminated freshwater (e.g. by swimming or boating) is an important clue. Histology of involved tissues is the gold standard for diagnosis. Observation of the spine and positive staining with Ziehl-Neelsen for *S. mansoni* are useful, but serology with ELISA and MRI imaging are also helpful.

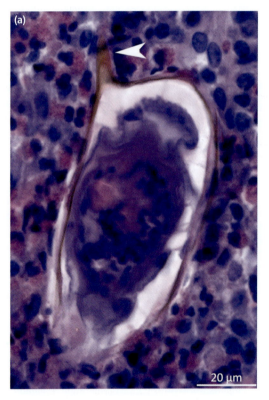
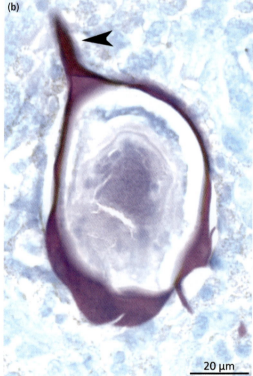

Figure 48.7 Schistosomiasis. (a) *Schistosoma mansoni* egg, displaying a lateral spine (arrowhead) and containing the miracidium. Hematoxylin and eosin (H&E) stain. (b) Eggshell positively stained by Ziehl-Neelsen; arrowhead shows lateral spine. Ziehl-Neelsen stain.

Paragonimiasis

Paragonimiasis is a foodborne parasitic zoonosis, endemic in many parts of Asia, Africa, and South America, and caused by ingestion of various fluke species of the genus *Paragonimus*. *Paragonimus* spp. are common parasites of crustacean-eating mammals. The adults live in the lungs and lay eggs, which develop into miracidia when they reach freshwater. Then, they penetrate various species of aquatic snails or crustaceans to produce larvae (metacercariae). Human infection occurs via ingestion of raw or undercooked freshwater crabs or crayfish, containing metacercariae. Metacercariae excyst in the small intestine, penetrate the abdominal cavity wall, and then migrate to the lungs, the principal target, in three to eight weeks.

More than 50 different species are described; 9 are known to cause infections in humans. *P. westermani* is the most important. About 23 million people are infected in the world, with 293 million people at risk [76, 77]. The main differential diagnosis to be excluded is tuberculosis.

Immature flukes rarely migrate to extrapulmonary sites including brain, spinal cord, liver, spleen, ovary, and subcutaneous tissue. Cerebral paragonimiasis is the most common and most serious extrapulmonary manifestation [78, 79], accounting for 2–27% of all *Paragonimus* infections [80]. Early symptoms include fever, headache, vomiting, seizures, and neck stiffness. Chronic symptoms include seizures, personality change, visual disturbance, chronic headache, motor weakness, and sensory deficit. Epilepsy is described in 37% of patients, probably because of marked inflammatory reaction to massive amounts of parasite protein released in degenerative lesions [79].

Macro- and microscopic appearances depend on the developmental stages: (i) the infiltrative or exudative stage causes meningoencephalitis and early necrotizing granulomas; (ii) then large well-encapsulated cystic granulomas form, with central necrosis containing eggs, surrounded by fibrosis with foreign body granulomas; and (iii) the late stage is characterized by cystic granulomas surrounded by a sclerotic layer because of organization of granulomas and calcification [81]. In the lesions, large $80 \times 50\,\mu m$ oval-shape unembryonated eggs can be found with apical opercula, a double shell, and no spicules (in contrast to *Schistosoma* eggs). An adult worm is only detected in the brain in about 10% of cases [82].

Diagnosis is based on clinical data, results of CT or MRI imaging in the lung, which can be mistaken for lung cancer or tuberculosis, serology, detection of eggs or the worm in sputum or bronchoalveolar lavage, and histopathology.

Infection by nematodes

Angiostrongylosis

Neuroangiostrongylosis is the result of the migration of larvae of *A. cantonensis*, also known as the rat lungworm, to the brain and is the most common cause of eosinophilic meningitis in humans [83]. Twenty-one *Angiostrongylus* spp. are currently recognized, but only *A. cantonensis* and *A. costaricensis* are known to be pathogenic for humans, the latter being responsible for human abdominal angiostrongylosis without CNS involvement [84]. Seventeen rodent species can be definitive hosts for *A. cantonensis*. They become infected by third-stage larvae when eating intermediate or paratenic hosts [83]. Larvae penetrate the intestinal wall and reach the bloodstream to be dispersed. In the brain, they molt in the subarachnoid space to become young adults (fifth-stage larvae) and then leave the CNS via the circulation into the pulmonary arteries. There, adults reach sexual maturity and females produce eggs, which hatch in terminal branches of the pulmonary arteries liberating first-stage larvae. These larvae penetrate alveoli and migrate to the pharynx where they are swallowed to finish their course in the rat's feces [85]. Intermediate hosts, mostly mollusks, get infected by ingesting rat feces or by active penetration of first-stage larvae through their tegument [86]. Paratenic hosts, such as lizards, frogs, freshwater shrimps, fish and crabs, eat mollusks and the third-stage larvae they contain. Humans are accidental hosts and become infected by consuming undercooked paratenic and intermediate hosts or fresh products contaminated with mollusks, all containing third-stage larvae [83].

This disease is traditionally endemic to Eastern Asia [87] but has extended to Southeast Asia, especially to Thailand, Pacific Islands, South and Central America, the Caribbean, United States, Australia, and even Europe. In total, 30 countries have reported neuroangiostrongylosis cases since the first identification in 1945 [88–94].

Clinical manifestations are mostly the result of increased intracranial pressure because of vasodilation in the subarachnoid space and brain parenchyma, decreased resorption of CSF, or brain edema [95, 96]. Patients have headache, neck stiffness, paraesthesia, muscle weakness, fever, vomiting, and nausea. In rare cases, severe neurological sequelae may appear, including coma, convulsion, epilepsy, mental impairment, poor memory, and even death [95, 97, 98]. Encephalitic angiostrongylosis is a rare generally fatal manifestation. Myelitis, sacral myeloradiculitis, polyradiculoneuritis, cerebral hemorrhage, and ocular symptoms have also been reported [83, 95, 99].

As clinical signs are not specific, diagnosis is difficult and relies on epidemiologic data, imaging, eosinophilia in CSF or blood, and increased protein concentration in CSF and serology, although no consensus exists [100–103]. It is extremely rare to find larvae in patients' CSF [83]; therefore, their absence cannot exclude neuroangiostrongylosis.

The differential diagnosis includes eosinophilic meningitis (e.g. gnathostomiasis, schistosomiasis, cysticercosis, toxocariasis, and hydatidosis), fungal infections (e.g. coccidioidomycosis, aspergillosis), bacterial infections (e.g. neurosyphilis, Rocky mountain spotted fever), viral infections (e.g. Coxsackievirus, Arenaviridae), neoplasms (e.g. chronic eosinophilic leukemia, mastocystosis), or drug effects (e.g. ibuprofen, ciprofloxacin, gentamicin, and rifampicin) [96, 104].

CNS lesions are due to migration tracts or inflammation. Macroscopic examination of brain and spinal cord is usually devoid of significant lesions [98, 105]. It is often impossible to correlate the larva migration tracts with the observed clinical symptoms [106].

The main histological changes in humans include eosinophilic and lymphocytic or plasmacytic meningitis, multiple microcavities, tortuous tracts and hemorrhages surrounded by inflammation and necrosis, granulomatous inflammation surrounding dead larvae especially in meninges, nerve roots, blood vessels, and perivascular spaces, and nonspecific vascular changes such as thrombosis and aneurysm formation [107, 108]. The lesions tend to be more severe in the cortex and hippocampus [109]. *A. cantonensis* is a nematode (see Figure 48.1 for the morphological criteria) with a thin polymyarian and coelomyarian musculature, typical intestine with microvillar border, and a uterus with thin-shelled ovoid eggs. First-stage larvae have a distinct kinked tail and small dorsal spines.

Without therapy, only few patients with mild disease recover spontaneously. Treatment is aimed at reducing inflammation and intracranial pressure, eradicating worms, and managing pain. Repeated lumbar punctures associated with analgesics (ibuprofen), mannitol or glycerol or fructose, and corticosteroids may be used to reduce intracranial pressure [95, 96, 110, 111] and limit headaches. Antihelminthics such as albendazole, mebendazole, flubendazole, and ivermectin are often used, although their efficacy is controversial [95]. Combined corticosteroid and antihelminthic therapy seems more effective [112, 113].

Gnathostomiasis

Gnathostomiasis is a foodborne zoonotic infection caused by *Gnathostoma* spp. nematodes. At least 13 species have been described. The most important is *Gnathostoma spinigerum,* but *Gnathostoma doloresi, Gnathostoma Hispidum,* and *Gnathostoma nipponica* have also been reported in human infections [114]. Adult worms reside in the gastric wall of the natural definitive host (e.g. pigs, cats, dogs, wild animals) and unembryonated eggs are passed in the feces. When the eggs hatch, larvae are ingested by a first-intermediate host (i.e. small crustacean), then by a second-intermediate host (i.e. fish, frog, snake), and eventually by the definitive host. The disease is endemic in Southeast Asia (most cases are reported from Thailand), South and Central America, and some areas of Africa [6].

Humans are accidental hosts and become infected after eating raw or undercooked freshwater fish, frogs, birds, or reptiles containing third-stage larvae or by drinking water contaminated by crustaceans. The main clinical symptoms are migratory subcutaneous swellings with eosinophilia. The parasite rarely reaches adult form and the lesions are the result of larval migration [115]. Once ingested, third-stage larvae penetrate the gastrointestinal wall and then spread to any organ. The brain and spinal cord can be directly reached by invading the neural foramina at the skull base or along nerve roots through the intervertebral foramina [115]. Once in the spinal cord, larvae can ascend and reach the brain; the secretion of matrix metalloproteinases plays a key role in the pathogenesis of *Gnathostoma* [116]. Cerebral gnathostomiasis is rare (1%) [117].

Clinical signs of severe headache, increased intracranial pressure, seizures, drowsiness, and coma vary depending on the larva migration [117]. The disease is severe; mortality rates from 7 to 12% have been reported [118].

Macroscopic lesions reflect mechanical damage because of larval migration: hemorrhagic tracts in the brain and spinal cord can be seen at autopsy [119] with subarachnoid hemorrhage and aneurysm. Microscopic lesions consist of necrotic tracts, edema, hemorrhages, and eosinophilic meningitis.

Diagnosis is based on clinical history, serological tests, CSF analysis, and imaging. The main differential diagnosis is *A. cantonensis*, which rarely causes severe disease with prominent spinal or cerebral involvement.

Neurotoxocariosis (visceral larva migrans)

Visceral larva migrans is caused by the migration of second-stage larvae of animal nematodes such as *Toxocara canis*, *Toxocara cati*, *Baylisascaris procyonis*, *Capillaria hepatica*, *Ascaris suum*, and *Ancylostoma* spp. in human viscera. In humans, migration is abortive because these nematodes are adapted to non-human hosts. *Toxocara canis* is a parasite of dogs and other canids, has a worldwide distribution, and is the most frequent agent that causes neurotoxocarosis [120, 121].

Humans are accidental hosts and get infected by ingesting embryonated eggs from soil via geophagy (eating soil), onychophagy (nail-biting), contaminated hands or consumption of raw fruits, vegetables, meat, and offals from paratenic hosts (i.e. birds, rabbits, giblets) [122–126]. The eggs hatch in the small intestine, liberating immature larvae [125], which penetrate the mucosa, enter the portal circulation toward the liver, lungs, and left heart to be disseminated via the bloodstream to muscles, optic nerves, and CNS in rare cases. Larvae do not develop to adults in humans [127]. The exact prevalence is difficult to assess because many infections are asymptomatic or undiagnosed. Children may be over-represented because of their tendency to put their fingers in their mouths or their playing habits [128]. Estimated seroprevalence is around 2–5% in urban areas, 14–37% in rural areas in the United States and Europe, reaching 39–93% in tropical regions [124, 126, 127, 129–132].

Patients usually present with a combination of general signs (i.e. hyperthermia, anorexia, body weight loss, malaise) with multiple organ involvement (i.e. lung, liver, eye, gastrointestinal tract, skin, heart, joints, and CNS) [122, 133, 134]. Symptoms depend on the parasite load, host sensitivity, affected tissue, previous exposure to larvae, and persistent sources of contamination [122, 135]. Neurotoxocariosis may manifest as eosinophilic meningitis [136], encephalitis or meningoencephalitis with or without vasculitis [137, 138], arachnoiditis, spinal cord lesions [139], and cognitive disorder [129].

The diagnosis is based on a combination of compatible clinical and imaging signs, presence of risk factors, eosinophilia in CSF or blood, high titers of antibodies against *Toxocara* spp. in CSF or blood, improvement after antihelmintic therapy and, most of all, absence of any alternative diagnosis [124].

Larvae are rarely present on histological sections; if present, they elicit a perivascular granulomatous inflammation. In most cases, only necrotic debris and eosinophils are found in the migration tracts, sometimes associated with vasculitis. Lesions are predominantly found in cerebral or cerebellar white matter [131, 140, 141].

There is no consensus on neurotoxocariosis therapy. Albendazole alone or with corticosteroids was described [127, 141, 142]. The best marker for post-treatment follow-up is the blood eosinophil count [126, 135]. Total recovery without any therapy has been reported [143, 144].

Neurotrichinosis

Neurotrichinosis, also called neurotrichinellosis, is caused by the migration of larvae of *Trichinella* spp. to the CNS. Transmission in animals is assumed to be through predatory consumption or scavenging of tissue from an infected animal. Nine species and three genotypes have been documented in the genus *Trichinella*. *Trichinella spiralis* is by far the most common species responsible for neurotrichinosis, followed by *Trichinella britovi;* there are rare reports of infection by *Trichinella madurelli, Trichinella pseudospiralis, Trichinella Nativa,* and *Trichinella nelson* [145]. Humans get infected by consuming undercooked contaminated meat (mainly pork, horse, and game). As many as 10 000 cases occur every year and the death rate can reach 0.2%. Fifty-five different countries have reported indigenous cases [146]. The incidence appears to depend on culinary habits. Trichinellosis often appears as outbreaks following consumption of infected meat from a common source, which is not always identified. Wild boar meat is currently the second-most important source after uncooked or undercooked pork. Outbreaks involving hunters and their families have been reported worldwide [147].

The life cycle of *Trichinella* spp. involves many mammal, bird, and reptile species. The gravid female worm settles in the intestinal mucosa, produces first-stage larvae that directly migrate into lymphatic and blood vessels to be transported to highly oxygenated muscles that they penetrate. Myocytes act as "nurse cells," allowing parasites to develop into infective muscle-stage larvae without molting, and they may survive locally for years (Figure 48.8). Calcification of the collagen capsule and the nurse cell may occur This state of arrested development is maintained until ingested by another host, in which gastric digestion liberates larvae, which then invade duodenal mucosa [148].

Neurotrichinosis is a rare complication. In the acute phase, patients exhibit disturbed consciousness, somnolence, apathy, unequal pupils, facial nerve paralysis, disorientation, memory and behavioral disturbance, and oculomotor dysfunction [145, 149].

The diagnosis is based on epidemiology, clinical manifestations, laboratory and serological tests, and imaging [6]. Larvae are rarely found on CNS histological sections; when present, they elicit a granulomatous and eosinophilic meningoencephalitis, glial hyperplasia, small hemorrhagic foci in white matter or arteriolar, and capillary thromboses with small ischemic lesions. Lesions may be found in gray and white matter, mainly in the cerebellum, pons, and spinal cord [150].

Treatment with corticosteroids is said to improve vasculitis-related symptoms and prevent complications; they should be combined with antihelminthics such as albendazole [146, 149]. The poor efficacy of treatment underlines the importance of prevention through mandatory veterinary examination of meat from potentially infected animals; Commission Implementing Regulation [EU] 2015/1375 of 10 August 2015 lays down rules on official controls for *Trichinella* in meat.

Filariases

Filariases rarely involve the CNS; a cerebral effect was described for *Loa* and only recently suggested for *Onchocerca volvulus*. On microscopy, adult Filarids display ridges, bosses, or annulations on their cuticle, lateral internal ridges, coelomyarian polymyarian muscles, and a very small intestine (Figure 48.9). Microfilariae can be detected in their uterus and in tissues [7].

Loa is a filarian parasite distributed in Central Africa (Nigeria, Cameroon, Central Africa Republic, Republic of Congo, Equatorial Guinea, Gabon) and transmitted by tabanid flies of the genus *Chrysops*. The adult worm migrates throughout subcutaneous tissue, occasionally crossing eye conjunctiva, moving to the eyeball, at a speed of <1 cm/min. Red itchy swellings ("Calabar edema") are suggestive of the disease. The microfilariae circulate in peripheral blood and are ingested by

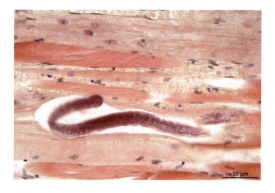

Figure 48.8 Skeletal muscle trichinosis. *Trichinella spiralis* larva in a skeletal myocyte (nurse cell). Hematoxylin and eosin (H&E) stain.

Helminth Infections of the CNS Chapter 48

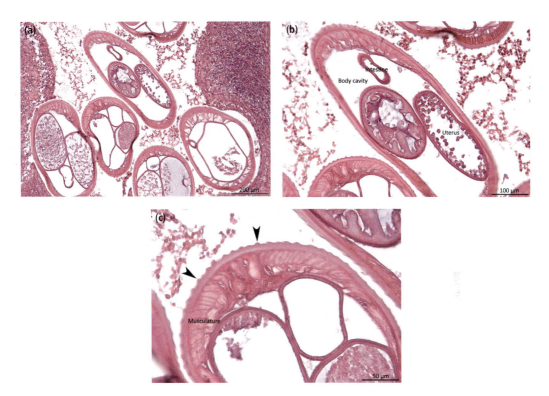

Figure 48.9 Filariasis. Nematodes displaying bosses on their cuticle (arrowheads), coelomyarian polymyarian muscles and a very small intestine: Filarids. Hematoxylin and eosin (H&E) stain.

the Chrysops to complete the life cycle. Patients with large numbers of microfilariae in blood are susceptible to severe adverse reactions when treatment causes extensive larval lysis. These reactions have led to cessation of mass treatment with ivermectin for the elimination of onchocerciasis or lymphatic filariasis because ivermectin is also active against *Loa* larvae [151]. Visceral lesions occur and encephalitis and meningitis has been described especially after diethylcarbamazine (DEC) and ivermectin treatment [152–154]. Histological lesions are characterized by occlusions of small blood vessels by microfilariae, associated with a mainly perivascular inflammatory reaction with microglial nodules.

Onchocerca volvulus, responsible for "river blindness," affects 17.7 million people worldwide in 34 countries (Africa, Middle East, South and Central America) [155]. Although microfilariae have never been seen in the CNS, there is increasing evidence that *O. volvulus* can be associated with epilepsy [156].

Strongyloidiasis

Strongyloidiasis, caused by the nematode *Strongyloides stercoralis,* affects 30–100 million people in 70 countries [157], mainly in tropical regions, but it can also occur in temperate climates. Human infection occurs when filariform larvae present in contaminated soil penetrate the skin, mostly in the feet. Larvae enter the venous circulation to reach the lungs and then the trachea and pharynx; they are swallowed and on reaching the small intestine they mature to adults and release eggs. After hatching, larvae are excreted in the feces. Oro-fecal infection is also described [158]. The peculiar property of this worm, compared with other nematodes, is that larvae reinvade the intestine or perianal skin, initiating an "autoinfection cycle," enabling persistence of *Strongyloides* infection for decades (up to 75 years in one case report [159]) and explaining the rises and falls of blood eosinophil counts.

People who are immunocompetent can control the disease, which remains mild or asymptomatic.

In contrast, in patients who are chronically infected and immunocompromised, a life-threatening syndrome can occur through "hyperinfection," characterized by overproliferation of larvae and dissemination to ectopic sites including the brain, associated with translocation of enteric bacteria that can cause sepsis [158]. It is extremely important to suspect the diagnosis and to prophylactically treat the infection, even if asymptomatic, in patients known to be at risk of strongyloidiasis reactivation.

Neuropathological findings in *S. stercoralis* infection include presence of larvae in the subarachnoid space [160], brain micro-infarcts [161], brain abscesses [162], necrotic foci, and granulomas with intraparenchymal parasitic larvae or larvae without an inflammatory reaction [163].

Genetic predisposition

Very few studies focus on the genetic susceptibility to CNS helminth infestations; most relate to the susceptibility to develop symptoms in NCC. In endemic areas, rarely more than 10% of infected people develop symptoms [164, 165], which vary from mild to life-threatening [166].

HLA genes [167], toll-like receptor 4 (TLR4) or intercellular adhesion molecule-1 (ICAM-1) [168] are directly linked to immunity. Regarding TLR4, Asp299Gly and Thr399Ile polymorphisms have been associated with symptomatic NCC, by modulating the Th-1/Th-2 axis [169]. Th-2 type immune response seems to favor asymptomatic disease, while a switch to Th-1 type leads to the development of symptoms [170].

Gluthatione S-transferase GST is a critical protein for protection from reactive oxygen species. Its genotypes GSTM1 and GSTT1 are associated with a higher susceptibility and increased risk for symptomatic disease in NCC, whereas GSTM3 and GSTP1 are protective [171].

Many other factors play a role in NCC symptom expression, including genetics, age, gender, immune status, and other geographic, occupational, and socioeconomic factors [172–174]. Apart from the latter, equivalent risk factors seem to predispose to neurotoxocariosis [175].

Animal models

Several models have been used to study NCC: different host species, routes of administration, infecting stages, and species. Up to now, none has recreated CNS infestation from oro-fecal contamination as occurs in humans.

The use of oncospheres of *T. solium* is difficult in rodents because the cysts are too large for rodent brains and could cause severe mass effect and inflammation [176]. Porcine models have been developed. Like humans, pigs are an intermediate host for *T. solium*, offering interesting perspectives for research on NCC pathophysiology and therapy.

Alternatives to infections with *T. solium* in rodents were developed. *Taenia crassiceps* and *Mesocestoides corti* can be injected intracranially at the metacestode stage, which is different to the oncosphere stage occuring in the natural disease in humans.

Hydrocephalus is a severe complication of NCC and is difficult to manage, mostly requiring surgery. Filho et al. proposed a model of NCC with hydrocephalus by suboccipital injection of parasites directly into rat cisterns [177].

For *Toxocara canis* research, rodents, particularly mice are used because they are a natural host, have similar manifestations to humans [178], and are useful to study neurotoxocariosis.

The gerbil may be an efficient model for neuroangiostrongylosis. Although they manifest more severe symptoms than humans, in the early phase of infection the immune responses are similar [179]. Mice and rats may also be used; BALB/c mice being more sensitive than rats or C57BL/10J and C57BL/6J mice [179–182].

For Trematodes, models of *S. mansoni* and *S. japonicum* infestation were described in mice [183] and rabbits [184], respectively.

Conclusions

CNS helminth infections are a worldwide health problem with large endemic areas and huge populations at risk, increasing because of immunosuppression and international travel. Diagnosis is difficult because clinical signs are non-specific, and tests are poorly specific. Histology is important for parasite identification, but biopsies of CNS are frequently impossible or very small, and the parasite may be absent in the stained sections. New improved diagnostic procedures including imaging and biomarkers should be considered particularly in endemic areas, to enable earlier more effective therapy.

References

1. Cox, F.E.G. (2000). History of human parasitology. *Clin. Microbiol. Rev.* 15: 595–612.
2. Crompton, D.W. (1999). How much human helminthiasis is there in the world? *J. Parasitol.* 85: 397–403.
3. Finsterer, J. and Auer, H. (2013). Parasitoses of the human central nervous system. *J. Helminthol.* 87: 257–270.
4. Jones, T., Hunt, R., and King, N. (1997). *Diseases Caused by Parasitic Helminths and Arthropods. Veterinary Pathology*, 6e, 1392. Baltimore: Lippincott Williams & Wilkins.
5. Lv, S., Zhang, Y., Steinmann, P. et al. (2010). Helminth infections of the central nervous system occurring in Southeast Asia and the Far East. *Adv. Parasitol.* 72: 351–408.
6. Dzikowiec, M., Góralska, K., and Błaszkowska, J. (2017). Neuroinvasions caused by parasites. *Ann. Parasitol.* 63: 243–253.
7. Gardiner, C.H. (1999). Identification of Metazoan and Protozoan. Paper presented at the 46th Annual AFIP/ARP. Washington DC (10 August 1999).
8. Coyle, C.M. (2014). Neurocysticercosis: an update. *Curr. Infect. Dis. Rep.* 16: 437.
9. Baird, R.A., Wiebe, S., Zunt, J.R. et al. (2013). Evidence-based guideline: treatment of parenchymal neurocysticercosis: report of the Guideline Development Subcommittee of the American Academy of Neurology. *Neurology* 80: 1424–1429.
10. Fogang, Y.F., Savadogo, A.A., Camara, M. et al. (2015). Managing neurocysticercosis: challenges and solutions. *Int. J. Gen. Med.* 8: 333–344.
11. Lerner, A., Shiroishi, M.S., Zee, C.-S. et al. (2012). Imaging of neurocysticercosis. *Neuroimaging Clin. N. Am.* 22: 659–676.
12. Escobar, A., Aruffo, C., Cruz-Sánchez, F., and Cervos-Navarro, J. (1985). Neuropathologic findings in neurocysticercosis. *Arch. Neurobiol. (Madr.)* 48: 151–156.
13. Singhi, P. and Suthar, R. (2015). Neurocysticercosis. *Indian J. Pediatr.* 82: 166–171.
14. Carabin, H., Ndimubanzi, P.C., Budke, C.M. et al. (2011). Clinical manifestations associated with neurocysticercosis: a systematic review. *PLoS Negl. Trop. Dis.* 5: e1152.
15. Gripper, L.B. and Welburn, S.C. (2017). Neurocysticercosis infection and disease-A review. *Acta Trop.* 166: 218–224.
16. Kimura-Hayama, E.T., Higuera, J.A., Corona-Cedillo, R. et al. (2010). Neurocysticercosis: radiologic-pathologic correlation. *Radiographics* 30: 1705–1719.
17. Del Brutto, O.H. (2012). Neurocysticercosis: a review. *Sci. World J.* 2012: 159821.
18. Callacondo, D., Garcia, H.H., Gonzales, I. et al. (2012). High frequency of spinal involvement in patients with basal subarachnoid neurocysticercosis. *Neurology* 78: 1394–1400.
19. Lucas, S., Bell, J., and Chimelli, L. (2008). Parasitic and fungal infections. In: *Greenfield's Neuropathology*, 8e (eds. S. Love, D.N. Louis and D.W. Ellison), 1473–1487. Taylor and Francis Group.
20. Adalid-Peralta, L., Arce-Sillas, A., Fragoso, G. et al. (2013). Cysticerci drive dendritic cells to promote in vitro and in vivo Tregs differentiation. *Clin. Dev. Immunol.* 2013: 981468.
21. Fleury, A., Cardenas, G., Adalid-Peralta, L. et al. (2016). Immunopathology in Taenia solium neurocysticercosis. *Parasite Immunol.* 38: 147–157.
22. Restrepo, B.I., Llaguno, P., Sandoval, M.A. et al. (1998). Analysis of immune lesions in neurocysticercosis patients: central nervous system response to helminth appears Th1-like instead of Th2. *J. Neuroimmunol.* 89: 64–72.
23. Escobar, A. (1983). The pathology of neurocysticercosis. In: *Cysticercosis of the Central Nervous System* (eds. E. Palacios, J. Rodriguez-Carbajal and J. Taveras), 27–54. Charles C Thomas: Springfield.
24. Del Brutto, V.J., Del Brutto, O.H., Ochoa, E., and García, H.H. (2012). Single parenchymal brain cysticercus: relationship between age of patients and evolutive stage of parasites. *Neurol. Res.* 34: 967–970.
25. Singh, G., Rajshekhar, V., Murthy, J.M.K. et al. (2010). A diagnostic and therapeutic scheme for a solitary cysticercus granuloma. *Neurology* 75: 2236–2245.
26. Sáenz, B., Ramírez, J., Aluja, A. et al. (2008). Human and porcine neurocysticercosis: differences in the distribution and developmental stages of cysticerci. *Tropical Med. Int. Health* 13: 697–702.
27. Saini, A.G., Vyas, S., and Singhi, P. (2017). Racemose neurocysticercosis. *J. Infect. Public Health* 10: 884–885.

28. Gupta, P., Agrawal, M., Sinha, V.D., and Gupta, A. (2015). Intraventricular racemose type neurocysticercosis with anterior interhemispheric fissure cyst: A rare case report. *J. Neurosci. Rural Pract.* 6: 234–237.
29. Mahale, R.R., Mehta, A., and Rangasetty, S. (2015). Extraparenchymal (Racemose) neurocysticercosis and its multitude manifestations: a comprehensive review. *J. Clin. Neurol.* 11: 203–211.
30. Zammarchi, L., Bonati, M., Strohmeyer, M. et al. (2017). Screening, diagnosis and management of human cysticercosis and Taenia solium taeniasis: technical recommendations by the COHEMI project study group. *Tropical Med. Int. Health* 22: 881–894.
31. Del Brutto, O.H., Rajshekhar, V., White, A.C. et al. (2001). Proposed diagnostic criteria for neurocysticercosis. *Neurology* 57: 177–183.
32. Teerasukjinda, O., Wongjittraporn, S., Tongma, C., and Chung, H. (2016). Asymptomatic giant intraventricular cysticercosis: a case report. *Hawaii J. Med. Public Health* 75: 187–189.
33. Venkat, B., Aggarwal, N., Makhaik, S., and Sood, R. (2016). A comprehensive review of imaging findings in human cysticercosis. *Jpn. J. Radiol.* 34: 241–257.
34. Webb, C.M. and White, A.C. (2016). Update on the diagnosis and management of neurocysticercosis. *Curr. Infect. Dis. Rep.* 18: 44.
35. Sako, Y., Takayanagui, O.M., Odashima, N.S., and Ito, A. (2015). Comparative study of paired serum and cerebrospinal fluid samples from neurocysticercosis patients for the detection of specific antibody to Taenia solium immunodiagnostic antigen. *Trop. Med. Health* 43: 171–176.
36. Zhang, Z., Fan, J., Dang, Y. et al. (2017). Primary intramedullary hydatid cyst: a case report and literature review. *Eur. Spine J.* 26: 107–110.
37. Duishanbai, S., Jiafu, D., Guo, H. et al. (2010). Intracranial hydatid cyst in children: report of 30 cases. *Childs Nerv. Syst.* 26: 821–827.
38. Karakoç, Z.C., Kasimcan, M.O., Pipia, A.P. et al. (2016). A life-threatening brainstem compression by cerebral Echinococcus granulosus. *Infez. Med.* 24: 62–66.
39. Izci, Y., Tüzün, Y., Seçer, H.I., and Gönül, E. (2008). Cerebral hydatid cysts: technique and pitfalls of surgical management. *Neurosurg. Focus.* 24: E15.
40. Nakao, M., Lavikainen, A., Yanagida, T., and Ito, A. (2013). Phylogenetic systematics of the genus Echinococcus (Cestoda: Taeniidae). *Int. J. Parasitol.* 43: 1017–1029.
41. Ito, A., Dorjsuren, T., Davaasuren, A. et al. (2014). Cystic echinococcoses in Mongolia: molecular identification, serology and risk factors. *PLoS Negl. Trop. Dis.* 8: e2937.
42. Hajhouji, F., Aniba, K., Laghmari, M. et al. (2016). Epilepsy: unusual presentation of cerebral hydatid disease in Children. *Pan Afr. Med. J.* 25: 58.
43. Chen, S., Li, N., Yang, F. et al. (2018). Medical treatment of an unusual cerebral hydatid disease. *BMC Infect. Dis.* 18: 12.
44. Taslakian, B. and Darwish, H. (2016). Intracranial hydatid cyst: imaging findings of a rare disease. *BMJ Case Rep.* 2016.
45. Kemaloğlu, S., Ozkan, U., Bükte, Y. et al. (2001). Growth rate of cerebral hydatid cyst, with a review of the literature. *Childs Nerv. Syst.* 17: 743–745.
46. El-Shamam, O., Amer, T., and El-Atta, M.A. (2001). Magnetic resonance imaging of simple and infected hydatid cysts of the brain. *Magn. Reson. Imaging* 19: 965–974.
47. Pluchino, F. and Lodrini, S. (1981). Multiple primitive epidural spinal hydatid cysts: case report. *Acta Neurochir.* 59: 257–262.
48. Talan-Hranilovic, J., Sajko, T., Negovetic, L. et al. (2002). Cerebral cysticercosis and echinococcosis: a preoperative diagnostic dilemma. *Arch. Med. Res.* 33: 590–594.
49. Krajewski, R. and Stelmasiak, Z. (1991). Cerebral hydatid cysts in children. *Childs Nerv. Syst.* 7: 154–155.
50. Umerani, M.S., Abbas, A., and Sharif, S. (2013). Intra cranial hydatid cyst: A case report of total cyst extirpation and review of surgical technique. *J. Neurosci. Rural Pract.* 4: S125–S128.
51. Lescano, A.G. and Zunt, J. (2013). Other cestodes: sparganosis, coenurosis and Taenia crassiceps cysticercosis. *Handb. Clin. Neurol.* 114: 335–345.
52. El-On, J., Shelef, I., Cagnano, E., and Benifla, M. (2008). Taenia multiceps: a rare human cestode infection in Israel. *Vet. Ital.* 44: 621–631.
53. Liu, Q., Li, M.-W., Wang, Z.-D. et al. (2015). Human sparganosis, a neglected food borne zoonosis. *Lancet Infect. Dis.* 15: 1226–1235.
54. Transurat, P. (1971). Sparganosis. In: *Pathology of Protozoal and Helminthic Diseases with Clinical Correlation* (ed. R.A. Marcia-Rojas), 585–591. Baltimore: Williams & Wilkins.
55. Wong, C.W. and Ho, Y.S. (1994). Intraventricular haemorrhage and hydrocephalus caused by intraventricular parasitic granuloma suggesting cerebral sparganosis. *Acta Neurochir.* 129: 205–208.
56. Shirakawa, K., Yamasaki, H., Ito, A., and Miyajima, H. (2010). Cerebral sparganosis: the wandering lesion. *Neurology* 74: 180.
57. Hong, D., Xie, H., Zhu, M. et al. (2013). Cerebral sparganosis in mainland Chinese patients. *J. Clin. Neurosci.* 20: 1514–1519.

58. Chamadol, W., Tangdumrongkul, S., Thanaphaisal, C. et al. (1992). Intracerebral hematoma caused by sparganum: a case report. *J. Med. Assoc. Thail.* 75: 602–605.
59. Lo Presti, A., Aguirre, D.T., De Andrés, P. et al. (2015). Cerebral sparganosis: case report and review of the European cases. *Acta Neurochir.* 157: 1339–1343.
60. Yu, Y., Shen, J., Yuan, Z. et al. (2016). Cerebral sparganosis in children: epidemiologic and radiologic characteristics and treatment outcomes: a report of 9 cases. *World Neurosurg.* 89: 153–158.
61. Deng, L., Xiong, P., and Qian, S. (2011). Diagnosis and stereotactic aspiration treatment of cerebral sparganosis: summary of 11 cases. *J. Neurosurg.* 114: 1421–1425.
62. Jeong, S.C., Bae, J.C., Hwang, S.H. et al. (1998). Cerebral sparganosis with intracerebral hemorrhage: a case report. *Neurology* 50: 503–506.
63. Holodniy, M., Almenoff, J., Loutit, J., and Steinberg, G.K. (1991). Cerebral sparganosis: case report and review. *Rev. Infect. Dis.* 13: 155–159.
64. Song, T., Wang, W.-S., Zhou, B.-R. et al. (2007). CT and MR characteristics of cerebral sparganosis. *AJNR Am. J. Neuroradiol.* 28: 1700–1705.
65. Steinmann, P., Keiser, J., Bos, R. et al. (2006). Schistosomiasis and water resources development: systematic review, meta-analysis, and estimates of people at risk. *Lancet Infect. Dis.* 6: 411–425.
66. Rose, M.F., Zimmerman, E.E., Hsu, L. et al. (2014). Atypical presentation of cerebral schistosomiasis four years after exposure to Schistosoma mansoni. *Epilepsy Behav. Case Rep.* 2: 80–85.
67. Houston, S., Kowalewska-Grochowska, K., Naik, S. et al. (2004). First report of Schistosoma mekongi infection with brain involvement. *Clin. Infect. Dis.* 38: e1–e6.
68. Liu, H., Lim, C.C.T., Feng, X. et al. (2008). MRI in cerebral schistosomiasis: characteristic nodular enhancement in 33 patients. *AJR Am. J. Roentgenol.* 191: 582–588.
69. Roberts, M., Cross, J., Pohl, U. et al. (2006). Cerebral schistosomiasis. *Lancet Infect. Dis.* 6: 820.
70. Camuset, G., Wolff, V., Marescaux, C. et al. (2012). Cerebral vasculitis associated with Schistosoma mansoni infection. *BMC Infect. Dis.* 12: 220.
71. Liu, L.X. (1993). Spinal and cerebral schistosomiasis. *Semin. Neurol.* 13: 189–200.
72. Carod Artal, F.J. (2012). Cerebral and spinal schistosomiasis. *Curr. Neurol. Neurosci. Rep.* 12: 666–674.
73. Ferrari, T.C.A. and Moreira, P.R.R. (2011). Neuroschistosomiasis: clinical symptoms and pathogenesis. *Lancet Neurol.* 10: 853–864.
74. Gryseels, B., Polman, K., Clerinx, J., and Kestens, L. (2006). Human schistosomiasis. *Lancet* 368: 1106–1118.
75. Carmichael, F.A. and Cowley, H.S. (1952). Schistosomiasis of the brain. *J. Neurosurg.* 9: 620–634.
76. Fischer, P.U. and Weil, G.J. (2015). North American paragonimiasis: epidemiology and diagnostic strategies. *Expert Rev. Anti-Infect. Ther.* 13: 779–786.
77. Keiser, J. and Utzinger, J. (2005). Emerging foodborne trematodiasis. *Emerg. Infect. Dis.* 11: 1507–1514.
78. Xia, Y., Ju, Y., Chen, J., and You, C. (2015). Cerebral paragonimiasis: a retrospective analysis of 27 cases. *J. Neurosurg. Pediatr.* 15: 101–106.
79. Chen, J., Chen, Z., Lin, J. et al. (2013). Cerebral paragonimiasis: a retrospective analysis of 89 cases. *Clin. Neurol. Neurosurg.* 115: 546–551.
80. Nomura, M., Nitta, H., Nakada, M. et al. (1999). MRI findings of cerebral paragonimiasis in chronic stage. *Clin. Radiol.* 54: 622–624.
81. Oh, S.J. (1969). Cerebral paragonimiasis. *J. Neurol. Sci.* 8: 27–48.
82. Kim, S.K. and Walker, A.E. (1961). Cerebral paragonimiasis. *Acta Psychiatr. Scand. Suppl.* 153: 1–85.
83. Barratt, J., Chan, D., Sandaradura, I. et al. (2016). Angiostrongylus cantonensis: a review of its distribution, molecular biology and clinical significance as a human pathogen. *Parasitology* 143: 1087–1118.
84. Spratt, D.M. (2015). Species of Angiostrongylus (Nematoda: Metastrongyloidea) in wildlife: a review. *Int. J. Parasitol. Parasites Wild* 4: 178–189.
85. Thiengo, S.C., de Simões R, O., Fernandez, M.A., and Maldonado, A. (2013). Angiostrongylus cantonensis and rat lungworm disease in Brazil. Hawaii. *J. Med. Public Health* 72: 18–22.
86. Morassutti, A.L., Thiengo, S.C., Fernandez, M. et al. (2014). Eosinophilic meningitis caused by Angiostrongylus cantonensis: an emergent disease in Brazil. *Mem. Inst. Oswaldo Cruz* 109: 399–407.
87. York, E.M., Butler, C.J., and Lord, W.D. (2014). Global decline in suitable habitat for Angiostrongylus (Parastrongylus) cantonensis: the role of climate change. *PLoS One* 9: e103831.
88. Eamsobhana, P., Gan, X.X., Ma, A. et al. (2014). Dot immunogold filtration assay (DIGFA) for the rapid detection of specific antibodies against the rat lungworm Angiostrongylus cantonensis (Nematoda: Metastrongyloidea) using purified 31-kDa antigen. *J. Helminthol.* 88: 396–401.
89. Eamsobhana, P., Lim, P.E., and Sen, Y.H. (2013). Genetic diversity of the rat lungworm, Angiostrongylus cantonensis, the major cause of eosinophilic meningitis. *Hawaii J. Med. Public Health* 72: 15–17.

90. Wang, Q.-P., Wu, Z.-D., Wei, J. et al. (2012). Human Angiostrongylus cantonensis: an update. *Eur. J. Clin. Microbiol. Infect. Dis.* 31: 389–395.
91. Beaver, P.C. and Rosen, L. (1964). Memorandum on the tirst report of Angiostrongylus in man, by Nomura and Lin, 1945. *Am. J. Trop. Med. Hyg.* 13: 589–590.
92. Iwanowicz, D.D., Sanders, L.R., Schill, W.B. et al. (2015). Spread of the Rat Lungworm (Angiostrongylus cantonensis) in Giant African Land Snails (Lissachatina fulica) in Florida, USA. *J. Wildl. Dis.* 51: 749–753.
93. Chan, D., Barratt, J., Roberts, T. et al. (2015). The prevalence of Angiostrongylus cantonensis/mackerrasae complex in molluscs from the Sydney Region. *PLoS One* 10: e0128128.
94. Teem, J.L., Qvarnstrom, Y., Bishop, H.S. et al. (2013). The occurrence of the rat lungworm, Angiostrongylus cantonensis, in nonindigenous snails in the Gulf of Mexico region of the United States. Hawaii. *J. Med. Public Health* 72: 11–14.
95. Murphy, G.S. and Johnson, S. (2013). Clinical aspects of eosinophilic meningitis and meningoencephalitis caused by Angiostrongylus cantonensis, the rat lungworm. *Hawaii J. Med. Public Health* 72: 35–40.
96. Graeff-Teixeira, C., da Silva, A.C.A., and Yoshimura, K. (2009). Update on eosinophilic meningoencephalitis and its clinical relevance. *Clin. Microbiol. Rev.* 22: 322–348.
97. Tseng, Y.-T., Tsai, H.-C., Sy, C.L. et al. (2011). Clinical manifestations of eosinophilic meningitis caused by Angiostrongylus cantonensis: 18 years' experience in a medical center in southern Taiwan. *J. Microbiol. Immunol. Infect.* 44: 382–389.
98. Wang, Q.-P., Lai, D.-H., Zhu, X.-Q. et al. (2008). Human angiostrongyliasis. *Lancet Infect. Dis.* 8: 621–630.
99. Hsu, J.-J., Chuang, S.-H., Chen, C.-H., and Huang, M.-H. (2009). Sacral myeloradiculitis (Elsberg syndrome) secondary to eosinophilic meningitis caused by Angiostrongylus cantonensis. *BMJ Case Rep.* https://doi.org/10.1136/bcr.10.2008.1075. Epub Aug 3, 2009.
100. Dorta-Contreras, A.J., Padilla-Docal, B., Moreira, J.M. et al. (2011). Neuroimmunological findings of Angiostrongylus cantonensis meningitis in Ecuadorian patients. *Arq. Neuropsiquiatr.* 69: 466–469.
101. Hu, X., Du, J., Tong, C. et al. (2011). Epidemic status of Angiostrongylus cantonensis in Hainan island, China. *Asian Pac J Trop Med* 4: 275–277.
102. Cowie, R.H. (2013). Pathways for transmission of angiostrongyliasis and the risk of disease associated with them. *Hawaii J. Med. Public Health* 72: 70–74.
103. Tsai, H.-C., Liu, Y.-C., Kunin, C.M. et al. (2003). Eosinophilic meningitis caused by Angiostrongylus cantonensis associated with eating raw snails: correlation of brain magnetic resonance imaging scans with clinical findings. *Am. J. Trop. Med. Hyg.* 68: 281–285.
104. Diaz, J.H. (2009). Recognizing and reducing the risks of helminthic eosinophilic meningitis in travelers: differential diagnosis, disease management, prevention, and control. *J. Travel. Med.* 16: 267–275.
105. Morton, N.J., Britton, P., Palasanthiran, P. et al. (2013). Severe hemorrhagic meningoencephalitis due to Angiostrongylus cantonensis among young children in Sydney, Australia. *Clin. Infect. Dis.* 57: 1158–1161.
106. Mengying, Z., Yiyue, X., Tong, P. et al. (2017). Apoptosis and necroptosis of mouse hippocampal and parenchymal astrocytes, microglia and neurons caused by Angiostrongylus cantonensis infection. *Parasit. Vectors* 10: 611.
107. Wang, L.-C., Jung, S.-M., Chen, C.-C. et al. (2006). Pathological changes in the brains of rabbits experimentally infected with Angiostrongylus cantonensis after albendazole treatment: histopathological and magnetic resonance imaging studies. *J. Antimicrob. Chemother.* 57: 294–300.
108. Lindo, J.F., Escoffery, C.T., Reid, B. et al. (2004). Fatal autochthonous eosinophilic meningitis in a Jamaican child caused by Angiostrongylus cantonensis. *Am. J. Trop. Med. Hyg.* 70: 425–428.
109. Luo, S., OuYang, L., Wei, J. et al. (2017). Neuronal apoptosis: pathological basis of behavioral dysfunctions induced by Angiostrongylus cantonensis in rodents model. *Korean J. Parasitol.* 55: 267–278.
110. Thanaviratananich, S., Thanaviratananich, S., and Ngamjarus, C. (2015). Corticosteroids for parasitic eosinophilic meningitis. *Cochrane Database Syst. Rev.* 10: CD009088.
111. Slom, T.J., Cortese, M.M., Gerber, S.I. et al. (2002). An outbreak of eosinophilic meningitis caused by Angiostrongylus cantonensis in travelers returning from the Caribbean. *N. Engl. J. Med.* 346: 668–675.
112. Chotmongkol, V., Sawadpanitch, K., Sawanyawisuth, K. et al. (2006). Treatment of eosinophilic meningitis with a combination of prednisolone and mebendazole. *Am. J. Trop. Med. Hyg.* 74: 1122–1124.

113. Diao, Z., Chen, X., Yin, C. et al. (2009). Angiostrongylus cantonensis: effect of combination therapy with albendazole and dexamethasone on Th cytokine gene expression in PBMC from patients with eosinophilic meningitis. *Exp. Parasitol.* 123: 1–5.
114. Nawa, Y. (1991). Historical review and current status of gnathostomiasis in Asia. *Southeast Asian J. Trop. Med. Public Health* 22 (Suppl): 217–219.
115. Katchanov, J., Sawanyawisuth, K., Chotmongkoi, V., and Nawa, Y. (2011). Neurognathostomiasis, a neglected parasitosis of the central nervous system. *Emerg. Infect. Dis.* 17: 1174–1180.
116. Uparanukraw, P., Morakote, N., Harnnoi, T., and Dantrakool, A. (2001). Molecular cloning of a gene encoding matrix metalloproteinase-like protein from Gnathostoma spinigerum. *Parasitol. Res.* 87: 751–757.
117. Germann, R., Schächtele, M., Nessler, G. et al. (2003). Cerebral gnathostomiasis as a cause of an extended intracranial bleeding. *Klin. Paediatr.* 215: 223–225.
118. Herman, J.S. and Chiodini, P.L. (2009). Gnathostomiasis, another emerging imported disease. *Clin. Microbiol. Rev.* 22: 484–492.
119. Boongird, P., Phuapradit, P., Siridej, N. et al. (1977). Neurological manifestations of gnathostomiasis. *J. Neurol. Sci.* 31: 279–291.
120. Chang, S., Lim, J.H., Choi, D. et al. (2006). Hepatic visceral larva migrans of Toxocara canis: CT and sonographic findings. *AJR Am. J. Roentgenol.* 187: W622–W629.
121. Beaver, P.C., Snyder, C.H., Carrera, G.M. et al. (1952). Chronic eosinophilia due to visceral larva migrans; report of three cases. *Pediatrics* 9: 7–19.
122. Noh, Y., Hong, S.-T., Yun, J.Y. et al. (2012). Meningitis by Toxocara canis after ingestion of raw ostrich liver. *J. Korean Med. Sci.* 27: 1105–1108.
123. Lee, I.H., Kim, S.T., Oh, D.K. et al. (2010). MRI findings of spinal visceral larva migrans of Toxocara canis. *Eur. J. Radiol.* 75: 236–240.
124. Jabbour, R.A., Kanj, S.S., Sawaya, R.A. et al. (2011). Toxocara canis myelitis: clinical features, magnetic resonance imaging (MRI) findings, and treatment outcome in 17 patients. *Medicine (Baltimore)* 90: 337–343.
125. Hoffmeister, B., Glaeser, S., Flick, H. et al. (2007). Cerebral toxocariasis after consumption of raw duck liver. *Am. J. Trop. Med. Hyg.* 76: 600–602.
126. Magnaval, J.F., Glickman, L.T., Dorchies, P., and Morassin, B. (2001). Highlights of human toxocariasis. *Korean J. Parasitol.* 39: 1–11.
127. Finsterer, J. and Auer, H. (2007). Neurotoxocarosis. *Rev. Inst. Med. Trop. Sao Paulo* 49: 279–287.
128. Deshayes, S., Bonhomme, J., and de La Blanchardière, A. (2016). Neurotoxocariasis: a systematic literature review. *Infection* 44: 565–574.
129. Bächli, H., Minet, J.C., and Gratzl, O. (2004). Cerebral toxocariasis: a possible cause of epileptic seizure in children. *Childs Nerv. Syst.* 20: 468–472.
130. Moiyadi, A., Mahadevan, A., Anandh, B. et al. (2007). Visceral larva migrans presenting as multiple intracranial and intraspinal abscesses. *Neuropathology* 27: 371–374.
131. Kazek, B., Jamroz, E., Mandera, M. et al. (2006). The cerebral form of toxocarosis in a seven-year-old patient. *Folia Neuropathol.* 44: 72–76.
132. Poulsen, C.S., Skov, S., Yoshida, A. et al. (2015). Differential serodiagnostics of Toxocara canis and Toxocara cati--is it possible? *Parasite Immunol.* 37: 204–207.
133. Cianferoni, A., Schneider, L., Schantz, P.M. et al. (2006). Visceral larva migrans associated with earthworm ingestion: clinical evolution in an adolescent patient. *Pediatrics* 117: e336–e339.
134. Macpherson, C.N.L. (2013). The epidemiology and public health importance of toxocariasis: a zoonosis of global importance. *Int. J. Parasitol.* 43: 999–1008.
135. Xinou, E., Lefkopoulos, A., Gelagoti, M. et al. (2003). CT and MR imaging findings in cerebral toxocaral disease. *AJNR Am. J. Neuroradiol.* 24: 714–718.
136. Gould, I.M., Newell, S., Green, S.H., and George, R.H. (1985). Toxocariasis and eosinophilic meningitis. *Br. Med. J.* 291: 1239–1240.
137. Rüttinger, P. and Hadidi, H. (1991). MRI in cerebral toxocaral disease. *J. Neurol. Neurosurg. Psychiatry* 54: 361–362.
138. Sommer, C., Ringelstein, E.B., Biniek, R., and Glöckner, W.M. (1994). Adult Toxocara canis encephalitis. *J. Neurol. Neurosurg. Psychiatry* 57: 229–231.
139. Russegger, L. and Schmutzhard, E. (1989). Spinal toxocaral abscess. *Lancet* 2: 398.
140. Jagannath, P.M., Venkataramana, N.K., Rao, S.A. et al. (2009). Recurrent cerebral larva migrans: A case report and review of literature. *J. Pediatr. Neurosci.* 4: 36–40.
141. Eberhardt, O., Bialek, R., Nägele, T., and Dichgans, J. (2005). Eosinophilic meningomyelitis in toxocariasis: case report and review of the literature. *Clin. Neurol. Neurosurg.* 107: 432–438.

142. Helsen, G., Vandecasteele, S.J., and Vanopdenbosch, L.J. (2011). Toxocariasis presenting as encephalomyelitis. *Case Rep. Med.* 2011: 503913.
143. Gorgulu, A., Albayrak, B.S., Gorgulu, E., and Tural, O. (2006). Postoperative cerebral abscess formation caused by Toxocara canis in a meningioma cavity. *J. Neuro-Oncol.* 77: 325–326.
144. Sick, C. and Hennerici, M.G. (2014). Expect the unexpected: a case of isolated eosinophilic meningitis in toxocariasis. *Case Rep. Neurol.* 6: 259–263.
145. Bruschi, F., Brunetti, E., and Pozio, E. (2013). Neurotrichinellosis. In: *Handbook of Clinical Neurology* (eds. H. Garcia, H. Tanowitz and O. Del Brutto), 243–249. Elsevier.
146. Moscatelli, G., Sordelli, N., Nora, S. et al. (2014). Neurotrichinosis in a pediatric patient. *Pediatr. Infect. Dis. J.* 33: 115–117.
147. Rostami, A., Gamble, H.R., Dupouy-Camet, J. et al. (2017). Meat sources of infection for outbreaks of human trichinellosis. *Food Microbiol.* 64: 65–71.
148. Gottstein, B., Pozio, E., and Nöckler, K. (2009). Epidemiology, diagnosis, treatment, and control of trichinellosis. *Clin. Microbiol. Rev.* 22: 127–145.
149. Pozio, E. (2007). World distribution of Trichinella spp. infections in animals and humans. *Vet. Parasitol.* 149: 3–21.
150. Taratuto, A.L. and Venturiello, S.M. (1997). Trichinosis. *Brain Pathol.* 7: 663–672.
151. Kamgno, J., Pion, S.D., Chesnais, C.B. et al. (2017). A test-and-not-treat strategy for onchocerciasis in Loa loa-endemic areas. *N. Engl. J. Med.* 377: 2044–2052.
152. Lukiana, T., Mandina, M., Situakibanza, N.H. et al. (2006). A possible case of spontaneous Loa loa encephalopathy associated with a glomerulopathy. *Filaria J.* 5: 6.
153. Boussinesq, M., Gardon, J., Gardon-Wendel, N., and Chippaux, J.-P. (2003). Clinical picture, epidemiology and outcome of Loa-associated serious adverse events related to mass ivermectin treatment of onchocerciasis in Cameroon. *Filaria J.* 2 (Suppl 1): S4.
154. Carme, B., Boulesteix, J., Boutes, H., and Puruehnce, M.F. (1991). Five cases of encephalitis during treatment of loiasis with diethylcarbamazine. *Am. J. Trop. Med. Hyg.* 44: 684–690.
155. Udall, D.N. (2007). Recent updates on onchocerciasis: diagnosis and treatment. *Clin. Infect. Dis.* 44: 53–60.
156. Colebunders, R., Mandro, M., Njamnshi, A.K. et al. (2018). Report of the first international workshop on onchocerciasis-associated epilepsy. *Infect. Dis. Poverty* 7: 23.
157. Siddiqui, A.A. and Berk, S.L. (2001). Diagnosis of Strongyloides stercoralis infection. *Clin. Infect. Dis.* 33: 1040–1047.
158. Greaves, D., Coggle, S., Pollard, C. et al. (2013). Strongyloides stercoralis infection. *BMJ* 347: f4610.
159. Prendki, V., Fenaux, P., Durand, R. et al. (2011). Strongyloidiasis in man 75 years after initial exposure. *Emerg. Infect. Dis.* 17: 931–932.
160. Owor, R. and Wamukota, W.M. (1976). A fatal case of strongyloidiasis with Strongyloides larvae in the meninges. *Trans. R. Soc. Trop. Med. Hyg.* 70: 497–499.
161. Neefe, L.I., Pinilla, O., Garagusi, V.F., and Bauer, H. (1973). Disseminated strongyloidiasis with cerebral involvement. A complication of corticosteroid therapy. *Am. J. Med.* 55: 832–838.
162. Masdeu, J.C., Tantulavanich, S., Gorelick, P.P. et al. (1982). Brain abscess caused by Strongyloides stercoralis. *Arch. Neurol.* 39: 62–63.
163. Morgello, S., Soifer, F.M., Lin, C.S., and Wolfe, D.E. (1993). Central nervous system Strongyloides stercoralis in acquired immunodeficiency syndrome: a report of two cases and review of the literature. *Acta Neuropathol.* 86: 285–288.
164. Cruz, M.E., Schantz, P.M., Cruz, I. et al. (1999). Epilepsy and neurocysticercosis in an Andean community. *Int. J. Epidemiol.* 28: 799–803.
165. Fleury, A., Gomez, T., Alvarez, I. et al. (2003). High prevalence of calcified silent neurocysticercosis in a rural village of Mexico. *Neuroepidemiology* 22: 139–145.
166. Del Brutto, O.H. and Sotclo, J. (2003). Foodborne Helminths: Taenia solium. In: *International Handbook of Foodborne Pathogens* (eds. O.R. Fennema, Y.H. Hui, M. Karel, et al.), 522–535. Marcel Dekker Inc: New York, Basel.
167. Del Brutto, O.H., Granados, G., Talamas, O. et al. (1991). Genetic pattern of the HLA system: HLA A, B, C, DR, and DQ antigens in Mexican patients with parenchymal brain cysticercosis. *Hum. Biol.* 63: 85–93.
168. Singh, A., Singh, A.K., Singh, S.K. et al. (2014). Association of ICAM-1 K469E polymorphism with neurocysticercosis. *J. Neuroimmunol.* 276: 166–171.
169. Verma, A., Prasad, K.N., Gupta, R.K. et al. (2010). Toll-like receptor 4 polymorphism and its association with symptomatic neurocysticercosis. *J. Infect. Dis.* 202: 1219–1225.
170. Prasad, A., Prasad, K.N., Gupta, R.K., and Pradhan, S. (2009). Increased expression of ICAM-1 among symptomatic neurocysticercosis. *J. Neuroimmunol.* 206: 118–120.

171. Singh, A., Prasad, K.N., Singh, A.K. et al. (2017). Human Glutathione S-Transferase enzyme gene polymorphisms and their association with neurocysticercosis. *Mol. Neurobiol.* 54: 2843–2851.
172. Flisser, A., Sarti, E., Lightowlers, M., and Schantz, P. (2003). Neurocysticercosis: regional status, epidemiology, impact and control measures in the Americas. *Acta Trop.* 87: 43–51.
173. Silva-Vergara, M.L., Prata, A., Netto, H.V. et al. (1998). Risk factors associated with taeniasis-cysticercosis in Lagamar, Minas Gerais State, Brazil. *Rev. Soc. Bras. Med. Trop.* 31: 65–71.
174. Vázquez-Flores, S., Ballesteros-Rodea, G., Flisser, A., and Schantz, P.M. (2001). Hygiene and restraint of pigs is associated with absence of Taenia solium cysticercosis in a rural community of Mexico. *Salud Publica Mex.* 43: 574–576.
175. Kayes, S.G. (1997). Human toxocariasis and the visceral larva migrans syndrome: correlative immunopathology. *Chem. Immunol.* 66: 99–124.
176. Verastegui, M.R., Mejia, A., Clark, T. et al. (2015). Novel rat model for neurocysticercosis using Taenia solium. *Am. J. Pathol.* 185: 2259–2268.
177. Hamamoto Filho, P.T., Zanini, M.A., Botta, F.P. et al. (2015). Development of an experimental model of neurocysticercosis-induced hydrocephalus. Pilot study. *Acta Cir. Bras.* 30: 819–823.
178. Janecek, E., Beineke, A., Schnieder, T., and Strube, C. (2014). Neurotoxocarosis: marked preference of Toxocara canis for the cerebrum and T. cati for the cerebellum in the paratenic model host mouse. *Parasit. Vectors* 7: 194.
179. Wei, Y., Hong, Q., Chen, D. et al. (2014). Permissibility of Mongolian gerbil for Angiostrongylus cantonensis infection and utility of this animal model for anthelmintic studies. *Parasitol. Res.* 113: 1687–1693.
180. OuYang, L., Wei, J., Wu, Z. et al. (2012). Differences of larval development and pathological changes in permissive and nonpermissive rodent hosts for Angiostrongylus cantonensis infection. *Parasitol. Res.* 111: 1547–1555.
181. Wang, J.J., Lee, J.D., Chang, J.H. et al. (1995). The susceptibility of five stains mice to infections with Angiostrongylus cantonensis. *Gaoxiong Yi Xue Ke Xue Za Zhi* 11: 599–603.
182. Sugaya, H. and Yoshimura, K. (1988). T-cell-dependent eosinophilia in the cerebrospinal fluid of the mouse infected with Angiostrongylus cantonensis. *Parasite Immunol.* 10: 127–138.
183. Silva, L.M., de Oliveira, C.N., and Andrade, Z.A. (2002). Experimental neuroschistosomiasis: inadequacy of the murine model. *Mem. Inst. Oswaldo Cruz* 97: 599–600.
184. Wang, P., Wang, D., Chen, S.-J. et al. (2011). Establishment of a cerebral schistosomiasis experimental model in rabbits. *Neurosci. Bull.* 27: 91–98.

Appendix

CASE EXAMPLE: *Schistosoma mekongi* Neuroschistosomiasis

Edward S. Johnson
Department of Laboratory Medicine and Pathology, University of Alberta, Edmonton, Alberta, Canada

Tourists and expatriates are an increasingly common group presenting with varied forms of neuroschistosomiasis. Compounding the complexity of their presentation is travel through a region endemic for a lesser-known species of schistosomiasis, a history of travel through multiple countries at different time periods, or concurrent coinfection [1]. This case example of a 25-year-old man is illustrative. While on a two month trip to Costa Rica and Panama, he experienced onset of a combination of neurological symptoms: paresthesias in the right arm and leg, dysphasia, and features of raised intracranial pressure. Initial investigations including abdominal ultrasound were unhelpful, but a series of radiological imaging studies of the brain revealed an enlarging mass in the left temporal lobe (Figure 48.10a). Open neurosurgical biopsy disclosed collections of confluent nodular masses of granulomas, with associated chronic inflammation, that contained aggregates of schistosome ova (Figure 48.10b–e). Analysis of these ova in tissue sections and minced tissue preparations (Figure 48.10f), identified them as belonging to *S. mekongi* species. On questioning, the patient stated two years previously he had swum in the Mekong River while traveling in Laos. His serology confirmed schistosome infection, which was also positive in two asymptomatic travel companions. However, no ova were found in a single fecal examination; rectal biopsy or snips were not done. He responded to a therapeutic course of praziquantel.

Even though clinically mimicking infection by *S. japonicum*, *S. mekongi* is a separate species with a distinctly characteristic ovum and different intermediate snail host, *Neotricula aperta*, that is restricted in habitat to the Mekong River Basin in Cambodia and Laos. In addition to this case [2], another presumed pseudotumoral *S. mekongi* neuroschistosomiasis in a traveler has been described [3], as have acute symptomatic and asymptomatic cases [1, 4, 5]. Points demonstrated by this example are:

- Neuropathologists are most likely to encounter schistosome infection of the brain in the pseudotumoral form.
- In this setting there is usually minimal evidence of hepato-intestinal disease, detection of ova in the feces being sparse or absent.
- Diagnosis is reliant on identification of ova in tissue sections or minced preparations from biopsy specimens, including rectal snips or biopsies.

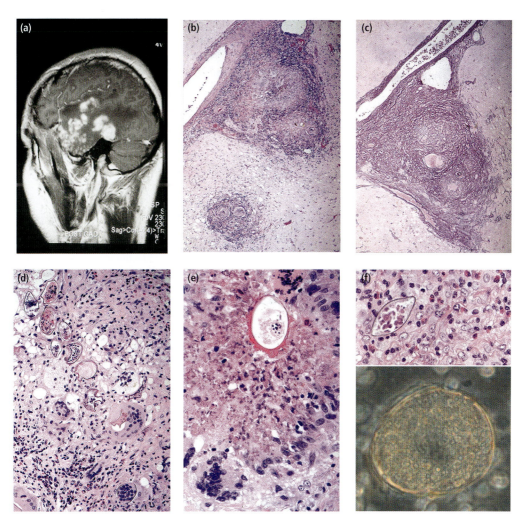

Figure 48.10 (a) T1 weighted postgadolinium magnetic resonance imaging (MRI) scan of brain, sagittal plane, showing marked expansion of the left temporal lobe by an edematous mass studded by multifocal, variously sized, irregular contrast-enhancing nodules. (b) Biopsy of the mass discloses multitudes of granulomatous nodules, often confluent, in the leptomeninges extending into the cerebral cortex and also isolated foci in the neural parenchyma (Hematoxylin and eosin [H&E]). (c) These granulomas evoke an intense sclerosing reaction with skeins of reticulin deposition (Gordon-Sweet reticulin). (d) Within the granulomas are deposits of numerous ova, some with necrotic embryos, surrounded by multinucleated foreign body giant cells. One giant cell has phagocytozed an ovum, leaving an empty shell (H&E). (e) An occasional dying ovum elicits an intense cell-mediated reaction because of leakage of histotoxic soluble egg antigen to cause caseous-like necrosis with peripheral palisading of epitheliod cells and giant cells (H&E). (f) Ovum in tissue section (top, H&E), with accompanying infiltrate of macrophages, chronic inflammatory cells, and eosinophils, compared to ovum in wet mount of minced tissue preparation from biopsy (bottom). The ovum is rounded, measuring 54 × 58 µm, and lacks a lateral or terminal spine, consistent with *S. mekongi* species. Source: courtesy of the authors from [2] by permission of Oxford University Press.

- Serological tests are sensitive for diagnostic confirmation but cannot distinguish between either different species or recurrent chronic infection.

The advent of molecular techniques employing different formats of polymerase chain reaction (PCR) analysis and target gene sequences, should enable timely diagnostic reporting, improved species identification, and diagnostic sensitivity [6, 7].

References

1. Campa, P., Develoux, M., Belkadi, G. et al. (2014). Chronic *Schistosoma mekongi* in a traveler – A case report and review of the literature. *J. Travel Med.* 21: 361–363.
2. Houston, S., Kowalewska-Grochowska, K., Naik, S. et al. (2004). First report of *Schistosoma mekongi* infection with brain involvement. *Clin. Infect. Dis.* 38: e1–e6.
3. Carmony, D., Nolan, C., and Allcutt, D. (2008). Intracranial *Schistosoma mekongi* infection. *Ir. Med. J.* 101: 315.
4. Leshem, E., Meltzer, E., Marva, E., and Schwartz, E. (2009). Travel-related schistosomasis acquired in Laos. *Emerg. Infect. Dis.* 15: 1823–1826.
5. Clerinx, J., Cnops, L., Huyse, T. et al. (2013). Diagnostic issues of acute schistosomiasis with *Schistosomasis mekongi* in a traveler: A case report. *J. Travel Med.* 20: 322–325.
6. Cnops, L., Tannich, E., Polman, K. et al. (2012). *Schistosoma* real-time PCR as diagnostic tool for international travellers and migrants. *Tropical Med. Int. Health* 17: 1208–1216.
7. Li, J., Zhao, G.-H., Lin, R.Q. et al. (2015). Rapid detection and identification of four major *Schistosoma* species by high-resolution melt (HRM) analysis. *Parasitol. Res.* 114: 4225–4232.

49 Brain Myiasis

Arnault Tauziede-Espariat[1,2]

[1] Department of Neuropathology, Sainte Anne Hospital, Paris, France
[2] Paris University, Paris, France

Definition

Myiasis is the term applied to the invasion of living human or other mammalian tissues by the larvae of dipterous insects of different genera and species. The term "myiasis" was first coined by Hope in 1840 [1]. The main reservoirs for this infection are rodents and large mammals, but cattle, horses and pigs are common hosts in rural areas, whereas humans are accidental hosts. In general, human cases have a close association with cattle [1]. In most cases, female flies are attracted to lay their eggs on the edges of open ulcers or wounds. From there, end-stage larvae penetrate the tissues and feed on necrotic flesh (i.e. are necrobiophagous). The life cycle of a fly commences with the egg stage and is followed by the larval stage, the pupal stage, and finally the adult fly.

Cutaneous myiasis is the most common presentation. However, visceral involvement has been described in various organs. Cerebral myiasis is exceptionally rare with no more than 15 cases reported. The first case of human cerebral myiasis was described by Froomin and Kaznelson in 1939 [1]. During their complete cycle in cattle, larvae reside for several weeks in the peridural space but very rarely reach the brain itself, except in the horse, where larvae find entry into the brain, causing serious neurological disorders. This may possibly also apply to humans.

Microbiological characteristics

Calliphora, *Musca*, and *Lucilia* species are common in myiasis. In the brain, the reported offending species have been *Hypoderma bovis* (four cases), *Phaenicia sericata* (two cases), *Hypoderma lineatum* (one case), *Callitroga americana* (1 case), *Dermatobia hominis* (one case), and *Musca domestica* (one case) and undetermined in three cases [2–5].

Epidemiology

Myiasis is more prevalent in humid tropical and subtropical regions, which are natural habitats for many fly species, so the majority of cases occur in developing countries. Poor hygiene, diabetes, immunocompromised status, and delay in seeking medical attention predispose to myiasis in humans [5]. The age of the reported patients ranged from 5 months to 75 years [5].

Clinical features

The severity of myiasis depends on the location of the infestation and the lesions and tissue inflammation. In the brain, the infestation has a predilection

Infections of the Central Nervous System: Pathology and Genetics, First Edition. Edited by Fabrice Chrétien, Kum Thong Wong, Leroy R. Sharer, Catherine (Katy) Keohane and Françoise Gray.
© 2020 John Wiley & Sons Ltd. Published 2020 by John Wiley & Sons Ltd.

for the frontal lobe (10/12 reported cases) [2–5]. Because the frontal lobe is the largest lobe and commonly involved in traumatic brain injuries, it is statistically most likely to be affected. Most of the brain cases of myiasis developed following trauma or brain surgery [2, 4, 5]. Routine blood tests are in general normal or reveal leukocytosis. On examination there is usually a local scalp defect with hypertrophied erythematous edges. Within the defect, the dura can be eroded, leaving exposed cortex. Lesions vary in size from 1 to 17 cm. In cases without a scalp defect, brain imaging shows a hypodense lesion with ringlike contrast enhancement. In those cases, the radiological diagnosis was hematoma.

Pathology

The diagnosis of myiasis is usually made by the surgeon who observes dense clusters of maggots embedded within the cerebrum. In some cases, there are active movements of maggots throughout the lesion and over the exposed cortical surface, and histology was not performed. Most cases only had investigation to identify the parasite. The brain around the larvae consists of hematoma without any particular histopathological features.

Treatment and conclusions

Cerebral myiasis is almost uniformly fatal, especially when a large area of the brain is affected. All but two of the reported cases had a fatal outcome [2–5]. There are frequent associated polymicrobial infections [5]. Wide debridement of adjacent normal brain, followed by prolonged treatment with broad-spectrum antibiotics are the gold standard of treatment.

This exceedingly rare neurologic infection, with less than 15 cases described worldwide, is caused by different fly genera and species. Poor living conditions, head trauma, or immunocompromised status are risk factors. In general, the diagnosis is made by a surgeon who sees larvae and maggots during an operation. Surgical debridement and prolonged antibiotic therapy may be effective, but the majority of reported cases have been fatal.

References

1. Kalelioglu, M., Akturk, G., Akturk, F. et al. (1989). Intracerebral myiasis from *Hypoderma bovis* larva in a child. *J. Neurosurg.* 7: 929–931.
2. Giri, S.A., Kotecha, N., Giri, D. et al. (2016). Cerebral myiasis associated with artificial cranioplasty flap: a case report. *World Neurosurg.* 661: e13–e16.
3. Navarro, J.N. and Alves, R.V. (2016). Postoperative cerebral myiasis: a rare cause of wound dehiscence in developing countries. *Surg. Neurol. Int.* 7: 69.
4. Cheshier, S.H., Bababeygy, S.R., Higgins, D. et al. (2007). Cerebral myiasis associated with angiosarcoma of the scalp: case report. *Neurosurgery* 61: E167.
5. Terterov, S., Taghva, A., MacDougall, M. et al. (2010). Posttraumatic human cerebral myiasis. *World Neurosurg.* 73: 557–559.

50 Emerging CNS Infections

Kum Thong Wong

Department of Pathology, Faculty of Medicine, University of Malaya, Kuala Lumpur, Malaysia

Abbreviations

AIDS	acquired immunodeficiency syndrome
CNS	central nervous system
EV	enterovirus
EVD	Ebola virus disease
MERS-CoV	Middle Eastern Respiratory Syndrome coronavirus
MRI	magnetic resonance imaging
NiV	Nipah virus
WNV	West Nile virus
ZIKV	Zika Virus

Definition

Emerging CNS infections, as defined herein, are infections involving the CNS that have newly emerged or re-emerged in the last two decades [1, 2]. These may be caused by newly recognized microbes (e.g. Nipah virus [NiV]) or re-emergence of known microbes resulting in an increased number of infections after a decline in incidence (e.g. West Nile virus ([WNV]) [3].

In this chapter, the major or significant emerging or re-emerging microbes that caused outbreaks or epidemics are highlighted, but there were also many smaller or rare outbreaks caused by other microbes. By no means exhaustive, Table 50.1 lists some of these outbreaks and epidemics. Many of these CNS infections were caused by viruses, but bacterial, fungal, and parasitic (protozoa) infections are recognized as well.

Newer and more advanced molecular techniques have helped speed up microbial identification and expedited diagnosis of outbreaks caused by both newly emerging and re-emerging microbes. With regard to *Plasmodium knowlesi* for example, because the peripheral blood film morphology of this malaria parasite resembles *Plasmodium malariae* or *Plasmodium falciparum,* its discovery as a fifth major *Plasmodium* responsible for human malaria was unknown for a long time until it was identified by molecular methods [4]. Furthermore, molecular techniques have also resulted in rapid identification of virulence genes and enabled molecular epidemiology (via phylogenetic analysis) to trace the source and spread of infections.

CNS pathology

Unfortunately, the pathology of many of these emerging CNS infections are underinvestigated and therefore not well understood, probably because human autopsy and biopsy materials are hard to come by. A more thorough understanding of the neuropathology, especially of newly emerging infections, will require more time, effort, and

---

Infections of the Central Nervous System: Pathology and Genetics, First Edition. Edited by Fabrice Chrétien, Kum Thong Wong, Leroy R. Sharer, Catherine (Katy) Keohane and Françoise Gray.
© 2020 John Wiley & Sons Ltd. Published 2020 by John Wiley & Sons Ltd.

Table 50.1 List of selected major and significant emerging CNS infections.

Microbe	Significant year(s) of emergence[a]	Main CNS disease and symptoms	CNS pathology[b]	Animal hosts, vectors involved	Person-to-person transmission	Main Region(s) involved[c]	Known or probable important factors or changes responsible for emergence	Significant potential for future outbreaks
Virus								
Nipah virus (NiV)	1998–1999	Encephalitic syndrome	Meningoencephalitis, vasculitis	Bat Pig Other domestic animals	Yes	Asia	Human • occupational hazard Environment • ecosystem and animal populations	Yes
West Nile virus (WNV)	1999	Encephalitic syndrome Acute flaccid paralysis	Meningoencephalomyelitis	Bird Mosquito	No	North America	Human • population movement and international travel Environment • climate and weather • ecosystem and animal populations	Yes
Powassan virus	Around 1999	Encephalitic syndrome	Meningoencephalomyelitis (single autopsy report)	Deer Tick	No	North America	Environment • climate and weather • ecosystem and animal populations	Yes
Enterovirus A71	1999	Encephalitic syndrome Acute flaccid paralysis	Meningoencephalomyelitis	None	Yes	Asia	Human • demography Environment • lack of public health services	Yes
Chikungunya virus (CHIKV)	2004	Encephalitic syndrome Myelopathy, etc.	Nonspecific features (single autopsy report)	Mosquito	No	Africa, Asia	Microbe • adaptation and mutation Environment • climate and weather	Yes

Zika virus (ZIKV)	2007	Microcephaly Congenital Zika syndrome	Microcephaly, craniofacial and brain malformations	Mosquito	Yes	Pacific Islands South America	Human • demography • population movement and international travel Environment • economic development and land use • ecosystem and animal populations • lack of public health services	Yes
MERS coronavirus	2012	Encephalitic syndrome	Unknown	Dromedary camel	Yes	Middle east	Human • population movement and international travel	Yes
Ebola virus	2014	Encephalitic syndrome	Unknown	Bat, Ape Monkey Other wild animals	Yes	West Africa	Microbe • adaptation and mutations Human • demography • population movement and International travel • behavior and cultural practices Environment • lack of public health services • poverty and social inequality • war and famine	Yes
Enterovirus D68	2014	Acute flaccid paralysis Encephalitic syndrome	Meningoencephalomyelitis (single autopsy report)	None	Yes	North America	Unknown	Yes
Bacteria								
Mycobacterium Tuberculosis (multi-drug resistant)	2000s	Meningitis	Tuberculous meningitis, tuberculoma	None	Yes	India, China, Russian Federation, Africa	Human • demography • inappropriate antimicrobial use	Yes

(continued)

Table 50.1 (Continued)

Microbe	Significant year(s) of emergence[a]	Main CNS disease and symptoms	CNS pathology[b]	Animal hosts, vectors involved	Person-to-person transmission	Main Region(s) involved[c]	Known or probable important factors or changes responsible for emergence	Significant potential for future outbreaks
Streptococcus agalactiae, Group B	2015	Meningitis	Unknown	Fish	No	Singapore	Human • behavior and cultural practices	No
Fungus								
Cryptococcus gattii	1999	Meningitis	Unknown	No	No	North America	Environment • climate and weather	Yes
Cryptococcus neoformans	2000s	Meningitis	Meningoencephalitis	Birds	No	Sub-Saharan Africa	Human • behavior and cultural practices Environment • lack of public health services	Yes
Exserohilum rostratum	2012	Meningitis Stroke	Meningitis, vasculitis	No	No	North America	Environment • technology and industry	No
Parasite								
Plasmodium falciparum artemisinin resistant	2000s	Cerebral malaria	Cerebral malaria	Mosquito	Yes	Southeast Asia	Microbe • adaptation and mutation Human • demography • inappropriate antimicrobial use	Yes
Plasmodium knowlesi	2004	Cerebral malaria[b]	Cerebral malaria (single autopsy report)	Monkey Mosquito	Yes	Southeast Asia	Human • demography Environment • economic development and land use • ecosystem and animal populations	Yes

[a] Except for definite documentation of the onset of distinct outbreaks and epidemics, some years are approximate only.
[b] Where CNS pathology based on confirmed cases has not been reported, it is stated as "unknown."
[c] Region(s) where emergence or re-emergence first started.

availability of study materials. Wider availability of neuroimaging has helped to confirm CNS involvement as suggested by clinical manifestations. In some cases, the types and distribution of lesions have been helpful where the pathology is unknown.

Among the newly emerging viruses, NiV caused severe neurological disease, and the neuropathology, consisting mainly of neuronal infection and vasculopathy, is now better understood (see Chapter 12). Rare neurological manifestations of confusion, coma, ataxia, and focal motor deficit associated with the novel Middle Eastern Respiratory Syndrome coronavirus (MERS-CoV) infection have been reported [5]. However, the CNS pathology is unknown. Brain magnetic resonance imaging (MRI) shows widespread and bilateral hyperintense lesions within the white matter, corpus callosum, basal ganglia, and subcortical areas of the cerebrum.

As far as re-emerging viruses are concerned, the main pathologies of WNV encephalitis (see Chapter 15) and Enterovirus A71 (EV-A71) encephalomyelitis (see Chapter 22) had already been characterized. The striking similarity of CNS lesions in Enterovirus D68 (EV-D68) to EV-A71 infection, as evidenced from imaging studies [6] and from a single autopsy report [7] suggest that the basic neuropathology may be similar (i.e. EV-D68 is neuronotropic). Although the pathology of re-emerging Powassan meningoencephalomyelitis is unknown, it probably does not differ from the closely related deer tick virus reported in a single autopsy [8] or from other tick-borne encephalitides (see Chapter 14). Zika virus (ZIKV) first re-emerged in the Pacific islands in 2007 and then in South America in 2014. The main CNS manifestations are microcephaly and a congenital syndrome in fetuses and newborns [9]. Autopsy studies have demonstrated craniofacial malformations, cerebral atrophy and maldevelopment, and diffuse calcifications (see Chapter 16). Viral antigens were localized to neuroglial cells and placental chorionic villi [10]. Numerous reports of re-emerging Chikungunya virus (CHIKV)-associated neurological complications, including meningoencephalitis and encephalomyelitis have been published [11] (see Chapter 20). The few brain MRI studies to date showed hyperintense white matter and cortical and subcortical lesions [12–14]. A single autopsy case reported so far merely demonstrated limited demyelination and mild perivascular lymphocytic infiltration in the basal ganglia, thought to be nonspecific features; so much more remains to be learned from further studies. Neurological manifestations in Ebola virus disease (EVD) have been increasingly reported [15, 16]. Given the potential for large and recurrent epidemics, much more should be discovered about neurological disease and CNS pathology associated with EVD. Limited brain MRI studies had demonstrated multiple white matter microvascular lesions [16]. Up to now, human CNS pathology is unknown, but in nonhuman primates, meningoencephalitis with glial nodules and viral antigen positivity have been described [17].

Emerging, multidrug resistant *Mycobacterium tuberculosis* is associated with tuberculous meningitis and parenchymal granulomata (see Chapter 36). Group B *Streptococcus agalactiae* infection in adults predominantly presented with meningoencephalitis, and brain MRI shows abnormalities in the subarachnoid space, ventricles, and parenchyma [18]. Presumably, the subarachnoid space lesions could represent the pyogenic meningitis typically seen in neonatal group B, serotype III, *S. agalactiae* infection (see Chapter 31). So far, these abnormalities have not been corroborated by pathological findings.

Cryptococcus neoformans and *Cryptococcus gattii* meningoencephalitis (see Chapter 44) have re-emerged under different circumstances. In sub-Saharan Africa, *C. neoformans* has been increasing as an opportunistic infection associated with acquired immunodeficiency syndrome (AIDS) because of poor availability of antiretroviral therapy, despite a falling incidence in many other regions where there is good access to treatment [19]. The re-emergence of *C. gattii*, mainly in patients who are immunocompetent, was first reported in Canada [20] but is now thought to have a global distribution [21]. The incidence of *C. gattii* could possibly be lower than *C. neoformans*, albeit its identification can be problematic if lab facilities are not equipped to distinguish it from the latter. *Exserohilum rostratum* re-emerged when contaminated methylprednisolone injections given into the epidural or paraspinal space caused a rare fungal meningitis (see Chapter 44) in a 2012 outbreak in the United States [22, 23].

As a re-emerging parasitic infection, *P. knowlesi* was fortuitously discovered in Borneo recently [4], even though it was known since the 1960s to infect monkeys as the natural host and humans as a zoonotic infection [24]. Based on the clinical presentations and a single autopsy case report [25], the pathology and pathogenesis is probably very similar to cerebral malaria caused by the more common *P. falciparum* (see Chapter 45). The newly emergent artemisinin-resistant *P. falciparum*, recently confirmed in Cambodia and other countries in Indochina, has raised alarm because it has serious implications for treatment, morbidity, and mortality of cerebral malaria [26].

Reasons for emerging CNS infections

There are numerous reasons for infections to continuously emerge and re-emerge. Some may be due to a single factor, but more likely, many factors may affect the complex interactions among microbes, human hosts (see Chapter 3), and the environment to cause CNS infections (Table 50.1) [27, 28]. Needless to say, alert health professionals need to recognize a previously unknown or rare CNS syndrome (e.g. EVD [15] or MERS-CoV [5]) to identify or confirm an emerging CNS infection.

Genetic adaption and mutations in microbes could enable human infections to emerge by altering their ability to infect new hosts, including human and intermediate hosts [27]. The CHIKV pandemic that started in Kenya in 2004 and then spread across the Indian Ocean to Asian countries was thought to be the result of a genomic mutation. The mutation increased CHIKV fitness in, and transmission by, *Aedes albopictus*, an otherwise infrequent and atypical mosquito vector for that virus [29]. A mutation in the prM protein of ZIKV has been found to be associated with microcephaly [30].

Susceptibility to drugs or microbial response to host immunity can also be altered by mutations [27]. Multidrug resistant and extensively drug-resistant *M. tuberculosis* infections defined as in vitro resistance to rifampicin or isoniazid, and other anti-TB drugs, respectively, continues to be widely reported in many countries [31]. Inevitably, this had led to the emergence of drug-resistant tuberculous meningitis [32, 33]. Mutations in the *katG, inhA,* and *rpoB* and many other genes have been found to be responsible [34]. Artemisinin-resistant *P. falciparum* is associated with *Kelch13* gene mutation [35].

However, in many emerging CNS infections, microbial genetic adaption and mutations may be difficult to identify or prove. Despite the well-known propensity of RNA viruses like EV-A71 and EV-D68 to rapidly mutate into quasispecies, so far no mutations have been unequivocally identified as neurovirulence determinants [36].

Numerous factors involving the human host could impact the emergence of CNS infections, including new susceptibility to infection, new treatments including organ transplants and biological agents, changes to human demography, human behavior and cultural practices, increased population movement and international travel, occupational hazard, inappropriate antimicrobial use, and even bioterrorism [27, 28].

New susceptibility to infection in the case of *C. neoformans*, involved AIDS-related immunosuppression. Comorbidities (e.g. older age, diabetes, cancer) that increase host susceptibility are well-recognized in WNV encephalitis [37]. Demographic changes in human population growth, density, and distribution could facilitate spread of infection or bring people in contact with new pathogens, animal hosts, or vectors. Human behavior and cultural practices increasing susceptibility to infection is well known and exemplified by the outbreak of *S. agalactiae* meningitis in adults from consuming contaminated raw fish [38]. The devastating EVD epidemic was partly exacerbated by certain high-risk burial practices according to local culture [39].

Facilitated by modern international travel, increased human population movement and transfer of intermediate hosts and arthropod vectors to and from faraway places has enabled microbes to spread around the world. WNV probably crossed the Atlantic Ocean to North America from the Middle East in this way [40], perhaps via intermediate hosts or vectors. On the other hand, CHIKV may have spread across the Indian Ocean from

Africa to Asia by patients who were viremic [41]. In the NiV outbreak in Malaysia, occupational hazard certainly played a key role because pig farmers were mainly infected from handling sick pigs [42]. Inappropriate antimicrobial use by human populations on a large scale often leads to drug resistance [28] and likely gave rise to drug-resistant *P. falciparum* [43] and *M. tuberculosis* [34].

Recent, often extreme changes to the human environment are probably the most important factors for emerging infections [27]. These interlinked changes include climate and weather changes, alteration to ecosystems and animal populations, economic development and land use, technology and industry, lack of public health services, poverty and social inequality, war and famine, and lack of political will [28].

Because zoonoses feature prominently in emerging infections (Table 50.1), changing climate and weather, ecosystems, and animal populations invariably play important roles. There is increasing recognition that global warming may have a strong impact and could encourage proliferation and wider distribution of arthropod vectors. For example, in the United States, increasing deer tick and mosquito populations have resulted in a higher incidence of Powassan virus encephalitis [44] and the phenomenal spread of WNV encephalitis, respectively [37]. The high incidence and circulation of *P. knowlesi* in Southeast Asia [4, 45] is likely related to human economic development and land use infringing on forests where the enzootic cycle between monkeys and the *Anopheles* mosquitoes had long existed. "Species" jump in this and other cases (Table 50.1) is an important phenomenon because the vast majority of emerging infections were zoonotic in origin [27, 28].

A serious lack of public health services would certainly result in emergence of any infection. In Africa, *C. neoformans* re-emergence is the result of the poor availability and delivery of antiretroviral therapy to patients with AIDS, whereas in the Western world, its incidence has already been declining [19]. Technology and industry advancing new therapies for various diseases may also have unintended effects on emerging infections. For example, *E. rostratum*-contaminated methylprednisolone injections given to patients as part of their treatment inadvertently led to iatrogenic meningitis. Failure of industrial standards and practices to ensure sterility of these pharmaceutical products played a critical role in this outbreak.

Multiple environmental factors combined with human factors to give rise to the unprecedented EBD epidemic in West Africa (i.e. Guinea, Liberia, Sierra Leone), which started in 2014 and went on to infect 28 000 people, killing more than 11 000 [39]. Apparently it took three months before the infection was diagnosed due to lack of public health services, including diagnostic lab facilities and doctors' inexperience because EVD had never been encountered there before [46]. Poverty and previous wars in these countries had already left public health facilities in a poor state. Severe shortage of healthcare workers and poor hospital supportive care contributed to the high morbidity and mortality. Moreover, human demographic changes due to migration driven by poverty and the need to find food or jobs, and urban overcrowding, human behavior, and cultural practices related to high-risk funeral and burial practices, all directly contributed to rapid and widespread person-to-person transmission. Finally, whether or not microbial genetic adaptation may have played a role is still unanswered.

Future perspective and conclusions

Undoubtedly, the human race will perpetually continue to be challenged by emerging CNS infections [3]. This is because, despite advances in treatment and vaccine development for disease prevention, uniquely, microbes can genetically adapt to ensure their continued infectivity and transmissibility to susceptible hosts. Moreover, most pathogens are zoonotic in nature, having derived from, or coevolved with, animals, and so are impossible to eradicate.

Almost all the emerging CNS infections listed in Table 50.1 have the potential for future outbreaks. Among the nonzoonotic human infections, EV-A71 and EV-D68, being spread via bodily fluids, will be impacted by environmental factors such as lack of public health services (e.g. poor sanitation and hygiene) and changes in human demography (e.g.

overcrowding). Improvements in these areas may help reduce future epidemics. Fortunately, effective EV-A71 vaccines should be available soon [47].

Emergence of drug-resistant CNS tuberculosis can be reduced by better detection methods and coverage, in addition to better patient compliance with treatment [48]. Improved availability and distribution of antiretroviral therapy should reduce the incidence of AIDS-related *C neoformans* infection in Africa over time. Artemisinin-resistant *P. falciparum* will likely pose a greater threat in the near future because its emergence seems inexorable. Hopefully, development of other effective antimalarial drugs may mitigate the situation. Conventional vector control through improved public health services and human behavior changes (e.g. sleeping under mosquito nets) may help reduce the spread of artemisinin-resistant *P. falciparum* malaria and other mosquito-borne emerging CNS infections like WNV and CHIKV.

The One Health approach to control zoonotic infections, whereby multiple sectors work together to control emerging infections has been recommended because the same microbes often infect animals and humans in the same ecosystem [48, 49]. It calls for different experts and professionals working in public health, animal and plant health, and the environment to mount systematic and coordinated efforts to deal with outbreaks. Epidemiological, laboratory, and research data should be widely shared to achieve this purpose. A similar multidisciplinary approach was applied to tackle the emergence of new variant Creutzfeldt Jakob Disease following the bovine spongiform encephalopathy epidemic in the United Kingdom. (Prion diseases are outside the scope of this book).

It is clear that emerging CNS infections do not respect international borders or the socioeconomic status of a country (Table 50.1). Many more studies are needed to understand these infections and the role of neuropathologists is pivotal to establish diagnosis and to investigate pathology and pathogenesis [50]. With better knowledge, we may be able to gain the upper hand in this ongoing "battle" against microbes by developing strategies and ways to manage, treat, and prevent emerging CNS infections, especially newly emerging infections.

References

1. Centers for Disease Control and Prevention (2014). *What are the "emerging" infectious diseases? EID journal background and goals*. https://wwwnc.cdc.gov/eid/page/background-goals (accessed 17 July 2019).
2. van Doorn, H.R. (2014). Emerging infectious diseases. *Medicine* 42 (60–63).
3. Fauci, A.S. and Morens, D.M. (2012). The perpetual challenge of infectious diseases. *N. Engl. J. Med.* 366: 454–461.
4. Singh, B. and Daneshvar, C. (2013). Human infections and detection of *Plasmodium knowlesi*. *Clin. Microbiol. Rev.* 26: 165–184.
5. Arabi, Y.M., Harthi, A., Hussein, J. et al. (2015). Severe neurologic syndrome associated with Middle East respiratory syndrome corona virus (MERS-CoV). *Infection* 43: 495–450.
6. Messacar, K., Schreiner, T.L., Maloney, J.A. et al. (2015). A cluster of acute flaccid paralysis and cranial nerve dysfunction temporally associated with an outbreak of enterovirus D68 in children in Colorado, USA. *Lancet* 385: 1662–1671.
7. Kreuter, J.D., Barnes, A., McCarthy, J.E. et al. (2011). A fatal central nervous system Enterovirus 68 infection. *Arch. Pathol. Lab. Med.* 135: 793–796.
8. Tavakoli, N.P., Wang, H., Dupuis, M. et al. (2009). Fatal case of deer tick virus encephalitis. *N. Engl. J. Med.* 360: 2099–2107.
9. Baud, D., Gubler, D.J., Schaub, B. et al. (2017). An update on Zika infetion. *Lancet* 390: 2099–2109.
10. Martines, R.B., Bhatnagar, J., Ramos, A.M.D.O. et al. (2016). Pathology of congenital Zika syndrome in Brazil: a case series. *Lancet* 388: 898–904.
11. Mehta, R., Gerardin, P., de Brito, C.A.A. et al. (2018). The neurological complications of Chikungunya virus: a systemic review. *Rev. Med. Virol.* 28: e1978.
12. Ganesan, K., Diwan, A., Shankar, S.K. et al. (2008). Chikungunya encephalomyeloradiculitis: report of 2 cases with neuroimaging and 1 case with autopsy findings. *Am. J. Neuroradiol.* 29: 1636–1638.
13. Chusri, S., Siripaitoon, P., Hirunpat, S., and Silpapojakul, K. (2011). Short report: case reports of neuro-Chikungunya in Southern Thailand. *Am. J. Trop. Med. Hyg.* 85: 386–389.
14. Robin, S., Ramful, D., Seach, F.L. et al. (2008). Neurologic manifestations of pediatric Chikungunya infection. *J. Child Neurol.* 23: 1028–1035.
15. Wong, G., Qiu, X., Bi, Y. et al. (2016). More challenges from Ebola: infection of the central nervous system. *J. Infect. Dis.* 214 (S3): s294–s296.

16. Billioux, B.J., Smith, B., and Nath, A. (2016). Neurological complications of Ebola virus infection. *Neurotherapeutics* 13: 461–470.
17. Larsen, T., Stevens, E.L., Davis, K.J. et al. (2007). Pathologic findings associated with delayed death in nonhuman primates experimentally infected with Zaire Ebola virus. *J. Infect. Dis.* 196 (S2): S323–S328.
18. Tan, K., Wijaya, L., Chiew, H.J. et al. (2017). Diffusion weighted MRI abnormalities in an outbreak of Streptococcus agalatiae serotype III, multilocus sequence type 283 meningitis. *J. Magn. Reson. Imaging* 45: 507–514.
19. Rajasingham, R., Smith, R.M., Park, B.J. et al. (2017). Global burden of disease of HIV-associated cryptococcal meningitis: an updated analysis. *Lancet Infect. Dis.* 17: 873–881.
20. Galanis, E. and MacDougall, L. (2010). Epidemiology of Cryptococcus gattii, British Columbia, Canada, 1999–2007. *Emerg. Infect. Dis.* 16: 251–257.
21. Springer, D.J. and Chaturvedi, V. (2010). Projecting global occurrence of *Cryptococcus gattii*. *Emerg. Infect. Dis.* 16: 14–20.
22. Kainer, M.A., Reagan, D., Nguyen, D.B. et al. (2012). Fungal infections associated with contaminated methylprednisolone in Tennessee. *N. Engl. J. Med.* 367: 2194–2203.
23. Ritter, J.M., Muehlenbachs, A., Blau, D.M. et al. (2013). Exserohilum rostratum infections associated with contaminated steroid injections. *Am. J. Pathol.* 183: 881–892.
24. Chin, W., Contacos, P.G., Coatney, G.R., and Kimball, H.R. (1965). A naturally acquired quotidian-type malaria in man tranferable to a monkey. *Science* 149: 865.
25. Cox-Singh, J., Hiu, J., Lucas, S.B. et al. (2010). Severe malaria- a case of fatal *Plasmodium knowlesi* infection with post mortem findings: a case report. *Malar. J.* 9: 10.
26. Ashley, E.A., Dhorda, M., Fairhurst, F.M. et al. (2014). Spread of Artemisinin resistance in Plasmodium falciparum malaria. *N. Engl. J. Med.* 371: 411–423.
27. Lederberg, J., Shope, R.E., and Oaks, S.C. (eds.) (1992). *Emerging Infections: Microbial Threats to Health in the United States*. Washington DC: National Academy Press.
28. Morens, D.M. and Fauci, A.S. (2013). Emerging infectious diseases: threats to human health and global stability. *PLoS Pathog.* 9: e1003467.
29. Tsetsarkin, K.A., Vanlandingham, D.L., McGee, C.E., and Higgs, S. (2007). A single mutation in Chikungunya virus affects vector specificity and epidemic potential. *PLoS Pathog.* 3: e201.
30. Yuan, L., Huang, X.Y., Lin, Y.Z. et al. (2017). A single mutation in the prM protein of Zika virus contributes to microcephaly. *Science* 358: 933–936.
31. World Health Organization (WHO) (2018). *WHO global tuberculosis report*. http://www.who.int/tb/publications/global_report/en (accessed 17 July 2019).
32. Wang, T., Feng, G.D., Pang, Y. et al. (2016). High rate of drug resistance among tuberculous meningitis cases in Shaaxi province, China. *Sci. Rep.* 6: 25251.
33. Patel, V.B., Padayatchi, N., Bhigjee, A.I. et al. (2004). Multidrug-resistant tuberculous meningitis in KwaZulu-Natal, South Africa. *Clin. Infect. Dis.* 38: 851–856.
34. Smith, T., Wolff, K.A., and Nyugen, L. (2013). Molecular biology of drug resistance in *Mycobacterium tuberculosis*. *Curr. Top. Microbiol. Immunol.* 374: 53–80.
35. Ariey, F., Witkowski, B., Amaratunga, C. et al. (2014). A molecular marker of artemisinin-resistant *Plasmodium falciparum* malaria. *Nature* 505: 50–55.
36. Ong, K.C. and Wong, K.T. (2005). Understanding Enterovirus 71 neuropathogenesis and its impact on other neurotropic enteroviruses. *Brain Pathol.* 15: 614–624.
37. Petersen, L.R., Brault, A.C., and Nasci, R.S. (2013). West Nile virus: review of the literature. *JAMA* 310: 308–315.
38. Chau, M.L., Chen, S.L., Yap, M. et al. (2017). Group B Streptococcus infections caused by improper sourcing and handling of fish for raw consumption, Singapore, 2015–2016. *Emerg. Infect. Dis.* 23: 1982–1990.
39. World Health Organization (WHO) (2015). *Emergencies preparedness, response. Factors that contributed to undetected spread of Ebola virus and impeded rapid containment*. https://www.who.int/csr/disease/ebola/one-year-report/factors/en (accessed 17 July 2019).
40. Sejvar, J.J. (2003). West Nile virus: an historical overview. *Ochsner J.* 5: 6–10.
41. Staples, J.E., Breiman, R.F., and Powers, A.M. (2009). Chikungunya fever: an epidemiological review of a re-emerging infectious disease. *Clin. Infect. Dis.* 49: 942–948.
42. Chua, K.B., Goh, K.J., Wong, K.T. et al. (1999). Fatal encephalitis due to Nipah virus among pig farmers in Malaysia. *Lancet* 354: 1257–1259.
43. Noedl, H., Se, Y., Socheat, D., and Fukuda, M.M. (2008). Evidence of Artemisin-resistant malaria in Western Cambodia. *N. Engl. J. Med.* 359: 2619–2620.
44. Fatmi, S.S., Zehra, R., and Carpenter, D.O. (2017). Powassan virus- a new reemerging tick-borne disease. *Front. Public Health* 5: 342.

45. Vythilingam, I., NoorAzian, Y.M., Tan, C.H. et al. (2008). Plasmodium knowlesi in humans, macaques and mosquitoes in peninsular Malaysia. *Parasit. Vectors* 1: 26.
46. World Health Organization (WHO) (2019). *WHO fact sheet on Ebola virus disease*. https://www.who.int/news-room/fact-sheets/detail/ebola-virus-disease (accessed 17 July 2019).
47. Yi, E.J., Shin, Y.J., Kim, J.H. et al. (2017). Enterovirus 71 infection and vaccines. *Clin. Exp. Vaccin. Res.* 6: 4–14.
48. World Health Organization (WHO) (2017). *One Health*. https://www.who.int/features/qa/onehealth/en (accessed 17 July 2019).
49. Centers for Disease Control and Prevention (CDC) (2018). *CDC One Health fact sheet*. http://www.cdc.gov/onehealth/basics/index.html (accessed 17 July 2019).
50. Wong, K.T. (2010). Emerging epidemic viral encephalitides with a special focus on henipaviruses. *Acta Neuropathol.* 120: 317–325.

Index

Note: Page numbers followed by f, t, and b indicate figures, tables, and boxes, respectively.

β2AR 288–289, 288f

ABM *see* acute bacterial meningitis
abscess
  actinomycosis 337–341
  amoebic 464
  brain 29, 36–40, 281, 310–311, 311–313f, 320, 320f
  community-acquired 29, 36–40
  epidural 282–283, 313–315, 321, 322f
  nocardiosis 343–347
  non-tuberculous mycobacterial infections 357–362
  post-operative 320–321
  subdural empyema 283, 311–313, 320, 321f
  see also brain abscess; epidural abscess; extradural abscess; surgical site infections
Acanthamoeba spp. 464, 465–466
acquired immune deficiency syndrome (AIDS)
  adenovirus meningoencephalitis 79, 80f
  animal models 225
  children 27, 221–222
  cryptococcosis 222, 426, 508t, 509–511
  cytomegalovirus 67
  diffuse poliodystrophy 220–221, 221f
  epidemiology 217
  highly active antiretroviral therapy complications 223–225
  neurological complications 218–223
  opportunistic infections 23–25, 222–223
  pathogenesis 225–227
  polyomavirus 85
  primary lesions 218–222
  secondary lesions 223
  Toxoplasma gondii 451–455, 544–545f
  treatment 223–225, 227
  varicella-zoster virus 56–58
  see also human immunodeficiency virus
actinomycosis 337–341
  clinical features 338–339
  diagnosis 338–339
  epidemiology 338
  microbiology 337–338
  pathology 339–340
  treatment 340
acute bacterial meningitis (ABM) 29–33, 280, 285t, 295–307
  adjunctive measures 33t
  antibiotics 32t
  clinical features 30–31, 298–299
  community acquired 29–33
  diagnosis 30–31, 280, 298–301
  differential diagnosis 300–301
  epidemiology 30, 285t, 296
  microbiology 296–298
  pathology 301–303
  pathophysiology 31
  prognostic factors 301
  treatment 31–33, 32–33t, 303–305
  vaccines 304–305
acute disseminated encephalomyelitis (ADEM) 251–255
  clinical features 252
  diagnosis 252
  epidemiology 252
  measles virus 95
  pathogenesis 254–255
  pathology 252–254, 253–254f
acute hemorrhagic leukoencephalitis (AHLE) 251, 255, 256f

Index

acute herpes simplex virus encephalitis 47–49, 47–48f
acute necrotizing encephalopathy (ANE) 251, 255, 256f
acyclovir 51–52, 61, 63
ADEM *see* acute disseminated encephalomyelitis
adenovirus (ADV) meningoencephalitis 77–82
  clinical features 78
  diagnosis 79
  epidemiology 78
  imaging studies 78
  pathogenesis 79–80
  pathology 79
  treatment 81
adenovirus encephalitis (ADVE) *see* adenovirus meningoencephalitis
adhesins, bacterial invasion 283–292, 286f, 288f, 290f
adjunctive measures, acute bacterial meningitis 33t
ADV *see* adenovirus
ADVE (adenovirus encephalitis) *see* adenovirus meningoencephalitis
AEE *see* alphaviral equine encephalomyelitis
aerosol sources, *legionella* 384b
African tick bite fever 275
African trypanosomiasis 7t, 467–469
AIDS *see* acquired immune deficiency syndrome
α-herpesviridae 43, 55–61
alphaviral equine encephalomyelitis (AEE) 183–187
  animal models 186
  clinical features 184–185
  epidemiology 184
  microbiology 183–184
  pathogenesis 186
  pathology 185–186, 185t
  treatment 186–187
amikacin 360
amoebiasis 7t, 463–466
  abscess 464
  granulomatous encephalitis 465–466
  keratitis 466
  primary meningoencephalitis 464–465

amoxicillin 303
anaplasmal tick-borne rickettsioses 275
Anaplasma phagocytophilum 5t, 272, 275
angiostrongylosis 476t, 487–488
ANI *see* asymptomatic neurocognitive impairment
animal hosts
  dengue virus 148–151, 149t
  flaviviruses 132–133, 136f, 148–151, 149t
  henipaviruses 14
  leishmaniasis 472
  Murray Valley encephalitis 148–151, 149t
  rabies 121–122
  St. Louis encephalitis virus 148–151, 149t
  Toxoplasma gondii 449–461
  trypanosomiasis 466, 469
  West Nile virus 148–151, 149t
  yellow fever virus 148–151, 149t
animal models
  acquired immune deficiency syndrome 225
  acute hemorrhagic leukoencephalitis 255
  adenovirus meningoencephalitis 79–80
  alphaviral equine encephalomyelitis 186
  Borrelia burgdorferi 372–373
  cytomegalovirus 72
  dengue virus 159, 160–161t
  flaviviruses 137–138, 143, 157–159, 160–161t, 173–174
  helminth infections 492
  henipavirus encephalitis 117–118
  hepatitis C & E viruses 180
  human immunodeficiency virus 225
  Japanese encephalitis virus 173–174
  John Cunningham virus 91
  legionellosis 388–389
  leptospirosis 375
  malaria 441–444
  measles virus 100–101
  Mycobacterium tuberculosis 355
  poliomyelitis 200
  polyomavirus 91

  rabies 125
  St. Louis encephalitis virus 159, 160–161t
  sarcoidosis 399
  tick-borne encephalitis virus 143
  Toxoplasma gondii 457–458
  Treponema pallidum 369–370
  West Nile virus 159, 160–161t
  yellow fever virus 159, 160–161t
antibiotics
  acute bacterial meningitis 32t, 303–304
  cerebral actinomycosis 340
  community acquired meningitis 32t
  legionellosis 390
  Listeria monocytogenes 32t
  Mycoplasma pneumoniae 268
  nocardiosis 346
  post-operative pyogenic infections 326
  Tropheryma whipplei 335
antiretroviral therapy (ART) 216, 217
apoptosis, sepsis-associated encephalopathy 16
arboviruses 132, 189
  Chikungunya virus 189–193, 506t, 509–512
  Zika virus 137, 163–168, 507t, 509–510
ART *see* antiretroviral therapy
artemisinin-resistant *Plasmodium falciparum* 508t, 510–512
artesunate 444–446
aseptic meningitis
  herpes simplex virus 50
  measles virus 95
aspergillosis 38, 421–423, 433t
asymptomatic carriers, human immunodeficiency virus 217–218
asymptomatic neurocognitive impairment (ANI) 218
atypical herpes simplex virus encephalitis 49–50
autoimmunity
  human T cell leukemia/lymphoma virus type 1 240
  Rasmussen encephalitis 262–263
autoinfection, strongyloidiasis 491
autolysis, *Streptococcus pneumoniae* invasion 287

Index

axonal damage
  human immunodeficiency virus 219–220
  sepsis-associated encephalopathy 16
azithromycin 360

Bacillus cereus 416
bacterial infections
  acute meningitis 29–33, 280, 285t, 295–307
  brain abscess 29, 36–40, 281, 320, 320f
  chronic meningitis 280–281
  classification 5–6t
  clinical presentation 280–283
  community-acquired brain abscess 29, 36–40
  emerging 507–508t
  epidural abscess 282–283, 313–315, 321, 322f
  following neurosurgical procedures 319–330
  inflammation 292
  invasion mechanisms 283–292
    Escherichia coli 291
    group B *streptococcus* 290–291, 290f
    Listeria monocytogenes 291–292
    Neisseria meningitidis 287–289, 288f
    Streptococcus pneumoniae 284–287, 286f
    Treponema pallidum 370
  mycotic aneurysm 315–316
  pyogenic 295–330
  septic embolism 315–316
  subdural empyema 283, 311–313, 320, 321f
  suppurative intracranial phlebitis 316–317, 317t
  transcystosis 284, 286–287, 286f, 287–291, 288f
  ventriculitis 283
  see also individual species...
bacterial meningitis (BM)
  acute see acute bacterial meningitis
  chronic 280–281
Balamuthia mandrillaris 464, 465–466
Basigin 283, 288–289, 288f, 289f

bat-to-human transmission
  henipaviruses 114
  rabies virus 124
Behçet disease/syndrome 263–264
Besnier–Boeck–Schaumann disease see sarcoidosis
beta-2 adrenergic receptor (β2AR) 288–289, 288f
β-herpesviridae 43–44, 65–76
biomarkers, sepsis-associated encephalopathy 13
BK virus (BKV) 84–85, 91
  see also John Cunningham virus; polyomavirus
blood-brain barrier (BBB), bacterial invasion 283–284, 286f, 288f, 290f
blood markers, sepsis-associated encephalopathy 13
BM see acute bacterial meningitis; bacterial meningitis, chronic
Borrelia burgdorferi (Lyme disease) 370–374
  chronic meningitis 281
  clinical features 371–372
  epidemiology 371
  historical perspectives 370–371
  microbiology 371
  pathogenesis 372–373
  pathology 372
  relapsing fever 373–374
  treatment 373–374
botulinum neurotoxin (BoNT) 414–416
boutonneuse fever 272, 275
brain abscess 29, 36–40, 281, 310–311, 311–313f, 320, 320f
  actinomycosis 337–341
  amoebic 464
  capsule development 310–311
  community-acquired 29, 36–40
  diagnosis 38
  epidemiology 36–37
  imaging 37–38
  immunodeficient patients 37
  nocardiosis 343–347
  non-tuberculous mycobacterial infections 357–362
  pathogenesis 37
  pathology 310–311, 311–313f
  post-operative 320, 320f

  treatment 39t, 40
  see also surgical site infections
brain myiasis 504
Brill-Zinsser disease 275
bronchitis 77
Brucella spp. 379–382
  chronic meningitis 281
  clinical features 380
  diagnosis 380
  epidemiology 379, 380
  genetic factors 381
  microbiology 379–380
  pathology/pathogenesis 380–381
  treatment 381
bulbar encephalitis, varicella-zoster virus 57
"burnt-out" lesions
  highly active antiretroviral therapy 223, 224f
  Rasmussen encephalitis 260–262, 261f
  varicella-zoster virus 58, 60f
burst suppression 13
bystander toxicity 240

candidiasis 427–428, 433t
capsule development, brain abscess 310–311
carbapenem, nocardiosis 346
cART see combined antiretroviral therapy
CbpA see choline-binding protein A
CD4 antigen 216
CD147 283, 288–289, 288f, 289f
CE see cystic echinococcosis
cefotaxime 303
cephalosporins 298, 346
cerebrospinal fluid (CSF) see laboratory tests and individual species diagnosis
cestodes 8t, 476t, 478–485
  coenurosis 476t, 484
  cystic echinococcosis 476t, 480–483, 483f
  neurocysticercosis 478–480, 481f, 482t
  sparganosis 476t, 484–485, 485f
Chagas disease 469–470
chickenpox see varicella-zoster virus
Chikungunya virus (CHIKV) 189–193, 506t, 509–512
  clinical features 190–191

517

Index

Chikungunya virus (CHIKV) (cont'd)
  diagnosis 191
  pathology 191
  pathophysiology 189–190
  treatment 191–192
  vaccines 192
choline-binding protein A
    (CbpA) 286–287
chronic herpes simplex virus
    encephalitis 49, 49f
chronic meningitis 280–281
chronic pachymeningitis *see*
    hypertrophic pachymeningitis
chronic Parechovirus A
    infections 247
cidofovir 72, 92
ciprofloxacin 360
clarithromycin 360
classic herpes simplex virus
    encephalitis 46–49
classifications 1–9, 3–4t, 4–6t, 6–7t,
    7–8t
  bacterial infections 4–6t
  enteroviruses 4–6t, 195–196
  flaviviruses 3–4t, 132
  fungal infections 6–7t, 420–421
  herpes simplex viruses 3t, 43–44
  mycoplasmal infections 4–6t,
      267, 272
  non-tuberculous mycobacterial
      infections 357–358
  parasitic infections 7–8t, 437,
      449, 463, 476–477t
  rickettsial infections 4–6t, 272
clindamycin 458
clinical features *see individual species
    and conditions...*
Clostridium botulinum 414–416
Clostridium difficile 416
Clostridium perfringens 414
Clostridium sordellii 416
Clostridium tetani 412–414
CMV *see* cytomegalovirus
coccidioidomycosis 428–429
coenurosis 476t, 484
coma, sepsis-associated
    encephalopathy 13
combined antiretroviral therapy
    (cART) 216
combined granulocytic and
    lymphocytic disorders,
    opportunistic 24

community-acquired acute bacterial
    meningitis 29–33
  see also acute bacterial meningitis
computed tomography (CT)
  brain imaging 37–38
  hypertrophic
      pachymeningitis 405
  Japanese encephalitis virus 171
  Mycoplasma pneumoniae
      268, 269f
  polyomavirus 86
  post-operative infections 326
  septic embolism 315
  Toxoplasma gondii 451–452
  West Nile virus 153
congenital Chagas disease 470
congenital immunodeficiency
    22–23, 26–27
congenital infections
  cytomegalovirus 66, 67–68, 72,
      73–74f
  Toxoplasma gondii 451, 452–453,
      456, 456f
congenital rubella syndrome (CRS)
    107–108, 109–110
corticosteroids
  acute bacterial meningitis 304
  Chikungunya fever 191–192
  post-operative pyogenic
      infections 326
cranial neuropathies, sarcoidosis
    395–396
croup 77
CRS *see* congenital rubella syndrome
cryptococcosis 425–427, 433t, 508t,
    509–511
  acquired immune deficiency
      syndrome 222, 426
  encephalitis 35
CSF (cerebrospinal fluid) *see under*
    laboratory tests and
    individual species diagnosis
cystic echinococcosis (CE) 476t,
    480–483, 483f
cysticercosis 478–480, 481f, 482t
cytokines
  bacterial infections 292
  cerebral malaria 442–443
cytomegalovirus (CMV) 65–76
  acquired immune deficiency
      syndrome 222
  animal models 72

clinical features 67–68
congenital infection 67–68, 72,
    73–74f
diagnosis 68–69
encephalitis 36
epidemiology 66
imaging studies 68
laboratory tests 68–69
latent infections 72
microbiology 66–67
neonates 66, 67–68, 72, 73–74f
pathology 66–67, 69–72
treatment 72–74
cytotoxic model, human T cell
    leukemia/lymphoma virus
    type 1 239

DAA *see* direct-acting antivirals
daclatasvir, hepatitis C virus 180
damage-associated molecular
    pattern molecules (DAMPs),
    sepsis-associated
    encephalopathy 15
DAMPs *see* damage-associated
    molecular pattern molecules
delirium, sepsis-associated
    encephalopathy 12–13, 15
dematiaceous molds 6t, 425, 433t
demyelination
  acute disseminated
      encephalomyelitis 251–255
  acute hemorrhagic
      leukoencephalitis 255
dengue virus (DENV) 147–162
  animal models 159, 160–161t
  clinical features 150t, 151–153
  epidemiology 132, 133f,
      148–151, 149t
  genetic factors 151
  laboratory tests 154
  pathogenesis 158–159, 158b
  pathology 150t, 157
  treatment 159
  vaccines 161
dexmedetomidine, sepsis-associated
    encephalopathy 15–16
diagnosis *see under* individual
    species or condition
diffuse nodular encephalitis,
    cytomegalovirus 69
diffuse poliodystrophy (DPD)
    220–221, 221f

Index

dimorphic fungi 7t, 428–430, 433t
  blastomycosis 7t, 429
  coccidioidomycosis 7t, 428–429
  histoplasmosis 7t, 429
  paracoccidioidomycosis 7t, 429–430
dipterous insects, myiasis 503–504
direct-acting antivirals (DAA), hepatitis C & E viruses 180–181
DNA replication inhibitors, acyclovir 51–52
dog-to-human transmission, rabies virus 124
doxycycline 273, 335
DPD *see* diffuse poliodystrophy
drug-resistant *Mycobacterium tuberculosis* 350, 354–355, 507t, 509, 510, 512
dysentery 416

early changes, human immunodeficiency virus 217
early neurosyphilis 365
Eastern equine encephalomyelitis (EEE) 183–187
  animal models 186
  clinical features 184–185
  epidemiology 184
  microbiology 183–184
  pathogenesis 186
  pathology 185–186, 185t
  treatment 186–187
Ebola virus disease (EVD) 507t, 509–511
EBV *see* Epstein–Barr virus
Echinococcus granulosus 476t, 480–483, 483f
Ehrlichia chaffeensis 5t, 272, 275
EL *see* encephalitis lethargica
electroencephalograms (EEG)
  alphaviral equine encephalomyelitis 184
  Japanese encephalitis virus 171
  sepsis-associated encephalopathy 13
electron microscopy (EM)
  herpes simplex virus encephalitis 48–49f
  Mycoplasma pneumoniae 268, 271f
  poliovirus 198, 198–199f

polyomavirus 88–89, 88–90f
Tropheryma whipplei 333–334, 334f
emerging infections 505–514
  major and significant 506–508t
  pathology 505–510
  reasons for 510–511
emetic toxins 416
EMPRINN *see* extracellular matrix metalloproteinase inducer
encephalitis
  adults 29, 33–36
  amoebiasis 464–466
  causative organisms 34t
  clinical features 34
  cryptococcosis 35
  cytomegalovirus 36
  epidemiology 33, 34t
  granulomatous amoebic 465–466
  henipavirus 113–119
  herpes simplex virus 34–35, 46–52
  HSV and VZV 34–35
  human herpesvirus 6 36
  immunocompromised patients 35–36
  Japanese 169–176
  John Cunningham virus 36
  measles inclusion body 99
  Murray Valley 147–162
  primary amoebic meningo- 464–465
  Rasmussen 259–263
  rubella virus 106–107
  St. Louis virus 147–162
  tick-borne virus 132, 133f, 138–144
  see also inflammation
encephalitis lethargica (EL) 264–265
encephalopathy
  Hashimoto 265
  sepsis-associated 11–20
Entamoeba histolytica 463–465
enterobacteriaceae, antibiotics 32t
enteroviruses (EV)
  A71 205–213, 506t, 509–512
  clinical features 208
  epidemiology 206–208, 506t, 509–512
  microbiology 205–206
  pathogenesis 209–211

  pathology 208–209, 209–210f
  treatment 211
  vaccines 211
  classification 195–196
  D68 507t, 509, 511–512
  poliovirus 195–204
epidemic louse-borne classic typhus 275–276
epidemiology *see* under individual species or condition
epidural abscess 282–283, 313–315, 321, 322f
  see also extradural abscess; surgical site infections
epilepsy, sepsis-associated encephalopathy 13
epiregulin (EREG) 26
Epstein–Barr virus (EBV) 61–63
  clinical features 61–63
  neuropathology 63
  treatment 63
Escherichia coli
  acute bacterial meningitis 297
  invasion mechanisms 291
ethambutol 360
EV *see* enteroviruses
EVD *see* Ebola virus disease
exanthem-producing febrile acute infections, rubella virus 106, 107f
excitotoxicity, sepsis-associated encephalopathy 15
Exserohilum rostratum 508t, 509–510
extensively drug-resistant *Mycobacterium tuberculosis* (XDR TB) 350
extracellular matrix metalloproteinase inducer (EMPRINN) 283, 288–289, 288f, 289f
extradural abscess 314–315

facilitated transport, bacterial invasion 284
factor H-binding protein (fHBP) 287
febrile respiratory illness 77
fHBP *see* factor H-binding protein
filariasis 490–491, 491f
flaviviruses (FV) 131–176
  animal hosts 132–133, 136f

Index

flaviviruses (FV) (cont'd)
  animal models 137–138, 143, 157–159, 160–161t, 173–174
  classification 132
  clinical features 137, 140–141, 150t, 151–153, 163, 164f, 170–172
  dengue virus 147–162
  epidemiology 139, 140f, 148–151, 149t, 170
  genetics 132, 134f, 139, 165–166
  historical perspectives 132, 134f, 138–139
  Japanese encephalitis virus 132, 133f, 169–176
  lifecycle 133, 135–136f
  microbiology 132, 134f, 139, 170
  Murray Valley encephalitis 147–162
  pathogenesis 137–138, 143, 157–159, 158b, 165–166, 173–174
  pathology 137, 141–143, 142f, 150t, 154–157, 163–164, 172–173, 172f
  St. Louis encephalitis virus 147–162
  tick-borne encephalitis 138–144
  treatment 138, 144, 159, 166, 174
  vaccines 138, 159–161, 174
  West Nile virus 147–162, 506t, 509–510
  yellow fever virus 147–162
  Zika virus 163–168, 507t, 509–510
flea-borne rickettsioses 276–277
focal cerebritis 310
folinic acid 458
food poisoning 416
foscarnet 36, 61, 63, 72
fungal infections 419–436
  animal models 431–434
  aspergillosis 421–423
  blastomycosis 429
  candidiasis 427–428
  classification 6–7t, 420–421, 433t
  coccidioidomycosis 428–429
  cryptococcosis 222, 426, 508t, 509–511
  dematiaceous molds 6t, 425
  diagnosis 421–424, 432f
  dimorphic 7t, 428–430, 433t
  emerging 508t

Exserohilum rostratum 508t, 509–510
  genetic factors 430–431
  histoplasmosis 429
  laboratory tests 433t
  molds 38, 421–425
  mucormycosis 424
  paracoccidioidomycosis 429–430
  pauciseptate hyaline molds 6t, 424–425
  risk factors 433t
  Scedosporium spp. 423–424
  septate hyaline molds 6t, 38, 421–424
  treatment 433t
  yeasts 7t, 425–428
furious rabies 125
FV *see* flaviviruses

GAE *see* granulomatous amoebic encephalitis
γ-herpesviridae 44, 61–63
ganciclovir 36, 63, 72
GBS *see* group B streptococcus; Guillain–Barré syndrome
general paresis of the insane (GPI) 366–368, 368–369f
genetic factors
  Brucella spp. 381
  congenital immunodeficiencies 26
  dengue virus 151
  fungal infections 430–431
  helminth infections 492
  malaria 26, 438–439
  measles virus 96
  Mycobacterium tuberculosis 26, 355
  poliovirus 198–199, 202
  postpolio syndrome 202
  Rasmussen encephalitis 260
  rubella virus 110
  sarcoidosis 398
  subacute sclerosing panencephalitis 97
  Tropheryma whipplei 334–335
  Zika virus 165–166
genetics *see* genomes
genomes
  actinomyces 337–338, 340
  alphaviral equine encephalomyelitis 183–184, 186
  Borrelia burgdorferi 371

Chikungunya virus 190
enterovirus A71 206–207, 211
flaviviruses 132, 134f
henipaviruses 113
human immunodeficiency virus 216–217
human T cell leukemia/lymphoma virus type 1 233
Japanese encephalitis virus 170
John Cunningham virus 84
Mycobacterium tuberculosis 350, 354–355
nocardiosis 345–346
Parechovirus A 243–244
poliovirus 196
tick-borne encephalitis 139
Toxoplasma gondii 456–457
Treponema pallidum 363
  see also microbiology
glutathione S-transferase (GST) 492
gnathostomiasis 477t, 488–489
GPI *see* general paresis of the insane
granulation tissue, brain abscess 311
granulocytic disorders, opportunistic infections 24
granulomatous amoebic encephalitis (GAE) 465–466
granulomatous herpes simplex virus encephalitis 50
gray matter pathologies
  human immunodeficiency virus 220–221, 221f
  John Cunningham virus 89, 90f
group B *streptococcus* (GBS)
  emerging 507t, 509
  invasion mechanisms 290–291, 290f
  meningitis 280, 297
  vaccines 305
GST *see* glutathione S-transferase
Guillain–Barré syndrome (GBS)
  arboviruses 191
  rubella virus 106
gumma, cerebral 366, 367f

HAART *see* highly active antiretroviral therapy
HAD *see* human immunodeficiency virus-associated dementia
Haemophilus influenzae type b (Hib)
  meningitis 280, 297
  vaccines 305

Index

HAM/TSP *see* human T cell leukemia/lymphoma virus type 1 associated myelopathy/tropical spastic paraparesis
HAND *see* human immunodeficiency virus-associated neurocognitive disorder
hand-foot-mouth disease (HFMD) 205–213
   epidemiology 206–208
   treatment 211
   vaccines 211
   see also enteroviruses, A71
Hashimoto encephalopathy 265
HCMV (human cytomegalovirus) *see* cytomegalovirus
Heerfordt's syndrome *see* sarcoidosis
helminth infections 8t, 475–502, 476–477t
   angiostrongylosis 476t, 487–488
   animal models 492
   cestodes 476t, 478–485
   classification 8t, 476–477t
   coenurosis 476t, 484
   cystic echinococcosis 476t, 480–483, 483f
   filariasis 490–491, 491f
   genetic factors 492
   gnathostomiasis 477t, 488–489
   nematodes 476–477t, 487–492
   neurocysticercosis 478–480, 481f, 482t
   neurotoxocariasis 477t, 489
   neurotrichinosis 477t, 489–490
   paragonimiasis 476t, 487
   pathology 476–477t, 478, 479f
   schistosomiasis 477t, 485–486, 500–502
   sparganosis 476t, 484–485, 485f
   strongyloidiasis 477t, 491–492
   trematodes 476t, 485–487, 500–502
Hendra virus (HeV) 113–119
   see also henipavirus encephalitis
henipavirus encephalitis 113–119
   animal models 117–118
   clinical features 114–115
   diagnosis 114–115
   epidemiology 113–114
   microbiology 113, 114f
   pathogenesis 117–118
   pathology 115–117, 116–117f
   relapsing 117
   treatment 118
hepatic encephalopathy 223
hepatitis C virus (HCV) 177–181
   animal models 180
   characteristics 178, 178t
   clinical features 179–180
   epidemiology 179
   historical perspectives 177–178
   microbiology 178–179
   pathogenesis 180
   pathology 180
   treatment 180
hepatitis E virus (HEV) 177–181
   animal models 180
   characteristics 178–179, 178t
   clinical features 179–180
   epidemiology 179
   historical perspectives 177–178
   microbiology 178–179
   pathogenesis 180
   pathology 180
   treatment 180–181
herpes simplex virus encephalitis (HSVE) 34–35, 46–52
   acute 47–49, 47–48f
   aseptic meningitis 50
   atypical 49–50
   chronic 49, 49f
   classic 46–49
   clinical approaches 34–35
   clinical features 46, 50–51
   granulomatous 50
   neonatal 50–51, 52f
   spinal cord disease 50
herpes viruses 43–76
   herpes simplex viruses (HSV) 43–54
   classification 43–44
   cytomegalovirus 65–76
   epidemiology 45
   Epstein–Barr virus 61–63
   historical perspective 44
   pathophysiology 44–45
   primary infections 44, 45–46
   spinal cord disease 50
   susceptibility factors 51
   treatment 51–52
   varicella-zoster virus 55–61
α-herpesviridae 43, 55–61
β-herpesviridae 43–44, 65–76
γ-herpesviridae 44
Heubner arteritis 366
HeV *see* Hendra virus
HFMD *see* hand-foot-mouth disease
HHV-5 (human herpesvirus-5) *see* cytomegalovirus
HHV-6 *see* human herpesvirus 6
Hib *see* Haemophilus influenzae type b
highly active antiretroviral therapy (HAART) 216
   associated CNS changes 223–225
   immune reconstitution inflammatory syndrome 25, 223–225, 226f
   and neurocognitive disorders 225, 227
   opportunistic infections 24–25
   varicella-zoster virus 58
hippocampus, Zika virus 164f, 165
histopathology *see* neuropathology; pathology
HIV *see* human immunodeficiency virus
HIVE *see* human immunodeficiency virus encephalitis
host-related factors 21–42
   adults 29–42
   children 26–27
   immune reconstitution inflammatory syndrome 25
   immunodeficiencies 22–25
   intrauterine infections 25–26
   neonates 26–27
   opportunistic infections 23–25, 27
   see also genetic factors; risk factors
HSV *see* herpes simplex viruses
HSVE *see* herpes simplex encephalitis; herpes simplex virus encephalitis
HTLV-1 *see* human T cell leukemia/lymphoma virus type 1
human cytomegalovirus (HCMV) *see* cytomegalovirus
human herpesvirus-5 (HHV-5) *see* cytomegalovirus
human herpesvirus 6 (HHV-6), encephalitis 36
human immunodeficiency virus-associated dementia (HAD) 218

Index

human immunodeficiency virus-associated neurocognitive disorder (HAND) 218, 225, 227
human immunodeficiency virus encephalitis (HIVE) 218–222, 220f, 227
human immunodeficiency virus (HIV) 215–229
  adenovirus meningoencephalitis 79, 80f
  animal models 225
  asymptomatic carriers 217–218
  children 221–222
  cryptococcosis 35, 222, 426, 508t, 509–511
  cytomegalovirus 67
  diffuse poliodystrophy 220–221, 221f
  early changes 217
  epidemiology 216–217
  highly active antiretroviral therapy recipients 223–225, 224f
  historical perspective 215–216
  immune reconstitution inflammatory syndrome 25
  John Cunningham virus 36
  microbiology 216
  Mycobacterium tuberculosis co-infection 354
  neurological complications 218–223
  opportunistic infections 24–25, 222–223
  pathogenesis 225–227
  polyomavirus 85
  primary lesions 218–222
  secondary lesions 223
  Toxoplasma gondii 451–455, 544–545f
  treatment 223–225, 227
  Treponema pallidum infections 367f, 368–369
  see also acquired immune deficiency syndrome
human immunodeficiency virus leukoencephalopathy (HIVL) 218–220, 227
human T cell leukemia/lymphoma virus type 1 associated myelopathy/tropical spastic paraparesis (HAM/TSP) 232t, 235–240
  clinical features 237–238
  epidemiology 235–237, 236f
  pathogenesis 238–240, 239f
  pathology 238–239
  risk factors 237
  treatment 240
human T cell leukemia/lymphoma virus type 1 (HTLV-1) 231–242
  associated diseases 232t
  epidemiology 234–237, 234f, 236f
  historical perspectives 232
  microbiology 232–233
  treatment 240
HvgA see hypervirulent GBS adhesin
hydrocephalus, Zika virus 164–165, 164f
hydrochloroquinine 335
hyperinfection, strongyloidiasis 492
hypertrophic pachymeningitis (HP) 403–409
  clinical features 404–405
  diagnosis 405
  epidemiology 404
  pathogenesis 407–408
  pathology 405–407
  treatment 408
hypervirulent GBS adhesin (HvgA) 291
hypocholinergia, sepsis-associated encephalopathy 15

ICAM-1, bacterial infections 292
IL see interleukin
imaging see computed tomography; diagnosis; magnetic resonance imaging
immune reconstitution inflammatory syndrome (IRIS) 25, 86, 90–91, 223–225, 226f
immunocompromised patients see immunodeficiency
immunocytochemistry
  herpes simplex virus encephalitis 47–49
  poliovirus 198, 198–199f
immunodeficiency
  acquired 23–25, 27
  brain abscess 282
  chronic Parechovirus A infections 247
  community-acquired brain abscess 37
  congenital 22–23, 26–27
  cryptococcosis 35, 426
  encephalitis 35–36
  primary 22–23, 26–27
  Toxoplasma gondii 451–452
  Tropheryma whipplei 334–335
  tuberculous meningitis 35–36
immunoglobulins
  anti-rabies 127
  see also intravenous immune globulin
immunohistochemistry
  rabies virus 127
  Rasmussen encephalitis 262
  Tropheryma whipplei 333
immunoprotective niches 370
incubation
  alphaviral equine encephalomyelitis 184
  enterovirus A71 208
  rabies virus 124
  Rickettsia 272
  tick-borne encephalitis 140
individual clinical presentation variations 21–28
  see also genetic factors; risk factors; single nucleotide polymorphisms
inducible nitric oxide synthase (iNOS) 15
infants
  cytomegalovirus 66, 67–68, 72, 73–74f
  infections 26–27
  rubella virus 107–110, 108–109f
  Toxoplasma gondii 451, 452–453, 456, 456f
  see also neonates
inflammation
  acute disseminated encephalomyelitis 251–255
  acute hemorrhagic leukoencephalitis 255
  bacterial infections 292
  cerebral malaria 443–444, 445f
  encephalitis lethargica 264–265
  Hashimoto encephalopathy 265

Index

immune reconstitution syndrome 25
John Cunningham virus 90–91
miscellaneous disorders 259–266
neuro-Behçet disease 263–264
physiology 445f
Rasmussen syndrome 259–263
sepsis-associated encephalopathy 13–15
see also encephalitis; encephalopathy
iNOS *see* inducible nitric oxide synthase
interleukins (IL) 13
intermediate hosts, henipaviruses 114
intra-axial neuro-Behçet syndrome 263–264
intracranial epidural abscess 313–314
intrauterine infections, pregnancies 25–26
intravenous immune globulin (IVIG)
  enterovirus A71 211
  Parechovirus A 248
invasion mechanisms
  bacterial infections 283–292
    Escherichia coli 291
    group B streptococcus 290–291, 290f
    Listeria monocytogenes 291–292
    Neisseria meningitidis 287–289, 288f
    Streptococcus pneumoniae 284–287, 286f
    Treponema pallidum 370
IRIS *see* immune reconstitution inflammatory syndrome
ischemic lesions, sepsis-associated encephalopathy 14
ivermectin 488, 491
IVIG *see* intravenous immune globulin

Japanese encephalitis virus (JEV) 169–176
  animal models 173–174
  clinical features 170–172
  diagnosis 170–172
  epidemiology 132, 133f, 170
  historical perspective 169
  lifecycle 136f
  microbiology 170
  pathogenesis 173–174
  pathology 172–173, 172f
  treatment 174
  vaccines 174
JCV *see* John Cunningham virus
JCVE *see* John Cunningham virus encephalitis
JEV *see* Japanese encephalitis virus
John Cunningham virus encephalitis (JCVE) 86, 89, 90f
John Cunningham virus (JCV) 36, 84–93
  animal models 91
  clinical features 85–87
  diagnosis 85–87
  epidemiology 85
  genome 84f
  gray matter pathologies 89, 90f
  inflammatory pathologies 90–91
  microbiology 84–85
  neuropathology 87–89, 87–90f
  pathogenesis 91
  progressive multifocal leukoencephalopathy 83–89, 87f
  treatment 91–92

Kaposi sarcoma 44
keratitis, *Acanthamoeba* 466

laboratory tests
  acute bacterial meningitis 299–300
  aspergillosis 422–423
  cerebral actinomycosis 338–339
  cerebral nocardiosis 344
  Chikungunya virus 191
  cytomegalovirus 68–69
  dengue virus 154
  enterovirus A71 208
  flaviviruses 137
  fungal infections 422–424, 433t
  henipaviruses 115
  hepatitis C & E viruses 179–180
  hypertrophic pachymeningitis 405
  Japanese encephalitis virus 171–172
  legionellosis 384, 386, 389t
  mucormycosis 424
  Murray Valley encephalitis virus 153–154
  Mycoplasma pneumoniae 268
  Parechovirus A 244–245, 247
  poliomyelitis 197
  post-operative infections 326
  rabies virus 125–126
  Rocky Mountain spotted fever 273
  rubella virus 108–109
  St. Louis encephalitis virus 153–154
  Scedosporium spp. 424
  Toxoplasma gondii 452
  Treponema pallidum 365
  Tropheryma whipplei 332
  West Nile virus 153–154
  yellow fever virus 154
  see also diagnosis
late cerebritis 310
late neurosyphilis 365
latent infections, cytomegalovirus 72
ledipasvir 180
legionellosis 383–391
  aerosol sources 384b
  clinical features 385–386, 387t
  diagnosis 385–386, 387t, 389t
  epidemiology 384–385
  laboratory tests 384, 386, 389t
  microbiology 384
  pathogenesis 388–389, 390b
  pathology 386–388
  risk factors 384–385, 385t
  treatment 390
leishmaniasis 8t, 472–473
leptomeningeal vasculitis 57, 59f
leptospirosis 374–375
lifecycles
  dipterous insects 503
  flaviviruses 133, 135–136f, 157–158, 158b
  malaria 438
  Toxoplasma gondii 450
lipoteichoic acid (LTA) 291
Listeria monocytogenes
  antibiotics 32t
  invasion mechanisms 291–292
  meningitis 280, 297–298
Loa 490–491, 491f
Löfgren syndrome *see* sarcoidosis
long-term cognitive dysfunctions, sepsis-associated 12

Index

long-term sequelae, cerebral
    malaria 444
louse-borne rickettsioses 275–276
LTA *see* lipoteichoic acid
lumbar puncture 280
Lyme disease *see* Borrelia burgdorferi
lymphocytes
    cerebral malaria 442
    opportunistic infections 24–25
lyssaviruses
    microbiology 122
    rabies 121–129
    species of 121–122

MA *see* mycotic aneurysm
MAC *see* Mycobacterium avium/
    intracellulare complex
macrocirculatory impairment,
    sepsis-associated 14
macroscopic findings
    hypertrophic pachymeningitis 405
    Rasmussen encephalitis 260
    Tropheryma whipplei 333
    Zika virus 164–165, 164f
magnetic resonance imaging (MRI)
    acute bacterial
        meningitis 298–299
    acute disseminated
        encephalomyelitis 252
    alphaviral equine
        encephalomyelitis 184
    brain abscess 281, 282f
    cerebral actinomycosis 338–339
    cerebral nocardiosis 344
    cytomegalovirus 68, 69
    enterovirus A71 208
    henipavirus encephalitis 114–115
    human T cell leukemia/lymphoma
        virus type 1 associated
        myelopathy/tropical spastic
        paraparesis 238
    hypertrophic pachymeningitis 405
    Japanese encephalitis virus
        171–172
    legionellosis 385–386
    Mycoplasma pneumoniae 268
    neuro-Behçet disease/
        syndrome 264
    neurosarcoidosis 394–395
    polyomavirus 86
    post-operative infections 326
    St. Louis encephalitis virus 153

septic embolism 315
Toxoplasma gondii 451–452
Tropheryma whipplei 332
West Nile virus 153
malaria 7t, 437–448
    animal models 441–444
    artemisinin resistance 508t,
        510–512
    childhood infections 26
    clinical features 439
    cytokines 442–443
    diagnosis 439
    epidemiology 438–439
    historical perspectives 438
    inflammation 443–444, 445f
    life cycle 438
    long-term sequelae 444
    lymphocytes 442
    microvascular dysfunction 441
    pathogenesis 440–444, 443f
    pathology 439, 440–442f
    platelets 442
    treatment 444–446
matrix metalloproteinases
    (MMPs) 289, 292
MBFVs *see* mosquito-borne
    flaviviruses
MDR TB *see* multidrug-resistant
    Mycobacterium tuberculosis
measles inclusion body encephalitis
    (MIBE) 95, 98–100, 101–102
measles virus (MV) 95–103
    animal models 100–101
    epidemiology 96
    measles inclusion body
        encephalitis 95, 98–100,
        101–102
    microbiology 96
    subacute sclerosing panencephalitis
        95, 97–98, 101
    treatment 101–102
    vaccines 101
Mediterranean spotted fever (MSF)
    272, 275
meningitis
    acute bacterial 29–33, 280, 285t,
        295–307
    aseptic 50
    chronic 280–281
    community-acquired 29–33
    post-operative 321
    tuberculous 35–36, 280–281

meningovascular neurosyphilis 366,
    366–367f
meningovascular sarcoidosis
    396–397
MERS-CoV *see* Middle Eastern
    Respiratory Syndrome
    coronavirus
metabolic abnormalities, acquired
    immune deficiency
    syndrome 223
MGNs *see* microglial nodules
MIBE *see* measles inclusion body
    encephalitis
microbiology
    acute bacterial meningitis
        296–298
    African trypanosomiasis 467–468
    alphaviral equine
        encephalomyelitis 183–184
    aspergillosis 421–442
    Borrelia burgdorferi 371
    Brucella spp. 379–380
    cerebral actinomycosis 337–338
    cerebral nocardiosis 343–347
    Chikungunya virus 189–190
    Clostridium botulinum 415
    Clostridium perfringens 414
    Clostridium tetani 413
    cytomegalovirus 66–67
    enterovirus A71 205–206
    flaviviruses 132, 134f
    henipaviruses 113, 114f
    hepatitis C & E viruses 178–179
    human immunodeficiency
        virus 216
    human T cell leukemia/lymphoma
        virus type 1 232–233
    Japanese encephalitis virus 170
    John Cunningham virus 84–85
    legionellosis 384
    measles virus 96
    Mycobacterium tuberculosis 350
    Mycoplasma pneumoniae
        267–268
    non-tuberculous mycobacterial
        infections 357–358
    Parechovirus A 243–244
    poliovirus 196
    polyomavirus 84–85
    post-operative pyogenic
        infections 323
    rabies 122

rubella virus 105–106
South American
    trypanosomiasis 469
subdural empyema 312
tick-borne encephalitis 139
Toxoplasma gondii 450
Treponema pallidum 363
see also molecular biology
microcephaly
    congenital rubella virus
        108f, 110
    Zika virus 164–165, 164f
microcirculatory impairment,
    sepsis-associated
    encephalopathy 14
microglia, sepsis-associated
    encephalopathy 15
microglial nodules (MGNs),
    cytomegalovirus 69,
    69–71f
microsporidiosis 7t, 470–472
microvascular dysfunction,
    malaria 441, 444f
Middle Eastern Respiratory
    Syndrome coronavirus
    (MERS-CoV) 507t, 509
minocycline 15
minor neurocognitive disorder
    (MND) 218
mite-borne rickettsioses 277
mitochondrial dysfunction, sepsis-
    associated
    encephalopathy 16
MMP-9 see tumor necrosis factor-
    soluble receptor decreased
    matrix metalloproteinase-9
MMPs see matrix metalloproteinases
MND see minor neurocognitive
    disorder
MOG see myelin oligodendrocyte
    glycoprotein
molds 6t, 38, 421–425
molecular biology
    flaviviruses 132, 134f
    John Cunningham virus 91
    see also genomes; microbiology
mononeuritis multiplex,
    cytomegalovirus 69, 71f
Morbilliviruses, measles virus
    95–103
mortality, sepsis-associated
    encephalopathy 12

mosquito-borne alphaviruses,
    equine encephalomyelitis
    183–187
mosquito-borne flaviviruses
    (MBFVs) 133, 136f
    dengue virus 147–162
    Japanese encephalitis virus 132,
        133f, 136f, 169–176
    Murray Valley encephalitis virus
        147–162
    St. Louis encephalitis
        virus 147–162
    West Nile virus 132, 133f, 136f,
        147–162, 506t, 509–510
    yellow fever virus 147–162
    Zika virus 163–168, 507t,
        509–510
MOTT (mycobacteria other than
    Mycobacterium tuberculosis)
    see non-tuberculous
    mycobacterial infections
mouse models, adenovirus
    meningoencephalitis 79–80
MRI see magnetic resonance
    imaging
MSF see Mediterranean spotted fever
MTB see *Mycobacterium tuberculosis*
mucormycosis 424, 433t
multidrug-resistant *Mycobacterium
    tuberculosis* (MDR TB) 350,
    507t, 509, 510, 512
multifocal leukoencephalitis
    acquired immune deficiency
        syndrome 223
    cytomegalovirus 67
    varicella-zoster virus 57, 58f, 59
murine endemic flea-borne typhus
    272, 276–277
Murray Valley encephalitis virus
    (MVEV) 147–162
    clinical features 150t, 151–152
    epidemiology 148–151, 149t
    laboratory tests 153–154
    pathogenesis 157–158, 158b
    pathology 150t, 156
    treatment 159
Mycobacterium avium/intracellulare
    complex (MAC) 358
Mycobacterium haemophilum
    358–360
Mycobacterium tuberculosis (MTB)
    349–356

chronic meningitis 280–281
clinical features 351–354
drug-resistant 350, 354–355, 507t,
    509, 510, 512
encephalitis 35–36
epidemiology 350, 354
historical perspectives 349–350
HIV co-infection 354
microbiology 350
spinal tuberculosis 353, 356
susceptibility polymorphisms 26
treatment 355–356
tuberculoma 353–354, 356
tuberculous meningitis 351–353,
    355–356
Mycoplasma hominis 4t, 272
Mycoplasma pneumoniae 267–271
    clinical features 4t, 268
    epidemiology 267
    microbiology 267–268
    pathology 268, 269–271f
    treatment 268
mycotic aneurysm (MA) 315–316
myelin oligodendrocyte glycoprotein
    (MOG), acute disseminated
    encephalomyelitis 252–255
myelitis, herpes simplex virus 50
myeloradiculopathy,
    cytomegalovirus 69, 71f
myiasis 503–504

NBS see neuro-Behçet disease/
    syndrome
NCC see neurocysticercosis
necrotizing encephalitis,
    cytomegalovirus 69, 69–71f
necrotizing multifocal
    leukoencephalopathy 14
necrotizing ventriculoencephalitis,
    cytomegalovirus 69, 69–70f
nectin 4 96
Neisseria meningitidis
    acute bacterial meningitis 29–33,
        280, 280t, 296–297
    antibiotics 32t
    epidemiology 30
    invasion mechanisms
        287–289, 288f
    vaccines 304–305
nematodes 8t, 476–477t, 487–492
    angiostrongylosis 476t, 487–488
    filariasis 490–491, 491f

Index

nematodes (cont'd)
  gnathostomiasis 477t, 488–489
  neurotoxocariasis 477t, 489
  neurotrichinosis 477t, 489–490
  strongyloidiasis 477t, 491–492
neonates 26–27
  Chagas disease 470
  cytomegalovirus 66, 67–68, 72, 73–74f
  herpes simplex virus 45, 50–51, 52f
  immunodeficiency 22–23, 26–27
  meningitis 280
  rubella virus 107–110, 108–109f
  Toxoplasma gondii 451, 452–453, 456, 456f
  varicella-zoster virus 60–61
neural progenitor cells (NPCs), Zika virus 165–166
neuro-Behçet disease/syndrome (NBS) 263–264
neuroborreliosis 370–374
  clinical features 371–372
  epidemiology 371
  historical perspectives 370–371
  microbiology 371
neurobrucellosis 379–382
  clinical features 380
  diagnosis 380
  epidemiology 379, 380
  genetic factors 381
  microbiology 379–380
  pathology/pathogenesis 380–381
  treatment 381
neurocysticercosis (NCC) 478–480, 481f, 482t
neuroendocrine sarcoidosis 397–398
neuroimaging *see* computed tomography; diagnosis; magnetic resonance imaging
neuroinflammatory processes, sepsis-associated encephalopathy 15
neuron-specific enolase (NSE) 13
neuropathology
  acquired immune deficiency syndrome 218–225
  adenovirus meningoencephalitis 79
  BK virus 91
  encephalitis lethargica 265
  enterovirus A71 208–209, 209–210f

Epstein–Barr virus 63
highly active antiretroviral therapy 223–225
measles inclusion body encephalitis 99–100
neonatal herpes simplex virus 51
neuro-Behçet disease/syndrome 264
polyomavirus 87–89, 87–90f
Rasmussen encephalitis 260–262, 261f
subacute sclerosing panencephalitis 98
varicella-zoster virus 57–58, 58–59f
Zika virus 163–165, 164f
see also pathology
neurosarcoidosis 393–401
  clinical features 395–398
  diagnosis 394–395
  genetic factors 398
  pathogenesis 399
  pathology 395–398
  treatment 399
neurosurgery
  community-acquired brain abscess 40
  management of infections 326
  post-operative pyogenic infections 319–330
neurosyphilis 281, 363–370
neurotoxicity
  adenovirus meningoencephalitis 79–80
  brain abscess 38
  sepsis-associated encephalopathy 16
neurotoxocariasis 477t, 489
neurotransmission impairment, sepsis-associated 15–16
neurotrichinosis 477t, 489–490
Nipah virus (NiV) 113–119, 506t
  see also henipavirus encephalitis
nitric oxide (NO), Japanese encephalitis virus 174
N-methyl-D-aspartate receptors (NMDARs), sepsis-associated encephalopathy 15
nocardiosis 343–347
  clinical features 344
  genetics 345–346
  microbiology 343–347

pathology 344–345, 345f
treatment 346
nonsteroidal anti-inflammatory drugs (NSAIDs), Chikungunya fever 191–192
non-tuberculous mycobacterial infections (NTM) 357–362
  classification 357–358
  microbiology 357–358
  Mycobacterium avium/intracellulare complex 358
  Mycobacterium haemophilum 358–360
  treatment 360–361
NSAIDs *see* nonsteroidal anti-inflammatory drugs
NSE *see* neuron-specific enolase
NTM *see* non-tuberculous mycobacterial infections

OIs *see* opportunistic infections
Onchocerca volvulus 490–491, 491f
opportunistic infections (OIs) 23–25, 23t
  acquired immune deficiency syndrome 222–223
  children 27
  polyomavirus 83–93
Orientia tsutsugamushi 5t, 272, 277
oxidative stress
  bacterial infections 292
  sepsis-associated 16

PAA *see* plasma anticholinergic activity
pachymeningitis *see* hypertrophic pachymeningitis
PAF *see* platelet-activating factor
PAM *see* primary amoebic meningoencephalitis
PAMPs *see* pathogen-associated molecular pattern molecules
pan drug-resistant *Mycobacterium tuberculosis* (PDR TB) 350
paracoccidioidomycosis 429–430
paragonimiasis 476t, 487
paralytic rabies 125
parasitic infections *see* helminth infections; protozoal infections
Parechovirus A (PeVA) 243–249
  acute adult infections 247–248

chronic infections 247
clinical features 245
diagnosis 244–245, 247
epidemiology 244
microbiology 243–244
pathology 245–247, 246–247f
treatment 248
parenchymatous neurosyphilis 366–368, 368–369f
parenchymatous sarcoidosis 397
paretic dementia 366–368, 368–369f
pathogen-associated molecular pattern molecules (PAMPs) 15
pathogenesis *see under individual species or condition*
Picornaviruses 243
pIgR *see* polymeric immunoglobulin receptor
pili
　group B streptococcus 291
　Neisseria meningitidis 288
plasma anticholinergic activity (PAA) 15
Plasmodium berghei Anka (PbA) 441, 444–445f
Plasmodium falciparum 7t, 437–448
　artemisinin resistance 508t, 510–512
Plasmodium knowlesi 508t, 510
platelet-activating factor (PAF), *Streptococcus pneumoniae* invasion 286–287
platelets, cerebral malaria 442
pleconaril, enterovirus A71 211
PML *see* progressive multifocal leukoencephalopathy
PMNL *see* polymorphonuclear leukocytes
pneumolysin 286–287
polioencephalitis 195–200
poliomyelitis 195–200
　clinical features 197
　diagnosis 197–198
　epidemiology 196–197
　laboratory tests 197
　microbiology 196
　pathogenesis 199–200
　pathology 198, 198–199f
　treatment 200
poliovirus (PV) 195–204
　animal models 200

clinical features 197, 200–201
diagnosis 197, 200–201
epidemiology 196–197, 200
genetic factors 198–199, 202
historical perspectives 195–196, 200
laboratory tests 197
microbiology 196
pathogenesis 199–200, 201–202
pathology 198, 198–199f
treatment 200, 202
poliovirus receptor-related 4 (PVLRL4) protein 96
polymeric immunoglobulin receptor (pIgR) 286
polymorphonuclear leukocytes (PMNL), bacterial infections 290–291, 292
polyomavirus 83–93
　animal models 91
　clinical features 85–87
　diagnosis 85–87
　epidemiology 85
　genomes 84f
　gray matter pathologies 89, 90f
　inflammatory pathologies 90–91
　microbiology 84–85
　neuropathology 87–89, 87–90f
　pathogenesis 91
　progressive multifocal leukoencephalopathy 83–89, 87f
　treatment 91–92
positron emission tomography (PET), Whipple disease 332
postexposure management, rabies 127
postinfection inflammatory conditions
　acute disseminated encephalomyelitis 251–255
　acute hemorrhagic leukoencephalitis 251, 255, 256f
postinfectious encephalitis, measles virus 95
post-operative pyogenic infections 319–330
　clinical features 323–326, 324–325t
　definitions 320–321
　diagnosis 326
　epidemiology 323

microbiology 323
risk factors 321, 323t
treatment 326
postpolio syndrome 200–202
Powassan virus 506t, 509, 511
predictive factors, sepsis-associated encephalopathy 12
pregnancies
　intrauterine infections 25–26
　meningitis 280
primary amoebic meningoencephalitis (PAM) 464–465
primary herpes simplex virus infections 44, 45–46
primary immunodeficiency 22–23, 26–27
primary lesions, human immunodeficiency virus 218–222
primary pathogens, features 23t
primary reservoirs, flaviviruses 133
prognostic factors *see* risk factors
progressive multifocal leukoencephalopathy (PML)
　acquired immune deficiency syndrome 222
　polyomavirus 83–89, 87f
progressive panencephalitis, rubella virus 107–108, 109–110
prophylaxis, flaviviruses 138
protozoal infections 7–8t, 437–474
　amoebiasis 463–466
　leishmaniasis 472–473
　malaria 437–448, 508t, 510–512
　microsporidiosis 470–472
　sarcocystosis 472
　Toxoplasma gondii 449–461
　trypanosomiasis 466–470
PV *see* poliovirus
PVLRL4 *see* poliovirus receptor-related 4 protein
pyogenic infections 295–330
　acute bacterial meningitis 29–33, 280, 285t, 295–307, 321
　brain abscess 29, 36–40, 281, 310–311, 311–313f, 320, 320f
　epidural abscess 282–283, 313–315, 321, 322f
　following neurosurgical procedures 319–330
　mycotic aneurysm 315–316

527

Index

pyogenic infections (cont'd)
   septic embolism 315–316
   subdural empyema 283, 311–313, 320, 321f
   suppurative intracranial phlebitis 316–317, 317t, 321, 322f
pyrimethamine 458

quinine 444

rabies virus (RABV) 121–129
   animal models 125
   clinical features 125
   diagnosis 125–126
   epidemiology 122–124, 123f
   historical perspectives 122
   laboratory tests 125–126
   microbiology 122
   pathogenesis 124–125
   pathology 126–127
   treatment 127–128
RABV *see* rabies virus
radiology
   hypertrophic pachymeningitis 405
   see also computed tomography; magnetic resonance imaging
RAN binding protein 2 255, 256f
rashes
   Rocky Mountain spotted fever 273
   rubella virus 106, 107f
Rasmussen syndrome/Rasmussen encephalitis (RS/RE) 259–263
   clinical features 260
   diagnosis 262–263
   epidemiology 260
   pathogenesis 262–263
   treatment 263
RE *see* Rasmussen syndrome/Rasmussen encephalitis
reactive oxygen species (ROS), bacterial infections 292
relapsing fever 373
relapsing henipavirus encephalitis 117
resveratrol, sepsis-associated encephalopathy 15
ribavirin 180, 211
Rickettsia 4t, 272–278
   African tick bite fever 275
   conorii 272, 275

   flea-borne 276–277
   louse-borne 275–276
   Mediterranean spotted fever 272, 275
   mite-borne 277
   prowazekii 272, 275–276
   rickettsii 272, 273
   Rocky Mountain spotted fever 273, 274f
   tick-borne 273–275
   typhi 272, 276–277
rifampicin 360
risk factors
   acute bacterial meningitis 30, 301
   Brucella spp. 381
   chronic persistent infections 27
   cytomegalovirus 66
   dengue virus 151
   fungal infections 433t
   herpes simplex virus 45, 51
   HTLV-1 associated myelopathy/tropical spastic paraparesis 237
   legionellosis 384–385, 385t
   malaria 26
   measles virus 96
   mucormycosis 424
   Murray Valley encephalitis virus 151
   Mycobacterium tuberculosis 26
   post-operative pyogenic infections 321, 323t
   rubella virus 106
   St. Louis encephalitis virus 151
   Tropheryma whipplei 334–335
   West Nile virus 151
   yellow fever virus 151
river blindness 490–491, 491f
RMSF *see* Rocky Mountain spotted fever
Rocky Mountain spotted fever (RMSF) 273, 274f
ROS *see* reactive oxygen species
RS *see* Rasmussen syndrome/Rasmussen encephalitis
rubella virus (RV) 105–111
   clinical features 106–109
   congenital 107–110, 108–109f
   encephalitis 106–107
   epidemiology 106
   exanthem-producing febrile acute infections 106, 107f

   genetic factors 110
   laboratory tests 108–109
   microbiology 105–106
   pathogenesis 110
   pathology 109–110
   progressive panencephalitis 107–108, 109–110
   treatment 110
Runyon classification 357–358

S100β protein 13
SAE *see* sepsis-associated encephalopathy
St. Louis encephalitis virus (SLEV) 147–162
   animal models 159, 160–161t
   brain imaging 153
   clinical features 150t, 151–152
   epidemiology 148–151, 149t
   laboratory tests 153–154
   pathogenesis 157–158, 158b
   pathology 150t, 156
   treatment 159
sample processing, brain abscess 40t
sarcocystosis 472
sarcoidosis 393–401
   animal models 399
   clinical features 395–398
   diagnosis 394–395
   epidemiology 394
   genetic factors 398
   pathogenesis 399
   pathology 395–398
   treatment 399
"scar" lesions, highly active antiretroviral therapy 223, 224f
Scedosporium spp. 423–424, 433t
Schaumann syndrome *see* sarcoidosis
schistosomiasis 477t, 485–486, 500–502
scrub typhus 272, 277
SCS *see* spinal cord sarcoidosis
secondary lesions, acquired immune deficiency syndrome 223
sepsis-associated encephalopathy (SAE) 11–20
   blood markers 13
   cell status 16
   clinical features 12–13
   definitions 12

epidemiology 12
ischemic processes 14–15
mortality 12
neurotoxicity 16
neurotransmission impairment 15–16
physiopathology 13–16
predictive factors 12
treatment 16–17, 17t
septate hyaline molds 6t, 38, 421–424
septic embolism 315–316
serine-rich repeat (Srr) proteins 291
Sfb *see* streptococcal fibronectin-binding protein
SFG *see* spotted fever group
shiga toxin (Stx) 416
Shigella dysenteriae 416
shingles *see* varicella-zoster virus
Simian virus 40 (SV40) 84
   see also John Cunningham virus; polyomavirus
single nucleotide polymorphisms (SNPs)
   dengue virus susceptibility 151
   measles virus susceptibility 96
   poliovirus susceptibility 199
sleeping sickness 467–469
SLEV *see* St. Louis encephalitis virus
Snail1 291
sofosbuvir, hepatitis C virus 180
South American trypanosomiasis 7t, 469–470
sparganosis 476t, 484–485, 485f
spinal cord disease, herpes simplex virus encephalitis 50
spinal cord sarcoidosis (SCS) 398
spinal epidural abscess 314–315, 321, 322f
spinal tuberculosis 353, 356
spirochetal infections 363–377
   borreliosis 281, 370–374
   leptospirosis 374–375
   neurosyphilis 281, 363–370
Spirometra mansion 476t, 484–485, 485f
spotted fever group (SFG) rickettsioses 272, 273–275
Srr *see* serine-rich repeat
SSPE *see* subacute sclerosing panencephalitis
staphylococcal food poisoning 416

steroids, hypertrophic pachymeningitis 408
streptococcal fibronectin-binding protein (Sfb) 291
streptococci, antibiotics 32t
Streptococcus agalactiae
   emerging 507t, 509
   invasion mechanisms 290–291, 290f
   meningitis 280, 297
   vaccines 305
Streptococcus pneumoniae
   acute bacterial meningitis 29–33, 280, 285t, 296
   antibiotics 32t
   epidemiology 30
   invasion mechanism 284–287, 286f
   vaccines 304
strongyloidiasis 477t, 491–492
Stx *see* shiga toxin
subacute sclerosing panencephalitis (SSPE), measles virus 95, 97–98, 101
subdural empyema 283, 311–313, 320, 321f
   clinical features 312–313
   epidemiology 312
   microbiology 312
   pathogenesis 312
   pathology 313
   see also surgical site infections
sulfadiazine 458
suppurative intracranial phlebitis 316–317, 317t, 321
suramin, enterovirus A71 211
surgical site infections (SSI) 319–330
   clinical features 323–326, 324–325t
   definitions 320–321
   diagnosis 326
   epidemiology 323
   microbiology 323
   risk factors 321, 323t
   treatment 326
susceptibility factors
   genetic factors 151
   herpes simplex virus (HSV) 51
   measles virus 96
   poliovirus 198–199
   Tropheryma whipplei 334–335
   see also genetic factors; risk factors

sustained virologic response (SVR), hepatitis C 180
SV40 *see* Simian virus 40
SVR *see* sustained virologic response
syphilis *see Treponema pallidum*

tabanid flies 490
tabes dorsalis 366–368, 369f
Taenia multiceps 476t, 484
Taenia solium 478–480, 481f, 482t
tapeworms 476t, 478–485
   see also cestodes
Tax protein 239
TB *see* tuberculosis
TBEV *see* tick-borne encephalitis virus
TBM *see* tuberculous meningitis
TeNT *see* tetanus neurotoxin
tetanus neurotoxin (TeNT) 412–414
third-generation cephalosporin 346
tick-borne encephalitis virus (TBEV) 132, 133f, 138–144
   animal models 143
   clinical features 140–141
   epidemiology 132, 133f, 139, 140f
   historical perspectives 138–139
   microbiology 139
   pathogenesis 143
   pathology 141–143, 142f
   treatment 144
tick-borne flaviviruses (TBFVs) 133, 136f, 138–144
TNF *see* tumor necrosis factor
Togaviridae
   Chikungunya virus 189–193, 507t, 509–512
   rubella virus 105–111
toll-like receptors, sepsis-associated encephalopathy 15
TORCH *see Toxoplasma gondii*, rubella, cytomegalovirus, and herpes simplex virus
toxin-induced diseases 411–418
   alternate 416
   direct toxins 412–414
   emetic 416
   indirect toxins 414–416
   physiopathology 417
Toxocara canis 477t, 489
Toxoplasma gondii 7t, 449–461
   clinical features 451–453
   congenital 451, 452–453, 456, 456f

529

Index

Toxoplasma gondii (cont'd)
  diagnosis 451–453
  differential diagnosis 452, 453
  epidemiology 450–451
  genetics 456–457
  immunocompromised patients 451–455, 544–545f
  microbiology 450
  pathogenesis 457–458
  pathology 453–456, 454–456f
  treatment 458
Toxoplasma gondii, rubella, cytomegalovirus, and herpes simplex virus (TORCH) 72
toxoplasmosis, acquired immune deficiency syndrome 222
transcystosis, bacterial invasion 284, 286–287, 286f, 287–291, 288f
transverse myelitis, varicella-zoster virus 57
treatment *see under* individual species or condition
trematodes 8t, 476t, 485–487, 500–502
Treponema pallidum (syphilis) 363–370
  chronic meningitis 281
  clinical features 365
  diagnosis 365–366
  epidemiology 364–365
  general paresis of the insane 366–368, 368–369f
  gumma, cerebral 366, 367f
  historical perspectives 363–364
  and HIV infections 367f, 368–369
  invasion mechanisms 370
  meningovascular pathology 366
  microbiology 363
  pathogenesis 369–370
  pathology 366–368, 366–369f
  persistence 370
  tabes dorsalis 366–368, 369f
  treatment 370
Trichinella spiralis 477t, 489–490
Tropheryma whipplei 331–336
  clinical features 332
  diagnosis 332–333
  epidemiology 331–332
  pathogenesis 334–335
  pathology 333–334

  treatment 335
tropical spastic paraparesis/HTLV-1 associated myelopathy (TSP/HAM) 232t, 235–240
  clinical features 237–238
  epidemiology 235–237
  pathogenesis 238–240, 239f
  pathology 238–239
  risk factors 237
  treatment 240
trypanosomiasis
  African 467–469
  South American 469–470
TSP/HAM *see* tropical spastic paraparesis/HTLV-1 associated myelopathy
tuberculoma 353–354, 356
tuberculosis (TB) 349–356
  chronic meningitis 280–281
  clinical features 351–354
  drug-resistant 350, 354–355, 507t, 509, 510, 512
  encephalitis 35–36
  epidemiology 350, 354
  historical perspectives 349–350
  HIV co-infection 354
  microbiology 350
  spinal tuberculosis 353, 356
  susceptibility polymorphisms 26
  treatment 355–356
  tuberculoma 353–354, 356
  tuberculous meningitis 351–353, 355–356
tuberculous meningitis (TBM) 35–36, 351–353
  diagnosis 351–353
  pathology 351, *352*
  treatment 355–356
tumor necrosis factor (TNF)-soluble receptor decreased matrix metalloproteinase-9 (MMP-9) 13
type 1 interferons, enterovirus A71 211
type IV pili (T4P) 288
typhus 275–277

ultrasound (US)
  cytomegalovirus 69
  neurosarcoidosis 394

uveoparotid fever *see* sarcoidosis

vaccines
  acute bacterial meningitis 304–305
  Chikungunya virus 192
  Clostridium perfringens 414
  Clostridium tetani 414
  dengue virus 161
  emerging 512
  enterovirus A71 211
  flaviviruses 138, 144, 159–161, 174
  Japanese encephalitis virus 174
  measles virus 101
  Parechovirus A 248
  rabies 127
  rubella virus 110
  tick-borne encephalitis 144
  varicella-zoster virus 61
  West Nile virus 161
  yellow fever virus 159–161
vacuolar myelopathy 223
valganciclovir 72
variations according to hosts 21–42
  adults 29–42
  children 26–27
  immune reconstitution inflammatory syndrome 25
  immunodeficiencies 22–25
  intrauterine infections 25–26
  neonates 26–27
  opportunistic infections 23–25, 27
  see also genetic factors; single nucleotide polymorphisms
varicella-zoster virus (VZV) 55–61
  "burnt-out" lesions 58, 60f
  clinical features 57, 60
  encephalitis 34–35
  epidemiology 56
  neonates 60–61
  neuropathology 57–58, 58–59f
  pathogenesis 59–61
  pathophysiology 60–61
  treatment 61
VCAM-1 292
vectors
  dengue virus 148–151, 149t
  flaviviruses 132–133, 136f, 148–151, 149t
  henipaviruses 14

leishmaniasis 472
Murray Valley encephalitis 148–151, 149t
rabies 121–122
St. Louis encephalitis virus 148–151, 149t
Toxoplasma gondii 449–461
trypanosomiasis 466, 469
West Nile virus 148–151, 149t
yellow fever virus 148–151, 149t
Venezuelan equine encephalomyelitis (VEE) 183–187
  animal models 186
  clinical features 184–185
  epidemiology 184
  microbiology 183–184
  pathogenesis 186
  pathology 185–186, 185t
  treatment 186–187
ventriculitis
  bacterial infections 283
  varicella-zoster virus 57, 59f
ventriculomegaly, Zika virus 164, 164f
viral encephalitis 34–35, 36
viral infections
  classification 3–4t
  emerging 506–507t
  see also specific viruses and syndromes...
virology
  Chikungunya virus 189–190
  Parechovirus A 243–244
  see also microbiology
visceral larva migrans 477t, 489
visceral leishmaniasis (VL) 472–473
VZV *see* varicella-zoster virus

Weil disease 375
Wernicke encephalopathy 223
Western equine encephalomyelitis (WEE) 183–187
  animal models 186
  clinical features 184–185
  epidemiology 184
  microbiology 183–184
  pathogenesis 186
  pathology 185–186, 185t
  treatment 186–187

West Nile virus (WNV) 147–162, 506t, 509–511
  animal models 159, 160–161t
  clinical features 150t, 151–152
  epidemiology 148–151, 149t, 506t, 509–511
  laboratory tests 153–154
  lifecycle 136f
  neuroimaging 153
  pathogenesis 157–158, 158b
  pathology 150t, 154–156, 155f
  treatment 159
  vaccines 161
Whipple disease (WD) 331–336
  clinical features 332
  diagnosis 332–333
  epidemiology 331–332
  pathogenesis 334–335
  pathology 333–334
  treatment 335
white matter pathologies, human immunodeficiency virus 219–220
wild poliovirus (WPV) 195–204
  epidemiology 196–197
  microbiology 196
  see also poliovirus
WNND (West Nile neuroinvasive disease) *see* West Nile virus
WNV *see* West Nile virus
WPV *see* wild poliovirus

XDR TB *see* extensively drug-resistant *Mycobacterium tuberculosis*

yeasts 425–428
  candidiasis 7t, 427–428
  cryptococcosis 7t, 35, 222, 425–427, 508t, 509–511
yellow fever virus (YFV) 147–162
  animal models 159, 160–161t
  clinical features 150t, 151–152
  diagnosis 150t, 151–152, 154
  epidemiology 132, 133f, 148–151, 149t
  laboratory tests 154
  pathogenesis 158, 158b
  pathology 150t, 156–157
  treatment 159
  vaccines 159–161

YFV *see* yellow fever virus

Zika virus (ZikV) 137, 163–168, 507t, 509–510
  clinical features 163, 164f
  epidemiology 5, 137, 507, 509–510, 509–1007t
  histopathology 165, 166–167f
  macroscopic findings 164–165, 164f
  pathogenesis 165–166
  pathology 163–164
  transmission 137
  treatment 166
zoonotic diseases
  African tick bite fever 275
  African trypanosomiasis 467–469
  alphaviral equine encephalomyelitis 183–187
  angiostrongylosis 476t, 487–488
  borreliosis 281, 370–374
  Brucella spp. 281, 379–382
  coenurosis 476t, 484
  cystic echinococcosis 476t, 480–483, 483f
  dengue virus 132, 133f, 147–162
  Ebola virus 507t, 509–511
  emerging 506–508t
  filariasis 477t, 490–491, 491f
  flaviviruses 131–176
  gnathostomiasis 477t, 488–489
  henipaviruses 113–119
  Japanese encephalitis virus 132, 133f, 136f, 169–176
  leishmaniasis 472–473
  leptospirosis 374–375
  malaria 437–448, 508t, 510–512
  microsporidiosis 470–472
  Murray Valley encephalitis virus 147–162
  myiasis 503–504
  neurocysticercosis 478–480, 481f, 482t
  neurotoxocariasis 477t, 489
  neurotrichinosis 477t, 489–490
  paragonimiasis 476t, 487
  rabies 121–129
  Rickettsia 272–278
  St. Louis encephalitis virus 147–162
  sarcocystosis 472

Index

zoonotic diseases (*cont'd*)
  schistosomiasis 477t, 485–486, 500–502
  South American trypanosomiasis 469–470
  sparganosis 476t, 484–485, 485f
  strongyloidiasis 477t, 491–492
  tick-borne encephalitis 132, 133f, 138–144
  toxoplasmosis 449–461
  trypanosomiasis 466–470
  West Nile virus 147–162, 506t, 509–510, 509–511
  yellow fever virus 132, 133f, 147–162
  Zika virus 137, 163–168, 507t, 509–510